PERCEPTUAL AND MOTOR SKILLS

ISSN 0031-5125   June 2004, Part 1

Multiple Rapid Automatic Naming Measures of Cognition: Normal Performance and Effects of Aging: JAMES M.
  JACOBSON, NIELS PETER NIELSEN, LENNART MINTHON, SIEGBERT WARKENTIN, AND ELISABETH H. WIIG 739
*An Examination of High School Students' Attitudes Toward Physical Education With Regard to Sex and Sport
  Participation:* CANAN KOCA AND GIYASETTIN DEMIRHAN 754
*Left:Right Differences in Psychophysical and Electrodermal Measures of Olfactory Thresholds and Their Relation
  to Electrodermal Indices of Hemispheric Asymmetries:* GÉRARD BRAND, JEAN-LOUIS MILLOT, LAURENCE
  JACQUOT, STÉPHANIE THOMAS, AND SONIA WETZEL 759
Effect on Truck Drivers' Alertness of a 30-min. Exposure to Bright Light: a Field Study: ULF LANDSTRÖM, TOR-
  BJÖRN ÅKERSTEDT, MARIANNE BYSTRÖM, BERTIL NORDSTRÖM, AND ROGER WIBOM 770
Perceived Building Density as a Function of Layout: JOHN ZACHARIAS AND ARTHUR STAMPS 777
Meaning: John Steinbeck's Work Examined: GLENN L. THOMPSON AND SARA KUNTO 785
Simple Reaction Tasks: ROLAND KALB, STEPHANIE JANSEN, UDO REULBACH, AND STEFANIE
  793
With Shyness Among Japanese and American University Students: TOSHIYUKI SAKURAGI 803

continued inside back cover

PERCEPTUAL AND MOTOR SKILLS

Perceptual and Motor Skills is published bimonthly, two volumes a year, the first with issues in February, April, and June, and the second with issues in August, October, and December, from Box 9229, Missoula, Montana, 59807-9229. Subscriptions are accepted only for full calendar years. A minimum of 2600 pages is planned for 2004. Subscription rate is $370.00 per year plus postage and handling ($25.00, outside USA $30.00). Single issues are $45.00 plus postage ($5.00, outside USA $25.00).

The purpose of this journal is to encourage scientific originality and creativity. Material of the following kinds is carried: experimental or theoretical articles dealing with perception or motor skills, especially as affected by experience; articles on general methodology; new material listings and reviews. All material of scientific merit will be taken in some form. An attempt is made to balance critical editing with specific suggestions from multiple referees of each paper as to changes. The approach is interdisciplinary, including such fields as perception, anthropology, physical education, physical therapy, orthopedics, time and motion study, and sports psychology. Four copies of an article should be submitted to one of the editors at Box 9229, Missoula, Montana 59807-9229. Each article must have a carefully prepared summary of appropriate length to aid readers and abstractors.

Publication is in order of receipt of proof from the authors. Authors pay for preprints, plus costs of figures and special composition, e.g., tables, mathematics. There are three publication arrangements.

(1) *Regular articles.* These are articles which require from 3 through 20 printed pages. Authors receive 200 preprints. Preprint charge is $27.50 per page in multiples of four pages. Additional preprints can be ordered.

(2) *Brief articles.* This arrangement is useful where the author does not intend to do further work in the area but feels that preliminary findings should be put on record, where it is expected that it will be several years before the final study is completed and reported, where the author submits a summary of a study accompanied by the full report for filing with the Archive for Psychological Data, or where a particular finding can be reported completely in one page. Authors receive 50 preprints. Preprint charge is $27.50. Additional preprints can be ordered.

(3) *Monograph supplements.* Certain papers printing to more than 20 pages are published as monograph supplements. These are distributed to subscribers of *Perceptual and Motor Skills* as parts of regular issues. Authors receive 200 preprints of the monographs with covers. Preprint charge is $27.50 per page in multiples of four pages. Additional preprints can be ordered.

Articles should be prepared carefully, following the form suggested for publications of the American Psychological Association (see 1983, 1994 revision, or earlier versions). During 2003 and 2004 either the old or the new APA form will be acceptable. Proof is mailed to the author within approximately three weeks of acceptance of the article, and preprints are mailed within approximately five weeks of receipt of proof from the author.

It is the policy of this journal to file raw data with the Archive for Psychological Data whenever possible. Authors should submit appropriate tables with their articles. In this way, a permanent file of data available to all researchers could be accumulated.

Responsibility for address changes rests with the subscriber. Claims for missing issues must be made within two months of publication.

Second Class Postage Paid at Missoula, Montana

PERCEPTUAL AND MOTOR SKILLS
ISSN 0031-5125

Vol. 98, No. 3, Part 1		June 2004
SENIOR EDITORS	R. B. Ammons and C. H. Ammons	Ammons Scientific, Ltd.
EDITORS	Bruce Ammons, Douglas Ammons, S. A. Isbell	

ASSOCIATE EDITORS

Marian Annett
University of Leicester

Clark D. Ashworth
NE Washington Family Counseling

Richard W. Bohannon
University of Connecticut

Willard L. Brigner
Appalachian State University

Josef Brožek
St. Paul, MN

Peter Brugger
University Hospital Zurich

Ross H. Day
La Trobe University, Bundoora

Robert Didden
Katholieke Universiteit Nijmegen

G. William Domhoff
University of California, Santa Cruz

Christopher C. Dunbar
Brooklyn College of CUNY

John Eliot
University of Maryland, College Park

H. J. Eysenck
University of London

Ann M. Filinger
Hagerstown, MD

Bernard Fine
Weston, MA

Robert Fudin
Long Island University

David M. Furst
San Jose State University

Richard Gajdosik
The University of Montana

K. O. Götz
Kunstakademie Düsseldorf

E. Rae Harcum
The College of William & Mary

Julian Hochberg
Columbia University

Alan S. Kaufman
Yale University School of Medicine

Johannes Kingma
University Hospital Groningen

Marcel Kinsbourne
Boston University

Muriel Lezak
Oregon Health Sciences University

Paul Naitoh
San Diego, California

Kent B. Pandolf
U.S. Army Research Institute

J. Timothy Petersik
Ripon College

Paul Roodin
SUNY College at Oswego

Leon E. Smith
St. Thomas University, Miami

Arthur E. Stamps III
Institute of Environmental Quality

D. L. Streiner
Baycrest Center for Geriatric Care

Stephan Swinnen
Katholieke Universiteit Leuven

Üner Tan
Cukurova University

James M. Vanderplas
Washington University

Min Q. Wang
University of Maryland

Paul R. Yarnold
Northwestern Univer. Medical School

Published bimonthly by Perceptual and Motor Skills, Box 9229, Missoula, Montana; printed by Ammons Scientific, Ltd., 1911-17 South Higgins Avenue, Missoula, Montana 59801-1911. Please address correspondence and changes of address to Box 9229, Missoula, Montana 59807-9229. POSTMASTER: Send address changes to *Perceptual and Motor Skills*, P.O. Box 9229, Missoula, Montana 59807-9229.

Copyright 2004   Perceptual and Motor Skills

Permission to Copy Material in this Journal

It is the policy of this journal to obtain and hold the copyrights for all articles published, with the exception of a very few articles or parts of articles in the public domain. Authors are allowed and encouraged to make copies of their articles for any scholarly purpose of their own. Other scholars are hereby given permission to make single or multiple copies of single articles for personal scholarly use without explicit written permission, providing that no such copies are sold or used for commercial purposes. We consider it the obligation of any user to acknowledge sources explicitly and to obtain permission of the authors if extensive use is to be made of materials or information contained in an article. Extensive use of copy privileges in such a way as to substitute for a subscription to this journal is not intended or permitted. Such use would be unethical and, in the long run, self-defeating, since it would destroy the very basis for publication.

These policies are proposed on a trial basis and will be followed until further notice.

C. H. Ammons, Editor

R. B. Ammons, Editor

January 1, 1978

Perceptual and Motor Skills has been printed on acid-free paper since 1962, Vol. 14, No. 1 (February). See the following references.

AMMONS, R. B., & AMMONS, C. H. Permanent or temporary journals: are PR and PMS stable? *Perceptual and Motor Skills*, 1962, 14, 281.

AMMONS, C. H., & AMMONS, R. B. Permanent or temporary journals: PR and PMS become stable. *Psychological Reports*, 1962, 10, 537.

Disclaimer

This Journal is not responsible for the statements of any contributor. Statements or opinions expressed in the journal reflect the views of the authors and not the Editors, Associate Editors, or special reviewers. Publication should not be construed as endorsement. Contributing authors are expected to follow ethical procedures and sound scientific principles.

MULTIPLE RAPID AUTOMATIC NAMING MEASURES OF COGNITION: NORMAL PERFORMANCE AND EFFECTS OF AGING[1]

JAMES M. JACOBSON

*Net Education Design, Inc.
Arlington, Texas*

NIELS PETER NIELSEN

Hvidovre Hospital, Copenhagen

LENNART MINTHON, SIEGBERT WARKENTIN

*Department of Psychiatry and Neuropsychiatric Clinic
University Hospital MAS, Malmo, Sweden*

ELISABETH H. WIIG

Knowledge Research Institute, Inc., Arlington, TX

Summary.—Rapid automatic naming tasks are clinical tools for probing brain functions that underlie normal cognition. To compare performance for various stimuli in normal subjects and assess the effect of aging, we administered six single-dimension stimuli (color, form, number, letter, animal, and object) and five dual-dimension stimuli (color-form, color-number, color-letter, color-animal, and color-object) to 144 normal volunteers who ranged in age from 15 to 85 years. Rapid automatic naming times for letters and numbers were significantly less than for forms, animals, and objects. Rapid automatic naming times for color-number and color-letter stimuli were significantly less than for color-form, color-animal, or color-object stimuli. Age correlated significantly with rapid automatic naming time for each single-dimension stimulus and for color-form, color-number, color-animal, and color-object stimuli. Linear regression showed that rapid automatic naming times increased with age for aggregated color stimuli, aggregated single-dimension stimuli, and aggregated dual-dimension stimuli. This age effect persisted in subgroups less than 60 years of age and greater than 60 years of age. We conclude that normal performance time is dependent on the task, with letter and number stimuli eliciting most rapid responses, and that most rapid automatic naming times increase with age.

Cognitive performance in a normal population is characterized by broad variance, due in part to the influence of hereditary and developmental factors, and also by education, practice, medical disease, medication, age, and a host of environmental factors (Stroop, 1935; Goetz, Jacobson, Murnane, Reid, Repperger, & Goodyear, 1989; Salthouse, 1991; Strauss, Loring, Chelune, Hunter, Hermann, Perrine, Westerveld, Trenerry, & Barr, 1995; Vendrell, Junque, Pujol, Jurado, Molet, & Grafman, 1995; Wechsler, 1997).

---

[1]Address enquiries to Elisabeth H. Wiig, Ph.D., Knowledge Research Institute, Inc., 7101 Lake Powell Drive, Arlington, TX 76016.

Thus, some individuals display clearly superior cognitive skills, while others display inferior, albeit normal skills. This broad normal variance, both between individuals and within individuals, complicates detection of disease states that impair cognitive performance (Callahan, Hendrie, & Tierney, 1995; Fox, Warrington, Freeborough, Hartikainen, Kennedy, Stevens, & Rossoor, 1996; Duncan & Siegal, 1998; Geerlings, Jonker, Bouter, Ader, & Schmand, 1999; Christensen, 2001). Because it is difficult to differentiate the early disease state from the preceding normal state, the disease is said to have an "insidious" onset.

Assessment for impaired cognitive ability has been based, most commonly, on observation or testing of cognitive content, such as memory and construction (Folstein, Folstein, & McHugh, 1975; Rosen, Mohs, & Davis, 1984; Molloy, Alemayehu, & Roberts, 1991; Siegerschmeidt, Mosch, Siemen, Forstl, & Bickel, 2002). Because aberration of content is both clearly recognizable and clearly abnormal, these observations or tests are useful to detect established dementia and differentiate it from the normal state. For instance, the Mini-Mental State Examination (Folstein, *et al.*, 1975) tests a subject's ability to perform serial subtraction, recall three words previously registered, name common objects, repeat a sentence, read text, write text, and copy geometric figures. The Alzheimer's Disease Assessment Scale cognitive subscale (Rosen, *et al.*, 1984) tests the subject's ability to speak, understand spoken speech, recall instructions, find words for spoken speech, follow simple commands, name simple objects, construct geometric figures, name common objects, and recall high-imagery words. Educated English-speaking adults with normal cognition usually perform these tasks without difficulty.

The current study examined normal performance for six single-dimension and five dual-dimension stimuli and extended the exploration of age-related differences in rapid automatic naming to assess how stimulus variability or age-effect influence performance.

Rapid Automatic Naming to Assess Cognitive Function

An alternative approach to assess cognitive function is to measure processing speed. Tests of processing speed use time, rather than content, as the outcome measure and include both reaction time and response time for various tasks (Stroop, 1935; Hick, 1952; Teichner, 1954; Teichner & Krebs, 1974; Repperger, Jacobson, Walbroehl, Michel, & Goodyear, 1985; Wiig, Nielsen, Minthon, & Warkentin, 2002). These methods are sensitive to even small changes in processing speed and have been used to examine the effects on cognition of epilepsy, executive function disorders, frontal lobe involvement, temporal-parietal lobe dysfunction, medication effect, and other neurological conditions (Goetz, *et al.*, 1989; Strauss, *et al.*, 1995; Vendrell, *et al.*, 1995).

Tasks based on rapid automatic naming of familiar competing stimuli are specialized measures of processing speed that allow evaluation of cognitive functions that underlie recognition, memory, reading, and language production. In this study, we examined six single-dimension (comprised of one cognitive test) and five dual-dimension (comprised of two single-dimension tests administered simultaneously) tests of rapid automatic naming included in the Alzheimer's Quick Test (Wiig, Nielsen, Minthon, & Warkentin, 2002). Although tests of processing speed, including rapid automatic naming, have potential as sensitive measures of cognitive performance, they have received less attention as a test for dementia because dementia is commonly considered an abnormality of cognitive content. Cognitive testing based on processing speed, rather than memory content, may allow for earlier detection of cognitive impairment.

Further, sustained rapid automatic naming causes redistribution of cerebral blood flow specific for the particular stimulus and task (Warkentin, Risberg, Nilsson, Karlson, & Graae, 1991). Color-form dual-dimension naming, for instance, consistently increases flow to temporal and parietal brain regions, while suppressing flow to frontal regions when tested in normal adults (Wiig, Nielsen, Minthon, & Warkentin, 2002; Wiig, Nielsen, Minthon, McPeek, Said, & Warkentin, 2002). Therefore, rapid automatic naming tasks have potential to serve as functional probes to measure normal and deteriorating cognitive function.

Processing Speed and Age

The literature concerning the relationship between age and cognitive performance is vast and covers a broad range of cognitive skills, competencies, and strategies (Frith, Friston, Liddle, & Frackowiak, 1991; Salthouse, 1991; Semel, Wiig, & Secord, 1995; Institute for the Study of Aging and International Longevity Center-USA, 2001). Both Botwinick and Thompson (1966) and Obrist (1953) reported that elderly patients had slower simple reaction time than younger patients to an auditory stimulus, but it was not clear that age *per se*, as opposed to disease or other factors, was the basis for the difference. However, Jacobson, Repperger, Goodyear, and Michel (1986) extended these observations to show that reaction time increased progressively by 1.49 msec. per year of age and that the effects of aging may be different for different neurological pathways. The effect of age on rapid automatic naming is less well described, but several recent findings suggest that rapid automatic naming times may increase with age.

Age differences have been observed in the regional cerebral blood flow levels in healthy and normal functioning men and women (Rodriguez, Warkentin, Risberg, & Rosadini, 1988). Since cerebral blood flow is influenced by rapid repetition of cognitive tasks, the decreased blood flow with age is consistent with decreased cognitive activity in anatomic areas that support the cognitive process.

A recent study of random generation of strings of letters also indicated age-related differences in the occurrence of alphabetical stereotypes (Van der Linden, Beerten, & Pesenti, 1998). Because avoidance of stereotypes represents a frontal lobe executive function, the finding supports age-related changes on other tasks influenced by executive functions such as attention, explicit working memory during a conscious search, and self-monitoring. The Alzheimer's Quick Test dual-dimension naming tasks challenge executive function, so an age-related change in performance times would not be unexpected. The Alzheimer's Quick Test, however, also challenges parietal-lobe mediation and implicit working memory for visual input.

Another clue that age influences rapid automatic naming, specific to postmenopausal women, is that the estrogen effect on brain-activation patterns, as assessed by functional magnetic resonance imaging, shows age-related differences during working memory tasks (Shaywitz, Shaywitz, Pugh, Fulbright, Skudlarski, Mencl, Constable, Naftolin, Palter, Marchione, Katz, Shankweiler, Fletcher, Lacadie, Keltz, & Gore, 1999). In an earlier study of 60 adolescents and adults (age range 17 to 68 years) with some of the Alzheimer's Quick Test naming tasks used here (Wiig, Nielsen, Minthon, McPeek, Said, & Warkentin, 2002), age was a factor in naming single-dimension colors and forms, but not in naming dual-dimension stimuli, consistent with prior observations that color-form naming times decreased monotonically in the age range from 6 to 15 years and then stabilized for ages 16 to 21 years (Wiig, Zureich, & Chan, 2000). However, the inability to detect an age-related difference in dual-dimension naming times in the age range from 17 to 68 years may have been due to the small sample.

Method

Subjects

Subjects, 81 men and 63 women ranging in age from 15 to 85 years, agreed to participate. Treatment of all participants was in accordance with the ethical standards of the American Psychological Association. All were speakers of American English and resided in the USA. In the sample, 24 were African American, 6 Asian, 29 Hispanic, and 86 Euro-American, so the sample rather closely represented the diversity found in the USA, according to the 2000 Census (U.S. Bureau of the Census, 2000). All adolescent subjects (ages 15 to 19 yr.) had completed at least 10 years of education, and all adult subjects had completed 12 years of education or obtained an equivalent degree.

Materials and Procedure

Five rapid automatic naming tasks (color-form, color-number, color-letter, color-animal, and color-object naming) featured in the Alzheimer's Quick Test: Assessment of Parietal Function (Wiig, Nielsen, Minthon, & Warkentin, 2002) were used as the experimental measures. Each rapid automatic naming task consists of three separate tests. Test 1 is a single-dimension test requiring subjects to state the color of 40 rectangular blocks (black, blue, green, or red). Test 2 is a single-dimension test requiring subjects to name 40 black visual stimuli consisting of forms (circle, square, line, triangle), numbers (2, 4, 5, or 7), letters (a, b, e, o, k, m, o, p, o, t), animals (spider, bird, snake, fish, rat, cat), or objects (pencil, table, chair, bed, shoe). Test 3 is a dual-dimension test in that the subject must both state the color and name of the stimulus. The dual-dimension tests are color-form, color-number, color-letter, color-animal, and color-object. The Alzheimer's Quick Test naming tasks are objective (based on total naming time), highly reliable ($r = .88$ to .96), and easy and quick to administer and interpret (3–5 minutes per task) (Wiig, Nielsen, Minthon, & Warkentin, 2002). There is no evidence of habituation, learning, or fatigue in repeated trials over 10 min.

The five tasks from the Alzheimer's Quick Test were administered in random order during individual sessions, by professionals trained in speech-language pathology. Since the color-naming test was repeated with each of the five tasks, color naming was performed five times. Each experimental task was preceded by three short, practice tasks to establish adequacy in naming the experimental stimuli, e.g., single colors, single forms, and color-form combinations. Rapid automatic naming times were measured using a digital stopwatch, and recorded in seconds and tenths of a second. Timing was begun immediately after the examiner finished saying, "Begin now!" and stopped immediately after the test taker named the last stimulus on the page.

Data and Statistical Analyses

The total time in seconds to name the 40 visual stimuli on each of the 15 test plates (three tests for each of five tasks) provided the measures for statistical analysis. The ratio between naming times for dual-dimension and single-dimension naming tests was calculated for each rapid automatic naming stimulus as

Ratio = Time for Dual-dimension Task/(Time for Single-dimension Color
+ Time for Single-dimension Stimulus) .

Test results were analyzed with SPSS for Windows, 1997. Descriptive statistics were calculated for each of the test measures and for subject. To examine the effect of learning on naming time comparison, analysis of variance was performed with the color measure for each task as the dependent variable. To compare performance time for each of the single-dimension test stimuli, analysis of variance was performed with each of the five single-dimension tasks as the dependent variable of response time. The relationship between age and each test was estimated by Pearson product-moment correlations. Linear regression was used to examine the relationship between multiple independent variables and a dependent variable, specifically the relationship between age and test performance.

RESULTS

Naming Time for Rapid Automatic Naming Tasks

Detailed statistical results are shown in Table 1 below. Naming time for single-dimension color ranged from 20.7 sec. ($SD = 3.1$) to 21.1 sec. ($SD = 3.1$) for the five replications of Test 1. Small differences between mean times were not significant ($F = .29$, ns), supporting previous reports that the color naming is not subject to learning effect (Wiig, Nielsen, Minthon, & Warkentin, 2002).

Naming time for single-dimension letters and numbers (Table 1) were significantly ($p < .05$) less than for single-dimension forms, animals, or objects. Single-dimension naming times correlated weakly ($r = .58$) but not significantly ($p > .20$) with syllable length (range: 40–67) for the specific single-dimension test.

TABLE 1
MEANS AND STANDARD DEVIATIONS FOR RAPID AUTOMATIC NAMING TASKS IN NORMAL SUBJECTS ($N = 144$)

Task	Test 1 (sec.) Color M	SD	Test 2 (sec.) Single Dimension M	SD	Test 3 (sec.) Dual Dimension M	SD	Test 3/Test 2 Ratio M	SD
Color-Form	20.91	3.31	24.18	4.50	48.43	8.21	1.08	.13‡
Color-Number	20.93	3.19	14.26	2.72*	41.04	6.75*	1.17	.14
Color-Letter	20.74	3.08	14.11	2.90*	42.03	6.62*	1.21	.14
Color-Animal	21.08	3.16	25.74	3.75	48.29	7.18	1.04	.10†
Color-Object	21.09	3.12	26.72	4.27	47.67	7.27	1.00	.11†

*$p < .05$ by analysis of variance compared Color-Form, Color-Animal, or Color-Object. †$p < .05$ by analysis of variance compared Color-Form, Color-Number, or Color-Letter. ‡$p < .05$ by analysis of variance compared Color-Number, Color-Letter, or Color-Animal, or Color-Object.

Naming times for the dual-dimension stimuli, i.e., combinations of color with the other single-dimension stimuli, were consistently greater than for each of the related single-dimension stimuli. In fact, the dual-dimension tests required about as much time as the sum of the two related single-dimension tests. Naming time for color-number and color-letter were significantly ($p < .05$) less than for color-form, color-animal, or color-object. Dual-dimension naming times correlated weakly ($r = .63$) but significantly ($p > .25$) with the syllable length (range: 90–117) of the specific dual-dimension test.

The mean calculated dual-dimension/single-dimension ratio was greater than unity for each rapid automatic naming task, reflecting that naming time for each dual-dimension test was slightly greater than the sum of the naming times for the two related single-dimension stimuli from which it was composed. The time ratios were similar for color-form, color-animal, and color-object combination naming (range: 1.00–1.08), and significantly ($p < .05$) less than for color-number and color-letter combination naming (1.17 and 1.21, respectively). Mean times for the 15 test measures did not differ significantly for men and women.

Age Effect on Rapid Automatic Naming Tasks

The relationships between age and naming times for each test were examined using Pearson coefficients of correlation. The coefficients of correlation are shown in Table 2 below. The correlations between age and the single-dimension color naming times for each of the five tasks (Test 1) were all positive ($r = .26$ to $.33$) and statistically significant ($p < .05$). For form, number, letter, animal, or object naming (Test 2) correlations between age and the stimulus were positive for each task. The correlations between age and dual-dimension naming times (Test 3) for color-form, color-number, color-animal, and color-object were significant ($p < .05$), albeit low ($r = .21$ to $.32$), while the correlation between age and color-letter naming times was not significant ($p > .06$).

TABLE 2
Coefficients of Correlation Between Age and Alzheimer's
Quick Test Naming Times or Ratios ($N = 144$)

Task	Age vs Test 1	Age vs Test 2	Age vs Test 3	Age vs Ratio
A. Color-Form	.33†	.35†	.21*	–.16
B. Color-Number	.27†	.10	.26*	.09
C. Color-Letter	.28†	.03	.07	–.12
D. Color-Animal	.30†	.16	.21*	.02
E. Color-Object	.26†	.32†	.32†	.22*

*$p < .05$. †$p < .001$.

To understand better the effect that aging has on naming times, we examined the linear relationship between age and rapid automatic naming times (Table 3). For Test 1 (Color), Test 2 (single-dimension), and Test 3 (dual-dimension), we aggregated naming times across the five Alzheimer's Quick Test tasks. Doing so decreases the strength of relationship (Pearson r) between age and the test compared to the results in Table 2 because aggregation increases the variance of the dependent variable, but it allows use of linear regression to estimate a coefficient for the independent variable (age) across the aggregate of stimuli to assess the effect that aging has on the naming time for the aggregated stimuli.

TABLE 3
Linear Relationship Between Age and Aggregated Rapid Automatic Naming Times

Age Group	n	Aggregated Rapid Automatic Naming Time	Constant B0	Coefficient B1	p	R	R^2
All	144	Color[a]	18.70	.06	<.01	.29	.08
		Single-dimension Stimulus[b]	19.52	.04	<.05	.10	.02
		Dual-dimension Stimulus[c]	41.64	.10	<.01	.21	.05
<60 yr.	125	Color[a]	19.02	.05	<.01	.18	.03
		Dual-dimension Stimulus[c]	42.64	.07	<.01	.11	.01
>60 yr.	19	Color[a]	13.18	.14	<.01	.33	.12
		Dual-dimension Stimulus[c]	20.30	.42	<.01	.32	.12

[a] Test 1 scores aggregated across five rapid automatic naming tasks. [b] Test 2 scores aggregated across five rapid automatic naming tasks. [c] Test 3 scores aggregated across five rapid automatic naming tasks.

The analysis showed a significant ($p < .001$) relationship between age and color naming time (Table 3), described by the equation: Color Naming Time = 18.70 + .06(Age). The coefficient of .06 suggests that color naming time could be expected to slow by .06 sec. per year or about 1 sec. for every 16 years of aging. The Pearson correlation was low ($r = .29$), compared to the results in Table 2 given the effect of aggregating data. The coefficient of determination (R^2) indicated that aging accounts for only 8.2% of the variance in color naming time, whereas other factors accounted for the remaining 91.8% of the variance.

Similarly, there was a significant ($p < .05$) linear relationship between age and the other single-dimension naming times, described by the equation: Single-dimension Naming Time = 19.52 + .04(Age). Thus, single-dimension stimulus naming time for form, number, letter, animal, and object would be expected to slow by about 1 sec. every 25 years.

As might be expected, since both color and other single-dimension stimulus naming times were related to age, there was a significant ($p < .001$) linear relationship between age and the dual-dimension naming time described by the equation: Dual-dimension Naming time = 41.64 + .1(Age). Thus, dual-dimension naming time would be expected to increase by 1 sec. every 10 years. Notably, the aging effect on the dual-dimension task (coefficient = .10) is equal to the combined coefficients for aging on single-dimension color naming and single-dimension stimulus naming (coefficients = .06 and .04, respectively).

There was no significant linear relationship between age and calculated test ratio for aggregated data. This result is expected, since any effect of aging would most likely affect both the numerator and denominator of the ratio about equally, thus an aging effect would not be apparent in the calculated ratio.

Our sample population included subjects over age 60. To reduce the possibility that undiagnosed dementia or preclinical dementia in those over 60 years of age influenced the linear regressions, we repeated the statistical analysis using only 125 subjects who were younger than 60 years old (Table 3). The relationship between age and color naming remained significant ($p < .001$) and is described by the equation: Color Naming Time = 19.02 + .05 (Age). Thus, our data show an age-related decrement of .05 sec. per year in color-naming time, even in an age range not usually subject to effects of dementia.

For the subjects 60 and over, there is a statistically significant ($p < .001$) increase in color-naming time amounting to 0.14 sec. per year or about 1 sec. every 7 years. There was no significant relationship between single-dimension naming time and age, for either age group. However, there was a significant small relationship, other than for color naming, between age and dual-dimension naming times for both the subset under age 60 ($r = .11$, $p < .01$) and over age 60 ($r = .32$, $p < .01$).

Discussion

In this study, we describe the performance of normal subjects for each of several rapid automatic naming measures of cognitive performance and the effect of age on performance. Each measure is based on processing speed, as reflected in total naming time, for a single-dimension or dual-dimension task. The findings reflect that processing and naming speed are dependent on the specific cognitive task. Further, the findings show a performance decrement with age, even within a subset of subjects less than 60 years old, in whom clinical dementia would be unusual. Since patients with established dementia demonstrate far greater decrements in processing speed —typically 10 to 40 sec. above normal limits (Nielsen, Warkentin, Jacobson, Minthon, & Wiig, 2003), the small cognitive decrement related to age is unlikely to interfere with detection of dementia. Because an expected decrement related to age can be estimated, a more rapid decrement may be an indicator of mild cognitive impairment, even in subjects without clinical symptoms.

Naming Time

This study shows that various tests of single-dimension rapid automatic naming, though similar in concept, have markedly different processing speeds. Naming times for number and letter differ significantly from naming time for form; and each of these three measures is significantly different than naming times for animal and object (Table 1). Our results are supported by an earlier study (Wiig, Nielsen, Minthon, McPeek, Said, & Warkentin, 2002), which showed that naming time for color was significantly different than for form, number, and letter, and that naming time for form was significantly different than for number or letter. The similarity in the studies supports the conclusion that differences in naming times are not artifacts caused by differences in sample size or age distribution.

Why naming time for number and letter required about 12 sec. less time than naming for form, animal, or object is not established. One logical hypothesis is that processing speed is influenced by syllable length of the specific task. However, the weak and insignificant correlation between syllable length and naming times leads to the conclusion that syllable length alone cannot account for the findings. Another hypothesis is that processing speed for certain cognitive functions may improve or be better maintained when used frequently and repetitively, resulting in greater automatization (Wiig, Nielsen, Minthon, McPeek, Said, & Warkentin, 2002). According to this hypothesis, recall of letters and numbers may occur so frequently and repetitively that this pathway develops preferentially, resulting in more rapid processing time. Alternatively, recall for names of numbers and letters may utilize shorter or more rapid cognitive pathways, resulting in shorter test times. This latter hypothesis is supported by preliminary cerebral blood flow findings that during number and letter naming, there is preferential activation of the occipital and posterior temporal areas but less activation of the parietal areas than during color-form naming (Warkentin, 2003).

Similarly, the current study shows that tests of dual-dimension rapid automatic naming differ depending on the stimuli involved. Naming of color-number and color-letter required less time than naming color-form, color-animal, or color-object combinations. Again, the difference may be due either to automatization or to use of different cognitive pathways. However, the time advantage for the dual-dimension color-number and color-letter tasks is only about 6 sec. It may be that duality of the testing imposes additional cognitive overhead that requires time or impairs the benefit of automaticity.

Additional cognitive overhead would be expected to add a constant time requirement, while impairment of automaticity would be expected to influence naming time proportionally to the extent of automatization. In our study, the dual-dimension/single-dimension ratio for each of the five stimuli (Table 1) was inversely related to the naming time on single-dimension testing. Thus, naming time for single-dimension letter was the lowest of any of the five stimuli and had the highest ratio, while naming time for single-dimension object was the highest and had the lowest ratio. The inverse relationship with naming time for a single-dimension stimulus suggests that the ratio is a measure of automatization rather than cognitive overhead. That automaticity accounts only partially for the advantage of number and letter naming times over other stimuli is consistent with automatization causing only part of the difference between single-dimension and dual-dimension naming times. The remainder may be due to additional cognitive overhead or differences in cognitive pathways.

Age Effect

This study used correlation indices to explore the effect of age on the naming times in a sample of 144 normal adults ranging in age from 15 to 85 years (Table 2). In an earlier study, Wiig, Nielsen, Minthon, McPeek, Said, and Warkentin (2002) used analysis of variance to examine the effects of age and sex in 60 subjects and found significant age-related effect on naming times for color, form, color-form, and color-letter but no significant sex-related differences. The findings in the current study support and extend the earlier conclusions.

For each of the five tasks, the single-dimension naming time for color correlated significantly with age ($r = .26$ to $.33$, $p = .001$). Although the coefficient of correlation is low, accounting for only 6.9% of the variation in color naming times, it is consistent for each of the five repetitions of the test.

There was a significant correlation between age and single-dimension naming time for form and object ($r = .35$ and $.32$, respectively) but not for number, letter, or animal. The reason that naming times for letter and number do not correlate with age is unknown. It has been hypothesized that automatization of the cognitive task may protect it from age effects or that frequent use of the cognitive skill prevents its age-related decrement. An alternative is that cognitive pathways used for recall of number and letter may be shorter and, therefore, reflect smaller magnitude of aging effects.

Our results indicate statistically significant correlations between age and naming times for all but one (color-letter) of the dual-dimension naming tasks. This is not surprising, since naming time for each of the second stimuli in the dual-dimension test (color, form, age, and object) correlated with age as single-dimension stimuli. These findings agree with those of the earlier, less comprehensive study (Wiig, Nielsen, Minthon, McPeek, Said, & Warkentin, 2002), with one exception. In the earlier study, age influenced color-letter naming, but not color-number naming. In this study, the opposite effects were noted, as age showed a significant effect on color-number naming but not on color-letter naming. This inconsistency suggests that the automaticity for color-number and color-letter naming may be sensitive to differences in the active use of the linguistic repertories for numbers and letters within the two samples.

Age effect was not apparent in the dual-dimension/single-dimension ratio, likely because the effect occurred about equally in both the numerator and the denominator of the ratio. This independence from aging effect suggests that the ratios may provide stable measures in normally aging populations. However, they may indicate changes in adults with temporoparietal dysfunction or pathology such as dementia of the Alzheimer's type, a hypothesis that needs validation.

Age Effect as Assessed by Regression

Normal cognitive function requires frequent use of all cognitive functions we assessed. To assess better the overall effect of aging on rapid naming, we aggregated stimulus naming times across the five tasks. This identified an increase in color naming time of .06 sec. per year, an increase in other single-dimension naming time of .04 sec. per year, and an increase in dual-dimension naming time of .10 sec. per year. Since dual-dimension naming time requires naming of both color and a second single-dimension stimulus, it seems reasonable that the aging decrement for dual-dimension naming (increased time) is equal to the sum for the color and other single-dimension stimulus naming times. Interestingly, the decrement with age for the dual-dimension task is almost identical to the decrement identified for an eye-hand reaction time task that required processing two bits of information (Repperger, *et al.*, 1985; Jacobson, *et al.*, 1986).

Rapid Automatic Naming and Diagnosis of Alzheimer's Disease

At present, diagnosis of Alzheimer's Disease remains a clinical diagnosis, based on clinical criteria and supported by cognitive function tests, each of which has a specific purpose and limitation. The Mini-Mental State Examination, for example, may be useful for office screening and follow-up to measure onset and relative severity of cognitive impairment, but it is affected by education, cultural background, literacy, and interpretation (Folstein, *et al.*, 1975; Molloy, *et al.*, 1991; Karlawish & Clark, 2003). Furthermore, research indicates that test-retest scores and interrater reliability are inadequate for monitoring dementia treatments (Bowie, Branton, & Holmes, 1999). The Alzheimer's Disease Assessment Scale, Cognitive subscale (Rosen, *et al.*, 1984) assesses selected aspects of cognitive performance, including elements of memory orientation, language, praxis, attention, and concentration in patients with varying severity of dementia; but administration requires about an hour and availability of highly trained medical professionals to administer and interpret the test.

Because they require special training for administration or interpretation or because they are influenced by education and training, neither the Mini-Mental State Examination nor Alzheimer's Disease Assessment Scale, Cognitive subscale is optimal for widespread screening for established Alzheimer's Disease. These tests measure grossly aberrant cognitive content rather than processing speed or working memory, which means they are less useful to detect early Alzheimer's Disease in the preclinical phase.

The Alzheimer's Quick Test color-form combination naming test shows promise as a methodology for general use to screen for clinical evidence of temporoparietal dysfunction of the Alzheimer's Disease type. Since rapid automatic naming tasks included in the Alzheimer's Quick Test are influenced by the subject's age, adjustment of the normal limit to account for age should be considered. Currently, the defined limits for Alzheimer's Quick Test are: Normal: < 60 sec., Questionable: 60–70 sec., Abnormal: > 70 sec. (Wiig, Nielsen, Minthon, & Warkentin, 2002). The age-related decrement (about 0.1 sec. per year) is small when compared to the decrement in Alzheimer's disease (10 to 30 sec. above normal), so age-related adjustment need not be considered except for very elderly persons. With global increases in the expected life span of adults (ISOA & ILC-USA, 2001), the Alzheimer's Quick Test limit of normality may, in the future, require an additional factor to account for very advanced age.

Administration of Alzheimer's Quick Test rapid automatic naming tests is simple, inexpensive, and independent of technical equipment or highly trained medical personnel. Further, as highly reliable measures based on processing speed, rapid automatic naming tests offer promise as a sensitive measure to detect preclinical cognitive impairment prior to development of clinically apparent symptoms. The present study defines normal performance for the Alzheimer's Quick Test of automatic naming and describes an age-related decrement in normal performance that is unlikely to limit use of Alzheimer's Quick Test rapid automatic naming tests for evaluation of cognitive performance.

REFERENCES

BOTWINICK, J., & THOMPSON, L. W. (1966) Components of reaction time in relation to age and sex. *Journal of Genetic Psychology*, 108, 175-183.

BOWIE, P., BRANTON, T., & HOLMES, J. (1999) Should the Mini-Mental State Examination be used to monitor dementia treatments? *The Lancet*, 354, 1527-1528.

CALLAHAN, C. M., HENDRIE, J. C., & TIERNEY, W. M. (1995) Documentation and evaluation of cognitive impairment in elderly primary care patients. *Annals of Internal Medicine*, 122, 422-429.

CHRISTENSEN, H. (2001) What cognitive changes can be expected with normal ageing? *Australian and New Zealand Journal of Psychiatry*, 35, 768-775.

DUNCAN, B. A., & SIEGAL, A. P. (1998) Early diagnosis and management of Alzheimer's disease. *Journal of Clinical Psychiatry*, 59, S15-S21.

FOLSTEIN, M. F., FOLSTEIN, S. E., & McHUGH, P. R. (1975) "Mini-mental state": a practical method for grading the cognitive state of patients for the clinician. *Journal of Psychiatric Research*, 12, 189-198.

FOX, N. C., WARRINGTON, E. K., FREEBOROUGH, P. A., HARTIKAINEN, P., KENNEDY, A. M., STEVENS, J. M., & ROSSOOR, M. N. (1996) Presymptomatic hyppocampal atrophy in Alzheimer's disease: a longitudinal MRI study. *Brain*, 119, 2001-2007.

FRITH, C. D., FRISTON, K., LIDDLE, P. F., & FRACKOWIAK, R. S. (1991) Willed action and the prefrontal cortex in man: a study with PET. *Proceedings of the Royal Society, London, B., Biological Science*, 244, 241-246.

GEERLINGS, M. I., JONKER, C., BOUTER, L. M., ADER, H. J., & SCHMAND, B. (1999) Association between memory complaints and incident Alzheimer's disease in elderly people with normal baseline cognition. *American Journal of Psychiatry*, 56, 521-527.

GOETZ, D. W., JACOBSON, J. M., MURNANE, J. E., REID, M. J., REPPERGER, D. W., & GOODYEAR, C. (1989) Prolongation of simple and choice reaction times in a double-blind comparison of twice-daily hydroxyzine versus terfenadine. *The Journal of Allergy and Clinical Immunology*, 84, 316-322.

HICK, W. E. (1952) On the rate of gain of information. *Quarterly Journal of Experimental Psychology*, 4, 11-26.

INSTITUTE FOR THE STUDY OF AGING & INTERNATIONAL LONGEVITY CENTER-USA. (2001) *Achieving and maintaining cognitive vitality with aging: workshop report*. New York: Authors.

JACOBSON, J. M., REPPERGER, D. W., GOODYEAR, C., & MICHEL, N. (1986) Effect of directional response variables on eye-hand reaction times and decision time. *Perceptual and Motor Skills*, 62, 195-208.

KARLAWISH, J. H. T., & CLARK, C. (2003) The diagnostic evaluation of elderly patients with mild memory problems. *Annals of Internal Medicine*, 138, 411-419.

MOLLOY, D., ALEMAYEHU, E., & ROBERTS, R. (1991) Reliability of a standardized Mini-Mental State Examination compared with the traditional Mini-Mental State Examination. *American Journal of Psychiatry*, 148, 102-105.

NIELSEN, N. P., WARKENTIN, S., JACOBSON, J. M., MINTHON, L., & WIIG, E. H. (2003) A comparison of AQT and MMSE for diagnosis of established Alzheimer's disease. (Working paper, Department of Clinical Physiology, Malmo University Hospital, Malmo, & Knowledge Research Institute, Arlington, TX)

OBRIST, W. D. (1953) Simple auditory reaction time in aged adults. *Journal of Psychology*, 35, 259-266.

REPPERGER, D. W., JACOBSON, J., WALBROEHL, G. S., MICHEL, N., & GOODYEAR, C. (1985) Design of a computerized device to measure simple reaction time/decision time. *Journal of Medical Engineering and Technology*, 9, 270-276.

RODRIGUEZ, G., WARKENTIN, S., RISBERG, J., & ROSADINI, G. (1988) Sex differences in regional cerebral blood flow. *Journal of Cerebral Blood Flow and Metabolism*, 8, 783-789.

ROSEN, W. G., MOHS, R. C., & DAVIS, K. L. (1984) A new rating scale for Alzheimer's disease. *American Journal of Psychiatry*, 141, 1356-1364.

SALTHOUSE, T. A. (1991) *Theoretical perspectives on cognitive aging*. Hillsdale, NJ: Erlbaum.

SEMEL, E. M., WIIG, E. H., & SECORD, W. A. (1995) *Clinical evaluation of language fundamentals–3*. San Antonio, TX: Psychological Corp.

SHAYWITZ, S. E., SHAYWITZ, B. A., PUGH, K. R., FULBRIGHT, R. K., SKUDLARSKI, P., MENCL, W. E., CONSTABLE, R. T., NAFTOLIN, F., PALTER, S. F., MARCHIONE, K. E., KATZ, L., SHANKWEILER, D. P., FLETCHER, J. M., LACADIE, C., KELTZ, M., & GORE, J. C. (1999) Effect of estrogen on brain activation patterns in postmenopausal women during working memory tasks. *The Journal of the American Medical Association*, 281, 1197-1202.

SIEGERSCHMEIDT, E., MOSCH, E., SIEMEN, M., FORSTL, H., & BICKEL, H. (2002) The clock drawing test and questionable dementia: reliability and validity. *International Journal of Geriatric Psychiatry*, 17, 1048-1054.

STRAUSS, E., LORING, D., CHELUNE, G., HUNTER, M., HERMANN, B., PERRINE, K., WESTERVELD, M., TRENERRY, M., & BARR, W. (1995) Predicting cognitive impairment in epilepsy: findings from the Bozeman Epilepsy Consortium. *Journal of Clinical and Experimental Neuropsychology*, 17, 909-917.

STROOP, J. R. (1935) Studies of interference in serial verbal reactions. *Journal of Experimental Psychology*, 18, 643-662.

TEICHNER, W. H. (1954) Recent studies of simple reaction time. *Psychological Bulletin*, 51, 128-149.

TEICHNER, W. H., & KREBS, M. J. (1974) Laws of visual choice reaction time. *Psychological Review*, 81, 75-98.

U.S. BUREAU OF THE CENSUS. (2000) *Current population survey, October 2000*. Washington, DC: U.S. Bureau of the Census.

VAN DER LINDEN, M., BEERTEN, A., & PESENTI, M. (1998) Age-related differences in random generation. *Brain and Cognition*, 38, 1-16.

VENDRELL, P., JUNQUE, C., PUJOL, J., JURADO, M. A., MOLET, J., & GRAFMAN, J. (1995) The role of prefrontal regions in the Stroop task. *Neuropsychologia*, 33, 341-352.

WARKENTIN, S. (2003) AQS assessment of temporo-parietal lobe function. Scientific Presentation to the European Union Consortium on Alzheimer's Disease, Liege, Belgium, April 11.

WARKENTIN, S., RISBERG, J., NILSSON, A., KARLSON, S., & GRAAE, E. (1991) Cortical activity during speech production: a study of regional blood flow in normal subjects performing a word fluency task. *Neuropsychiatry: Neuropsychology, and Behavioral Neurology*, 4, 305-316.

WECHSLER, D. (1997) *Wechsler Adult Intelligence Scale–Third Edition*. San Antonio, TX: Psychological Corp.

WIIG, E. H., NIELSEN, N. P., MINTHON, L., MCPEEK, D., SAID, K., & WARKENTIN, S. (2002) Parietal lobe activation in rapid, automatized naming by adults. *Perceptual and Motor Skills*, 94, 1230-1244.

WIIG, E. H., NIELSEN, N. P., MINTHON, L., & WARKENTIN, S. (2002) *Alzheimer's Quick Test: assessment of parietal function*. San Antonio, TX: Psychological Corp.

WIIG, E. H., ZUREICH, P., & CHAN, H. H. (2000) A clinical rationale for assessing rapid automatized naming in children with language disorders. *Journal of Learning Disabilities*, 33, 359-374.

Accepted January 30, 2004.

AN EXAMINATION OF HIGH SCHOOL STUDENTS' ATTITUDES TOWARD PHYSICAL EDUCATION WITH REGARD TO SEX AND SPORT PARTICIPATION [1]

CANAN KOCA

Sport Sciences Department
Baskent University, Ankara

GIYASETTIN DEMIRHAN

School of Sport Sciences and Technology
Hacettepe University

Summary.—This study assessed attitudes of high school students toward physical education with regard to sex and sport participation. A total of 440 sport participants (175 girls and 265 boys) and of 427 nonsport participants (227 girls and 200 boys), all of whom were 15 yr. old, voluntarily participated. The Attitudes Toward Physical Education Scale was administered to assess participants' attitudes toward physical education. The results of 2 × 2 (Sex × Sports Participation) analysis of variance indicated a significant difference in attitudes toward physical education between sport participants and nonsport participants, with the former scoring higher, and a difference between boys and girls, with boys scoring higher. However, there was no significant interaction between sex and sports participation on attitudes toward physical education. In general, sport participants had more favorable Attitudes Toward Physical Education scores than nonsport participants, and high school boys scored significantly higher than girls. There was a significant difference in Attitudes Toward Physical Education scores between female and male high school students, with boys having more favorable attitude scores.

The recent increase in research on students' attitudes toward physical education may be attributed to the influence of attitudes on later participation in physical activities outside of school (Carlson, 1995; Portman, 1995; Ennis, 1996) and on students' achievement in physical education (Silverman, 1993; Graham, 1995; Lee, 1997; Subramaniam & Silverman, 2000), as well as for developing curriculum content (Cothran & Ennis, 1998). Silverman and Subramaniam (1999) argued that, if attitude influences participation in most activities, a better understanding of how it affects perceptions and feelings toward physical education could provide valuable information to teachers, coaches, and parents.

Such information may help physical educators in their understanding of the teaching-learning process and class environment in physical education, feedback on effective instructional methods, curriculum content, and teaching-learning environments. According to Strand and Scantling (1994), the following factors influence students' attitudes toward physical education: the facilities, curriculum content, teachers' behavior, class atmosphere, and stu-

---

[1]Address correspondence to Canan Koca, Başkent Üniversitesi, Sağlık Bilimleri Fakültesi, Spor Bilimleri Bölümü, Bağlıca Kampüsü, Eskişehir Yolu 20 km. 06530, Ankara, Turkey or (canank@baskent.edu.tr) or (giyasettin.demirhan@hacettepe.edu.tr).

dents' perceptions. Studies undertaken to examine the role of teachers' and students' attitudes toward physical education generally support the view that teachers have an important role in providing appropriate learning opportunities and experiences that cultivate positive attitudes in students toward subject matter in physical education (Figley, 1985; Harrison & Blakemore, 1989; Luke & Sinclair, 1991). In other studies, program content was an important component in students' attitudes (Rice, 1988; Aicinena, 1991; Browne, 1992; Luke & Cope, 1994).

A number of studies have also compared girls' and boys' attitudes toward physical education and sport. Boys reported more positive attitudes toward physical activities that were challenging and had an element of risk (Smoll & Schutz, 1980; Folsom-Meek, 1992), whereas girls reported more favorable attitudes toward physical activities emphasizing aesthetics (Smoll & Schutz, 1980; Birtwistle & Brodie, 1991; Hicks, Wiggins, Crist, & Moode, 2001).

The present study further extends previous research by focusing specifically on sport participation and sex differences in Turkish students' attitudes toward physical education. Based on the previous research, the first hypothesis was that boys would exhibit a higher mean attitude score than girls. We examined the influence of sport participation on students' attitudes toward physical education. Therefore, the second hypothesis was that sport participants would exhibit a higher mean attitude score than nonsport participants.

Method

Participants

Participants were 867 students from eight high schools which represented middle socioeconomic status and were located in the center of Ankara, Turkey. A total of 440 sport participants [175 girls ($M_{age}=15.0$, $SD=0.4$) and 265 boys ($M_{age}=15.0$, $SD=0.4$)] and of 427 nonsport participants [227 girls ($M_{age}=15.0$, $SD=0.4$) and 200 boys ($M_{age}=15.0$, $SD=0.3$)] voluntarily participated. The majority of sport participants were members of school athletic teams, and the remainder were members of amateur sports clubs outside school.

Measures

A short questionnaire was administered to obtain demographic information and The Attitudes Toward Physical Education Scale to assess attitudes.

Attitudes Toward Physical Education Scale.—The Attitudes Toward Physical Education, developed by Demirhan and Altay (2001), was applied to all participants. This paper-and-pencil self-report questionnaire used a 5-point Likert-type scale asking the respondent to indicate attitudes using anchors of 1: Strongly Disagree and 5: Strongly Agree for 24 items. Total possible scores ranged from 24 to 120. A score of 24 represents the most negative attitude; 25–48 indicates a relatively negative attitude, 49–72 neutral attitude, 73–94 relatively positive attitude, and 95–120 the most positive attitude. The Cronbach coefficient alpha reliability was .93; the intraclass correlation coefficient was .85, and the scale validity coefficient was .83.

Data Collection

Permission was requested and granted from the Ministry of Education to conduct the study in schools. All participants completed the inventories in their classroom setting which were collected from them by the researcher.

Data Analysis

A 2 × 2 (Sex × Sport Participation) univariate analysis of variance assessed mean differences in attitudes toward physical education between sport participants and nonsport participants and between girls and boys.

RESULTS AND DISCUSSION

The means and standard deviations by sex for Attitudes Toward Physical Education scores are in Table 1. Mean attitude scores of boys, both sport participants and nonsport participants, were higher than those of girls, both sport participants and nonsport participants. With respect to our first hypothesis, the results of 2 × 2 (Sex × Sport Participation) analysis of variance indicated a significant mean difference in attitudes toward physical education between these male and female high school students ($F_{1,863} = 4.12$, $p < .05$). In addition, Table 1 presents the means and standard deviations for sport participation according to Attitudes Toward Physical Education scores. Both female and male sport participants had higher mean attitude scores than female and male nonsport participants.

TABLE 1
MEANS AND STANDARD DEVIATIONS OF HIGH SCHOOL STUDENTS' ATTITUDES TOWARD PHYSICAL EDUCATION SCORES

Sex	Group	n	M	SD
Girls	Sport Participants	175	3.35	0.56
	Nonsport Participants	227	3.20	0.55
Boys	Sport Participants	265	3.47	0.54
	Nonsport Participants	200	3.24	0.49

With respect to the second hypothesis, a significant difference in attitudes toward physical education between sport participants and nonsport participants ($F_{1,863} = 27.70$, $p < .01$) was noted, but there was no significant interaction for sex by group ($F_{1,863} = 1.33$, $p > .05$).

The purpose of this study was to assess attitudes of high school students toward physical education by sex and sport participation.

With respect to our first hypothesis, boys had a higher mean Attitudes Toward Physical Education score than girls. This finding confirms the findings of previous studies (Smoll & Schutz, 1980; Birtwistle & Brodie, 1991; Anderssen, 1993; Tannehill, Romar, O'Sullivan, England, & Rosenberg, 1994; Quaterman, Harris, & Chew, 1996). Although the age of participants and questionnaire differed from those of the present study, similar findings were also obtained by Hicks and his colleagues (2001). Those researchers examined sex differences in Grade 3 students' attitudes toward physical activity by using a multidimensional scale. Girls had significantly more positive attitudes than boys in the aesthetic domain.

The present findings also supported the second hypothesis that sport participants would have a higher mean attitude score than nonsport participants. The high school students who participated in out-of-school activities regularly had a higher mean attitude score than students who did not participate in any out-of-school activities. In addition, Anderssen (1993) reported similar results, indicating that physically active students perceived physical education more favorably than less active students. This finding provides valuable information for teachers, since provision of physical activities, which increase students' fitness and skill through extracurricular physical activities and those in school, have an important association in a more positive attitude in students toward physical education.

Two limitations of this study should be noted. Firstly, the inventory is one-dimensional. Further research is needed to examine attitudes toward physical education, using an adaptation for the Turkish population of multidimensional attitude inventories from the literature, or a multidimensional inventory for the Turkish population should be developed. The second limitation is the sample. Although this study provided some insight into Turkish students' attitudes toward high school physical education, the sample of 9th graders in high school was small and limited to one grade. Further research is recommended with students from other grades.

REFERENCES

AICINENA, S. (1991) The teacher and student attitudes toward physical education. *The Physical Educator*, 48(1), 28-32.

ANDERSSEN, N. (1993) Perception of physical education classes among young adolescents: do physical education classes provide equal opportunities to all students? *Health Education Research*, 8, 167-179.

BIRTWISTLE, G. E., & BRODIE, D. A. (1991) Children's attitudes towards activity and perceptions of physical education. *Health Education Research*, 6, 465-478.

BROWNE, J. (1992) Reasons for selection or non-selection of physical education studies by year 12 girls. *Journal of Teaching in Physical Education*, 11, 402-410.

CARLSON, T. B. (1995) We hate gym: student alienation from physical education. *Journal of Teaching in Physical Education*, 14, 467-477.

COTHRAN, D. J., & ENNIS, C. D. (1998) Curricula of mutual worth: comparisons of students' and teachers' curricular goals. *Journal of Teaching in Physical Education*, 17, 307-326.

Demirhan, G., & Altay, F. (2001) [Attitudes scale of high school first graders towards physical education and sport: II]. *Spor Bilimleri Dergisi*, 12(2), 9-20.

Ennis, C. D. (1996) Students' experiences in sport-based physical education: (more than) apologies are necessary. *Quest*, 48, 453-456.

Figley, G. E. (1985) Determinants of attitudes toward physical education. *Journal of Teaching in Physical Education*, 4, 229-240.

Folsom-Meek, S. L. (1992) A comparison of upper elementary school children's attitudes toward physical activity. (ERIC Document Reproduction Service No. ED 350 297)

Graham, G. (1995) Physical education through students' eyes and in students' voices: introduction. *Journal of Teaching in Physical Education*, 14, 364-371.

Harrison, J., & Blakemore, C. (1989) *Instructional strategies for secondary school physical education*. Dubuque, IA: Brown.

Hicks, M. K., Wiggins, M. S., Crist, R. W., & Moode, F. M. (2001) Sex differences in Grade three students' attitudes toward physical activity. *Perceptual and Motor Skills*, 93, 97-102.

Lee, A. M. (1997) Contribution of research on student thinking in physical education. *Journal of Teaching in Physical Education*, 16, 262-277.

Luke, M. D., & Cope, L. D. (1994) Student attitudes toward teacher behaviour and program content in school physical education. *The Physical Educator*, 51, 57-66.

Luke, M. D., & Sinclair, G. (1991) Gender difference in adolescents' attitudes toward school physical education. *Journal of Teaching in Physical Education*, 11, 31-46.

Portman, P. A. (1995) Who is having fun in physical education classes? Experiences of six grade students in elementary and middle schools. *Journal of Teaching in Physical Education*, 14, 445-453.

Quaterman, J., Harris, G., & Chew, R. M. (1996) African-American students' perceptions of the value of basic physical education activity programs at historically black colleges and universities. *Journal of Teaching in Physical Education*, 15, 188-204.

Rice, P. L. (1988) Attitudes of high school students toward physical education activities, teachers and personal health. *The Physical Educator*, 45, 94-99.

Silverman, S. (1993) Student characteristics, practice, and achievement in physical education. *Journal of Educational Research*, 87, 54-61.

Silverman, S., & Subramaniam, P. R. (1999) Student attitude toward physical education and physical activity: a review of measurement issues and outcomes. *Journal of Teaching in Physical Education*, 19, 97-125.

Smoll, F. L., & Schutz, R. W. (1980) Children's attitudes toward physical activity: a longitudinal analysis. *Journal of Sport Psychology*, 2, 137-147.

Strand, B., & Scantling, E. (1994) An analysis of secondary student preferences towards physical education. *Physical Educator*, 51, 119-129.

Subramaniam, P. R., & Silverman, S. (2000) Validation of scores from an instrument assessing student attitude toward physical education. *Measurement in Physical Education and Exercise Science*, 4, 29-43.

Tannehill, D., Romar, J. E., O'Sullivan, M., England, K., & Rosenberg, D. (1994) Attitudes toward physical education: their impact on how physical education teachers make sense of their work. *Journal of Teaching in Physical Education*, 13, 406-420.

Accepted February 13, 2004.

LEFT:RIGHT DIFFERENCES IN PSYCHOPHYSICAL AND ELECTRODERMAL MEASURES OF OLFACTORY THRESHOLDS AND THEIR RELATION TO ELECTRODERMAL INDICES OF HEMISPHERIC ASYMMETRIES [1]

GÉRARD BRAND, JEAN-LOUIS MILLOT, LAURENCE JACQUOT, STÉPHANIE THOMAS, AND SONIA WETZEL

Laboratoire de Neurosciences
Université de Franche Comté

Summary.—The study of lateralization processes in olfaction in human subjects has given rise to many contradictory findings. Indeed, sensorial cerebral asymmetry in olfaction depends on several factors (nature of task, quality of stimulus, characteristics of subjects, etc.) and could be also related to differences between the nostrils. In this field, few studies have assessed simultaneously the left–right nostril differences and the hemispheric asymmetry. The present work dealt with this question in the same population with the same odorants, procedures, and stimulations. Seven different concentrations of four specific odorants (two pleasant and two unpleasant) were used by single nostril stimulation with 30 dextral subjects (20 women and 10 men). Threshold detection in unilateral stimulation was investigated using electrodermal response to confirm the first psychophysic measure. Moreover, bilateral recordings of electrodermal activity (EDA) with unilateral stimulation were used as a measure of functional hemispheric asymmetry. Analysis showed no differences between the two nostrils for the threshold detection regardless of the method used (psychophysic or EDA response). However, most subjects presented a constant direction of electrodermal asymmetry whichever nostril was stimulated and whichever odorant stimulus used. The constant bilateral differences in EDA recordings are discussed in terms of asymmetrical activation of the hemispheres.

Initial research of Toulouse and Vaschide (45, 46) in olfaction suggested that left:right nostril, i.e., peripheral, differences are linked to hemispheric asymmetry. Subsequently, functional cerebral asymmetry in olfaction and peripheral differences has been carefully studied but has still not been fully clarified (5, 14). Recent research about peripheral differences is still contradictory. Experiments have not found any systematic lateral differences in detection-threshold tasks (4, 32) or in test scores for odor memory (8). Zatorre and Jones-Gotman (49) found the right nostril discriminated odors better. Other studies have shown an asymmetry of the peripheral receptors in relation to handedness (9, 24, 41, 48); right-handers seem to perform better with the left nostril whereas left-handers seem to perform better with the right nostril. However, there are other factors that appear to confound these

---

[1]Address enquiries to Dr. G. Brand, Laboratoire de Neurosciences, Université de Franche Comté, Place Leclerc, 25000 Besançon, France.

assessments, such as peripheral differences depending on nasal airflow (29), smelling behavior (36), or unilateral neglect in sensory input (3).

The data regarding hemispheric asymmetry have not been consistent. Research concerning the pathological aspects, especially in epileptic patients, found no significant differences in the olfactory detection thresholds between subjects with hemisphere lesions and controls (2, 19). In normal subjects, some studies have reported that chemosensory evoked potentials are of larger amplitude in the right than the left hemisphere, regardless of the side of nose stimulated (28, 30, 31). With positron emission tomography (PET) Zatorre, *et al.* (50) measured cerebral blood flow using the bolus H_2O technique during two PET scans, a control task and an activation task in which subjects smelt one odorant. They found a functional asymmetry with a focus of activation located in the right orbitofrontal cortex corresponding to Brodmann's Area 11.

This experiment was done (a) to explore further the nature of laterality differences in olfactory threshold sensitivity, measured both psychophysically and, indirectly, via alterations in odor-induced electrodermal activity and (b) to assess whether left:right differences, if present, correlate with left:right differences in hemispheric function, as measured by an electrodermal technique. This one is a psychophysiological response frequently used for observation in olfaction and has been a good indicator for analysing olfactory mechanisms (47). The first part of this work focuses on peripheral lateralization and uses the electrodermal response as an indicator of the detection threshold associated with a traditional method using psychophysical tests. The second part of this work evaluates hemispheric asymmetry using bilateral EDA recordings which show good reliability over time (39, 42). Much research (26, 27) has shown the usefulness of bilateral EDA recordings for cerebral functional asymmetry. When asymmetry is clearly shown by bilateral EDA recordings (in tonic or phasic measures), it reflects an asymmetry in the functioning of the cerebral hemispheres (23). Constancy in the direction of EDA asymmetry has been found by several researchers who presented the lateralization of electrodermal activity as a function of differential activation of hemispheres (10, 11, 18, 21, 34, 35, 38).

In a previous experiment using bilateral EDA recordings with unilateral stimulation using a pleasant odorant (lavender) in suprathreshold concentrations, Brand, *et al.* (6) found a functional asymmetry in a group of right-handed subjects. Two-thirds of the subjects appeared to have a left hemispheric dominance and one-third a right hemispheric dominance. Following these findings, the present study was designed to examine whether there are EDA differences in detection thresholds between the two nostrils and between monorhinal and birhinal stimulations and if there were variations related to the nature of the stimulus and more particularly the hedonic valence (pleasant/unpleasant) as some (35) have suggested.

Method

Subjects

Thirty undergraduate student volunteers (20 women and 10 men) participated. Their ages ranged from 20 to 27 years (*M* age 23 yr.). All subjects were dextrals (father and mother also dextral). The lateralization for both feet and hands was assessed by an adapted version of the Waterloo Questionnaire (16). All subjects were free of head colds or nasal allergies at the time of the tests.

Odorant Stimuli

Four specific odorants frequently used in olfactory research (with a good stability over time) were tested: two pleasant odorants *isoamyl acetate* (IA) [$C_7H_{14}O_2$ Mol.Wt.: 130.2] and *citral* (C) [$C_{10}H_{16}O$ Mol.Wt.: 152.2], and two unpleasant odorants *triethylamine* (T) [$C_6H_{15}N$ Mol.Wt.: 101.2] and *thioglycolic acid* (TA) [$C_2H_4O_2S$ Mol.Wt.: 92.11]. The dilutions for isoamyl acetate and citral were prepared in distilled water and those for triethylamine and thioglycolic acid were prepared in mineral oil. The concentrations were 0.1%, 0.5%, 1%, 2%, 5%, 10%, and 25%. The presentation in ascending order was alternated with pleasant and unpleasant odorants and the concentration range tested in accord with Devos, *et al.* (12): isoamyl acetate (0.13–32.55), thioglycolic acid (0.09–23.02), citral (0.15–38.05), triethylamine (0.10–25.30). The odorant stimulus in liquid form was presented in a bottle (7.5 cm high, 1 cm in diameter at the opening) filled with 4 ml of liquid. The bottle was presented to the subject during normal breathing for 3 sec. at a distance of 1 cm from the nostril, using a holder to avoid any olfactory or thermic interference with the experimenter's hand.

Procedure

The subjects were seated in a comfortable armchair in a quiet room (room temperature ranged from 19 to 21°C). The olfactory stimuli were delivered to one nostril, and the other nostril was blocked with a nose plug. The side tested first was randomized. The intertrial interval was random, ranging between 1 and 2 min. The tests of the second nostril began after a 5-min. period with normal breathing. During the olfactory experiments, visual cues were excluded by the use of blacked-out goggles, and auditory cues were excluded by a soundproof headphone. Also, the breathing cycle of the subjects was recorded with a Minigraph Lafayette Instrument (Model 76107 equipped with pneumo-bellows) and monitored to present the odor at the outset of inspiration and to check that the amplitude of inspiration did not change during the experiment. The experiment had to be run in two separate sessions (psychophysical tests and EDA recordings).

For psychophysical measures, the instructions were: "As soon as you perceive a smell raise your right hand." This procedure was used to have a similar situation in both psychophysical measures and EDA recordings. For EDA recordings, when the electrodes were in position, the subject was told not to move and asked to relax. Skin potential was recorded from each hand with an Alvar Electronic Polygraph (Model Praxigraph II TR) equipped with low-level DC preamplifiers. The active electrode was placed on the palmar surface and the reference electrode on the dorsal surface of the hand. Both hands were prepared by rubbing with alcohol and dried, then the conductive gel (Reegarpha) and standard electrodes were used according to the recommendations of Fowles, et al. (22). The skin potential response, expressed in microVolts, was used for data analyses. The response was considered when the minimal threshold of response latency was lower than 700 msec., the maximal threshold was higher than 3 sec., and the amplitude of the response was higher than 50 microVolts. The experiment began with two control bilateral auditive stimuli (440 Hz, 60 dB, 1 sec.; time interval of 2 min.).

Analysis of Data

The detection threshold was reached when two consecutive responses to two successively increased concentrations were obtained for an odorant. A threshold score from 0 (minimal concentration) to 7 (maximal concentration) was allotted to each odorant according to the concentration for which the first response was recorded (the maximum score being allotted to the weakest concentration). An overall score ranging between 0 to 28 (the sum of the four scores) was allotted to each subject for global detection of the four odorants for each nostril and each detection method (psychophysical test or EDA response). As the EDA recording was bilateral, the threshold was reached when a response was obtained on one or the other hand or both hands (minimum 50 µV). A threshold score ranging between 0 to 14 (the sum of both scores) was allotted to both the two pleasant and the two unpleasant odorants.

The bilateral skin potential was measured for the first response obtained for an odorant. For a specific odorant, the analysis retained only the cases where an EDA response was obtained for both nostrils. The comparative results between the two nostrils were treated in relation to the direction of asymmetry. The direction of asymmetry, right>left or left>right (R>L or L>R) was considered when the amplitude obtained on one hand was higher than 50 µV in relation to the other hand.

Student t tests (paired and independent) and the Spearman rank correlation coefficient were used for statistical analyses.

RESULTS

Threshold Detection

Overall results for the four odorants (Table 1).—First, a comparative analysis between the two nostrils showed that the detection thresholds were not significantly different for either the psychophysical measures ($t = 1.07$, ns) or the EDA responses ($t = .97$, ns). Second, the overall threshold scores for each nostril were positively correlated for the psychophysical tests ($r = .51$) and for the EDA responses ($r = .71$). Thus, the subjects who had a high threshold for one nostril also had a high threshold for the other nostril. Third, the overall threshold scores for both methods were positively correlated with either the right nostril ($r = .57$) or the left nostril ($r = .61$). Thus, the subjects who had a high threshold with one detection method also had a high threshold with the other. Regarding the overall threshold score for the four odorants and for all the subjects, the mean threshold score was higher for the psychophysical measure than for the EDA responses whatever the nostril. The statistical analysis indicated that these results were significant for the right ($t = 4.75$, $p < .0001$) and the left nostrils ($t = 4.13$, $p < .01$).

TABLE 1
Olfactory Threshold Detection (For Four Odorants in Unilateral Stimulation) Obtained by Psychophysical Method and Electrodermal Response

Measure	Right Nostril M	SD	Left Nostril M	SD	t	r
Psychophysical Detection	23.5	3.42	22.5	4.07	1.07	.51
Electrodermal Response	16.9	2.62	18.4	2.89	0.97	.71
t	4.72*		4.13*			
r	.57		.61			

*$p < .01$.

Analysis in relation to sex.—A comparative analysis for men and women showed that the detection thresholds were not significantly different whichever detection method and whichever nostril. The results of the analysis for the 20 women were similar to those obtained for the whole sample. The psychophysical detection threshold scores were higher than the EDA scores for the right nostril ($t = 2.43$, $p < .02$) and not significantly different for the left ($t = 1.86$, ns, although significance was $p < .08$). There was no significant difference between the two nostrils for the psychophysical tests ($t = .95$, ns) or the EDA method ($t = .14$, ns). The results of the analysis for the 10 men were similar to those obtained for the whole sample and those obtained for the female sample. The psychophysical detection threshold scores were higher than the EDA scores for the right ($t = 4.77$, $p < .001$) and the left ($t = 3.68$, $p < .005$) nostrils. There was no significant difference between the two nostrils for the psychophysical tests ($t = 1.19$, ns) or the EDA responses ($t = 1.14$, ns).

Analysis of the hedonic valence.—For pleasant odorants (Table 2), there were no significant threshold score differences between the two nostrils for either the psychophysical tests ($t=1.20$, ns) or the EDA responses ($t=0.52$, ns). The threshold scores obtained for the psychophysical tests were significantly higher than those for the EDA, for the right ($t=4.62$, $p<.0001$) and the left ($t=2.94$, $p<.006$) nostrils. The results were the same for both sexes. For these two odorants with a positive hedonic valence, there was no significant difference between the male and female populations whichever nostril and whichever detection method.

TABLE 2
OLFACTORY THRESHOLD DETECTION (FOR TWO PLEASANT ODORANTS IN UNILATERAL STIMULATION) OBTAINED BY PSYCHOPHYSICAL METHOD AND ELECTRODERMAL RESPONSE

Measure	Right Nostril M	SD	Left Nostril M	SD	t
Psychophysical Detection	12.7	1.82	12.1	2.11	1.20
Electrodermal Response	9.5	1.46	9.5	1.73	0.52
t	4.62*		2.94*		

*$p<.01$.

For unpleasant odorants (Table 3), there was no significant threshold score difference between the two nostrils for either the psychophysical tests ($t=1.46$, ns) or the EDA responses ($t=1.40$, ns). The threshold scores obtained for the psychophysical tests were significantly higher than those for the EDA responses, for the right ($t=3.51$, $p<.001$) and the left ($t=2.41$, $p<.01$) nostrils. The results were the same for both sexes. For these two odorants with a negative hedonic valence, there was no significant difference between the male and female populations regardless of nostril and or detection method used.

TABLE 3
OLFACTORY THRESHOLD DETECTION (FOR TWO UNPLEASANT ODORANTS IN UNILATERAL STIMULATION) OBTAINED BY PSYCHOPHYSICAL METHOD AND ELECTRODERMAL RESPONSE

Measure	Right Nostril M	SD	Left Nostril M	SD	t
Psychophysical Detection	10.9	1.65	10.0	1.31	1.46
Electrodermal Response	7.8	1.24	8.8	1.47	1.40
t	3.51*		2.41*		

*$p<.01$.

Bilateral Skin Potential

For isoamyl acetate, 22 subjects had a bilateral electrodermal response for each nostril. Among these, 20 subjects (90%) had the same direction of asymmetry whichever nostril was stimulated: 15 subjects (75%) systematically had a higher amplitude for the right hand, and 5 subjects (25%) systematically had a higher amplitude for the left hand. For thioglycolic acid,

22 subjects had a bilateral electrodermal response for each nostril. Among these, 21 subjects (95%) had the same direction of asymmetry whichever nostril was stimulated: 15 subjects (71%) systematically had a higher amplitude for the right hand, and 6 subjects (29%) systematically had a higher amplitude for the left hand. For citral, 11 subjects had a bilateral electrodermal response for each nostril. These 11 subjects had the same direction of asymmetry whichever nostril was stimulated: 6 subjects (55%) systematically had a higher amplitude for the right hand, and 5 subjects (45%) systematically had a higher amplitude for the left hand. For triethylamine, 19 subjects had a bilateral electrodermal response for each nostril. Among these, 18 subjects (95%) had the same direction of asymmetry whichever nostril was stimulated: 12 subjects (67%) systematically had a higher amplitude for the right hand, and 6 subjects (33%) systematically had a higher amplitude for the left hand.

Overall, whatever the odorant, there was agreement with the direction of asymmetry (between 90% and 100%). A higher proportion of the subjects had a right-hand dominance (from 57% for citral in the right nostril condition to 72% for thioglycolic acid in the right nostril condition) over the left hand, independently of the type of odorant or the hedonic valence (Table 4). An analysis based on the subjects who presented two EDA responses for an odorant, i.e., one in the right and one in the left nostril condition, showed a strong concordance in the direction of asymmetry (20/22 for isoamyl acetate, 21/22 for thioglycolic acid, 11/11 for citral, and 18/19 for triethylamine). Moreover, when a subject showed dominance of the EDA response on one particular hand for an odorant, the results would be generally the same for the other odorants: the 10 subjects who had a bilateral electrodermal response for both nostrils for the four odorants, individually had the same direction of the asymmetry for the four odorants. It was the same for the seven subjects who responded to three odorants and the four subjects who responded to two odorants.

TABLE 4
Percent Bilateral Electrodermal Asymmetries (Right Hand > Left Hand or Left Hand > Right Hand) For Both Nostrils During Four Odorant Threshold Stimulations

Isoamyl Acetate				Thioglycolic Acid			
Right Nostril		Left Nostril		Right Nostril		Left Nostril	
R>L	L>R	R>L	L>R	R>L	L>R	R>L	L>R
68	32	65	35	72	28	63	37

Citral				Triethylamine			
Right Nostril		Left Nostril		Right Nostril		Left Nostril	
R>L	L>R	R>L	L>R	R>L	L>R	R>L	L>R
57	43	66	34	62	38	61	39

The higher amplitude of the response on a particular hand for olfactory stimulations (right nostril or left nostril) was not linked to the results obtained for auditory stimulation whatever the odor. Thus, for each subject the direction of asymmetry was not the same with auditory and olfactory stimulation.

Discussion

The results for peripheral lateralization showed no differences in threshold detection regardless of the stimulus odorant and the method of detection (psychophysical or EDA response). Thresholds obtained by the EDA response were greater than the thresholds obtained by psychophysical method, and from a methodological point of view, these results are relevant because they support the finding there is no difference between the right and left sides of the nose. However, as justified in the Introduction, the threshold detection method used in this experiment was less elaborated than the classical psychophysical procedure, and the findings could be further confirmed by an extended experimental collecting of data. It has been evidenced for some considerable time that, when the detection method was based only on psychophysical tests, these methods can give questionable results, i.e., the number of false alerts (17) on a task on which the subjects have to decide between the presence or absence of an odorant. Our results are in agreement with those of Zatorre and Jones-Gotman (49), Betchen and Doty (4) using phenyl ethyl alcohol, Kölega (32) using amyl acetate, and Eskenazi, *et al.* (19) using butanol. The ipsilateral relation between nasal and hand dominance was not supported, contrary to the data of Yougentob, *et al.* (48) concerning olfactory detection thresholds.

The results for hemispheric asymmetry showed that whichever hemisphere is stimulated, the unilateral olfactory stimulation corresponded to the skin potential response amplitude of one hand more than the other, and for most of the subjects it was always the same side. This constancy in the direction of asymmetry did not depend on the recording conditions, according to the results of the control bilateral auditive stimulation. If one considers methodological problems in bilateral electrodermal research (handedness of subjects, quality of stimulus, and recording conditions) (37), the olfactory result may still indicate differential hemispheric activity and support the results of Brand, *et al.* (6) for suprathreshold stimulation using a lavender odor. The directional asymmetry was not linked to odor and hedonic valence, i.e., pleasant/unpleasant, contrary to what has been observed for other sense organs, for which the emotional valance of the stimulus also plays a role in hemispheric asymmetry (35). Our finding is in contrast with the observation of Brauchli, *et al.* (7) who found higher autonomic arousal in response to unpleasant versus pleasant odorants, as well as with the findings of Alaoui, *et al.* (1) who suggested that differences in skin potential were linked to the hedonic valence of the odorant stimulation.

Different authors have suggested that cerebral asymmetries for the sense organs other than olfaction appear in tasks that require "cognitive activity" and that the simple process of detection is not lateralized (35). In olfaction, this fact seems to be supported by the studies of Eskenazi, *et al.* (19, 20) and Bellas, *et al.* (2). However, our results indicate that olfactory threshold detection may well be lateralized. In general, other factors such as the nature of the olfactory stimulus can influence cerebral dominance mainly in relation to its trigeminal component [most odorants simultaneously stimulate the two systems; olfactory by CN I and trigeminal by CN V in the nasal cavity (15)], but this was not the case in the present study because the trigeminal impact of odorants was minimal at perithreshold concentrations.

This study showed that hemispheric asymmetry can be found without any coincident difference at the peripheral receptors. This result needs to be clarified with a larger sample of subjects and could open the way to further research. Some authors have reported that the monorhinal stimulations could affect olfactory performances (4, 8, 25), and other factors may influence lateral differences. For instance, in the present study no sex difference was found, but some studies have reported differences for threshold tasks (13, 33). In the same way many factors which were not taken into account in this study could play a role in lateral differences and be worthy of investigation, i.e., handedness (24), age (9), and, in a more general way, individual differences (40, 43, 44).

REFERENCES

1. ALAOUI-ISMAÏLI, O., VERNET-MAURY, E., DITTMAR, A., DELHOMME, G., & CHANEL, J. Odor hedonics: connection with emotional response estimated by automatic parameters. *Chemical Senses*, 1997, 22, 237-248.
2. BELLAS, D. N., NOVELLY, R. A., & ESKENAZI, B. Olfactory lateralization and identification in right hemisphere lesion and control patients. *Neuropsychologia*, 1989, 27, 1187-1191.
3. BELLAS, D. N., NOVELLY, R. A., ESKENAZI, B., & WASSERSTEIN, J. The nature of unilateral neglect in the olfactory sensory system. *Neuropsychologia*, 1988, 26, 45-52.
4. BETCHEN, S. A., & DOTY, R. L. Bilateral detection thresholds in dextral and sinistrals reflect the more sensitive side of the nose, which is not lateralized. *Chemical Senses*, 1998, 23, 453-457.
5. BRAND, G. Olfactory lateralization in human: a review. *Clinical Neurophysiology*, 1999, 29, 495-506.
6. BRAND, G., MILLOT, J. L., & HENQUELL, D. Olfaction and hemispheric asymmetry: unilateral stimulation and bilateral electrodermal recordings. *Neuropsychobiology*, 1999, 39, 160-164.
7. BRAUCHLI, P., RÜEGG, P. B., ETZWEILER, F., & ZEIER, H. Electrocortical and autonomic alteration by administration of a pleasant and unpleasant odor. *Chemical Senses*, 1995, 20, 505-515.
8. BROMLEY, S. M., & DOTY, R. L. Odor recognition memory is better under bilateral than unilateral test conditions. *Cortex*, 1995, 31, 25-40.
9. CAIN, W. S., & GENT, J. F. Olfactory sensitivity: reliability, generality and association with aging. *Journal of Experimental Psychology*, 1991, 17, 382-391.

10. COMPER, P., & LACROIX, J. M. Further evidence of lateralization in the electrodermal system as a function of relative hemispheric activation. *Psychophysiology*, 1981, 18, 149. [Abstract]
11. DE BONIS, M., & FREIXA I BAQUÉ, E. Stress, verbal activity and bilateral electrodermal response. *Neuropsychobiology*, 1980, 6, 249-259.
12. DEVOS, M., PATTE, F., ROUAULT, J., & LAFFORT, P. *Standardized human olfactory thresholds.* Oxford, UK: Cambridge, Univer. Press, 1990.
13. DOTY, R. L., APPLEBAUM, S., ZUSHO, H., & SETTLE, R. G. Sex differences in odor identification ability: a cross-cultural analysis. *Neuropsychologia*, 1985, 23, 667-672.
14. DOTY, R. L., BROMLEY, S. M., MOBERG, P. J., & HUMMEL, T. Laterality in human nasal chemoreception. In S. Christman (Ed.), *Cerebral asymmetries in sensory and perceptual processing.* Amsterdam: North Holland, 1997. Pp. 497-542.
15. DOTY, R. L., BRUGGER, W. E., JURS, P. C., ORNDORFF, M. A., SNYDER, P. J., & LOWRY, L. D. Intranasal trigeminal stimulation from odorous volatiles: psychometric responses from anosmic and normal humans. *Physiology & Behavior*, 1978, 20, 175-185.
16. ELIAS, L., BRYDEN, M. P., & BULMAN-FLEMING, B. Footedness is a better predictor than is handedness of emotional lateralization. *Neuropsychologia*, 1998, 36, 37-43.
17. ENGEN, T. The effect of expectation on judgements of odor. *Acta Psychologia*, 1972, 36, 450-458.
18. ERWIN, R. J., MCCLANAHAN, B. A., & KLEINMAN, K. M. Effects of level of arousal and type of task on bilateral skin conductance asymmetry and conjugate lateral eye movements. *Pavlovian Journal of Biological Sciences*, 1980, 15, 292-298.
19. ESKENAZI, B., CAIN, W. S., NOVELLY, R. A., & FRIEND, K. B. Olfactory functioning in temporal lobe epilepsy patients. *Neuropsychologia*, 1983, 21, 365-374.
20. ESKENAZI, B., CAIN, W. S., NOVELLY, R. A., & MATTSON, R. Odor perception in temporal lobe epilepsy patients with and without temporal lobectomy. *Neuropsychologia*, 1986, 24, 553-562.
21. FEDORA, O., & SCHOPFLOCHER, D. Bilateral electrodermal activity during differential cognitive hemispheric activation. *Psychophysiology*, 1984, 21, 307-311.
22. FOWLES, D. C., CHRISTIE, M. J., & EDELBERG, R. Publication recommendations for electrodermal measurements. *Psychophysiology*, 1981, 18, 232.
23. FREIXA I BAQUÉ, E., CATTEU, M. C., MIOSSEC, Y., & ROY, J. C. Asymmetry of electrodermal activity: a review. *Biological Psychology*, 1984, 18, 219-239.
24. GILBERT, A. N., GREENBERG, M. S., & BEAUCHAMP, G. K. Sex, handedness and side of nose modulate human odor perception. *Neuropsychologia*, 1989, 27, 505-511.
25. HORNUNG, D. E., LEOPOLD, D. A., MOZELL, M. M., SHEEHE, P. R., & YOUGENTOB, S. L. Impact of left and right olfactory abilities on binasal olfactory performance. *Chemical Senses*, 1990, 15, 233-237.
26. HUGDHAL, K. Hemispheric asymmetry and bilateral electrodermal recordings: a review of the evidence. *Psychophysiology*, 1984, 21, 371-393.
27. HUGDHAL, K. Bilateral electrodermal asymmetry: past hopes and future prospects. *International Journal of Neuroscience*, 1988, 39, 33-44.
28. HUMMEL, T., & KOBAL, G. Differences in human evoked potentials related to olfactory or trigeminal chemosensory activation. *Electroencephalography and Clinical Neurophysiology*, 1992, 84, 84-89.
29. KLEIN, R., PILON, D., PROSSER, S., & SHANNAHOFF-KHALSA, D. Nasal airflow asymmetries and human performance. *Biological Psychology*, 1986, 23, 127-137.
30. KOBAL, G., HUMMEL, T., & PAULI, E. Correlates of hedonic estimates in the olfactory evoked potential. *Chemical Senses*, 1989, 14, 718. [Abstract]
31. KOBAL, G., HUMMEL, T., & VAN TOLLER, S. Differences in chemosensory evoked potentials to olfactory and somatosensory chemical stimuli presented to left and right nostrils. *Chemical Senses*, 1992, 17, 233-244.
32. KÖLEGA, H. S. Olfaction and sensory asymmetry. *Chemical Senses and Flavour*, 1979, 4, 89-95.
33. KÖLEGA, H. S. Sex differences in olfactory sensitivity and the problem of the generality of smell acuity. *Perceptual and Motor Skills*, 1994, 78, 203-213.

34. LACROIX, J. M., & COMPER, P. Lateralization in the electrodermal system as a function of cognitive/hemispheric manipulation. *Psychophysiology*, 1979, 16, 116-129.
35. MEYERS, M. B., & SMITH, B. D. Cerebral processing of nonverbal affective stimuli: differential effects of cognitive and affective sets on hemispheric asymmetry. *Biological Psychology*, 1987, 24, 67-84.
36. MILLOT, J. L., & BRAND, G. Behavioral lateralization during spontaneous smelling tasks. *Perceptual and Motor Skills*, 2000, 90, 444-450.
37. MIOSSEC, Y., CATTEAU, M. C., FREIXA I BAQUÉ, E., & ROY, J. C. Methodological problems in bilateral electrodermal research. *International Journal of Psychophysiology*, 1985, 2, 247-256.
38. MYSLOBODSKY, M. S., & RATTOK, J. Bilateral electrodermal activity in waking man. *Acta Psychologica*, 1977, 41, 273-282.
39. NAVETEUR, J., & SEQUEIRA-MARTINHO, H. Reliability of bilateral differences in electrodermal activity. *Biological Psychology*, 1990, 31, 47-56.
40. O'CONNELL, R. J., STEVENS, D. A., AKERS, R. P., COPPOLA, D. M., & GRANT, A. J. Individual differences in the quantitative and qualitative responses of human subjects to various odors. *Chemical Senses*, 1989, 14, 293-302.
41. PENDSE, S. G. Hemispheric asymmetry in olfaction on a category judgement task. *Perceptual and Motor Skills*, 1987, 64, 495-498.
42. SCHULTER, G., & PAPOUSEK, U. Bilateral electrodermal activity: reliability, laterality and individual differences. *International Journal of Psychophysiology*, 1992, 13, 199-213.
43. STEVENS, D. A., & O'CONNELL, R. J. Individual differences in thresholds and quality reports of human subjects to various odors. *Chemical Senses*, 1991, 16, 57-67.
44. STEVENS, J. C., CAIN, W. S., & BURKE, R. J. Variability of olfactory thresholds. *Chemical Senses*, 1988, 13, 643-653.
45. TOULOUSE, E., & VASCHIDE, N. L'asymétrie sensorielle olfactive. *Comptes-Rendus Hebdomadaires de la Société de Biologie*, 1899, 51, 785-787.
46. TOULOUSE, E., & VASCHIDE, N. L'asymétrie sensorielle olfactive. *Revue Philosophique*, 1900, 49, 176-187.
47. VAN TOLLER, C., KIRK-SMITH, M., WOOD, N., LOMBARD, J., & DODD, G. H. Skin conductance and subjective assessments associated with the odour of 5-alpha-androstan-3-one. *Biological Psychology*, 1983, 16, 85-107.
48. YOUGENTOB, S. L., KURTZ, D. B., LEOPOLD, D. A., MOZELL, M. M., & HORNUNG, D. E. Olfactory sensitivity: is there laterality? *Chemical Senses*, 1982, 7, 11-21.
49. ZATORRE, R. J., & JONES-GOTMAN, M. Right-nostril advantage for discrimination of odors. *Perception & Psychophysics*, 1990, 47, 526-531.
50. ZATORRE, R. J., JONES-GOTMAN, M., EVANS, A. C., & MEYER, E. Functional localization and lateralization of human olfactory cortex. *Nature*, 1992, 360, 339-340.

Accepted February 23, 2004.

EFFECT ON TRUCK DRIVERS' ALERTNESS OF A 30-MIN. EXPOSURE TO BRIGHT LIGHT: A FIELD STUDY [1]

ULF LANDSTRÖM

National Institute for Working Life
Umeå, Sweden

TORBJÖRN ÅKERSTEDT

National Institute for Psychosocial Factors
and Health, Stockholm Sweden

MARIANNE BYSTRÖM, BERTIL NORDSTRÖM

National Institute for Working Life
Umeå, Sweden

ROGER WIBOM

National Institute for Working Life
Solna, Sweden

Summary.—Reduced alertness is common during night driving. Light treatment may constitute one countermeasure to reduce sleepiness. To test this idea six professional drivers participated in this study in which they self-administered a 30-min. light treatment during a break in the middle of a night drive of about 9 hours. Two experimental conditions were used, including light exposures with a light box and a light visor. There was a control condition. Alertness was measured on a 100-mm visual analogue scale. No significant effect of light was found, but ratings of sleepiness increased significantly through the night drive. The experimental light treatment was not correlated with any increased wakefulness compared to the drivings where no extra light exposures were carried out.

Sleepiness is an important causative factor in road accidents (Harris, 1977; Maycock, 1996; Horne & Reyner, 1999; National Transportation Safety Board, 1999). Both night driving and time at the wheel have been implicated (Hamelin, 1987), as well as sleep apnea (Stoohs, Guilleminault, Itoi, & Dement, 1994).

EEG studies of truck drivers have shown that late night driving is characterized by increased activity in the theta (4–8 Hz) and alpha (8–12 Hz) bands (Kecklund & Åkerstedt, 1993). The EEG changes associated with feelings of increased sleepiness and reduced driving performance have also been documented in driving simulators (Reyner & Horne, 1998).

Different measures to counteract sleepiness have been tested in laboratory as well as field studies. Increased wakefulness has been observed after napping as well as after consumption of coffee (Horne & Reyner, 1996). The waking effect of exercise has been reported very small (Horne & Foster, 1995), whereas positive effects have been found after noise exposure (Landström, Englund, Nordström, & Åström, 1998). In laboratory studies also bright light has improved alertness, performance, or EEG indicators of alertness (Campbell & Dawson, 1990; Badia, Myers, Boecker, & Culpepper,

---

[1]Please address correspondence to Ulf Landström, National Institute for Working Life, Box 7654, S-907 13 Umeå, Sweden.

1991; Myers & Badia, 1993; Heitmann, Stampi, Lerman, Burke, & Moore-Ede, 1995; Wright, Badia, Myers, & Plenzler, 1997; Foret, Daurat, & Tirilly, 1998; Caajochen, Zeitzer, Czeisler, & Dijk, 2000; Avery, Kizer, Bolte, & Hellekson, 2001). The latter effects have been arousal effects, apart from the well-known effect on the phase of the biological clock (Czeisler, Richardson, Zimmerman, Moore-Ede, & Weitzman, 1981).

An interesting question is whether a moderate exposure to bright light, applied during a break in driving a vehicle at night, could improve alertness. An effect might then occur with an arousal effect or an effect on the melatonin balance. The duration of the exposure would then have to be rather short to be acceptable to commercial driving.

The present study was designed to test whether a short (30-min.) exposure to bright light would affect the subjective sleepiness of the truck drivers during night driving. Two different types of light exposures were included in the study, one commercial visor type of exposure and one new constructed light-box exposure.

Method

Participants

Six healthy truck drivers, all men, ages 30 to 60 years, participated. They were recruited from local truck companies and did not receive any economic compensation for their participation. They all had experience driving the particular route and had a well-established driving schedule.

Design of Study

The study started in early December and ended early March, i.e., the time of the year with the longest periods of driving in the dark. The drivers were informed about the procedure, provided the equipment, and given instructions. The task was to drive a truck 500 km during the night from Umeå in northern Sweden to Stockholm. Three different conditions were used in a counterbalanced design: a light box, a light visor, and a control condition during which no extra light exposure was carried out. The light exposure was given during the first, legally required, 45-min. break after about 4.5 hr. of driving. Each condition was repeated 10 times each. The exposure was set to 30 min., with 15 min. of readaptation to driving in the dark. The control conditions involved exactly the same procedure but without additional light exposures. Before and after the exposure the drivers filled out rating scales of sleepiness. The drivers were asked not to consume coffee during their drive or to take any naps.

Each trip started at about 17.00 hr. The box conditions ended at 02.18 ± .35, the visor conditions at 2.94 ± .47, and the control conditions at 3.20 ± .66. These differences were not significant. Prior sleep length before the box condition was 7.89 ± .28 hr., the visor condition 8.35 ± .31 hr., and the control condition 8.06 ± .16 hr. The differences in sleep length before the tests were not significant.

Evaluation of Wakefulness

The drivers were asked to fill out a questionnaire with background data and questions about driving hours and pauses. During the drive a 100-mm rating scale for fatigue was marked at the start, before the break, after the break, as well as every hour after the break.

All drivers contributed 10 drives to each condition. After participation in all 30 drives, the drivers were asked to answer a new questionnaire dealing with aspects as interference with safety, comfort, and practical use of the light system as a measure against drivers' fatigue.

Light Exposures

Two different light-exposure devices were used. One consisted of a light box, which was placed on the steering wheel in front of the driver, and the other was a commercial light visor, which was worn on the head. The box, which was made of wood, was 50 cm high, 40 cm wide, and 10 cm deep. Four miniature lights (Phillips TL 8/84 full colour) were mounted on the box's plywood base. The vehicle's cigarette lighter outlet was used for electricity. The operator was of a HF type intended for 24 V. The top of the box was an opal-like white sheet of acrylic plastic. During exposure, the driver looked at the sheet, which had a luminance of 2000 candela/m^2. At a distance of 50 cm from the sheet, the illuminance was 1000 Lux.

The light visor was of the make Bio Brite and was manufactured in the USA. It was similar in appearance to a hat with a visor. Under the visor, in front of each eye, was mounted a miniature bulb (krypton) equipped with a reflector. The lamps (2.4 V 0.7 A), which were equipped with UV filters and a filter which suppressed the red end of the light spectrum, could be adjusted to illuminate the optic fundus. Built into the light visor was a voltage converter and a control equipment which enabled the light intensity to be varied and which was set to a predetermined level. The cigarette lighter outlet was used for current. The luminance, during the exposures, was 2500 candela/m^2. The illuminance 5 cm from the light source was measured as 600 Lux.

The light visor was of a commercial type while the light box was designed exclusively for this study. The light exposure was validated in laboratory test experiments prior to the field study (Åkerstedt, Landström, Byström, Nordström, & Wibom, 2003) and yielded a significant effect on subjective alertness.

Statistical Analyses

Data were analysed using a two-factor analysis of variance for repeated measures using all 12 points. A second analysis of variance was carried out using the four points immediately before the break and the three points immediately subsequent to the break. All results were corrected for imbalance of the variance—covariance matrix using the procedure of Huyn-Feldt (see epsilon values). The latter essentially involves a reduction in the degrees of freedom according to the sphericity of the data.

Results

The results of the study are summarized in Table 1 and Fig. 1. Table 1 shows a significant effect of time for the 12-point analyses, but no effect of condition and no interaction. The 4-point analysis showed no significant term. As can be seen from Fig. 1, sleepiness clearly increased as a function of the driving hours.

TABLE 1
F Ratios For Box and Visor Conditions vs Respective Control Conditions

	Condition $F_{1,5}$	Time $F_{5,55}$	Condition · Time $F_{5,55}$	Huyhn-Feldt Correction (%)
Box 12	3.57	3.89†	0.56	99/99/61
Visor 12	0.20	4.07†	1.56	99/57/31
Box 4	1.81	1.42	1.38	23/28/30
Visor 4	1.40	3.10	1.92	99/99/61

Note.—Huyhn-Feldt correction of degrees of freedom for imbalance of the variance-covariance matrix – in % for each factor of the analysis. F ratios with degrees of freedom. †$p < .001$.

The waking effect was also judged by the drivers on the basis of their answers to the question, "Did you think that the light exposure had a positive effect on your wakefulness?" In only five of the cases did the drivers say yes; in 17 cases the answer was no; in 18 applications no answer was given to the question. In the majority of the applications, the increase in wakefulness estimated by the drivers themselves indicates that they on average did not feel they had become more awake given the light exposure.

In most of the answers (85 of 120), no proposals for changes to the light exposure system were given; 24 gave no answer, 9 answered "don't know." In one case the answer was yes (the whole cab should be better lit).

In 114 of 120 applications, it was stated that the light exposure had no negative effect on driving safety. In four cases no answer was given. In two of the applications, the answer was yes.

Discussion

These results show that subjective sleepiness of the drivers gradually increased over the driving period. The light intervention, however, did not show any significant effects.

A significant waking effect of a 30-min. exposure has recently been de-

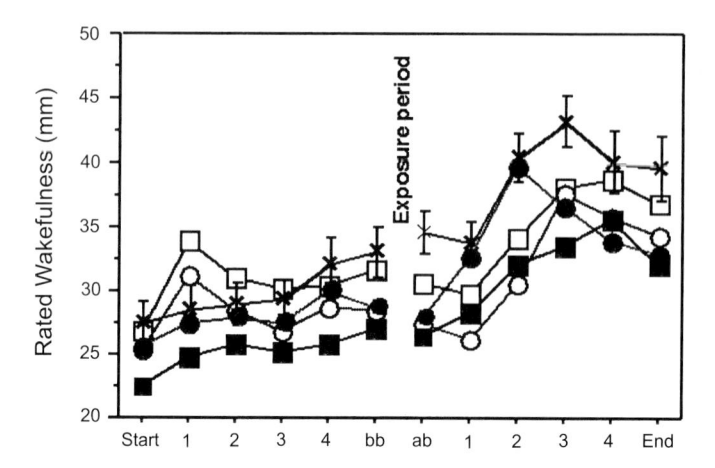

FIG. 1. Changes in rated wakefulness during the four experimental conditions and the control [light box (□), light visor (○), dark visor (●), dark box (■), control (×)] from experiment with light box. Start = start of driving (time defined in text), bb = before break, ab = after break, end = end of driving (time defined in text). The interval between the ratings was 1 hr., except for the ratings carried at the positions bb, ab, and end, which varied depending on when the pauses were taken and the driving hours.

scribed in a laboratory study carried out by the research group (Åkerstedt, et al., 2003). That study was, however, fully controlled for external influences, and it is possible that the present field study provided too much background variation to permit any effects of light exposure.

Another reason for the lack of effects may be the short duration of the exposure. Laboratory studies of the effects of light treatment on alertness have generally used a very long duration of exposure (Campbell & Dawson, 1990; Badia, et al., 1991; Myers & Badia, 1993; Heitmann, et al., 1995; Wright, et al., 1997; Foret, et al., 1998; Caajochen, Zeitzer, Czeisler, & Dijk, 2000; Avery, et al., 2001). However, if several hours of exposure are necessary to accomplish effects, light treatment as a countermeasure in driving is not a viable alternative.

Also, intensity could have been increased to obtain effects. The present intensity, however, represents the normal level for routine light treatment (Dijk, Boulos, Eastman, Lewy, Campbell, & Terman, 1995). Higher levels under self-treatment conditions might involve risks.

One may also speculate about insufficient compliance by the drivers. This does not seem likely from the spontaneous reports of the drivers and the good relationship between the experimenters and the drivers. Another possibility is that a larger number of subjects may have brought out significant results. On the other hand the F ratios of the interaction terms were quite low, and a large number of subjects would have been required while the effect on alertness would still have remained modest.

A negative result can never demonstrate that an effect truly does not exist; the obtained data only suggest that the present approach to light treatment does not have sustained effect of postexposure light treatment. This should not be taken to mean that other types of applications of light might not be used as countermeasures against sleepiness.

The focus of interest in the present analysis was on the interaction term; however, an expected development of sleepiness across the nighttime drive could be observed as previously described by Kecklund and Åkerstedt (1993). This development does not seem to have been affected by the break itself since the four-point analysis across pre-postbreak data yielded no significant effect of time. No control condition without a break, however, was included in the design.

It should be emphasized that the present study did not employ performance measures, which might have been affected. One might also speculate that light exposures were carried out too early, but should have been adopted later during the night.

REFERENCES

Åkerstedt, T., Landström, U., Byström, M., Nordström, B., & Wibom, R. (2003) Bright light as a sleepiness prophylactic: a laboratory study of subjective ratings and EEG. *Perceptual and Motor Skills*, 97, 811-819.

Avery, D. H., Kizer, D., Bolte, M. A., & Hellekson, C. (2001) Bright light therapy of subsyndromal seasonal affective disorder in the workplace: morning vs. afternoon exposure. *Acta Psychiatria Scandinavia*, 103, 267-274.

Badia, P., Myers, B., Boecker, M., & Culpepper, J. (1991) Bright light effects on body temperature, alertness, EEG and behavior. *Physiology and Behaviour*, 50, 1-10.

Caajochen, C., Zeitzer, J. M., Czeisler, C. A., & Dijk, D-J. (2000) Dose-response relationship for light intensity and ocular and electroencephalographic correlates of human alertness. *Behaviour and Brain Research*, 115, 75-83.

Campbell, S. S., & Dawson, D. (1990) Enhancement of nighttime alertness and performance with bright ambient light. *Physiology and Behaviour*, 48, 317-320.

Czeisler, C. A., Richardson, G. S., Zimmerman, M. C., Moore-Ede, M. C., & Weitzman, E. D. (1981) Entrainment of human circadian rhythms by light-dark cycles. *Photochemistry and Photobiology*, 34, 239-247.

Dijk, D-J., Boulos, Z., Eastman, C., Lewy, A., Campbell, S., & Terman, M. (1995) Light treatment for sleep disorders: consensus report: II. Basic properties of circadian physiology and sleep regulation. *Journal of Biological Rhythms*, 10, 113-125.

Foret, J., Daurat, A., & Tirilly, G. (1998) Effect of bright light at night on core temperature, subjective alertness and performance as a function of exposure time. *Scandinavian Journal of Work Environmental Health*, 24, 115-120.

Hamelin, P. (1987) Lorry driver's time habits in work and their involvement in traffic accidents. *Ergonomics*, 30, 1323-1333.

Harris, W. (1977) Fatigue, circadian rhythm and truck accidents. In R. R. Mackie (Ed.), *Vigilance*. New York: Plenum. Pp. 133-147.

Heitmann, A., Stampi, C., Lerman, S. E., Burke, P. E., & Moore-Ede, M. (1995) *Effectiveness of moderately bright control-room lighting in improving operator alertness and performance at night: a pilot study at a chemical plant.* Cambridge, MA: Institute for Circadian Physiology.

Horne, J., & Reyner, L. (1999) Vehicle accidents related to sleep: a review. *Occupational Environmental Medicine*, 56, 289-294.

Horne, J. A., & Foster, S. C. (1995) Can exercise overcome sleepiness? *Sleep Research*, 24A. [Abstract]

HORNE, J. A., & REYNER, L. A. (1996) Counteracting driver sleepiness: effects of napping, caffeine and placebo. *Psychophysiology*, 33, 306-309.

KECKLUND, G., & ÅKERSTEDT, T. (1993) Sleepiness in long distance truck driving: an ambulatory EEG study of night driving. *Ergonomics*, 36, 1007-1017.

LANDSTRÖM, U., ENGLUND, K., NORDSTRÖM, B., & ÅSTRÖM, A. (1998) Laboratory studies of a sound system that maintains wakefulness. *Perceptual and Motor Skills*, 86, 147-161.

MAYCOCK, G. (1996) Sleepiness and driving: the experience of UK car drivers. *Journal of Sleep Research*, 5, 229-237.

MYERS, B. L., & BADIA, P. (1993) Immediate effects of different light intensities on body temperature and alertness. *Physiology and Behaviour*, 54, 199-202.

NATIONAL TRANSPORTATION SAFETY BOARD. (1999) *Evaluation of U.S. Department of Transportation: efforts in the 1990s to address operation fatigue.* (Safety Report NTSB/SR-99/01) Washington, DC: National Transportation Safety Board.

REYNER, L. A., & HORNE, J. A. (1998) Falling asleep whilst driving: are drivers aware of prior sleepiness? *International Journal of Legal Medicine*, 111, 120-123.

STOOHS, R. A., GUILLEMINAULT, C., ITOI, A., & DEMENT, W. C. (1994) Traffic accidents in commercial long-haul truck drivers: the influence of sleep-disordered breathing and obesity. *Sleep*, 17, 619-623.

WRIGHT, K. P., JR., BADIA, P., MYERS, B. L., & PLENZLER, S. C. (1997) Combination of bright light and caffeine as a countermeasure for impaired alertness and performance during extended sleep deprivation. *Journal of Sleep Research*, 6, 26-35.

Accepted February 2, 2004.

PERCEIVED BUILDING DENSITY AS A FUNCTION OF LAYOUT[1]

JOHN ZACHARIAS AND ARTHUR STAMPS

*Department of Geography, Planning and Environment
Concordia University*

Institute of Environmental Quality

Summary.—This paper addresses two issues in the subjective measurement of density, (a) whether perceived density is influenced by the sizes and spacing of buildings and (b) whether perceived density is influenced by surface details. Two experiments were conducted. Stimuli in Exp. 1 were 9 photomontages of rows of residential buildings. Factors were (a) building surface area (at low, medium, and high levels) and (b) layout (many small buildings and small gaps to few large buildings and large gaps, in three levels). Amount of visible building surface area accounted for 63% of variance of scaled impressions of density, while layout accounted for 15% of variance. Stimuli in Exp. 2 were grey boxes with the same factors of building surface area and layout. Scaled impressions of density of buildings and boxes correlated at .95, suggesting that surface detail had a minor effect in perceived density.

In everyday conversation people refer to how much crowding or packing, including levels of urban building density. People readily affirm their ability to distinguish the densities of urban environments. Planners manipulate the limits to building density, usually defined as total floor space divided by site area, a relationship that is difficult to visualize. Typically, projects are presented to the interested public as sets of elevations, where one typically views a faithfully rendered image of a building proposal in its immediate building environment. At identical scales, simulations depict the proposed buildings in context where an estimate of density would require a visual estimation of total volume of building. Debate often surrounds the level or relative level of apparent urban density (Churchman, 1999). In the visual representation, as in reality, change in density necessitates a change in the size of building frontages, if spacing remains constant. A constant density can be maintained while varying the space between buildings, thus driving up the height. Such simultaneous manipulations of real building projects are routinely executed, although it is unclear how public perception of density is simultaneously related to actual density and spacing. Urban density can be represented by the visible amount of building. Layout can be represented by the spacing between buildings, or simultaneously by the size of the space and the height of the building at constant density.

---

[1]Address enquiries to J. Zacharias, Ph.D., Urban Studies Program, Department of Geography, Planning and Environment, Concordia University, 1455 de Maisonneuve Boulevard West, Montréal (Québec) H3G 1M8 Canada or A. Stamps, Ph.D., Institute of Environmental Quality, 290 Rutledge Street, San Francisco, CA 94110.

People can discriminate size when direct comparisons are allowed. Visual strategies such as averaging an array of objects can result in impressive accuracy in the estimation of size—75% accuracy was achieved with 6–8% diameter difference (Chong & Treisman, 2003). Viewing a set of objects allows more accurate estimates of size than when the objects are viewed one at a time. People are apparently scanning the set of objects to judge average size, then estimating variations from average (Ariely, 2001). When the objects are very different in size, there is a tendency to exaggerate the difference. For example, observers exaggerated the height of a four-story building by approximately 25% when comparing it with lampposts and parking meters (Chapanis & Manken, 1967). An individual may scan a single elevation to obtain an estimate of density that can be compared to other remembered environments or can scan two such elevations to judge the difference, if any, between their densities.

While people have ability to discriminate small differences in size, there are also consistent discrepancies between perceived and actual estimates attributable to optical effects. The quantitative, predictable discrepancy between the conscious percept and the physical stimulus was attributed early to proprioceptive feedback from eye movements interacting with the conscious experience of the visual stimulus (von Helmholtz, 1856). For example, the division of a block into smaller elements makes it appear larger than an undifferentiated block of the same size—the Oppel-Kundt effect. Spehar and Gillam (2002) recently demonstrated that the Poggendorff illusion could be reduced by manipulating lines in the representation. Individually such effects can be attributed to specific visual elements but in combination produce a new illusion that is not the summation of the individual ones (Bulatov, Bertulis, & Strogonov, 2001). The size of identical rooms was perceived as different in upper and lower stories of the same building (Kaya & Erkip, 2001), while a single room was perceived to change in size when the dimensions were altered while maintaining the same floor area (Munakata & Oi, 1997).

Discrepancies between actual and perceived density may be attributed to direct optical effect or visual memory of other building environments. This investigation concerns the existence of a discrepancy between perceived and actual density in typical elevation presentations of building environments. More specifically, the effect of gaps between buildings and architectural detail on estimates of density is examined. There were two hypotheses: H_1: increasing gaps between buildings of equal façade area will decrease estimations of density; H_2: the effect depends on the extent of building coverage in the picture plane and not facade elements or landscaping.

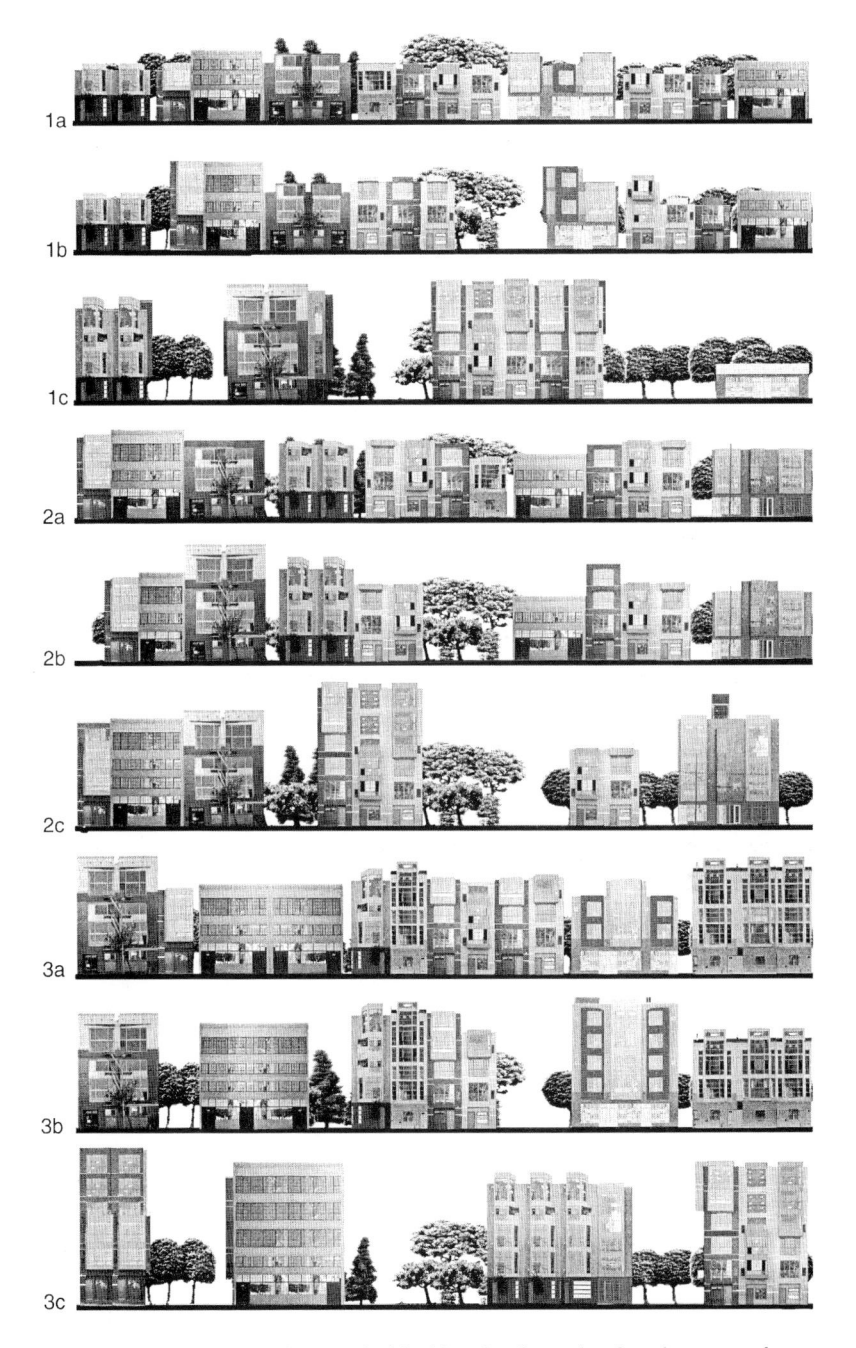

FIG. 1. Stimuli: layouts of photographed building façades as distributed across surface area

Experiment 1

Method

Stimuli.—Photographs were taken of the fronts of buildings in an urban neighborhood. The photographs were corrected for parallax and a set of façades was assembled from parts of photographed buildings. Although parallax had a very minor role in preference compared with complexity and height (Stamps, 1993b), it is much more difficult to estimate size with a parallax effect (Chapanis & Manken, 1967). There was an attempt to distribute the sampled elements across the picture plane (Fig. 1). The surface area covered by building frontages was held to three levels while the width of the gap between buildings also had three levels. Descriptive data are shown in Table 1.

TABLE 1
AREAS AND GAPS IN PHOTOMONTAGES AND BOXES

Photomontage Stimulus	Building Area	Cumulative Gap	Value	Box Stimulus	Box Area	Cumulative Gap	Value
a1	115.1	121.0	−.350	a1	107.9	171.4	−.278
a2	100.0	352.6	−.382	a2	100.0	220.3	−.664
a3	101.5	810.5	−.623	a3	103.6	234.6	−.772
b1	130.8	152.6	.179	b1	128.4	142.8	.212
b2	134.7	410.5	−.070	b2	129.5	171.4	.222
b3	141.4	736.8	−.331	b3	123.3	214.2	−.286
c1	180.7	100.0	.870	c1	155.4	100.0	.725
c2	167.9	473.7	.530	c2	154.1	134.6	.525
c3	153.7	836.8	.184	c3	152.2	173.4	.318

Nine stimuli were produced in the following array. Three levels of density were represented as three levels of surface area covered by building frontages. The size of the gap between buildings was also manipulated at three levels, leading to higher buildings as gaps increased in size. The two physical measures of density were then combined for nine combinations of density and gap. Size of gap varies with building height, such that the proportions of buildings change as the size of the gap changes. It is reasonable to assume that humans would assimilate both height and gap by scanning the elevation. This combined effect is referred to hereafter as layout.

The first experiment was conducted in a senior university course, using digital projection in a darkened room and 19 respondents. They were asked to select successively one of two elevations presented together that appeared to be at higher density, for a total of 36 pairs.

Results

The main analysis was done using the multifactor model for comparative judgement (Bock & Jones, 1968, pp. 187-207) and the angular response function, appropriate for a quantitative approach to the measurement of density (Bock & Jones, 1968, pp. 71-75). These results are reported as analyses of variance, including the proportions of variance attributable to the two variables. Contrasts between stimuli within levels of density are reported along with significance with respect to all nine stimuli. Effect sizes are also reported for responses to individual stimuli, for reasons given by Rosenthal and Rosnow (1991). The observed proportions are transformed into angular deviates, suitable for analysis of the response to quantitative measures of physical density, and for the analysis of variance and estimates of effect size. It was not thought that order was significant, so both experiments used the same alpha-numeric sequence for the presentation.

Table 2 presents the analysis of variance. Physical density and layout account, respectively, for about 63% and 15% of perceived density.

TABLE 2
ANALYSIS OF VARIANCE USING AN ANGULAR RESPONSE FUNCTION

Source of Variation	df	SS	MS	F	a	$\bar{\omega}^2$
Levels of physical density	2	12.60	6.30	53.9	5e-5	.631
Levels of layout	2	3.12	1.56	13.3	.002	.147
Residual	32	3.74	.12			
Total	34	19.46				

Hypothesis 1 was that larger spaces between the buildings with more visible vegetation reduced the impression of density in participants, even though buildings increased in height. For example, 1c should be perceived as less dense than 1b, while 1b should be perceived as less dense than 1a. Thus Hypothesis 1 predicted nine contrasts. Contrasts were calculated, and effect sizes (d) were estimated (Table 3 and Fig. 2). The graph shows a general decline in perception of density as the space between buildings increases and the buildings get higher. The smallest effect size falls into Cohen's category (1988) for an effect too small to be seen with the naked eye; the other eight effect sizes are medium ($d \approx .5$) to large ($d \approx .8$) in Cohen's (1988) system. However, only four contrasts are significant at $p < .05$, reflecting an underpowered experiment.

EXPERIMENT 2

In Exp. 1, open space, the amount of visible greenery and the number of building clusters all covaried. Such covariance could be said to represent the real environment; however, one or more of the variables may have contributed to lower perceived density. To focus on the effect of measured physical density and number of units, the second experiment involved objects without building references. Building clusters were replaced with simple boxes inside a frame. The areas covered by the boxes and the number of-

TABLE 3
CONTRASTS AMONG PHOTOMONTAGE STIMULI

Density	Gap Width	Stimulus	M	Contrast	Sig?	d
High	Small	3a	.870			
	Medium	3b	.530	.340	yes	.09
	Small	3a	.870			
	Large	3c	.184	.686	yes	2.02
	Medium	3b	.530			
	Large	3c	.184	.346	yes	1.02
Medium	Small	2a	.179			
	Medium	2b	−.070	.249	no	.73
	Small	2a	.179			
	Large	2c	−.331	.510	yes	1.50
	Medium	2b	−.070			
	Large	2c	−.331	.261	no	.77
Low	Small	1a	−.350			
	Medium	1b	−.382	.032	no	.09
	Small	1a	−.350			
	Large	1c	−.623	.273	no	.80
	Medium	1b	−.382			
	Large	1c	−.623	.241	no	.71

Note.—"Density" is the level of the density factor; "Gap width" is the legel of the layout factor. "Mean" is the scaled perception of density for the stimulus, averaged over participants. "Contrast" is the contrast between means for two stimuli. "Sig?" is whether the alpha level for the contrast was significant for an overall alpha, .05, and for nine simultaneous claims. "*d*" is the standardized mean contrast (the mean contrast divided by the square root of *mse* in the analysis of variance).

boxes replicated the arrangement in Exp. 1. The proportions attributed to each choice were also examined under the surface response function. The relationship between the sets of responses is addressed in Hypothesis 2.

Method

   Stimuli.—A second set of nine stimuli consisted of grey, cubic boxes set on a black line inside a black frame. The area in grey boxes as a proportion of the whole corresponded to the levels represented in the photomontage, while the gaps between buildings varied in number and corresponding size.

   Participants.—There were 30 new participants for this experiment, recruited from the student population. The nine stimuli were presented in pairs on poster boards to individual participants, who were asked to identify the stimulus that appeared to represent higher density.

   It was hypothesized that the visual content of the buildings or the silhouette of the building was not being examined for judging relative density but the coverage of buildings on the picture plane. Choice data from Exp. 2 were analysed with the Bock and Jones model.

Results

   The scaled values for perceived density are shown in Table 1. The cor-

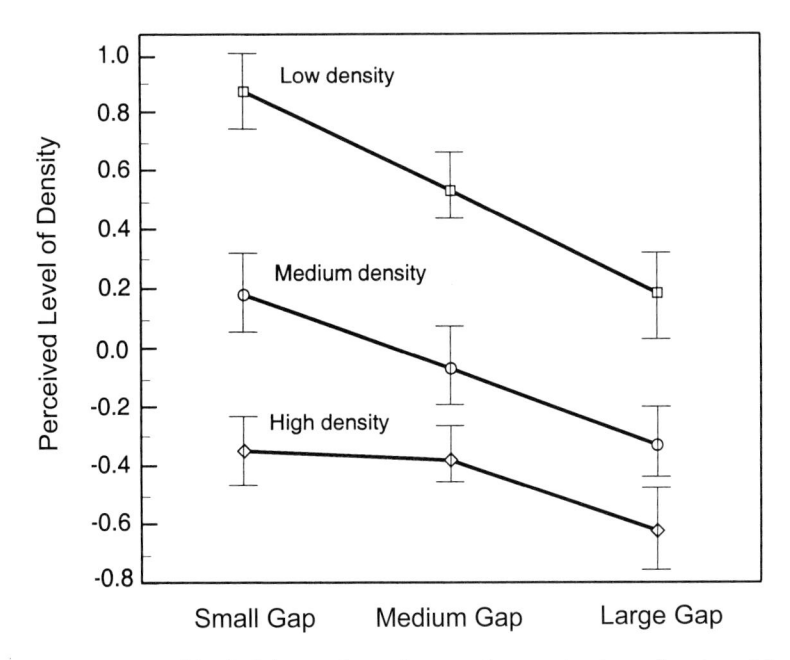

FIG. 2. Perceived level of density (linear deviates of proportions) as a function of the gap between buildings in photomontages

relation of perceived density between the two experiments was .95, indicating that perceived density is a function of the extent of building coverage, number of buildings, and building spacing and height, rather than architectural details, the silhouette of individual building groups, or landscaping.

Conclusion

Participants readily distinguished building density that varied in level by about 25% but referred to other pictorial elements in comparing density between individual stimuli. The gap between buildings resulted in a decrease in perceived density. While gap covaried with building height, it is logical to assume that it is the greater space between buildings which accounts for the lowered impression of density. The decrease in perceived density for the same physical density results in medium to large effects for eight of the nine stimuli. A more powerful experiment with a larger group of respondents would be required to draw definitive conclusions although the effect and its direction are clear in these experiments.

Elevations are commonly used to represent projects and elicit public opinion; thus it is important to work with this form of representation. On the other hand, density as measured and practised in urban planning is a three-dimensional concept. Linear increases in density in two-dimensional stimuli result in nonlinear increases in density when the elevation is rotated through 90°. Failing an effective way to represent three dimensions which allows for comparison, the elevation view remains the next best option. As such, it is a good surrogate for real environments where environmental preference is concerned. The correlation between preferences for photomontages and slides showing the whole block face was .93 (Stamps, 1993b). The cumulative correlation for preference in real environments and preference for static color images of real environments is .83, with $n = 553$ scenes (Stamps, 1993a). If evaluation of the desirability of an environment operates in much the same way as the evaluation of density, then elevations might well be an appropriate way to represent density.

Additional work should include a more powerful experiment of the same sort. Following that, the vegetation in the stimuli should be quantitatively varied to measure its possible role in the impression of lower density. Note that in the present study, the vegetation was identical in all photomontage stimuli, although only portions of the vegetation were visible between and above buildings. Secondly, it is of interest to vary the relative difference in height of buildings firstly because greater variation makes visual averaging more difficult and secondly to test the relationship between complexity and perceived density.

REFERENCES

ARIELY, D. (2001) Seeing sets: representation by statistical properties. *Psychological Science*, 12, 157-162.

BOCK, R., & JONES, L. (1968) *The measurement and prediction of judgment and choice.* San Francisco, CA: Holden-Day.

BULATOV, A., BERTULIS, A., & STROGONOV, V. (2001) Distortions on length perception in a combination of illusionary figures. *Human Physiology*, 27, 274-283.

CHAPANIS, A., & MANKEN, D. A. (1967) The vertical-horizontal illusion in a visually rich environment. *Perception & Psychophysics*, 2, 249-255.

CHONG, S. C., & TREISMAN, A. (2003) Representation of statistical properties. *Vision Research*, 43, 393-404.

CHURCHMAN, A. (1999) Disentangling the concept of density. *Journal of Planning Literature*, 13, 389-411.

COHEN, J. (1988) *Statistical power analysis for the behavioral sciences.* Hillsdale, NJ: Erlbaum.

HELMHOLTZ, H., VON. *Handbuch der Physiologischen Optik.* Leipzig: Voss. Part I (1856). Part II (1860). Part III (1866). (Transl. and republished, New York: Dover, 1962)

KAYA, N., & ERKIP, F. (2001) Satisfaction in a dormitory building: the effects of floor height on the perception of room size and crowding. *Environment and Behavior*, 33(1), 35-53.

MUNAKATA, J., & OI, N. (1997) Spaciousness of interiors with different views through a window. *Proceedings of the International Conference on Environment-Behavior Studies for the 21st century, Tokyo, 4-6 November.* Pp. 521-524.

ROSENTHAL, R., & ROSNOW, R. L. (1991) *Essentials of behavioral research: methods and data analysis.* New York: McGraw-Hill.

SPEHAR, B., & GILLAM, B. (2002) Modal completion in the Poggendorff illusion: support for the depth-processing theory. *Psychological Science*, 13, 306-312.

STAMPS, A. E. (1993a) Simulation effects on environmental preference. *Perceptual and Motor Skills*, 80, 668-670.

STAMPS, A. E. (1993b) Validating contextual urban design photoprotocols: replication and generalization from single residences to block faces. *Environment and Planning B: Planning and Design*, 20, 693-707.

Accepted February 16, 2004.

FROM PHONEMES TO MEANING: JOHN STEINBECK'S WORK EXAMINED [1]

GLENN L. THOMPSON AND SARA KUNTO

University of Ottawa

Summary.—Two novels were selected from two distinct periods in John Steinbeck's career, and text samples from each were pooled according to era. Using quantitative measures of text emotion, between-sample and norm-relative comparisons were computed to evaluate *a priori* expectations regarding differences in the use of implicit emotional information. These hypotheses reflected abstract characteristics that transcend the focus of a single novel. Analysis of word-based measures did not yield the between-sample differences expected. Rather, the hypotheses were supported by distinct patterns of phoneme distribution. The findings confirm and extend previous work by demonstrating that authors of prose manipulate the emotional quality of phonemes, and that the associated patterns can occur at a more abstract level than previously demonstrated.

Previous research has demonstrated the value of analysing the style of various English texts using objective measures of complexity (Whissell, 1998, 1999; Whissell & Sigelman, 2001) and of connotative meaning (Whissell, 1994, 2000, 2001; Whissell & Sigelman, 2001). Such analyses can successfully differentiate between authors (Whissell, 1994), and they are also sensitive to the within-author differences that occur across works (Whissell, 2001). This line of inquiry demonstrates that writers manipulate subtle cues when communicating with their audiences. These patterns are most convincingly identified when within-author comparisons and norm-relative information are combined, since strategic changes on the part of the writer and estimates of sensitivity to these changes are thereby assessed (Whissell, 2000).

The term connotative meaning refers to the emotional information associated with particular linguistic units (e.g., for words or individual phonemes) that is not dependent on an explicit definition. Typically, this concept is quantified by averaging ratings of word emotionality from human subjects along two orthogonal dimensions of emotional space (Whissell, 2000). Specifically, a continuum of "pleasantness" lies on one axis, while a continuum of "activation" is described by the other. Forty-five degree rotation produces two additional dimensions of emotion, and the eight resulting radii

---

[1]We thank Cynthia Whissell for use of her text analysis program and her helpful comments. In addition, we acknowledge the contribution of Lissa Sanchioni for her help in proofreading this paper and thank anonymous reviewers for their helpful comments. Please address correspondence to Glenn L. Thompson, School of Psychology, University of Ottawa, 145 Jean-Jacques Lussier, P.O. Box 450, Station A, Ottawa, Canada, K1N 6N5 or e-mail (gthom044@uottawa.ca).

define the categories of an emotional circumplex (Whissell, 2000). The radii labels are intended to be literal and are Pleasant, Unpleasant, Active, Passive, Sad, Cheery, Nasty, and Soft. Associations between these word classes and the occurrence of particular phonemes may then be discerned, but multiple etiologies are thought to be at the root of this relationship (Whissell, 2000, 2001). For example, the phoneme corresponding to the letters /ee/ occurs often in words rated as pleasant but also elicits muscular activity which is involved in a speaker's "smiling."

These ratings and classifications have been reliably associated with human performance. Among other known effects, objectively defined word emotionality affects recall in serial list (Lamarche & Campbell, 1993) and paired-associate (Howard-Voyer & Whissell, 1994) tasks. Similarly, the emotion associated with phonemes mediates the production and classification of nonsense text (Whissell, 2000). Not surprisingly, analysis of poetry (Whissell, 2001), of novels (Whissell, 1994, 1998), and of text sampled from specific prose contexts (Whissell, 2000) indicate that authors exploit this sensitivity to connotative meaning. However, the phoneme-use strategies that may be adopted by authors of prose at the level of a novel or several novels remain unexplored.

Although there is no shortage of worthy subjects for objective analysis in English literature, certain authors, such as John Steinbeck, have produced bodies of work that provide an especially interesting challenge for objective text analysis. Since literary critics identified Steinbeck's prose as characterized by a poetic style (Haft, 1995; Serafin, 1999), one might expect his novels to be saturated with connotative meaning and especially that related to sound. This assumption is especially relevant given Steinbeck's tendency to "feel" rather than to intellectualize that which he observed (Nelson, 1967). Also of interest is Steinbeck's tendency to explore general themes across several novels (Nelson, 1967; McWilliams, 1970; Haft, 1995; Serafin, 1999). Most notably, the periods of the 1930s and 1960s are respectively identified as homogeneous. Based on the above, Steinbeck's work seems ideally suited for evaluating the hypothesis that an author of prose can manipulate implicit emotional cues to convey abstract information to readers.

Evaluating the truth of this contention requires specific hypotheses. Two sources of information may be consulted for this purpose. One might look to Steinbeck's focus on the negative aspect of the *Zeitgeist*, or spirit of the times (Nelson, 1967; McWilliams, 1970), to formulate *a priori* hypotheses concerning his use of connotative meaning in different time periods. Alternatively, one can look to critical descriptions of the mood and themes or settings of novels from different eras. This information may legitimately be invoked as justification for hypotheses within this context because a manipulation by the author is being verified. The conclusions are thus valid regardless of whether the critics made use of connotative meaning in drawing their conclusions. When comparing the two sources of information, the face validity of critical descriptions seems preferable to the more arbitrary inferences based on general negative aspects of different eras. In practice, both strategies lead to similar sets of hypotheses. At any rate, the question is not whether novels of an era share similar emotional characteristics, but whether the attributes discussed below have been communicated using the emotional quality of phonemes.

Steinbeck's early work has been described as sad and nostalgic (McWilliams, 1970; Haft, 1995; Serafin, 1999). Since the labels of the emotional circumplex are quite general, nostalgia is loosely classified as a Soft characteristic for present purposes. Based on these descriptions, Sad as well as Soft words and phonemes should be used more prevalently in Steinbeck's early work. The same sources note the agricultural influence in the region and on Steinbeck's work and his focus on nature. When compared to an urban lifestyle, this setting and theme would be defined by a slow pace. This trend that dominated Steinbeck's early work might translate into use of Passive words and phonemes. The Sad, Soft, and Passive categories are proximal to each other within the emotional circumplex continuum, a fact that provides convergent validity for these expectations.

Steinbeck's focus changed in his later work. The 1960s novels are more reflective of the moral decay (Nelson, 1967) and the desegregation issues Steinbeck observed in America as a whole (Nelson, 1967); a larger number of Active, Unpleasant, and Nasty words and phonemes is therefore expected. The proximity of these radii within the emotional circumplex leads to the more general expectation that novels from both eras will occupy general but distinct regions of emotional space as a function of the defining trends noted above. Tolerance for generality may be required since the information being manipulated is so subtle that phonemes belonging to adjacent radii are sometimes confounded (Whissell, 2000).

Method

Text samples from two of John Steinbeck's randomly selected California novels, *Tortilla Flat* (1935) and *Of Mice and Men* (1937), were compared with samples from two of his randomly selected later works, *The Winter of Our Discontent* (1961) and *Travels with Charley: In Search of America* (1962), on measures of linguistic complexity, connotative meaning of words, and connotative meaning of phonemes. Six-page samples were selected randomly from each of the four books and were entered into a text analysis program developed by Whissell at Laurentian University. Previous experience with this type of analysis indicates that the chosen sampling strategy provides a good balance between obtaining results that are representative of the population in question and preserving the meaningfulness of significance tests (C. Whissell, personal communication, October, 2001).

Measures of connotative meaning for words included mean Pleasantness rating, Activation rating, and the proportional use of Very Pleasant, Very Active, Very Unpleasant, Very Passive, Cheery, Sad, Nasty, and Soft words (Whissell, 2001). The phonemic measures are based on the concordance of a particular phoneme with one of the basic word types (Whissell, 2000). What follows is a brief description of the measures used. The development of these measures and their validity are discussed at length elsewhere (Whissell, 1994, 1998, 2000, 2001).

All lexical norms were obtained from the new Dictionary of Affect which is currently under construction by Whissell. The corpus contains 8,742 English words collected from a wide variety of sources such as essays, newspapers, discussions, stories, children's literature, and the Kučera and Francis database. The new dictionary contains entries for approximately 90% of words within written text. From 1996 to 1998, over 200 volunteers rated these entries along the dimensions Pleasantness and Activation (3-point Likert scale). The only ratings of word emotion and normative usage that are available are modern. This kind of concern reflects a limitation of the present analysis, and many others, e.g., the Kučera and Francis frequency norms collected in 1967 are ubiquitously cited in recent articles.

As discussed in the Introduction, the two original dimensions were rotated 45° which increased the number of dimensions to four. For example, a word that is rated as Active and Unpleasant is classified as Nasty when the matrix is rotated. The resulting eight radii defined the categories that were used to classify words and estimate the emotional quality of phonemes. Whissell (2000) chose to use the 41 basic phonemes that define the mid-American accent in her analysis. The frequency with which these phonemes occurred within particular classes of words was then computed and their place within the emotional circumplex identified. In all, the patterns of occurrence associated with 34 phonemes were deemed interpretable. These classifications were subsequently replicated four times using different databases (Whissell, 2000), supporting their validity.

In this study, all lexical measures were compared across early and late samples using F ratios, and text means were also compared to normative usage (Whissell, 1998, 2001) by calculating confidence intervals. Phoneme comparisons were made using contingency χ^2 analyses for between-group comparisons, and z scores were employed for comparisons to the normative sample of phoneme use (Whissell, 2000).

The two sets of comparisons, i.e., between-group and normative, are warranted, since each provides unique information concerning the samples. Phoneme norms are based on a corpus of a third of a million words, which amounts to 1.25 million phonemes. The source of the word-based norms is discussed above. Norm-relative comparisons are less risky since the associated parameters are stable. Further, since the relationships being discussed are interpreted in terms of a pattern, and predictions were made *a priori*, the present analyses were conducted using the 5% alpha criterion adopted in related work (Whissell, 1994, 2000). The complexity of the text samples was also analysed, but these results will not be discussed here since they are not relevant to the principal hypotheses.

Results

Table 1 summarizes the means and results for the analyses involving word-based and phoneme-based estimates of text emotion. No differences in word-emotion pattern were discovered between the text samples. With regards to the normative sample, 95% confidence intervals indicated that

TABLE 1
Word-based Measures of Linguistic Complexity and Emotion
For Early (E) and Late (L) Steinbeck Samples

Linguistic Measure	Mean Early	Mean Late	Late vs Early	Samples vs Norm
Dictionary of Affect			95% Confidence Intervals	
Pleasantness	1.83	1.84	ns	E&L < norm
Activation	1.65	1.65	ns	E&L < norm
Very High Pleasantness	.05	.05	ns	L < norm
Very High Activation	.03	.04	ns	ns
Very Low Pleasantness	.04	.04	ns	ns
Very Low Activation	.20	.20	ns	ns
Cheery	.03	.04	ns	E&L < norm
Sad	.05	.06	ns	ns
Nasty	.03	.03	ns	ns
Soft	.05	.05	ns	ns
Phonoemotional Analysis			Z Scores	
Pleasant	21.5	19.7	‡ −	E = +4.40
Unpleasant	23.8	25.3	† +	L = +3.82
Active	30.7	32.5	† +	E = −3.28, L = −6.17
Passive	42.5	41.8	ns	E = +4.22, L = +3.71
Cheerful	29.0	28.8	ns	ns
Sad	22.3	20.7	† −	E = +6.74, L = +3.62
Nasty	34.0	35.6	* +	E = −3.70
Soft	27.4	26.0	* −	E = +3.22

Note.—ns denotes no significant difference. The + or − symbols indicate the direction of the effect from the Early to Late sample or relative to the norm. *$p < .05$. †$p < .01$. ‡$p < .001$.

Pleasantness and Activation scores, as well as Cheery word use, were below normative levels for both the early and late samples. Very Pleasant word use fell below the normative comparison for the later novels.

Levels of Pleasant phoneme ($\chi_1^2 = 9.09$, $p = .002$) were significantly lower in the later publication interval, while those for Unpleasant phoneme ($\chi_1^2 = 6.50$, $p = .01$) were significantly higher. Z-score tests indicated that the level of Pleasant phoneme for the early works was significantly above the normative mean, while Unpleasant phoneme use was significantly above the normative sample for Steinbeck's later works. Use of Active phonemes ($\chi_1^2 = 7.89$, $p = .005$) was more pronounced in the later novels but remained below the norm for both time periods. The use of Sad phonemes was less prominent in the later novels ($\chi_1^2 = 8.39$, $p = .004$) but was greater than the norm for both samples of Steinbeck's work. Nasty phoneme ($\chi_1^2 = 5.64$, $p = .02$) use increased, and conversely Soft phoneme ($\chi_1^2 = 5.25$, $p = .02$) use decreased across eras. Compared to the norm, Nasty phoneme use was significantly below the mean in Steinbeck's early works, and these same works were significantly above the mean for Soft phonemes. As is often the case with this type of analysis, the effect sizes for all measures are small ($< .10$).

Discussion

Contrary to predictions, connotative word meaning, as measured by the Dictionary of Affect, did not reflect the particularities critics associate with Steinbeck's early and later novels. No significant between-sample differences were observed. Measures of word emotion did, however, provide hypothesis-supporting results in that Pleasantness and Cheerfulness were below the norm for both time periods. This finding no doubt reflects the negative focus attributed to Steinbeck in the Introduction. Further, an unexpected consistency across eras was observed with passive words. Both samples fell below the norm for Activation when this was predicted for the early sample only. This overall lack of active words may reflect a passive style of writing inherent in Steinbeck's work.

Despite Steinbeck's characteristic negative focus, differences were expected between the early and later groups. The expected differences were found when phoneme emotion, rather than word emotion, was examined (see Table 1). Considering the poetic nature of Steinbeck's prose (Haft, 1995; Serafin, 1999), it is not surprising that the expected differences in tone were discovered in the more poetic arena of sound. The marked dissociation between the patterns of word and phoneme use was nonetheless unexpected.

As predicted, words from the 1930s novels sounded more Soft and more Sad than those from the 1960s novels, and the 1930s samples were also significantly above the mean on these measures. An additional finding, which makes sense *a posteriori*, is that the 1930s samples were more Pleasant than either the 1960s samples or the norm. The Pleasant category is adjacent to the Soft category, i.e., the one that was predicted, in the emotional circumplex, which speaks to their similarity. The additional pleasantness may also tie in with the notion that Steinbeck would paint his childhood region (California) with a softer brush than that used to illustrate 1960s America.

As expected, the 1960s samples were significantly different from the earlier samples, and the norm, in both Activation and Unpleasantness. Further, the 1960s samples were significantly Nastier, a measure that reflects both high Activation and Unpleasantness, than the 1930 novels. The results support the hypothesis that samples drawn from the later novels would be relatively Nasty and Active. It was hypothesized that both samples would be Unpleasant but only the later sample was significantly below the norm on that phoneme measure. In sum, when phoneme use was considered, the bulk of the results were supportive of the original hypotheses in that both samples occupy the regions of emotional space specified in the Introduction.

A stable trait in Steinbeck's writing is evident as Passivity and Sadness in both words and phonemes when compared to the norm. It would seem that rather than the hypothesized overall Unpleasant emotion, Steinbeck made use of its passive variation, i.e., Sadness, to convey the negativity he sought to explore. Perhaps Sadness was used to convey regret at losing older and, perhaps to Steinbeck, more noble ways of life. These constants in Steinbeck's style make the norm-relative comparisons more difficult to interpret.

The within-author comparisons involving phoneme use indicate that the author is attempting to convey different emotional information to his audience in each era. For instance, the analysis tells us that Steinbeck used Unpleasant phonemes more often in the samples taken from the 1960s work. Similarly, the norm-relative comparisons provide a crude estimate of the sensitivity of his audience to this manipulation (but see Method). In this case, the frequency of Unpleasant phonemes was significantly above the norm. In the present analysis, no other emotional category provided a combination of results that was as neatly interpretable. This fact tempers the claims that can be made with respect to the sensitivity of the audience to Steinbeck's multinovel manipulations. Of course, a reader who is familiar with Steinbeck's work may be sensitive to the differences between eras.

At any rate, the sensitivity of the audience is not as relevant as the detection of a manipulation by the author. Previous phonoemotional work pooled samples of text from specific types of written descriptions (Whissell, 2000) or pooled homogeneous types of poems (Whissell, 2001). The predictors of phoneme use described here are not nearly as concrete. Consider the fact that multinovel samples from two eras of Steinbeck's career were pooled, and the patterns of phoneme use were predicted with reasonable success on the basis of abstract concepts. The implication is that emotional expression via phoneme use occurs even when the intension of the author is very abstract. Of course, the evidence presented here should be considered preliminary. Stronger claims can be made once similar results have been obtained with additional authors of prose, or favourable experimental evidence is collected.

Despite a certain stability in style, the results presented here support the notion that phonemes were used by Steinbeck to provide nuance for his works, whether by design or by unconscious choice, and that these differences can be predicted with reasonable success on the basis of critical descriptions of his work and the era or region he described. If the information provided by simple phonemes is indeed within the realm of human sensitivity (Whissell, 2000, 2001), then their use by authors of prose may provide an overall impression of time and place which is conveyed without recourse to explicit semantic knowledge.

REFERENCES

HART, J. D. (Ed.) (1995) *The Oxford companion to American literature.* (6th ed.) New York: Oxford Univer. Press.

HOWARD-VOYER, C., & WHISSELL, C. (1994) Emotional descriptors of words as predictors of recall in a paired-associate task. *Perceptual and Motor Skills*, 78, 1187-1192.

LAMARCHE, S., & CAMPBELL, M. (1993) A memory advantage for serial lists composed of active words. *Perceptual and Motor Skills*, 77, 748-751.

MCWILLIAMS, C. (1970) A man, a place, a time: John Steinbeck and the long agony of the great valley in an age of depression, oppression, frustration and hope. *American West*, 7, 4-8, 39-40, 62-64.

NELSON, H. S. (1967) Steinbeck's politics then and now. *Antioch Review*, 27, 118-133.

SERAFIN, S. R. (Ed.) (1999) *The Continuum encyclopaedia of American literature.* New York: Continuum.

WHISSELL, C. (1994) A computer program for the objective analysis of style and emotional connotatives of prose: Hemmingway, Galsworthy and Faulkner compared. *Perceptual and Motor Skills*, 79, 815-824.

WHISSELL, C. (1998) A parsimonious technique for the analysis of word-use patterns in English texts and transcripts. *Perceptual and Motor Skills*, 86, 595-613.

WHISSELL, C. (1999) Linguistic complexity of abstracts and titles in highly cited journals. *Perceptual and Motor Skills*, 88, 76-86.

WHISSELL, C. (2000) Phonoemotional profiling: a description of the emotional flavour of English texts on the basis of the phonemes employed in them. *Perceptual and Motor Skills*, 91, 617-648.

WHISSELL, C. (2001) The emotionality of William Blake's poems: a qualitative comparison of Songs of Innocence with Songs of Experience. *Perceptual and Motor Skills*, 92, 459-467.

WHISSELL, C., & SIGELMAN, L. (2001) The times and the man as predictors of emotion and style in the inaugural addresses of U.S. presidents. *Computer and the Humanities*, 35, 255-272.

Accepted February 19, 2004.

SEX DIFFERENCES IN SIMPLE REACTION TASKS[1]

ROLAND KALB, STEPHANIE JANSEN, UDO REULBACH, STEFANIE KALB

Department of Psychiatry and Psychotherapy
University of Erlangen–Nuremberg

Summary.—Many anatomical and brain mapping studies show a higher bilateral symmetry of female brains and a higher asymmetry of male brains so correlations between simple visual and auditory, left- and right-hand reaction times were examined for such sex differences. 20 healthy women and 20 men were tested in two sessions. For women all six response times correlated with each other significantly in Session A, but in Session B there were only two significant interhemispheric correlations. This represented different changes in visual and auditory reaction times between Sessions A and B. Men showed the same pattern in both sessions: a significant correlation between the interhemispheric visual reaction times and one between auditory reaction times. Women showed a total correlation pattern in Session A and an interhemispheric correlation pattern in Session B. This was interpreted as a transition between a holistic information-processing strategy in Session A and an analytic strategy in Session B. Men showed an analytic strategy in both sessions.

The brains and behavior of men and women are different. Many studies have shown these evolutionary differences are advantageous (Kimura, 1992). Anatomical studies have suggested that females' brains show greater symmetry than males' (Wada, Nanbu, Kadoshima, Jiang, Koshino, & Hashimoto, 1996) as has often been reported in the sexual dimorphism of the corpus callosum (Allen, Richey, Chai, & Gorski, 1991; Holloway, Anderson, Defendini, & Harper, 1993). This greater bilateral symmetry of females' brains and greater asymmetry of male brains has been confirmed in fMRI studies. On mental-rotation tasks (Jordan, Wustenberg, Heinze, Peters, & Jancke, 2002) women exhibited more bilateral activations, and men showed significant asymmetrical activation of brain areas. On verbal and manual tasks men showed slightly larger laterality effects than women (Medland, Geffen, & McFarland, 2002). Gur, Turetsky, Matsui, Yan, Bilker, Hughett, and Gur (1999) used MRI to investigate the sex differences in brain gray and white matter in healthy young adults. In men the percentage of gray matter was higher in the left hemisphere, the percentage of white matter was symmetric, and the percentage of corticospinal fluid was higher in the right. Women showed no asymmetries. The MRI results of Yucel, Stuart, Maruff, Velakoulis, Crowe, Savage, and Pantelis (2001) suggested that in normal male brains, there were morphological asymmetries at both the global and local levels which are less apparent in female brains. Pujol, Lopez-Sala, Deus, Cardoner,

---

[1]Address correspondence to Prof. Dr. Roland Kalb, Department of Psychiatry and Psychotherapy, University of Erlangen–Nuremberg, Schwabachanlage 6, 91054 Erlangen, Germany or e-mail (Roland.Kalb@psych.imed.uni-erlangen.de).

Sebastian-Galles, Conesa, and Capdevila (2002) found with MRI that leftward asymmetry in frontal and temporal regions occurred in both sexes, although hemisphere differences were significantly larger for men. Good, Johnsrude, Ashburner, Henson, Friston, and Frackowiak (2001) used voxel-based morphometry (VBM) to examine human brain asymmetry and the effects of sex and handedness on brain structure. Males showed increased leftward asymmetry within Heschl's gyrus and the planum temporale over females. Functional MRI was used to investigate sex differences in brain activation during a paradigm similar to a lexical-decision task. Women showed a more symmetrical pattern in language-related areas (Rossell, Bullmore, Williams, & David, 2002). Vikingstad, George, Johnson, and Cao (2000) studied fMRI during language tasks. For males, activation during language primarily lateralized to the left, and for females, approximately half had left lateralization of activation and the other half had bilateral activation. Their data indicate that a previous view of female bilateral hemispheric dominance for language simplifies the complexity of cortical language distribution. Amunts, Jancke, Mohlberg, Steinmetz, and Zilles (2000) used *in vivo* MR morphometry to analyze interhemispheric asymmetric activation in the depth of the central sulcus in the region of cortical hand representation. No interhemispheric asymmetric activation was found for females. Anatomical asymmetry was associated with handedness only for males, but not females, suggesting sex differences in the cortical organization of hand movements.

The ERP results of Johnson, McKenzie, and Hamm (2002) reported the notion that visuospatial processing in mental rotation is more bilaterally organized in females. Camposano and Lolas (1992) have used auditory evoked potentials to show that women have less anatomical brain asymmetry, larger corpus callosum involvement, and more bilateral representation of specific functions.

A comparative study of visual and auditory reaction times in males and females showed significant sex differences in reaction times (Misra, Mahajan, & Maini, 1985), with males responding faster than females and the difference being significant mainly in auditory reaction times on the left side. Using cognitive sex differences in speed and problem-solving strategies on computerized neuropsychological tasks, Klinteberg, Levander, and Schalling (1987) reported that boys were significantly faster than girls on most reaction time subtasks. This speed advantage for men has been noted by many other authors (Misra, *et al.*, 1985; Nicholson & Kimura, 1996; Dane & Erzurumluoglu, 2003). However, other authors have found no significant sex differences on simple reaction tasks (Sanders, 1971). The results of Mikhelashvili-Browner, Yousem, Wu, Kraut, Vaughan, Oguz, and Calhoun (2003) suggested that sex seemed to be little related to fMRI brain activation when they compared performance on a simple reaction-time task.

Summing up, there were many anatomical and brain-mapping studies which showed a higher bilateral symmetry of female brains and a higher asymmetry of male brains. However, no reaction-time studies had examined sex differences in symmetry for different reaction times. To investigate these symmetries four different reaction times had to be measured and their intercorrelations with each other examined.

Method

We investigated a group of 40 healthy subjects, who were recruited from among medical students and staff members. All subjects were screened for history of neurologic, psychiatric, or medical problems, as well as current medication use (except birth control pills in younger women and hormonal replacement therapy in postmenopausal women). The group included 20 females (20–45 years; M age = 26.8 ± 5.6 yr.) and 20 males (20–48 years; M age = 26.7 ± 6.3 yr.). To exclude disturbing factors, persons with vision or hearing problems or any musculoskeletal complaints were not included. Thirty-seven subjects were right-handed, and three subjects were left-handed. All subjects took part voluntarily in the examination. The study was approved by the local ethics committee at the University of Erlangen–Nuremberg. Informed consent was obtained according to the Declaration of Helsinki.

We measured simple reaction times, auditory and visual, right hand and left hand in a first 1-hr. Session A and repeated the whole procedure in a second 1-hr. Session B some days later. The stimuli were presented with a random interstimulus time of 2.5 sec. on the average. Before starting the subject received instructions from the supervisor and had the chance to practice the tasks five times. Only the hand needed for the test was allowed to remain on the keyboard. The keys had to be pressed as fast and accurately as possible when the stimulus appeared. The order of the tasks was counterbalanced: half of the subjects performed the auditory tasks first and half of the subjects the visual tasks first. The four different reaction times of one session were not measured simultaneously but successively: the four reaction tasks (left hand, right hand, visual, and auditory tasks) were performed one after the other. The correlations among successive tasks imply a temporal stability of reaction times within the measure time.

For the auditory response tasks, the test person sat in front of a PC wearing a headset. The eyes were closed. For the simple auditory task, 100 homogeneous tones (frequency: 100 Hz, duration: 55 msec.) appeared successively on the person's right ear, which had to be responded to by pressing a key with the right index finger. Then the same procedure was applied to the left side. The stimuli appeared at the person's left ear and had to be responded to with the left index finger.

For the visual response tasks, the test person sat in front of a laptop and fixated an arrow in the center of the screen. The arrangement of the tasks was the same as for the auditory tasks. The simple visual task consisted of 100 homogeneous stimuli (circles appearing under a numeral 1). The person pressed a key with the right index finger as quickly as possible. Then the same procedure was applied to the left side under equivalent conditions.

In the end there were four simple mean reaction times for each subject and each session. We calculated the median reaction time for the 100 trials of each task performed by a subject. Then the mean values for each task and each sex group were calculated. For comparisons between the mean values of each group and between the mean values of each session a two-sided Mann-Whitney U test and the Wilcoxon signed-ranks test were used. The Pearson correlation coefficient was calculated. Significance was set at $\alpha = .05$. Data were analyzed using SPSS™ Version 11.0.1.

Results and Discussion

There were no significant sex differences for mean simple reaction times of these young adults, in Sessions A and B. The differences between mean reaction times of Sessions A and B were not significant, although, in Session A women responded faster than men, and in Session B men responded faster on the auditory tasks and women on the visual tasks. These findings were not, however, significant ($p > .05$). The test-retest reliability was high for all measured reaction times (Pearson correlation coefficients).

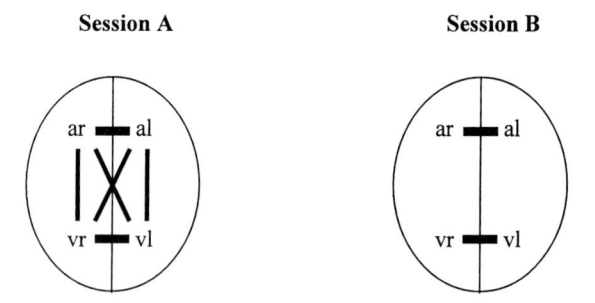

Fig. 1. Women show a total symmetry in Session A and a mirror symmetry in Session B (ar = reaction time, auditory, right-hand, etc.)

The pattern of correlations of the median reaction times showed clear sex differences (Figs. 1 and 2). For women all six reaction times correlated with each other significantly in Session A. In Session B there were only two significant interhemispheric correlations—between the two mean auditory reaction times and between the two visual reaction times. The correlation pattern in both sessions for men was the same and a significant interhemispheric value for visual reaction times and also for auditory reaction times. The correlation coefficients and the significance levels are shown in Table 1.

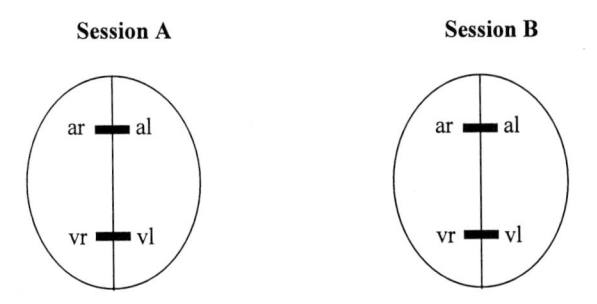

FIG. 2. Men show a mirror symmetry in both sessions

TABLE 1
SEX DIFFERENCES IN PEARSON CORRELATIONS BETWEEN REACTION TIMES AND SIGNIFICANCE

	Women r	Women p	Men r	Men p
Auditory right/left hand A	.83	<.01	.79	<.01
Visual right/left hand A	.97	<.01	.82	<.01
Auditory/visual right hand A	.49	<.05	.07	ns
Auditory/visual left hand A	.51	<.05	.34	ns
Auditory right/visual left hand A	.48	<.05	.27	ns
Auditory left/visual right hand A	.47	<.05	.10	ns
Auditory right/left hand B	.83	<.01	.84	<.01
Visual right/left hand B	.88	<.01	.66	<.01
Auditory/visual right hand B	.40	ns	.22	ns
Auditory/visual left hand B	.28	ns	.33	ns
Auditory right/visual left hand B	.30	ns	.16	ns
Auditory left/visual right hand B	.35	ns	.27	ns

For men the auditory and visual median reaction times changed in the same way from Session A to B, whereas in women the visual reaction times did not change much while the auditory median reaction times changed a lot. This opposite change in auditory and visual reaction times in women led to the audiovisual decorrelation between the two sessions. In Fig. 3 the opposite changes in auditory and visual median reaction times can be seen. Because the difference in auditory reaction times of Sessions A and B deviated from the difference of visual reaction times of Sessions A and B, the correlation was not significant (Fig. 3). By contrast, the correlation remained constant for women when the right-hand auditory differences between Sessions A and B and the left-hand auditory differences between Sessions A and B did not deviate (Fig. 4).

Young adults showed no significant sex differences in simple reaction times in this study. This lack of significant sex differences in reaction times

TABLE 2
Sex Differences in Mean Reaction Times by Modality and 95% Confidence Intervals (CI)

Reaction Time (msec.)	Women M	SD	95% CI	Men M	SD	95% CI
Auditory/right hand A	211	40	192 230	214	43	194 234
Auditory/left hand A	218	40	199 236	219	42	199 239
Visual/right hand A	244	59	216 271	254	51	230 278
Visual/left hand A	258	53	233 283	262	38	244 280
Auditory/right hand B	208	28	194 221	205	30	191 219
Auditory/left hand B	215	24	204 226	206	30	192 220
Visual/right hand B	229	45	208 250	235	33	219 250
Visual/left hand B	253	42	233 273	250	26	237 261

had been reported earlier (Sanders, 1971; Mikhelashvili-Browner, et al., 2003); however, sex differences have been found in many other studies. The reason for these inconsistent findings could be related to the different mean ages in these studies.

Nevertheless, comparison of correlations for the different reaction times showed distinct sex differences at least in Session A. Women showed six significant intra- and interhemispheric correlations in Run A and two interhemispheric correlations in Run B. Men showed two interhemispheric correlations in both sessions. That means women had four significant correlations more than men in Session A, two additional intrahemispheric audiovisual correlations and two additional interhemispheric audiovisual correlations. In contrast to the above fMRI studies men and women showed the same bilateral symmetry. But women had an increased number of interhemispheric correlations: they showed two additional interhemispheric audiovisual correlations, and they had two additional intrahemispheric audiovisual correlations. These additional significant intrahemispheric audiovisual correlations in Session A for women had not been described in previous studies. The increased interhemispheric symmetry in women, relative to men, has been reported in many structural and functional brain studies (see above).

This change in the female correlation pattern between Session A and Session B was due to an opposite development of the visual and auditory reaction times. Women were relatively stable in their visual reaction times, but their auditory reaction times changed. A possible explanation would be a

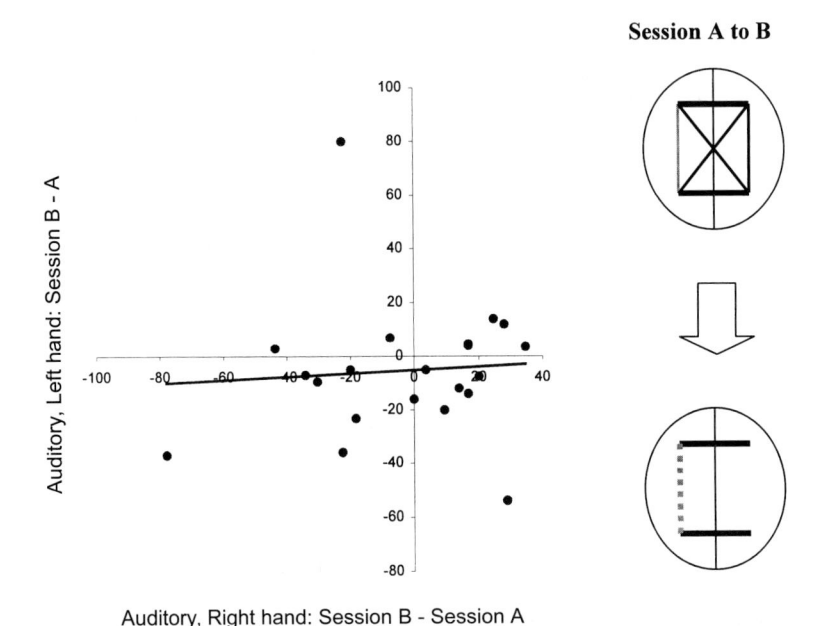

FIG. 3. In women the auditory and visual changes between Sessions A and B are asymmetrical, i.e., they do not change in the same way so the line is not a 45° inclination.

different implicit learning in the two modalities. Men could perform the transition from the maximal correlation pattern to the purely bilateral pattern early in Session A, while women would do this step at the end of Session A or the beginning of Session B. However, an increase in many reaction times between Sessions A and B is an argument against this possibility.

There must be a factor which affects the auditory modality other than the visual modality, a factor which affects the two auditory reaction times in the same way and affects the two visual reaction times in the same way but which does not affect the auditory times in the same way as the visual times would have shaped the males' correlation pattern early in Session A and does so for the female correlation pattern later in Session B. This "audiovisual decorrelation factor" stops holistic information processing for the benefit of specialized, analytic information processing. However, no reports could be found which confirm sex differences in holistic/analytic stimulus processing. After all, reports support the development from holistic to analytic information processing. Sakurai and Sugimura (1990) examined the holistic and analytic modes in classification learning of young children. They found that with increasing training trials, the number of subjects who used the analytic mode increased while the number who used the holistic mode de-

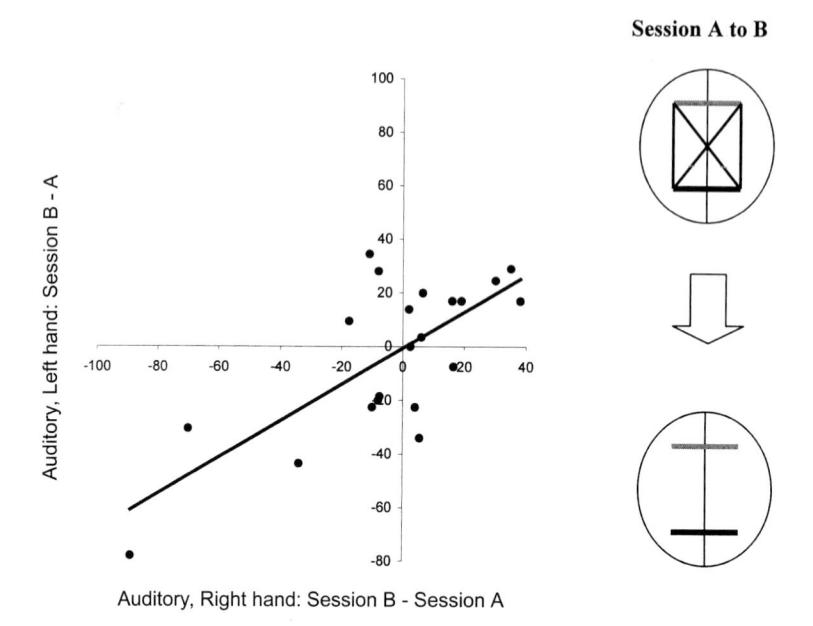

FIG. 4. In women the auditory changes are symmetrical. The correlation between the two auditory reaction times of Session A is the same as that between the two auditory reaction times of Session B ($r = .72$, $p < .001$).

creased. Ward (1983) had reported that holistic, integral processing preceded analytic dimensional processing.

The underlying neurobiological mechanism which switches between holistic and analytic information processing is not known. Possibly there are sex-related differences in neurotransmitters which shape the sex differences of human behavior. Molodtsova (1999) observed in the amygdala a hemispheric asymmetry of the 5-HT involvement, due to right-hemispheric changes in 5-HT metabolism, only in male rats. In females, an increase in 5-HT level was found in the left and right amygdalas in response to an irrelevant stimulus. These data suggest that serotonergic neurotransmitter mechanisms may be an important factor in determining hemispheric and sex differences in selective attention. Wisniewski (1998) gave converging evidence from various studies that sex steroid hormones are important for influencing cortical asymmetry. Although a mechanism has not yet been identified, testosterone would be the most likely candidate to influence cortical dominance.

Our study has shown that reaction time tasks for women and men need to be studied separately as different cognitive strategies in Session A and the same strategy in Session B were used. However, we investigated a range of young adults to middle-aged adults so we cannot generalize from these results to old age.

REFERENCES

Allen, L., Richey, M., Chai, Y., & Gorski, R. (1991) Sex differences in the corpus callosum of the living human being. *Journal of Neuroscience*, 11, 933-942.

Amunts, K., Jancke, L., Mohlberg, H., Steinmetz, H., & Zilles, K. (2000) Interhemispheric asymmetry of the human motor cortex related to handedness and gender. *Neuropsychologia*, 38, 304-312.

Camposano, S., & Lolas, F. (1992) Effects of stimulation intensity, gender and handedness upon auditory evoked potentials. *Arquivos de Neuro-Psiquiatria*, 50, 43-49.

Dane, S., & Erzurumluoglu, A. (2003) Sex and handedness differences in eye-hand visual reaction times in handball players. *International Journal of Neuroscience*, 113, 923-929.

Good, C. D., Johnsrude, I., Ashburner, J., Henson, R. N., Friston, K. J., & Frackowiak, R. S. (2001) Cerebral asymmetry and the effects of sex and handedness on brain structure: a voxel-based morphometric analysis of 465 normal adult human brains. *NeuroImage*, 14, 685-700.

Gur, R. C., Turetsky, B. I., Matsui, M., Yan, M., Bilker, W., Hughett, P., & Gur, R. E. (1999) Sex differences in brain gray and white matter in healthy young adults: correlations with cognitive performance. *Journal of Neuroscience*, 19, 4065-4072.

Holloway, R., Anderson, P., Defendini, R., & Harper, C. (1993) Sexual dimorphism of the human corpus callosum from three independent samples: relative size of the corpus callosum. *American Journal of Physiology and Anthropology*, 92, 481-498.

Johnson, B. W., McKenzie, K. J., & Hamm, J. P. (2002) Cerebral asymmetry for mental rotation: effects of response hand, handedness and gender. *NeuroReport*, 13, 1929-1932.

Jordan, K., Wustenberg, T., Heinze, H., Peters, M., & Jancke, L. (2002) Women and men exhibit different cortical activation patterns during mental rotation tasks. *Neuropsychologia*, 40, 2397-2408.

Kimura, D. (1992) Sex differences in the brain. *Scientific American*, 267, 118-125.

Klinteberg, B., Levander, S., & Schalling, D. (1987) Cognitive sex differences: speed and problem-solving strategies on computerized neuropsychological tasks. *Perceptual and Motor Skills*, 65, 683-697.

Medland, S., Geffen, G., & McFarland, K. (2002) Lateralization of speech production using verbal/manual dual tasks: meta-analysis of sex differences and practice effects. *Neuropsychologia*, 40, 1233-1239.

Mikhelashvili-Browner, N., Yousem, D. M., Wu, C., Kraut, M. A., Vaughan, C. L., Oguz, K. K., & Calhoun, V. D. (2003) Lack of sex effect on brain activity during a visuomotor response task: functional MR imaging study. *American Journal of Neuroradiology*, 24, 488-494.

Misra, N., Mahajan, K., & Maini, B. (1985) Comparative study of visual and auditory reaction time of hands and feet in males and females. *Indian Journal of Physiology and Pharmacology*, 29, 213-218.

Molodtsova, G. F. (1999) [Sexual and interhemispheric differences in the involvement of serotonin from the hippocampus and amygdaloid body in the processing of new and repeatedly presented information in rats]. *Zhurnal Vysshei Nervnoi Deiatelnosti Imeni I.P. Pavlova*, 49, 408-415.

Nicholson, K. G., & Kimura, D. (1996) Sex differences for speech and manual skill. *Perceptual and Motor Skills*, 82, 3-13.

Pujol, J., Lopez-Sala, A., Deus, J., Cardoner, N., Sebastian-Galles, N., Conesa, G., & Capdevila, A. (2002) The lateral asymmetry of the human brain studied by volumetric magnetic resonance imaging. *NeuroImage*, 17, 670-679.

Rossell, S. L., Bullmore, E. T., Williams, S. C., & David, A. S. (2002) Sex differences in functional brain activation during a lexical visual field task. *Brain and Language*, 80, 97-105.

Sakurai, T., & Sugimura, T. (1990) [Holistic and analytic modes in classification learning of young children]. *Shinrigaku Kenkyu [The Japanese Journal of Psychology]*, 61, 219-226.

Sanders, A. F. (1971) *Psychologie der Informationsverarbeitung*. Bern: Verlag Hans Huber.

Vikingstad, E. M., George, K. P., Johnson, A. F., & Cao, Y. (2000) Cortical language lateralization in right handed normal subjects using functional magnetic resonance imaging. *Journal of Neurological Science*, 175, 17-27.

WADA, Y., NANBU, Y., KADOSHIMA, R., JIANG, Z., KOSHINO, Y., & HASHIMOTO, T. (1996) Interhemispheric EEG coherence during photic stimulation: sex differences in normal young adults. *International Journal of Psychophysiology*, 22, 45-51.

WARD, T. B. (1983) Response tempo and separable-integral responding: evidence for an integral-to-separable processing sequence in visual perception. *Journal of Experimental Psychology: Human Perception and Performance*, 9, 103-112.

WISNIEWSKI, A. B. (1998) Sexually-dimorphic patterns of cortical asymmetry, and the role for sex steroid hormones in determining cortical patterns of lateralization. *Psychoneuroendocrinology*, 23, 519-547.

YUCEL, M., STUART, G. W., MARUFF, P., VELAKOULIS, D., CROWE, S. F., SAVAGE, G., & PANTELIS, C. (2001) Hemispheric and gender-related differences in the gross morphology of the anterior cingulate/paracingulate cortex in normal volunteers: an MRI morphometric study. *Cerebral Cortex*, 11, 17-25.

Accepted February 4, 2004.

ASSOCIATION OF CULTURE WITH SHYNESS AMONG JAPANESE AND AMERICAN UNIVERSITY STUDENTS [1]

TOSHIYUKI SAKURAGI

Gustavus Adolphus College

Summary.—Previous cross-cultural studies of shyness have generally reported a higher level of shyness among adults in Japan than in the United States. This study examined two aspects of culture potentially related to different levels of shyness among the Americans and the Japanese: complementary relationship orientation, a tendency to maximize the status difference during communication, and family interdependence, a dependent tendency between a child and a parent. The survey included the 13-item version of Cheek's Shyness Scale and Sakuragi's Complementary Relationship Orientation Scale, and the Family Interdependence Scale. Analysis of responses by 166 American university students (76 men, 90 women) and 187 Japanese (81 men, 106 women) indicated that complementary relationship orientation was significantly related to shyness for both the Americans and the Japanese. No significant relationship, however, was found between scores on family interdependence and shyness.

Despite the growing number of studies of shyness, cross-cultural (cross-national) studies of shyness are still relatively rare. An early study was the Stanford Shyness Project (Zimbardo, 1977), with one of the most remarkable results of the survey being the prevalence of shyness in Japan: 60% of the Japanese (ages 18–21 years) reported being currently shy, while 42% of the Americans did so. Zimbardo (1977, p. 212) also noted that three-fourths of the Japanese sample viewed shyness as a "problem," over 90% reported having labeled themselves as shy in the past or currently, and more than any of the other nationalities studied, the Japanese reported feeling shy in virtually all social situations.

Communication apprehension is a cognate construct of shyness, and its self-report measures—the Personal Report of Communication Apprehension for College Students (McCroskey, 1978) and its variations—have also led to a handful of studies directly comparing Americans and Japanese students. The studies by Klopf and Cambra (1979) and McCroskey, Gudykunst, and Nishida (1985) indicated that Japanese had higher scores on communication apprehension than Americans. Keaten, Kelly, and Pribyl (1997) assessed communication apprehension among Japanese elementary and secondary students and compared the results with normative scores on apprehension among a comparable population in the United States. Although the comparison indi-

---

[1]Address correspondence to Toshiyuki Sakuragi, Department of Modern Foreign Languages, Gustavus Adolphus College, 800 W. College Avenue, St. Peter, MN 56082-1498.

cated minimal differences between Japanese and American students in Grades K–12, Keaten, *et al.* (1997) noted a significant increase of communication apprehension among the 7th–9th grade Japanese students. These results point to the possibility that later-developing, self-conscious shyness as opposed to early developing, fearful shyness (Buss, 1980, 1986) may be largely accountable for the different scores on measures of shyness reported by Japanese and American adults.

Common to these cross-cultural studies of shyness and communication apprehension is their descriptive orientation; the primary purpose of these studies is simply to compare Japanese and Americans (and other cultural groups in some cases). A recent exception is the study by Jackson, Flaherty, and Kosuth (2000), who attempted an empirical examination of the relationship of individualism–collectivism, measured by the Individualism–Collectivism Scale (Hui, 1988), with shyness, measured by the Shyness Scale (Cheek & Buss, 1981), among Japanese female and American female students. However, the result was contrary to their expectation: they found a *negative* correlation between collectivism and shyness ($r = -.29$). A methodological issue that may have contributed to this unexpected result is their use of Hui's Individualism–Collectivism Scale (1988), which has produced inconsistent results in previous cross-cultural studies.[2] Furthermore, there has been a growing concern in recent years that a diffuse concept such as individualism–collectivism (cf. Hofstede, 1980) is a poor independent variable unless its links with behavior are specified in terms of mediating variables, and that in the absence of refined intervening variables, "what" in culture "causes" behavior is often not clear (Kagitcibasi, 1994).

This study, therefore, was an attempt to identify more specific aspects of culture that may explain the difference between Japanese and Americans in shyness.

Complementary Relationship Orientation

The concern about "Who am I supposed to be in this situation?" rather than "How can I be me in this situation?" has often been identified as a salient cognitive characteristic of shy persons in previous studies (see Cheek & Briggs, 1990, for a summary of such studies). Zimbardo (1977), who called Japan "the model of a shyness-generating society" (p. 213), identified the Japanese culture's emphasis on producing "proper" behavior for

---

[2]A group of instruments developed in a series of studies by Triandis and his colleagues (e.g., Hui, 1984; Triandis, Leung, Villareal, & Clark, 1985; Hui & Triandis, 1986; Triandis, Bontempo, Villareal, Asai, & Lucca, 1988) has produced results contrary to common expectations in several cross-cultural studies. For example, the American samples scored higher on collectivism than the samples from Hong Kong and People's Republic of China (Hui, 1988; Triandis, McCusker, & Hui, 1990).

one's social role and status as a potential cause of shyness. Miyake and Yamazaki (1995) also suggested "ranking-consciousness" as a possible antecedent to shyness among the Japanese.

To capture how much such role or status consciousness would characterize communication, the term "symmetrical or complementary relationship orientation" is used in the present study. According to Watzlawick, Bavelas, and Jackson (1967), an interpersonal relationship can be characterized either as symmetrical or as complementary. In a symmetrical relationship, the partners tend to mirror each other's behavior and reinforce equality, whereas in a complementary relationship one partner's behavior complements that of the other, reinforcing difference in status.

Although Watzlawick, et al. (1967) have postulated that symmetrical and complementary relationships are a universal aspect of human communication, both cultures and individuals are likely to vary in their emphasis on each type of interpersonal relationship. Therefore, symmetrical or complementary relationship orientation is defined as how much an individual or a cultural group tends to minimize or maximize the status difference during communication. At the cultural level, the United States and Japan appear to differ considerably in their orientation with symmetrical relationships more commonly observed in the United States than in Japan, while complementary relationships are more common in Japan than in the United States (Ishii, 1987).

As to the possible connection to shyness, individuals who are oriented toward complementary relationship tend to pay more attention to differences in status and attempt to adapt their communicative behavior to convey their recognition of the differences. The frequent use of honorific expressions in Japanese language is an example of such communicative adaptation. This adaptation is likely to be cognitively taxing to these individuals, and this burden, coupled with their fear of making mistakes, may contribute to shyness. Therefore, the following hypothesis was advanced for the present study: there is a positive correlation between complementary relationship orientation and shyness.

Family Interdependence

One of the difficulties with examining a relationship between individualism–collectivism and shyness is the variety of potential ingroups to consider. Hui's inventory (1988), for example, has a set of items focusing on "neighbor" as a kind of ingroup. Neighbors, however, are unlikely to be considered as an ingroup by urban residents in Japan or in the United States. To address this problem, the present study attempted to facilitate operationalization of individualism–collectivism by limiting the kind of ingroup for consideration to family—more specifically, to parent-child relationships. This cultural variable of "family interdependence" has the following three components: how much a person's self-concept is separate from his parent or child (*Self Identification with Child or Parent*), how much a person is willing to make emotional or economic sacrifices for his child or parent (*Self-sacrifice for Child or Parent*), and how much a person is inclined to foster independence or dependence of his child or parent (*Promotion of Independence or Dependence*).

Family, particularly parent-child relationships, was chosen as the target ingroup, for it is probably one of the most fundamental kinds of ingroup for most people. Cheek and Briggs (1990), for example, identified similar factors in the home environment, such as attachment, parental support, and sibling relationships, as promising targets for research on the development of the self-conscious type of shyness. Zimbardo (1977) apparently saw a link between a dependent tendency and shyness in Japanese culture, as he identified *amae* ("passive dependence") as an important concept for explaining shyness among the Japanese. According to Doi (1973), who proposed *amae* as a distinguishing characteristic of the Japanese, it is rooted in the young child's dependency on the mother. Miyake and Yamazaki (1995) also identified the incomplete mother-child separation, overprotective parents, and the resultant *amae* exhibited by the child as the common family characteristics of the cases of *taijin-kyoufu* (delusional social phobia) among the Japanese.

Empirical studies of the relationship between parenting styles and social withdrawal, however, have produced inconsistent results for American samples (see Mills & Rubin, 1993, for a review of these studies). It is also curious that Zimbardo (1977) considered "rugged individualism" and related traits to be possible sources of shyness among the Americans. Given the conflicting accounts of the relationship between familial factors and shyness, the following research question was advanced for the present study: what is the relationship between family interdependence and shyness?

Method

Participants

Altogether, 182 university students in the United States and 192 university students in Japan participated in the study. The participants in the United States were students enrolled in an introductory mass communication course, a course in comparative ethnic group relations, and a Japanese language course at a university in a midwestern state. The participants in Japan were 130 students enrolled in communications studies courses at a university in Chiba and 62 students enrolled in speech-communication courses and English language courses at a university in Kyushu. All the universities involved in this study are located in a city or suburban setting.

Among the participants in the United States, 14 individuals indicated that their native language was not English or that the United States was not the country that they had lived in for the longest period of their lives. These individuals were eliminated from the analysis, for the present study focused on American and Japanese cultural groups. Also, two cases whose responses were incomplete were eliminated from the American sample. From the Japanese sample, five cases were eliminated for incomplete responses. After the elimination of these cases, the American sample consisted of 166 individuals (76 men, 90 women, M age = 21.5 yr.), and the Japanese sample consisted of 187 individuals (81 men, 106 women, M age = 20.3 yr.).

Measures

Complementary Relationship Orientation.—The Complementary Relationship Orientation Scale (Sakuragi, 1994) has 10 items which tap the importance a person places on the difference in age or status and the person's tendency to adapt communicative behavior according to the difference. The participants responded to each item using a 5-point Likert-type scale with anchors of 1 = Not at all characteristic of me and 5 = Very much characteristic of me. The English and the Japanese versions of the Complementary Relationship Orientation Scale were constructed simultaneously; the ease of creating the English and Japanese versions was taken into consideration when the idea for each item was examined. This method circumvents the issue of decentering in cross-cultural research (e.g., Brislin, 1976). The English version of the scale is given in Appendix A (p. 812).

Family Interdependence.—The Family Interdependence Scale (Sakuragi, 1994) consists of 14 items in which various situations relating to a relationship between a parent and a child are presented. In each situation, a behavioral choice that reflects either a dependent or independent orientation is presented, and the participants are asked to respond to the behavioral choice using a 5-point Likert-type scale with anchors of 1 = Strongly disagree and 5 = Strongly agree. The English and the Japanese versions of the Family Interdependence Scale were constructed simultaneously. The English version of the scale is given in Appendix B (p. 813).

Shyness.—Shyness was measured by the 13-item version of the Shyness Scale (Cheek, 1983, as reported by Robinson, Shaver, & Wrightsman, 1991), which was created by adding four negatively phrased items to the original 9-item Shyness Scale (Cheek & Buss, 1981). This scale was chosen for the present study primarily because of its appropriateness for the Japanese sample and relative ease of translation into Japanese. Some evidence for the reliability and validity of the Shyness Scale for the Japanese population was provided by Aikawa (1991). The Shyness Scale was translated into Japanese for the Japanese sample by this author, and the translation was then checked by another bilingual.

Analyses

The analyses explored group comparisons and correlational analyses. To compare the American and Japanese samples on Shyness, Complementary Relationship Orientation, and Family Interdependence, t tests were conducted. Pearson correlation coefficients were computed to test the hypothesis and to examine their interrelations. When one or both cultural variables correlated significantly with Shyness, analysis of covariance was conducted to examine the extent of the group difference accounted for by the cultural variable(s).

Results

Cronbach alpha for the Complementary Relationship Orientation Scale was .77 for the American and .79 for the Japanese sample; for the Family Interdependence Scale, .73 for the American and .66 for the Japanese sample; and for the Shyness Scale .78 for the American and .86 for the Japanese sample.

Comparison of the Americans and the Japanese on the three measures produced results consistent with those of previous studies: the Japanese scored significantly higher on Complementary Relationship Orientation ($t = 8.85$, $p < .001$), Family Interdependence ($t = 11.57$, $p < .001$), and Shyness ($t = 4.34$, $p < .001$) than the Americans. These results represent evidence for the validity of the measures used for the present study. The means and standard deviations are summarized in Table 1.

TABLE 1
MEANS AND STANDARD DEVIATIONS ON MEASURES FOR TWO CULTURAL GROUPS

Measure	Americans M	Americans SD	Japanese M	Japanese SD
Family Interdependence	35.37	6.86	43.52	6.31
Complementary Relationship Orientation	30.06	6.15	35.77	5.93
Shyness	32.38	9.63	36.71	8.98

To examine the relations of cultural variables with scores for Shyness, Pearson correlation coefficients were computed. As predicted, Complementary Relationship Orientation was significantly positively related to Shyness for both the Americans ($r = .25$, $p < .005$) and the Japanese ($r = .20$, $p < .005$). No significant correlation, however, was found between Family Interdependence and Shyness for either of the national groups. These results are summarized in Table 2.

Since a significant correlation was found between Complementary Relationship Orientation and Shyness, analysis of covariance was conducted to examine the extent to which Complementary Relationship Orientation could

TABLE 2
Intercorrelations Between Scales For American and Japanese Groups

Scale	Complementary Relationship Orientation	Shyness
Americans ($n = 166$)		
Family Interdependence	.24*	.02
Complementary Relationship Orientation		.25*
Japanese ($n = 187$)		
Family Interdependence	.06	−.03
Complementary Relationship Orientation		.20*

*$p < .005$.

account for the difference in shyness scores between the American and the Japanese samples. The analysis of covariance model on nationality differences in Shyness with Complementary Relationship Orientation as a covariate was fitted to the data. This model was then compared with the base model without the covariate. The comparison indicated the introduction of

TABLE 3
Analysis of Covariance For Model 1: Model of Shyness by Nationality With Complementary Relationship Orientation (COMP) as Covariate and Model 2: Base Model Without Covariate

Source	Type III SS	df	MS	F
Model 1				
Corrected Model	3177.972[a]	2	1588.986	19.30†
Intercept	6125.562	1	6125.562	74.40†
COMP	1532.519	1	1532.519	18.61†
Nationality	395.528	1	396.528	4.82*
Error	28817.212	350	82.335	
Total	456477.000	353		
Corrected Total	31995.184	352		
$R^2 = .099$ (Adjusted $R^2 = .094$)[a]				
Model 2				
Corrected Model	1645.452[b]	1	1645.452	19.03†
Intercept	419846.472	1	419846.472	4855.60†
Nationality	1645.452	1	1645.452	19.03†
Error	30349.732	351	86.466	
Total	456477.000	353		
Corrected Total	31995.184	352		
$R^2 = .051$ (Adjusted $R^2 = .049$)[b]				

*$p < .05$. †$p < .001$.

Complementary Relationship Orientation as a covariate resulted in a 76% reduction of the effect of nationality (from the sum of squares of 1645.45 to 396.52). The results for these models are shown in Table 3.

Discussion

This study was done to identify some aspects of culture associated with shyness among university students in the United States and Japan. Analyses indicated that complementary relationship orientation is a useful variable for explaining the "cultural difference" in shyness between these American and Japanese students.

The present study did not advance our understanding of the relationship between family environment and shyness, as no significant correlation was found between scores on Family Interdependence and Shyness either for the Americans or for the Japanese. In addition to addressing the shortcomings of the measure used in the present study, e.g., the relatively low internal consistency of the Family Interdependence Scale, researchers may explore alternative theoretical models for the relationship between family environment factors and shyness. It may be useful, for example, to utilize a curvilinear model such as the one postulated in the circumplex model of family systems (Olson, 1979; Olson, McCubbin, Barnes, Larsen, Muxen, & Wilson, 1989).

REFERENCES

AIKAWA, A. (1991) A study of the reliability and validity of a scale to measure shyness as a trait. *Japanese Journal of Psychology*, 62, 149-155.

BRISLIN, R. W. (1976) Comparative research methodology: cross-cultural research. *International Journal of Psychology*, 11, 215-229.

BUSS, A. H. (1980) *Self-consciousness and social anxiety.* San Francisco, CA: Freeman.

BUSS, A. H. (1986) A theory of shyness. In W. H. Jones, J. M. Cheek, & S. R. Briggs (Eds.), *Shyness: perspectives on research and treatment.* New York: Plenum. Pp. 39-46.

CHEEK, J. M. (1983) The Revised Cheek and Buss Shyness scale. Unpublished manuscript, Wellesley College, Wellesley, MA.

CHEEK, J. M., & BRIGGS, S. R. (1990) Shyness as a personality trait. In W. R. Crozier (Ed.), *Shyness and embarrassment: perspectives from social psychology.* Cambridge, UK: Cambridge Univer. Press. Pp. 315-338.

CHEEK, J. M., & BUSS, A. H. (1981) Shyness and sociability. *Journal of Personality and Social Psychology*, 41, 330-339.

DOI, T. (1973) *The anatomy of dependence.* Tokyo: Kodansha International.

HOFSTEDE, G. (1980) *Culture's consequences: international differences in work-related values.* (Abridged ed.) Newbury Park, CA: Sage.

HUI, C. H. (1984) Individualism–collectivism: theory, measurement, and its relation to reward allocation. (Doctoral dissertation, Univer. of Illinois at Urbana-Champaign) *Dissertation Abstracts International*, 45, 3656.

HUI, C. H. (1988) Measurement of individualism–collectivism. *Journal of Research in Personality*, 22, 17-36.

HUI, C. H., & TRIANDIS, H. C. (1986) Individualism–collectivism: a study of cross-cultural researchers. *Journal of Cross-Cultural Psychology*, 17, 225-248.

ISHII, S. (1987) Taijin kankei to ibunka komyunikeesyon [Interpersonal relations and intercultural communication]. In G. Furuta (Ed.), *Ibunka komyunikeesyon [Intercultural communication].* Tokyo: Yuhikaku. Pp. 121-140.

JACKSON, T., FLAHERTY, S. R., & KOSUTH, R. (2000) Culture and self-presentation as predictors of shyness among Japanese and American female college students. *Perceptual and Motor Skills*, 90, 475-482.

KAGITCIBASI, C. (1994) Individualism–collectivism: theory, method, and applications. In U.

Kim, H. C. Triandis, C. Kagitcibasi, S. Choi, & G. Yoon (Eds.), *Individualism and collectivism: theory, method, and applications*. Thousand Oaks, CA: Sage. Pp. 52-65.

KEATEN, J., KELLY, L., & PRIBYL, C. B. (1997) Communication apprehension in Japan: grade school through secondary school. *International Journal of Intercultural Relations*, 21, 319-343.

KLOPF, D. W., & CAMBRA, R. E. (1979) Communication apprehension among college students in America, Australia, Japan, and Korea. *Journal of Psychology*, 102, 27-31.

MCCROSKEY, J. C. (1978) Measures of communication bound anxiety. *Speech Monographs*, 45, 192-203.

MCCROSKEY, J. C., GUDYKUNST, W. B., & NISHIDA, T. (1985) Communication apprehension among Japanese students in native and second language. *Communication Research Reports*, 2, 11-15.

MILLS, R. S., & RUBIN, K. H. (1993) Socialization factors in the development of social withdrawal. In K. H. Rubin & J. B. Assendorpf (Eds.), *Social withdrawal, inhibition, and shyness in childhood*. Hillsdale, NJ: Erlbaum. Pp. 117-148.

MIYAKE, K., & YAMAZAKI, K. (1995) Self-conscious emotions, child rearing, and child psychopathology in Japanese culture. In J. P. Tangney & K. W. Fischer (Eds.), *Self-conscious emotions: the psychology of shame, guilt, embarrassment, and pride*. New York: Guilford. Pp. 488-504.

OLSON, D. H. (1979) Circumplex model of marital and family systems: 1. Cohesion and adaptability dimensions, family types, and clinical applications. *Family Process*, 18, 3-28.

OLSON, D. H., MCCUBBIN, H. I., BARNES, H. L., LARSEN, A. S., MUXEN, M. J., & WILSON, M. A. (1989) *Families: what makes them work*. (Updated ed.) Newbury Park, CA: Sage.

ROBINSON, J. P., SHAVER, P. R., & WRIGHTSMAN, L. S. (Eds.) (1991) *Measures of personality and social psychological attitudes*. San Diego, CA: Academic Press.

SAKURAGI, T. (1994) Family independence/dependence and symmetrical/complementary relationship orientation as cultural values: their measurement and relation to communicative predispositions. (Doctoral dissertation, Univer. of Minnesota) *Dissertation Abstracts International*, 55, 3352.

TRIANDIS, H. C., BONTEMPO, R., VILLAREAL, M. J., ASAI, M., & LUCCA, N. (1988) Individualism and collectivism: cross-cultural perspectives. *Journal of Personality and Social Psychology*, 54, 323-338.

TRIANDIS, H. C., LEUNG, K., VILLAREAL, M., & CLARK, F. (1985) Allocentric vs ideocentric tendencies: convergent and discriminant validation. *Journal of Research in Personality*, 19, 395-415.

TRIANDIS, H. C., MCCUSKER, C., & HUI, C. H. (1990) Multimethod probes of individualism and collectivism. *Journal of Personality and Social Psychology*, 59, 1006-1020.

WATZLAWICK, P., BAVELAS, J. B., & JACKSON, D. D. (1967) *Pragmatics of human communication: a study of interactional patterns, pathologies, and paradoxes*. New York: Norton.

ZIMBARDO, P. G. (1977) *Shyness: what it is, what to do about it*. Reading, MA: Addison-Wesley.

Accepted February 24, 2004.

APPENDIX A

Complementary Relationship Orientation Scale (Sakuragi, 1994)

Please read each item carefully and decide to what extent it is characteristic of your feelings and behavior. Fill in the blank to the left of each item by choosing one of the following numbers.

1 = Not at all characteristic of me
2 = Not very characteristic of me
3 = Slightly characteristic of me
4 = Fairly characteristic of me
5 = Very much characteristic of me

_____ 1. When interacting with someone older than myself, I watch my language and behavior.
_____ 2. When I interact with individuals of higher status (e.g., my teachers), I watch my language and behavior.
_____ 3. When I meet someone for the first time, I want to know if he or she is older than I so that I can talk in a proper manner.
_____ 4. I talk and behave differently when I interact with individuals of higher status (e.g., my teachers) than when I interact with individuals of equal status (e.g., my classmates).
_____ 5. I believe that it is wrong to treat my teacher as if he or she is my friend.
_____ 6. The fact that someone is older than I does not affect the way I talk to him or her. (R)
_____ 7. The fact that someone is of higher status than I (e.g., my teacher) does not affect the way I talk to him or her. (R)
_____ 8. It is easier for me to talk with someone if I know whether or not he or she is older than I am.
_____ 9. I find it strange to refer to my former teacher as "my friend," even if I have known him or her for a long time.
_____ 10. If I find out that a person is older than I while talking to him or her, I change my behavior and language to be more polite.

Note.—(R) indicates item is reverse scored.

APPENDIX B

Family Interdependence Scale (Sakuragi, 1994)

Listed below are a number of statements to which I would like your reactions. Please fill in the blank to the left of each item by choosing one number from the scale printed below.

1 = Strongly disagree
2 = Disagree
3 = Neutral
4 = Agree
5 = Strongly agree

_____ 1. It is selfish for a couple with a young child(ren) to get a divorce.
_____ 2. Parents are not responsible for their children's debts. (R)
_____ 3. It is wrong for parents to sell their belongings to their children.
_____ 4. One has the responsibility to live with his or her elderly parent.
_____ 5. Adult children should send a part of their salary to their parents even if they don't live with their parents.
_____ 6. Parents are responsible for acts of juvenile delinquency committed by their children.
_____ 7. A couple who are not satisfied with their marriage should get a divorce even if they have a young child(ren). (R)
_____ 8. If a young person hits someone with his or her car and causes an injury, his or her parents should apologize to the victim.
_____ 9. It is wrong for parents to have their children write an I.O.U. when they lend money to their children.
_____ 10. When parents buy a new car, they should just give their old car, rather than sell it, to their children, if their children want it.
_____ 11. A couple with a small child should not go out for a movie by themselves leaving their child in someone else's care.
_____ 12. Parents should not be blamed when their children commit a crime. (R)
_____ 13. A person has an obligation to take care of his or her elderly parent.
_____ 14. A couple who want to get a divorce should wait until their child(ren) grow up.

Note.—(R) indicates item is reverse scored.

FINNO-UGRIANS, BLOOD TYPES, AND SUICIDE: COMMENT ON VORACEK, FISHER, AND MARUSIC[1]

DAVID LESTER

Center for the Study of Suicide

AND

SERGEI V. KONDRICHIN

Minsk, Belarus

Summary.—In a sample of 20 European nations, the distribution of blood types provided a better explanation for the association of longitude with suicide rates than did the percentage of Finno-Ugrian ethnic group.

Voracek, Fisher, and Marusic (2003) reported that European suicide rates vary with latitude and longitude and that this may reflect a spatial variation in the Finno-Ugrian population primarily composed of Finns and Hungarians; however, they did not include the Finno-Ugrian percentage as a variable in their study. This Comment notes that there are many other variables which correlate with suicide rates and may be mediating the association between suicide rates and latitude/longitude. For example, Lester (1987) found that the suicide rate in European nations was associated with the proportion of people with Type O blood in the nations.

The pattern of associations of blood type, suicide rate, latitude, and longitude parallel those for percentage of Finno-Ugrians, suicide, latitude, and longitude. In a sample of 20 European nations with blood-type distributions available from Mourant, Kopec, and Domaniewska-Sobczak (1976), the 1970 suicide rate was associated with the percentage of Finno-Ugrians and the percentage with Type O blood (Pearson $r = .55$ and $-.62$, respectively, one-tailed $p < .01$). Latitude was not associated with the percentage of Finno-Ugrians or Type O people ($r = .22$ and $.02$, respectively); however, longitude was associated with the percentage of Type O people ($r = -.73$, $p < .001$) but not with the percentage of Finno-Ugrians ($r = .37$).

Thus, the distribution of blood types may provide a better explanation of the variation of suicide rates with longitude than the percentage of the Finno-Ugrian ethnic group in these nations. There may, of course, be many other possible mediating variables.

REFERENCES

LESTER, D. (1987) National distribution of blood groups, personal violence (suicide and homicide), and national character. *Personality and Individual Differences*, 8, 575-576.

MOURANT, A. E., KOPEC, A. C., & DOMANIEWSKA-SOBCZAK, K. (1976) *The distribution of human blood groups and other polymorphisms.* New York: Oxford Univer. Press.

VORACEK, M., FISHER, M. L., & MARUSIC, A. (2003) The Finno-Ugrian suicide hypothesis. *Perceptual and Motor Skills*, 97, 401-406.

Accepted March 5, 2004.

---

[1]Address enquiries to David Lester, Ph.D., Center for the Study of Suicide, RR41, 5 Stonegate Court, Blackwood, NJ 08012-5356 or e-mail (lesterd@stockton.edu).

HANDEDNESS AND WRITING PERFORMANCE[1]

F. VLACHOS AND F. BONOTI

University of Thessaly

Summary.—The present study investigated possible differences in left- and right-handers' writing performance. An equal number of left- and right-handed Greek children ($N = 182$) ages 7 to 12 years were examined using the Greek adaptation of Luria-Nebraska's neuropsychological battery in spontaneous writing, copying, and writing to dictation. Analysis showed a significant effect of age in writing performance and writing speed, while handedness was not significantly related to writing performance or writing speed. However, the incidence of right-handers was slightly higher among proficient writers, whereas the left-handers were clearly overrepresented among poor writers. The results are discussed on the grounds of neuropathological as well as hormonal-developmental theories of handedness.

The handedness of a human being is assumed to be the expression of an inborn, innate lateralization of the cerebral hemispheres where one side dominates. In the neural system the tracts are "crossed." Thus, a dominant right cerebral hemisphere results in a dominant left hand, and a dominance of the left cerebral hemisphere is responsible for right-handedness.

Since there are asymmetric neural subsystems involved in the organization of movement (Kimura, 1982; Previc, 1991; Katanoda, Yoshikawa, & Sugishita, 2001), it is possible that the population of children, who are often described as dysgraphic, dyspraxic, clumsy, or poorly coordinated, may have different laterality profiles that reflect a disturbance of these complex neuromotor subsystems (see Armitage & Larkin, 1993). For example, it has been repeatedly found that in right-handers a loss of the ability to write with either hand (agraphia) is associated with left-hemispheric lesions (see Roeltgen, 1985, for a review). This relationship between agraphia and left-hemispheric lesions suggests that the left hemisphere plays a critical role in the control of writing.

Also, some research indicates an increased incidence of nonright-handedness among children with neurodevelopmental disorders or learning disabilities (for a review see Flannery & Liederman, 1995; Previc, 1996). More specifically, writing difficulties are the most frequently mentioned problems in children with Developmental Coordination Disorder (DSM-IV; American Psychiatric Association, 1994) or clumsiness (Schoemaker, 1992), while Wa-

---

[1]Please direct requests for reprints to Dr. F. Vlachos, Department of Special Education, University of Thessaly, Argonafton & Filellinon str., Volos 38 221, Greece or e-mail (fvlachos@uth.gr).

ber and Bernstein (1994) found that dysgraphia—the failure of normal development of writing skills—is a common complaint among learning-disabled children. The common feature of dysgraphic children is that even with the proper amount of instruction and practice, they do not make sufficient progress in the acquisition of the fine motor task of handwriting. In a comprehensive review of handwriting research, Graham and Weintraub (1996) pointed out that the writing of students who have learning disabilities or a handwriting problem is not as legible as that of students who are good handwriters. Poor handwriting is identified by problems in the spacing alignment and relative size of letters. These problems are typically motor in nature and are not related to poor spelling or other psycholinguistic problems (Hamstra-Bletz & Blöte, 1993; Smits-Engelsman & Van Galen, 1997).

A review of the literature indicates that the empirical data which examine the relation between handedness and handwriting is contradictory. Some researchers argue that right- and left-handers do not differ in writing speed and in qualitative characteristics of writing (Simner, 1984; Ziviani, 1984; Ziviani & Elkins, 1986; Tarnopol & de Feldman, 1987; Mergl, Tiggers, Schroter, Moller, & Hegerl, 1999). However, Graham and Miller (1980) support that right-handers write faster than left-handers, while Suen (1983) found that the right-handers' letters are more readable than those of left-handers. According to Graham, Berninger, Weintraub, and Schafer's conclusions (1998), although the handwriting of right-handers is as readable as that of left-handers, the efficiency of the two groups is different, with right-handers writing faster than left-handers. The authors report that this might be attributed to a different way of writing between the two groups or to teachers' possible disregard of the needs of left-handed students (Graham, et al., 1998). However, Meulenbroek and Van Galen (1989) suggested that handedness does not seem to have a significant influence on the efficiency of writing in terms of speed and fluency. They studied spatial and dynamic characteristics of handwriting, and only small spatial variations in letter slant and size were observed in left-handers, apparently explained as ergonomic adaptations to the specific position of the hand.

The present study was conducted for three reasons. First, the above mentioned studies provide inconclusive results concerning the relationship of handedness and writing performance. Second, previous research has also shown that right- and left-handers differ in directionality when drawing horizontal lines, i.e., right-handers draw the horizontal lines moving from left to right while left-handers from right to left (Scheirs, 1990; Glenn, Bradshaw, & Sharp, 1995), a process that might affect writing performance. Third, there is no relevant empirical data concerning left- and right-handed Greek children's writing performance. This should be of interest due to the differentiated Greek and Latin writing symbols, allowing additional assessment of the source of the differences in writing between left- and right-handed children.

Various theories have been put forward to explain the emergence of lateral dominance, which commonly refers to the ability to use one side of the body more efficiently than the other, and its implications in cognitive development and learning (Annett, 1985; Satz, Orsini, Saslow, & Henry, 1985; Geschwind & Galaburda, 1987). Although these theoretical approaches differ from each other, they allow a number of hypotheses to be formulated. The aim of the present study is to test several hypotheses concentrating on aspects of handwriting of left- and right-handed children. More specifically, our attempt was to interpret possible differences in writing performance between left- and right-handers based on the modest version of the neuropathological left-handedness theory (Satz, *et al.*, 1985; Bishop, 1990; Coren & Halpern, 1991), as well as on the hormonal-developmental theory (Geschwind & Galaburda, 1987).

According to the theoretical account of pathological left-handedness, a subgroup of left-handers suffer from a condition that involves an early injury to the left hemisphere of the brain and atypical hemispheric speech representation. Thus, nonclinical left-handers include a proportion of potentially pathological people, who might present impaired performance on various cognitive tasks as presumably the pathology stems from the left hemispheric damage (Satz, *et al.*, 1985; Bishop, 1990; Coren & Halpern, 1991). On the other hand, the hormonal-developmental theory postulates that there is a fundamental link between abnormal development of the left hemisphere, reduced dextrality, various learning disorders, immune disorders, and other medical conditions, which is forged by the prenatal influence of fetal testosterone in the developing nervous system (Geschwind & Galaburda, 1987).

The hypotheses stated for the present study were based on the two aforementioned models. More specifically, the statement that the left-handers' group includes more pathological cases (as the neuropathological theory assumes, Satz, *et al.*, 1985) led us to predict that their average writing performance would be poorer than that of right-handers (Hypothesis 1). Additionally, the delayed development of the left hemisphere in left-handers, as proposed by Geschwind and Galaburda (1987), leads to the hypotheses that there is a different pattern of performance across age groups for left- vs right-handers (Hypothesis 2); and there would be a preponderance of left-handed children among the poor writers (Hypothesis 3), that is, among children who perform more than two standard deviations below the mean of their age (O'Hare & Brown, 1989).

Method

Participants

An equal number of left-handed and right-handed children aged 7 to

12 years (*N*=182; 91 left-handed, 91 right-handed) participated in this study. The participants were selected from the school population of Volos, Greece, with permission of the Greek Ministry of Education. All of these children were in regular school placement and did not have a history of major medical illness, psychiatric illness, developmental disorder, or significant visual or auditory impairments, according to the medical reports of their schools.

The 182 participants were pairs matched by age, sex, and hand preference. The first age group was comprised of 70 children attending the second grade of primary school (the average age was 7.7 yr.), the second age group was comprised of 64 children attending fourth grade (average age 9.6 yr.), and the third age group was composed of 48 children attending sixth grade (average age 11.6 yr.). Girls constituted 42.9% (*n*=78) of the sample and boys 57.1% (*n*=104). The imbalance between sexes reflected the larger percentage of boys among left-handers and the procedure we used during sample collection (see details below). The 91 left-handed children were selected from a pool of about 1,200 primary school students.

Materials and Procedure

The children were tested for hand preference before moving on to the main test procedure. Handedness was defined according to the items of the Edinburgh Handedness Inventory (Oldfield, 1971) which has been previously used in other studies (Vlachos & Karapetsas, 1996). Also, the Science Citation Index indicates that it has been the most widely used inventory in the literature. The questionnaire is comprised of 10 items pertaining to hand preference in writing, drawing, throwing a ball, use of scissors, toothbrush, knife (without fork), spoon, broom (upper hand), striking a match, and opening a box. The right-handed children were randomly selected from the same classes (as the student following each left-hander according to the alphabetic order of the class register) and were tested for hand preferences using the same 10 criteria before the main test procedure. Examiners asked the children with which hand they performed each of the tasks of the questionnaire and wrote down the answer. Pupils who showed right- (or left-) hand preference for all the items were considered right-handed (or left-handed).

The writing skills of the students were examined individually with the writing scale of the Greek adaptation of Luria-Nebraska's neuropsychological battery (Golden, 1981). More specifically, students were examined using three writing tasks. During spontaneous writing the students were asked to write their full names as well as that of their mother. The students were also asked to copy small and capital letters, phonemes, words, and sentences from a placard. Then they were asked to write to dictation single letters, words, and sentences. Finally, in another task the speed of handwriting was measured by asking the children to write the word "excursion" (in Greek) as often as possible within a time space of 20 sec.

Scoring

Children's productions were evaluated on the three writing tasks depending on the placement of letters (if they leaned in the horizontal line of the examination sheet or if they were found above or under this line), their form (if it corresponded to the classic form of the letter or if there was confusion between small and capital letters) and their composition (if their size and their place in the word was correct). Based on the above criteria, three individual marks for each writing task were calculated, while their sum gave the total score for the writing. The scores differed depending on the student's age and ranged from 0 (no error) to 4 for each of the individual writing tasks and from 0 to 12 for the total score.

Writing speed was calculated as a decimal number, with the whole number (digit) indicating the complete words and the decimals the proportion of the number of letters in the incomplete word "excursion."

Children's scripts were scored independently by two judges, using the scoring criteria mentioned above. Agreement between the two raters was 91% for spontaneous writing, 95% for copying, and 93% for writing to dictation.

RESULTS

Table 1 presents the mean writing performance scores and standard deviations for the three age groups. The mean scores were 2.05 for the right-handed children and 2.76 for the left-handed children. Standard deviations ranged from 2.41 to 3.24, respectively.

TABLE 1
WRITING PERFORMANCE SCORES BY AGE AND HANDEDNESS GROUP

Group	Age Range (yr.)	n	Right-handed ($n=91$) M	SD	Left-handed ($n=91$) M	SD	Total ($N=182$) M	SD
Second Grade	7–8	70	2.43	2.32	3.37	3.65	2.90	3.07
Fourth Grade	9–10	64	2.44	2.72	2.84	2.94	2.64	2.82
Sixth Grade	11–12	48	1.00	1.82	1.75	2.82	1.38	2.38
Total		182	2.05	2.41	2.76	3.24	2.41	2.87

Scores were evaluated by 3 × 2 (age × handedness) mixed effects model analysis of variance. Although the analysis of variance showed a statistically significant main effect for age ($F_{2,176}=35.81$, $p<.05$) indicating that writing performance improved with age, the effect size was small to modest as established by Cohen (1988). The partial η^2 was just .049, which means that the factor age by itself accounted for only 4.9% of the overall (effect + error) variance, but there was sufficient power (.765) to detect true differences. No significant effect for handedness ($F_{1,176} = 2.74$, $p = .10$, $\eta^2 = .015$, $power = .377$) nor any interaction effects were found.

Attempting to investigate the proportion of left-handers among students who had different writing performance, we divided our sample into three subgroups by writing performance scores. Since the mean children's performance on this writing test was 2.41, with a standard deviation of 2.87, the Proficient subgroup consisted of the children who performed over the mean (0 to 2.41). In the Intermediate subgroup were included children whose performance was up to two standard deviations above the mean (scores of 2.42 to 8.15), and in the Poor writers' subgroup were children with the worst performance in writing (scores of 8.16 to 12), that is, two standard deviations above the mean. This final subgroup was the lowest 5% of normal distribution and can be considered as a clinical population (O'Hare & Brown, 1989; Gubbay & de Klerk, 1995) which needs remedial work on its handwriting skills. Table 2 displays the frequencies and the handedness ratios in the three subgroups of proficient, intermediate, and poor writers.

TABLE 2
Distribution of Left- and Right-handers in Three Subgroups of Writers

Writing Performance	Left-handed f	%	Right-handed f	%	Total f	%	Handedness Ratio*
Proficient	55	30.2	62	34.1	117	64.3	0.89
Intermediate	28	15.4	28	15.4	56	30.8	1.00
Poor	8	4.4	1	0.5	9	4.9	8.00
Total	91	5.0.	91	50.0	182	100.0	100.00

*LH:RH.

The cross-tabulation of writing categories with handedness had a statistically significant relationship ($\chi^2 = 5.99$, $df = 2$, $p < .05$). As can be seen in Table 2, the incidence of right-handedness is slightly elevated among proficient writers. On the other hand, there is a clear overrepresentation of left-handers among poor writers. This finding was associated with a medium to large effect size (W = .36), indicating the extent to which the two handedness populations do not overlap. Results of the power analysis indicated there was sufficient power (> .80) to detect actual differences.

A 3 × 2 (age × handedness) analysis of variance computed on the writing speed measures yielded a statistically significant main effect of age ($F_{2,176} = 30.65$, $p < .001$) which means that older children were faster on the writing task than younger children (mean writing speed for the second grade group = 3.44, $SD = 1.51$; for the fourth grade group $M = 4.45$, $SD = 1.36$; and for the sixth grade group $M=5.59$, $SD=1.56$). This significant difference was associated with a large effect size and power ($\eta^2=.258$, $power=1.000$). The same analysis, however, did not indicate a main effect of handedness ($F_{1,176}=3.81$, $p=.062$, $\eta^2=.021$, $power=.493$) (M writing speed for the left-handers$=4.16$, $SD=1.61$; for the right-handers $M=4.58$, $SD=1.77$) or an interaction of age × handedness. Thus, we can conclude that writing speed differences were not significantly related to handedness.

Discussion

The present study investigated the relationship of handedness to Greek children's writing skills and evaluated right- and left-handers' writing performance with regard to the hypotheses based on neuropathological and hormonal-developmental theories of handedness. Specifically, based on the neuropathological theory (Satz, *et al.*, 1985; Bishop, 1990; Coren & Halpern, 1991), we predicted differences between right- and left-handed children in writing performance. The data in this study do not offer empirical support for this account. Although writing performance of right-handed children was better than that of their left-handed schoolmates (see Table 1), this difference did not reach statistical significance. Given the sample size, the size of the observed effect, and the small power, there was not enough chance of identifying a handedness effect as statistically significant. Therefore, a repetition of the study with a larger sample size may be worthwhile.

The second hypothesis of the present study arose from Geschwind and Galaburda's (1987) hormonal developmental theory. According to this hypothesis the prediction was that the delay of left hemisphere maturation in left-handed individuals assumed to be due to a higher level of testosterone may also be evident in writing ability in younger and older left-handed children. The results showed a statistically significant relation between age and writing performance regardless of hand preference, but no significant effect of handedness. However, our retrospective effect size and power analysis suggest that the difference in writing performance between handedness groups could be practically important. Although we found no statistically significant difference among right- and left-handers in mean writing performance, the results fell short of statistical significance ($p=.10$). This lack of statistical significance may be a result of the relatively small effect size and the relatively low power, so it is important to consider the possibility of a Type II error when interpreting the results. Careful observation of the mean scores (Table 1) shows that right-handed children performed better than their matched left-handed peers in every age group. This table also indicates that age-related improvement of writing performance seems to occur at a different rate in right- and left-handed children. Right-handers did not show differences in writing performance between the second and fourth graders but a remarkable improvement in performance among sixth graders. On the other hand, left-handers showed a more gradual improvement in their performance across the three age groups. These data may suggest that there is a delay of left hemisphere maturation in left-handers that extends beyond primary school age. Further longitudinal evidence is needed to assess this suggestion.

Our third hypothesis predicted an increased incidence of left-handers among poor writers, based on the hormonal-developmental theory which correlated abnormal left-hemisphere development with learning disorders and nonright-handedness. Indeed, we found an elevated proportion of left-handers among poor writers, defined as children who had an average writing performance two standard deviations or more away from the mean, and so could be considered as having severe difficulties in writing. Given that in Greece most of the students with moderate learning difficulties are in regular school placement, and previous research (Waber & Bernstein, 1994; Graham & Weintraub, 1996) has shown that most of these children experience handwriting problems, it is possible that some of them were included in our sample, especially in the poor writers' subgroup.

Overall, the results of this study indicate that there is no strong effect of handedness on handwriting skills (performance and speed) as measured. Handwriting skills undergo significant development during childhood which is not significantly related to handedness, at least in the general population. These findings support most previous studies which have not yielded differences between right- and left-handers in qualitative characteristics of writing as well as in writing speed (Simner, 1984; Ziviani, 1984; Ziviani & Elkins, 1986; Tarnopol & Feldman, 1987; Meulenbroek & Van Galen, 1989; Mergl, et al., 1999) and importantly, indicate that the effect of handedness on writing performance is not affected by the alphabet used, i.e., Greek vs Latin script.

Furthermore, although differences in directionality of movements have been repeatedly found between handedness groups during the drawing process (Scheirs, 1990; Glenn, et al., 1995), this does not seem to affect writing performance substantially. This is also supported by findings which suggest that handedness has no significant effect on kinematic handwriting parameters, such as mean writing pressure (Mergl, et al., 1999).

The results showed an increased incidence of left-handers among poor writers, as well as an overrepresentation of right-handers among the students with proficient performance. This finding supports researchers (Natsopoulos, Kiosseoglou, Xeromeritou, & Alevriadou, 1998) who suggested that left-handers consist of heterogeneous subgroups of subjects at either extreme of abilities with significantly more subjects performing worse and significantly fewer subjects performing better compared to right-handers. The above argument seems to reinforce theoretical claims (Satz, et al., 1985; Bishop,

1990) about the inclusion of a proportion of potentially pathological persons among nonclinical left-handers, even if they do not present overt neuromotor abnormalities. This might be the reason Gaillard and Satz (1989) suggested that the association between handedness and abilities depends on whether the cohort is selected from the general school population or from a clinic. In the first case null results are usually reported. In contrast, studies based on clinical samples have often reported a significant effect of handedness.

REFERENCES

AMERICAN PSYCHIATRIC ASSOCIATION. (1994) *Diagnostic and statistical manual of mental disorders.* (4th ed.) Washington, DC: Author.

ANNETT, M. (1985) *Left, right, hand and brain: the right shift theory.* Hillsdale, NJ: Erlbaum.

ARMITAGE, M., & LARKIN, D. (1993) Laterality, motor asymmetry and clumsiness in children. *Human Movement Science*, 12, 155-177.

BISHOP, D. (1990) *Handedness and developmental disorders.* Oxford, UK: Blackwell.

COHEN, J. (1988) *Statistical power analysis for the behavioral sciences.* (2nd ed.) Hillsdale, NJ: Erlbaum.

COREN, S., & HALPERN, D. F. (1991) Left-handedness: a marker for decreased survival fitness. *Psychological Bulletin*, 109, 90-106.

FLANNERY, K., & LIEDERMAN, J. (1995) Is there really a syndrome involving the concurrence of neurodevelopmental disorder, talent, non-right handedness and immune disorder among children. *Cortex*, 31, 503-515.

GAILLARD, F., & SATZ, P. (1989) Handedness and reading disability. *Archives of Clinical Neuropsychology*, 4, 63-69.

GESCHWIND, N., & GALABURDA, A. M. (1987) *Cerebral lateralization: biological mechanisms, associations, and pathology.* Cambridge, MA: MIT Press.

GLENN, S. M., BRADSHAW, K., & SHARP, M. (1995) Handedness and the development of direction and sequencing in children's drawings of people. *Educational Psychology*, 15, 11-21.

GOLDEN, C. J. (1981) *Diagnosis and rehabilitation in clinical neuropsychology.* Springfield, IL: Thomas.

GRAHAM, S., BERNINGER, V., WEINTRAUB, N., & SCHAFER, W. (1998) Development of handwriting speed and legibility in grades 1–9. *The Journal of Educational Research*, 92, 42-52.

GRAHAM, S., & MILLER, L. (1980) Handwriting research and practice: a unified approach. *Focus on Exceptional Children*, 13, 1-16.

GRAHAM, S., & WEINTRAUB, N. (1996) A review of handwriting research: progress and prospects from 1980 to 1994. *Educational Psychology Review*, 8, 7-87.

GUBBAY, S., & DE KLERK, N. (1995) A study and review of developmental dysgraphia in relation to acquired dysgraphia. *Brain and Development*, 17, 1-8.

HAMSTRA-BLETZ, L., & BLÖTE, A. (1993) A longitudinal study on dysgraphic handwriting in primary school. *Journal of Learning Disabilities*, 26, 689-699.

KATANODA, K., YOSHIKAWA, K., & SUGISHITA, M. (2001) A functional MRI study on the neural substrates for writing. *Human Brain Mapping*, 13, 34-42.

KIMURA, D. (1982) Left-hemisphere control of oral and brachial movements and their relation to communication. *Philosophical Translations of the Royal Society of London*, B298, 135-149.

MERGL, R., TIGGERS, P., SCHROTER, A., MOLLER, H. J., & HEGERL, U. (1999) Digitized analysis of handwriting and drawing movements in healthy subjects: methods, results and perspectives. *Journal of Neuroscience Methods*, 90, 157-169.

MEULENBROEK, R., & VAN GALEN, G. (1989) Variations in cursive handwriting performance as a function of handedness, hand posture and gender. *Journal of Human Movement Studies*, 16, 239-254.

NATSOPOULOS, D., KIOSSEOGLOU, G., XEROMERITOU, A., & ALEVRIADOU, A. (1998) Do the hands talk on mind's behalf? Differences in language ability between left- and right-handed children. *Brain and Language*, 64, 182-214.

O'HARE, A. E., & BROWN, J. K. (1989) Childhood dysgraphia: Part 2. A study of hand function. *Child Care Health Development*, 15(3), 151-166.
OLDFIELD, R. (1971) The assessment and analysis of handedness: the Edinburgh inventory. *Neuropsychologia*, 9, 97-113.
PREVIC, F. (1991) A general theory concerning the prenatal origins of cerebral lateralization in humans. *Psychological Review*, 98, 299-334.
PREVIC, F. (1996) Nonright-handedness, central nervous system and related pathology, and its lateralization: a reformulation and synthesis. *Developmental Neuropsychology*, 12, 443-515.
ROELTGEN, D. (1985) Agraphia. In K. Heilman & E. Valenstein (Eds.), *Clinical neuropsychology*. New York: Oxford Univer. Press. Pp. 63-89.
SATZ, P., ORSINI, D., SASLOW, E., & HENRY, R. (1985) The pathological left-handedness syndrome. *Brain and Cognition*, 4, 27-46.
SCHEIRS, J. (1990) Relationships between the direction of movements and handedness in children. *Neuropsychologia*, 28, 743-748.
SCHOEMAKER, M. M. (1992) Physiotherapy for clumsy children: an effect evaluation study. Unpublished Ph.D. dissertation, Univer. of Groningen, The Netherlands.
SIMNER, M. L. (1984) The grammar of action and reversal errors in children's printing. *Developmental Psychology*, 20, 136-142.
SMITS-ENGELSMAN, B., & VAN GALEN, G. (1997) Dysgraphia in children: lasting psychomotor deficiency or transient developmental delay. *Journal of Experimental Child Psychology*, 67, 164-184.
SUEN, C. Y. (1983) Handwriting generation, perception and recognition. *Acta Psychologica*, 54, 295-312.
Tarnopol, M., & de Feldman, N. (1987) Handwriting and school achievement: a cross-cultural study. In J. Alston & J. Taylor (Eds.), *Handwriting theory, research, and practice*. London: Croom Helm. Pp. 190-212.
VLACHOS, F., & KARAPETSAS, A. (1996) Visuomotor organization and memory in the right-handed and the left-handed child: a comparative neuropsychological approach. *Child Neuropsychology*, 2, 204-212.
WABER, D., & BERNSTEIN, J. (1994) Repetitive graphmotor output in learning-disabled and nonlearning-disabled children: the repeated test. *Developmental Neuropsychology*, 10(1), 51-65.
ZIVIANI, J. (1984) Some elaborations on handwriting speed in 7-14-year-olds. *Perceptual and Motor Skills*, 58, 535-539.
ZIVIANI, J., & ELKINS, J. (1986) Effects of pencil grip on handwriting speed and legibility. *Educational Review*, 38, 247-257.

Accepted February 25, 2004.

ELEVATED NOCICEPTIVE THRESHOLDS IN RATS WITH MULTIFOCAL BRAIN DAMAGE INDUCED WITH SINGLE SUBCUTANEOUS INJECTIONS OF LITHIUM AND PILOCARPINE[1]

M. A. GALIC

Laurentian University

Summary.—To quantify the variability in thermal pain perception of rats with chemically induced brain injury following subcutaneous lithium and pilocarpine administration, 9 female Wistar rats were subjected to a nociceptive (hotplate) paradigm. At approximately 200 days of age, subjects were injected subcutaneously with 3 mEq/kg of lithium chloride followed 4 hr. later by 30 mg/kg of the cholinergic agonist pilocarpine to generate lesions that mimic human temporal lobe (limbic) epilepsy. Over 2 trials 4 of 9 subjects exhibited thermal latencies that exceeded 60 sec. while the remaining subjects obtained mean latencies of 13.40 sec. before demonstrating the criterion nociceptive response. These findings suggest that the multifocal neuronal necrosis subsequent to single peripheral injections of lithium and pilocarpine, followed by the neuroleptic, acepromazine, may significantly augment pain thresholds in certain rats within experimentally epileptic populations.

Rats in which limbic epilepsy had been induced by a single systemic injection of lithium and pilocarpine, exhibit flinch (pain) thresholds to electric shock (in milliamps), substantially above that of normal rats (Fleming, Persinger, & Koren, 1994). This antinociceptive effect has been correlated histologically, with the amount of quantitative necrosis within the claustrum, anterior portion of the paraventricular nucleus of the thalamus, mediodorsal thalamus, and lateral amygdala (Persinger, Peredery, Bureau, & Cook, 1997), when animals were treated with acepromazine (25 mg/kg) following lithium and pilocarpine. However, within these experimentally epileptic populations, observations indicate marked variance in thermal responding whose source is speculated as involving differential patterns of neuronal reorganization following seizure induction. This study was done to identify the magnitude of the proportions of sensitivities to pain produced by a thermal device (hotplate) in a rodent model of epilepsy.

In the present study, 9 female Wistar rats approximately 200 days of age were injected subcutaneously with 3 mEq/kg of lithium chloride followed 4 hr. later by 30 mg/kg of pilocarpine to mimic the neuropatholophysiology found in human temporal lobe (limbic) epileptics. Following the first episode of forelimb clonus, rearing, and falling (overt seizure display), seizures were attenuated with 25 mg/kg of acepromazine. Each rat was re-

---

[1]The author thanks Dr. M. A. Persinger for comments on this manuscript. Please send correspondence to M. A. Galic, Behavioural Neuroscience Laboratory, Department of Biology, Laurentian University, Sudbury, ON, Canada P3E 2C6.

moved from its home cage 80 days later, transported to the experimental room, and placed on a hotplate (Omnitech) maintained at 55° ± 1°C to assess the latency to nociceptive (thermal) threshold. The criterion for terminating a trial was two licks of the rear foot pads in any combination. This was followed by immediate removal from the chamber and return to home cage. A stopwatch was used to measure thermal latencies and recorded to the nearest 0.01 sec. Any animal that remained on the hotplate for more than 60 sec., but without demonstrating the criterion behavior, was removed from the apparatus and assigned this value. This procedure was repeated 3 days later, and latency to the nociceptive behavior was again recorded. Food and water were available *ad libitum*. The light:dark cycle was 12:12 with light onset at 0800 hr. local time. Ambient temperature was controlled between 20° and 21°C.

For both hotplate trials, separate cluster analysis and one-way analysis of variance (with SPSS) were performed. The mean thermal latencies for four of the nine subjects was 60 sec. ($SD=0$) which differed significantly ($F = 201.7$, $p < .001$) from the five remaining subjects who had a mean latency of 13.40 sec. ($SD=6.4$). It is inferred that subjects with higher hotplate latencies have a lower perception of thermally induced pain. Additional one-way analysis of variance showed no statistically significant differences between trials ($p > .05$). There were also no significant differences for body weights of those animals which displayed the elevated response compared to others.

This experiment supported previous findings that rats receiving the lithium-pilocarpine and acepromazine combination frequently respond differentially to painful stimuli compared to controls (Fleming, *et al.*, 1994). These differences suggest that in spite of relatively predictable and consistent patterns of brain damage that ensue following systemic injections of lithium and pilocarpine and then the atypical neuroleptic acepromazine, as previously confirmed by Bureau, Peredery, and Persinger (1994), the subtle differences in neuronal loss/regeneration can produce conspicuously variable responses to pain stimuli.

Further investigation is required to explain the variability in responsiveness among clinically epileptic populations with seemingly "equivalent" diagnoses, yet markedly different experiences of pain or painful stimuli as reported by Ostrowsky, Magnin, Ryvlin, Isnard, Guenot, and Mauguiere (2002).

REFERENCES

BUREAU, Y. R. J., PEREDERY, O., & PERSINGER, M. A. (1994) Concordance of quantitative damage within the diencephalon following systemic pilocarpine (380 mg/kg) or lithium (3 mEq/kg) pilocarpine (30 mg/kg) induced seizures. *Brain Research*, 648, 265-269.

FLEMING, J. L., PERSINGER, M. A., & KOREN, S. A. (1994) Magnetic pulses elevate nociceptive thresholds: comparisons with opiate receptor compounds in normal and seizure-induced brain-damaged rats. *Electro- and Magnetobiology*, 13, 67-75.

OSTROWSKY, K., MAGNIN, M., RYVLIN, P., ISNARD, J., GUENOT, M., & MAUGUIERE, F. (2002) Representation of pain and somatic sensation in the human insula: a study of responses to direct electrical cortical stimulation. *Cerebral Cortex*, 12, 376-385.

PERSINGER, M. A., PEREDERY, O., BUREAU, Y. R. J., & COOK, L. L. (1997) Emergent properties following brain injury: the claustrum as a major component of a pathway that influences nociceptive thresholds to foot shock in rats. *Perceptual and Motor Skills*, 85, 387-398.

Accepted March 6, 2004.

DIAGNOSING ESTIMATE DISTORTION DUE TO SIGNIFICANCE TESTING IN LITERATURE ON DETECTION OF DECEPTION [1]

M. T. BRADLEY AND G. STOICA

University of New Brunswick, Saint John

Summary.—Studies journals typically report or feature results significant by statistical test criterion. This is a bias that prevents obtaining precise estimates of the magnitude of any underlying effect. It is severe with small effect sizes and small numbers of measurements. To illustrate the problem and a diagnosis technique, results of published studies on the detection of deception are graphed. The literature contains large effect sizes affirming that deceptive responses in contrast to truthful responses are associated with more reactive Skin Resistance Responses. These effect sizes when graphed on the x-axis against n on the y-axis are distributed as funnel graphs. A subset of studies show support for predicted small to medium effects on different physiological measures, individual differences, and condition manipulations. These effect sizes graphed by sample ns follow negative correlations, suggesting that effect sizes from published values of t, F, and z are exaggerations.

By now it is broadly understood that significance testing has caused problems for the progress of science in psychology. Sterling (1959) documented a strong tendency to publish articles reporting results that are statistically significant. Greenwald (1975) named this practice "publication bias" and noted some negative consequences such as significant findings persist uncorrected in the literature, measurement is reduced to the yes/no status of suggesting that findings exist or do not, and when magnitude estimates are of interest, there is a high probability that statistically significant findings are overestimates. This review treated the published literature in the Detection of Deception/Information area in a meta-analytic fashion but then graphically analysed the results to gauge the magnitude of the distortion of estimates resulting from statistical significance testing.

Estimates of distortion are important for any summary of information across studies but are particularly important in this time when meta-analytic approaches (Lipsey & Wilson, 2001) purport to give accurate numeric summaries of literatures. Bradley (2000) listed five conditions under which the published literature on a given phenomena will be distorted and consist of exaggerated estimates. These exaggerated estimates, often represented as an aggregate of differences between means calculated in some standard effect size form, will, if derived under the following conditions, be larger than the

---

[1]Address correspondence to M. T. Bradley, Department of Psychology, P.O. Box 5050, University of New Brunswick, Saint John, New Brunswick E2L 4L5, Canada.

pect of the area investigated, may fit into small, medium, and large effect-size categories, (3) the author is familiar with this literature. In theory, any area with reasonable to good experimental designs could be selected for the analyses modeled in this paper.

In this area, F, t, and r statistics are available to reflect differences amongst groups or on continua. We converted these statistics to *eta* as a standardized effect-size measure to reflect: (1) polygraph test score differences between guilty and innocent participants using Skin Resistance Responses (SRRs), (2) the same difference using other physiological measures, and (3) differences due to psychological factors. As mentioned, it is incidental to the purpose of this paper that the examples are from the area of the detection of deception, but it was surmised that the range of effect sizes and the issues covered provide exemplars for many areas of experimental psychology.

Since the examples are from the detection literature, it is necessary to sketch out a few general terms. In laboratory studies, participants are "guilty" and "informed" through the enactments of a "mock crime" or by having information and imagining they are guilty. They are examined on one of two types of tests. The Control Question Test (Reid & Inbau, 1977) directly addresses issues of whether or not participants are guilty of the crime: "Did you steal the diamond?" The Guilty Knowledge Test (Lykken, 1959) focuses on information only guilty suspects could know through exposure to or commission of the "mock crime": "The stolen jewel was a/an: emerald, sapphire, ruby, diamond?" Expectations and supportive literature suggest that skin-resistance response differences between guilty and innocent participants on either of these types of tests are large. Virtually all published laboratory studies report differences, and anecdotal information suggests that lie-detection demonstrations can be successfully conducted in such settings as the classroom. In sum, the effect is robust or large.

With physiological measures other than the skin resistance responses, such as respiration or heart rate, there is uncertainty as to the contribution of these measures in discriminating between guilty and innocent participants. The expectation is that differences with these measures are of medium size. Psychological variables, whether related to individual differences measures or blocking variables such as sex or induced cognitive state changes through conditions or through drugs, are generally thought to modify detection in a small way.

It was predicted that graphs generated on each of these three categories of results graphed with study ns on the y-axis and effect sizes calculated from tests of significance on the x-axis would differ in form from each other given their underlying true effect sizes. That is, published studies that find a significant difference with a small n when the true difference is small report an exaggeration. With large ns precise estimates are given even with significance criteria imposed. It was expected that if the true difference is small, then a strong negative correlation between ns and the effect sizes would be found. When the true value is of medium size, the correlation would be more in the medium negative range. The graph of estimates by n from studies of a true large effect size was predicted to form a funnel curve, with the results of small n studies being more variable and large n studies less variable. The correlation would approach zero. A zero correlation occurs with true effects that are large because it is unlikely that any studies, even those with small samples, will not reject the null hypothesis.

Method

The detection literature was sampled. Experimental studies from major reviews were included as well as a few available works postdating reviews. F, t, and r values associated with the magnitudes of mean differences between groups were converted to a standardized metric, eta. Bruning and Kintz (1987) have outlined the conversion of F to eta and since $t^2 = F$, t-test values were readily converted. Also, r is the absolute value of eta so dropping the sign converts r to eta. Five graphs with eta on the x-axis and sample size on the y-axis were plotted and presented: 30 Control Question Tests and 20 Guilty Knowledge Test effect sizes on skin resistance response findings; 13 cardiovascular and 12 respiration results combined over both types of tests; 64 effect sizes from both tests on factors related to psychological variables.

Results and Discussion

Figs. 1 and 2 are graphs for two tests with skin resistance response data on the Control Question Test and the Guilty Knowledge Test. The Control

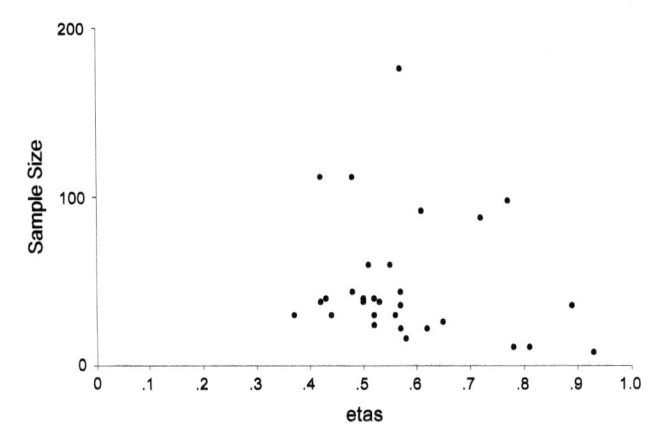

FIG. 1. *Etas* for Control Question Tests with skin resistance response measures (M eta = .58, SD = .14; r = .16, obs = 30)

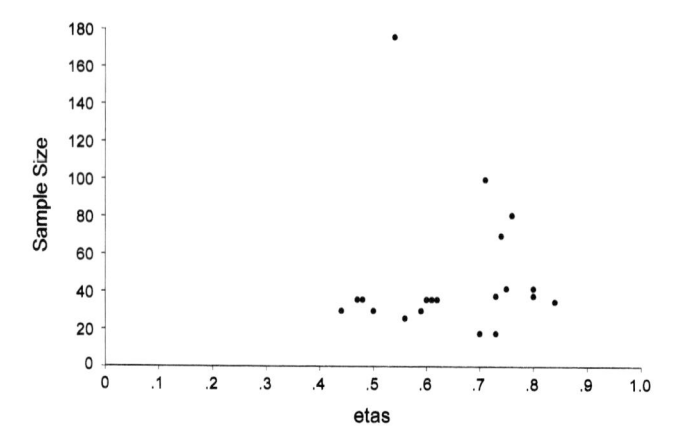

Fig. 2. Etas for Guilty Knowledge Tests with skin resistance response measures (M eta = .65, SD = .12; r = .00, obs = 20)

Question Test average *eta* is .58 (SD = .14), and r = −.16 between n and *eta*. For the Guilty Knowledge Test the average *eta* is .64 (SD = .12), and r = 0.

Figs. 3 and 4 are graphs for cardiovascular and respiration measures. For cardiovascular measures, the average eta = 0.44 (SD = .17), and r = −.44. For respiration, eta = .46 (SD = .12), and r = −.13.

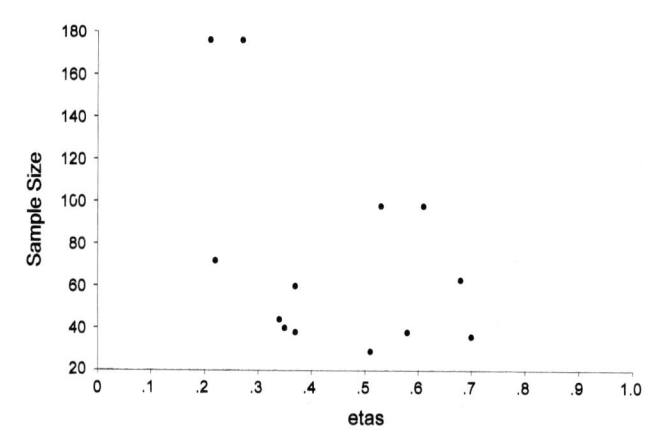

Fig. 3. Etas for detection tests from studies reporting cardiovascular measures (M eta = .44, SD = .17; r = −.44, obs = 13)

Fig. 5 depicts the n and *eta*s for subtle blocking variables and psychological effects. The average eta = .44 (SD = .13), and r = −.77.

Adjustment in the average *eta* for any given graphed set of values was

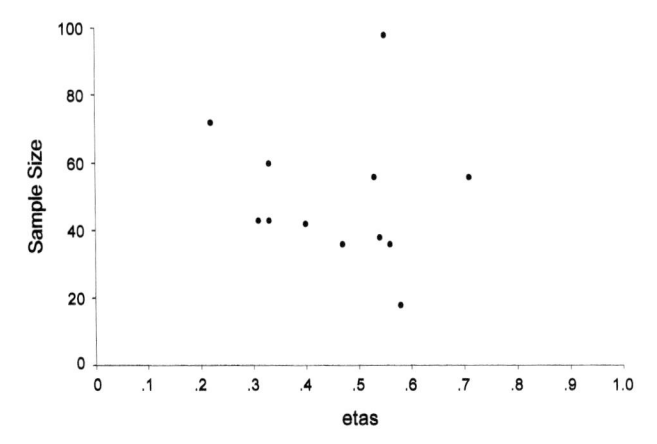

Fig. 4. *Eta*s for detection tests from studies reporting respiration measures (*M eta* = .46, *SD* = .12; *r* = .13, obs = 12)

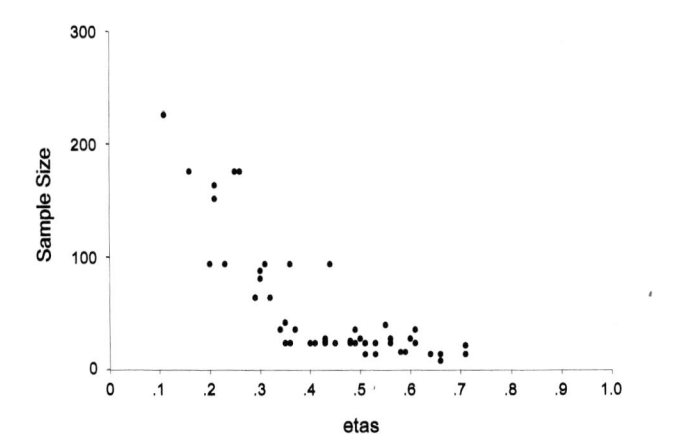

Fig. 5. *Eta*s from detection results modified due to psychological variables (*M eta* = .44, *SD* = .13; *r* = −.77, obs = 64)

made. The proportion of variance accounted for (r^2) derived from the appropriate correlation was multiplied by the average *eta* and then the resulting value was subtracted from the average *eta*. These *eta* values adjusted by the correlations are depicted in Table 1.

The hypotheses are supported. Correlations were large and negative when effect sizes were expected to be small and approached zero as true effect sizes were expected to increase. The graphs showed that *eta*s reported from studies on two types of tests commonly used in the detection area, the

TABLE 1
Original Adjusted *eta* Estimates For Tests, Measures, and Psychological Variables

Source of Estimate	eta Average	Adjusted
Skin resistance response (Control Question Test)	0.58	0.56
Skin resistance response (Guilty Knowledge Test)	0.65	0.65
Respiration	0.46	0.45
Cardiovascular responses	0.44	0.36
Psychological factors	0.44	0.18

Control Question Test and the Guilty Knowledge Test with skin-resistance response measures, approximate funnel graphs. Estimates from small samples vary widely but because the effect is inherently large, few or no small sample estimates are excluded from the published literature. The variance decreases with medium-sized samples but is still centered on the same mean, and finally the singular large sample estimate in each graph closely approximates the mean in the Control Question Test graph. It is reasonable to conclude that the average *eta*s for these tests accurately reflect their true value.

Distortion is apparent in the data for cardiovascular measures. The reported effects are overestimates. The table shows that adjustment of the mean of reported *eta*s by r^2 lowers the effect-size estimate. Respiration results present a conundrum. The current results suggest that respiration measures are effective and are being accurately measured. If, however, the single point on the graph associated with both a large sample and a large effect size is removed as an outlier because it neither fits the expectation of a funnel shape nor the transformation to a linear regression line, the correlation reflects distortion. The subsequent adjustment by r^2 reduces respiration results to about the same level as that found for cardiovascular studies.

The *eta*s calculated from studies on psychological effects show large overestimates. Many of these *eta*s exceed the average value for basic detection results, even though the text of articles examining these effects predict small or modest effects, and there were no indications in the literature that any small samples were unusual populations predicted to yield large differences. It is in the realm of small effect sizes with small numbers of measurements illustrated here that statistical testing most seriously distorts measurement (Bradley & Gupta, 1997).

The overall results show that statistical testing has mixed effects on the subject matter under scrutiny. If the underlying effect is large, statistical testing with a rigorous significance level will not cause much or any distortion. The worst that can happen is that small sized samples will result in widely varying estimates that will be misunderstood as to their true context. For example, in the detection literature there is a heated but from our perspective misguided debate over the effectiveness of the Control Question Test. Some believe it is a poor technique for discriminating between guilty and innocent suspects so it cannot be admitted for court use and should not be used by the police for interrogations (Lykken, 1981). Others suggest it is a highly accurate and effective interrogation tool and seek admission of polygraph results in court (Raskin, 1978). It is clear from the distribution of *eta*s that advocates and detractors are focusing on different tails of the distribution. In the context of studies with small samples which yield widely varying estimates, data supports both positions but, of course, the overall mean and the more precise estimates from large samples suggest a substantial effect but with plenty of room for error in individual cases. In all probability, the current practice by the police and legal system of seeking little input from experimental psychologists and using the polygraphs as an interrogation aid that is generally disallowed in court is reasonable given the average of estimates. A researcher interested in controversial therapies or drug effects might discover a similar distribution of effects. We speculate that each new adequately done study that yields significant results tends to be treated as definitive for a group on one side of the argument and a challenge for the group on the other side. Our portrayal of data suggests that each new estimate is just another estimate in a family or distribution of estimates.

The danger of statistical testing with small to medium effect sizes is that a percentage of published small sample studies will suggest a measure, treatment, or procedure is effective whereas another sizeable percentage of studies will suggest that it is not the case. A "Now you see it, now you don't" effect is created. A significant result is treated as a 1 whereas insignificant results are treated as 0. Thus, introductions to studies either directly or through inference contain inaccurate statements suggesting that one researcher reported an effect, whereas another researcher did not. In actual fact, each researcher had estimates that fit on a regular funnel graph of estimates, but, if the power is inadequate, only the exaggerated estimate is published and available in the literature. The potentially accurate but nonsignificant estimate is either not reported or treated as if nothing resulted from the study. A remedy is to publish all estimates regardless of statistical significance. In this way over time, a family of estimates would be created with the average suggesting the true effect size.

In the literature we reviewed, a majority of studies used polygraphs capable of measuring respiration and heart rate. The reports, however, typically mention these measures explicitly when they are involved in significant findings but do not when there is no significance. This has two effects on the literature, (a) researchers are encouraged by some positive reports to keep revisiting an issue and with sporadic success become confused, and (b) if they calculate power empirically, that power will be inadequate because it is based on reported exaggerations. Therefore, most researchers will not find significance and have no influence on the area whereas a "lucky" one or few will report the latest Type I error or exaggeration. As long as this situation prevails, the outlook for a cumulative, accurate, precise measurement in psychology is dim.

A goal of a scientific psychology is to produce accurate, precise measurements of phenomena. Over the past 50 years, this goal has been subverted to the production of statistically significant results. Significant effect-size measures and accurate effect sizes are not the same and diverge widely as power becomes more inadequate. The focus has been on significance, rather than accurate measurement. The focus needs to be on measurement and not on statistical significance. The results of adequate measurement procedures are primary. Statistical likelihood information is nice, but secondary. Studies submitted for publication would have to be judged primarily on measurement, and experimental procedures and results would have to be related to reasonable theory. Statistical probability estimates could give an indication of the chance of replication, but that is a more limited role. That is, any given result could have happened by chance 1 in 20 times or 1 in 10 or 1 in 5 times. The imperative from that information is to do the study again and cumulate the results.

Should the past 50 years of research done under significance testing rules of acceptance for publication be thrown out and we start over? No, but the way literatures on a topic are viewed could be changed. The most recent significant study should not be considered definitive. The new study simply gives one more estimate in a series of estimates. If significance testing has distorted the distribution of estimates, the distortion is predictable and can be measured. Understanding this problem gives the solution. The magnitude of distortion is gauged by a negative correlation between effect sizes and sample size. Thus, examination and diagnosis of past literature can still yield valuable estimates. To reiterate: (1) problems created by statistical testing are minuscule for inherently large effects, (2) if true effect sizes are small to moderate, then effect-size estimates can be assembled and techniques such as the correlation/variance method explained in this paper can be used, or the true number of experimental attempts could be estimated (Bradley & Gupta, 1997), or a variety of other methods could be used to make more appropriate estimates for the past literature (Bradley, et al., 2002).

Final Comment

Accurate measurements of mean differences are more important than likelihood estimates for those differences. Accurate estimates can be achieved in two ways, by large sample sizes or by the accumulation of measured differences in the form of a distribution from studies with small samples.

Minimizing or treating statistical likelihood estimates as interesting but secondary information would result in a shift in emphasis towards judging a study by adequacy of design. Greater attention to theory could be paid, and refinement of measurement techniques could lead to a reduction of error variance. The "Now you see it, now you don't" statistical significance approach would be supplanted by a scientific approach based on cumulative measurement and replication.

Literatures can be examined conveniently by correlating *eta* values (derived from F, t, or r) on the y-axis with sample sizes on the abscissa. A negative correlation suggests that the average *eta* is exaggerated.

REFERENCES[a]

BALLOON, K. D., & HOLMES, D. S. (1979) Effects of repeated examinations on the ability to detect guilt with a polygraphic examination: a laboratory experiment with a real crime. *Journal of Applied Psychology*, 64, 316-322.*

BARLAND, G. H., & RASKIN, D. C. (1975) An evaluation of field techniques in detection of deception. *Psychophysiology*, 12, 321-330.*

BEGG, C. B. (1994) Publication bias. In H. Cooper & L. V. Hedges (Eds.), *The handbook of research synthesis*. New York: Russell Sage Found. Pp. 400-409.

BEIJK, J. (1980) Experimental and procedural influences on differential electrodermal activity. *Psychophysiology*, 17, 274-278.*

BRADLEY, M. T. (2000) Quantitative review and quality diagnosis of detection of deception studies. *Canadian Psychology*, 41(2a), 101. [Abstract]

BRADLEY, M. T., & AINSWORTH, D. (1984) Alcohol and psychophysiological detection of deception. *Psychophysiology*, 21, 63-67.*

BRADLEY, M. T., & CULLEN, M. C. (1993) Polygraph lie detection on real events in a laboratory setting. *Perceptual and Motor Skills*, 73, 1051-1058.*

BRADLEY, M. T., & GUPTA, R. D. (1997) Estimating the effect of the file drawer problem in meta-analysis. *Perceptual and Motor Skills*, 85, 719-722.

BRADLEY, M. T., & JANISSE, M. P. (1981a) Accuracy demonstrations, threat and detection of deception: cardiovascular, electrodermal and pupillary measures. *Psychophysiology*, 21, 683-689.*

BRADLEY, M. T., & JANISSE, M. P. (1981b) Extraversion and the detection of deception. *Personality and Individual Differences*, 2, 99-103.*

BRADLEY, M. T., & KLOHN, K. I. (1987) Machiavellianism, the Control Question Test and the detection of deception. *Perceptual and Motor Skills*, 64, 747-757.*

BRADLEY, M. T., MACDONALD, P., & FLEMING, I. (1989) Amnesia, feelings of knowing, and the Guilty Knowledge Test. *Canadian Journal of Behavioral Science*, 21, 224-231.*

BRADLEY, M. T., MACLAREN, V. V., & BLACK, M. E. (1996) The Control Question Test in polygraphic examinations with actual controls for truth. *Perceptual and Motor Skills*, 83, 755-762.*

BRADLEY, M. T., & RETTINGER, J. (1992) Awareness of crime-relevant information and the Guilty Knowledge Test. *Journal of Applied Psychology*, 77, 55-59.*

BRADLEY, M. T., SMITH, D., & STOICA, G. (2002) A Monte-Carlo estimation of effect size distortion due to significance testing. *Perceptual and Motor Skills*, 95, 837-842.*

BRADLEY, M. T., & WARFIELD, J. F. (1984) Innocence, information, and the Guilty Knowledge Test in the detection of deception. *Psychophysiology*, 21, 683-689.*

BRUNING, J. L., & KINTZ, B. L. (1987) *Computational handbook of statistics*. Glenview, IL: Scott, Foresman.

COHEN, J. (1992) A power primer. *Psychological Bulletin*, 112, 155-159.

---

[a] References marked with an asterisk indicate studies included in the meta-analysis.

CUTROW, R. J., PARKS, A., NELSON, L., & THOMAS, K. (1972) The objective use of multiple physiological indices in the detection of deception. *Psychophysiology*, 9, 578-588.*

DAWES, R. M., LANDMAN, J., & WILLIAMS, M. (1984) Discussion on meta-analysis and selective publication bias. *American Psychologist*, 39, 75-78.

DAWSON, M. E. (1980) Physiological detection of deception: measurement of responses to questions and answers during countermeasure maneuvers. *Psychophysiology*, 17, 8-17.*

DRISCOLL, L. E., HONTS, C. R., & JONES, D. (1987) The validity of the positive control physiological detection of deception technique. *Journal of Police Science and Administration*, 115, 46-50.*

ELAAD, E. (1993) The role of guessing and verbal response type in psychophysiological detection of concealed information. *The Journal of Psychology*, 127, 455-464.*

ELAAD, E. (1997) Polygraph examiner awareness of crime-relevant information and the Guilty Knowledge Test. *Law and Human Behavior*, 1, 107-120.*

ELAAD, E., & BEN-SHAKHAR, G. (1989) Effects of motivation and verbal response type on psychophysiological detection of information. *Psychophysiology*, 26, 442-451.*

FOREMAN, R. F., & McCAULEY, C. (1986) Validity of the positive control polygraph test using the field practice mode. *Journal of Applied Psychology*, 71, 691-698.*

GIESEN, M., & ROLLISON, M. A. (1980) Guilty knowledge versus innocent associations: effects of trait anxiety and stimulus context on skin conductance. *Journal of Research in Personality*, 14, 1-11.*

GREENWALD, A. G. (1975) Consequences of prejudice against the null hypothesis. *Psychological Bulletin*, 82, 1-20.

GUDJONSSON, G. H. (1982) Some physiological determinants of electrodermal responses to deception. *Personality and Individual Differences*, 3, 381-391.*

HEDGES, L. V. (1992) Modeling publication selection effects in meta-analysis. *Statistical Science*, 7, 246-255.

HONTS, C. R., DEVITT, M. K., WINBUSH, M., & KIRCHER, J. C. (1996) Mental and physical countermeasures reduce the accuracy of the concealed knowledge test. *Psychophysiology*, 33, 84-92.*

HONTS, C. R., HODES, R. L., & RASKIN, D. C. (1985) Effects of physical counter-measures on the physiological detection of deception. *Journal of Applied Psychology*, 70, 177-187.*

HONTS, C. R., RASKIN, D. C., & KIRCHER, J. C. (1985) Effects of socialization on the physiological detection of deception. *Journal of Research in Personality*, 19, 373-385.*

HONTS, C. R., RASKIN, D. C., & KIRCHER, J. C. (1994) Mental and physical countermeasures reduce the accuracy of polygraph tests. *Journal of Applied Psychology*, 79, 252-259.*

HOROWITZ, S. W., KIRCHER, J. C., HONTS, C. R., & RASKIN, D. C. (1997) The role of comparison questions in physiological detection of deception. *Psychophysiology*, 34, 108-115.*

HORVATH, F. (1988) The utility of control questions and the effects of two control question types in field polygraph techniques. *Journal of Police Science and Administration*, 16, 198-209.*

IACONO, W. G., BOISVENU, G. A., & FLEMING, J. A. (1984) Effects of diazepam and methylphenidate on the electrodermal detection of guilty knowledge. *Journal of Applied Psychology*, 69, 289-299.*

IACONO, W. G., CERRI, A. M., PATRICK, C. J., & FLEMING, J. A. E. (1992) Use of antianxiety drugs as countermeasures in the detection of guilty knowledge. *Journal of Applied Psychology*, 77, 60-64.*

JANISSE, M. P., & BRADLEY, M. T. (1980) Deception, information and the pupillary response. *Perceptual and Motor Skills*, 50, 746-750.*

KIRCHER, J. C., & RASKIN, D. C. (1988) Human versus computerized evaluations of polygraph data in a laboratory setting. *Journal of Applied Psychology*, 73, 291-302.*

LIGHT, R. J., & PILLEMER, D. B. (1984) *Summing up: the science of reviewing research.* Cambridge, MA: Harvard Univer. Press.

LIPSEY, M. W., & WILSON, D. B. (2001) *Practical meta-analysis.* (Applied Social Research Methods Series, Vol. 49) London: Sage.

LYKKEN, D. T. (1959) The GSR in the detection of guilt. *Journal of Applied Psychology*, 43, 385-388.*

LYKKEN, D. T. (1981) *A tremor in the blood: uses and abuses of the lie detector.* New York: McGraw-Hill.

O'TOOLE, D., YUILLE, J. C., PATRICK, C. J., & IACONO, W. G. (1994) Alcohol and the physiological detection of deception: arousal and memory influences. *Psychophysiology,* 31, 253-263.*

PATRICK, C. J., & IACONO, W. G. (1991) A comparison of field and laboratory polygraphs in the detection of deception. *Psychophysiology,* 28, 632-638.*

PODLESNEY, J. A., & TRUSLOW, C. M. (1993) Validity of an expanded-issue (Modified General Question) polygraph technique in a simulated distributed-crime-roles context. *Journal of Applied Psychology,* 78, 788-797.*

RASKIN, D. C. (1978) Scientific assessment of the accuracy of detection of deception. *Psychophysiology,* 15, 344-359.

REID, J. E., & INBAU, F. E. (1977) *Truth and deception: the polygraph ("Lie Detection") technique.* Baltimore, MD: Williams & Wilkins.

ROSENTHAL, R. (1979) The "file drawer problem" and tolerance for null results. *Psychological Bulletin,* 86, 638-641.

SEDLMEIER, P., & GIGERENZER, G. (1989) Do studies of statistical power have an effect on the power of studies? *Psychological Bulletin,* 105, 309-316.

SMITH, M. L. (1980) Publication bias in meta-analysis. *Evaluation in Education,* 4, 22-24.

STELLER, M., HAENERT, P., & EISELT, W. (1987) Extraversion and the detection of information. *Journal of Research in Personality,* 21, 334-342.*

STERLING, T. D. (1959) Publication decisions and their possible effects on inferences drawn from tests on significance or vice versa. *Journal of the American Statistical Association,* 54, 30-34.

STERN, R. M., BREEN, J. P., WATANABE, T., & PERRY, B. S. (1981) Effect of feedback of physiological information on responses to innocent associations and guilty knowledge. *Journal of Applied Psychology,* 66, 677-681.*

WAID, W. M., ORNE, E. C., COOK, M. R., & ORNE, M. T. (1978) Effects of attention, as indexed by subsequent memory, on electrodermal detection of deception. *Journal of Applied Psychology,* 63, 728-733.*

WAID, W. M., ORNE, E. C., & ORNE, M. T. (1981) Selective memory for social information, alertness, and physiological arousal in the detection of deception. *Journal of Applied Psychology,* 66, 224-232.*

WAID, W. M., & ORNE, M. T. (1980) Individual differences in electrodermal lability and the detection of information and deception. *Journal of Applied Psychology,* 65, 1-8.*

WAID, W. M., & ORNE, M. T. (1982) The physiological detection of deception. *American Scientist,* 70, 402-409.*

WAID, W. M., ORNE, M. T., & WILSON, S. K. (1979a) Effects of level of socialization on electrodermal detection of deception. *Psychophysiology,* 16, 15-22.*

WAID, W. M., ORNE, M. T., & WILSON, S. K. (1979b) Socialization, awareness, and the electrodermal response to deception and self-disclosure. *Journal of Abnormal Psychology,* 88, 663-666.*

Accepted February 16, 2004.

CORSI'S BLOCK-TAPPING TASK: STANDARDIZATION AND LOCATION IN FACTOR SPACE WITH THE WAIS–R FOR TWO NORMAL SAMPLES OF OLDER ADULTS[1]

ARISTIDE SAGGINO, MICHELA BALSAMO, ANNA GRIECO,
MARIA ROSARIA CERBONE, AND NICLA NICOLINA RAVIELE

Università degli Studi "G. d'Annunzio" di Chieti-Pescara

Summary.—Corsi's block-tapping task and WAIS–R were administered to two Italian samples of 200 normal older adults (aged 65–74 years and 75–100 years). Corsi's reliabilities and standardization data are shown. Additionally, Corsi's location in the factor space of cognitive abilities represented by the 11 WAIS–R subtests is presented. Corsi's test seems to be a reliable one for older Italians. It seems also to be a measure of general intelligence in those 65–74 years of age and a measure of the Freedom from Distractibility factor in subjects 75 years and older.

The Corsi's block-tapping task (Corsi, 1972) is one of the most important nonverbal tests used in neuropsychological research and in the assessment of spatial memory of brain-damaged patients. Corsi (1972) developed the block-tapping task as a spatial alternative to procedures assessing memory for verbal sequences, as represented by the digit span task. At present, this task is usually included as a component of a major neuropsychological battery and has recently been adapted to a number of computerized formats (Berch, Krikorian,& Huha, 1998).

The age range to which it has been applied extends from children to older adults. Clinical populations studied to date have included Korsakoff's and Alzheimer's patients, the mentally retarded, learning-disabled children, and those with other neurological disorders (Berch, *et al.*, 1998).

The Corsi's block-tapping task has been used for a variety of purposes: to assess deficits in short-term nonverbal memory (De Renzi, Faglioni, & Previdi, 1977, cit. by Berch, *et al.*, 1998), to investigate sex differences (Orsini, Grossi, Capitani, Laiacona, Papagno, & Vallar, 1987; Capitani, Laiacona, Ciceri, & Gruppo Italiano per lo Studio Neuropsicologico dell'Invecchiamento, 1991), to clarify theoretical conceptions of visuospatial memory (Berch, *et al.*, 1998).

Orsini, *et al.* (1987) demonstrated that visuospatial immediate memory span, which is about four items in a normal subject, declines after the late

---

[1]The authors gratefully acknowledge the comments and the suggestions of Professor Arthur R. Jensen on earlier drafts of this article. This research was in part presented with some differences at the A.I.A.M.C. XI Congress, Palermo, Italy, 3–6 October 2001 and at the AIP Experimental Psychology Congress, Bari, Italy, 22–25 October, 2003. Address correspondence to A. Saggino, Università "G. d'Annunzio" di Chieti-Pescara, Facoltà di Psicologia, Via dei Vestini-66100 Chieti, Italy or e-mail (a.saggino@unich.it).

sixties and is affected by age, education, and sex differences, with male subjects scoring better. They also presented normative data both for normal Italian children and adults. They used a different administration and scoring procedure. The Corsi's score (spatial span score) was represented by the longest sequence the subject correctly recalled on three out of five trials. Similar results were obtained by Orsini, Chiacchio, Cinque, Cocchiaro, Schiappa, and Grossi (1986).

According to Berch, *et al.* (1998), Corsi's test has been used in research with different administration procedures and display characteristics. Furthermore, only a few studies have provided norms for the test. Therefore, Berch, *et al.* (1998) maintain that it is essential to establish definite display and administration procedures and collect normative data on different populations.

The aims of the present paper were the following: first, to provide Corsi's preliminary normative data on normal older Italian adults (aged 65–74 and 75–100 years); second, to study validity of Corsi's test across location in the factor space of cognitive abilities as identified by the 11 subtests of the Wechsler Adult Intelligence Scale–Revised (WAIS–R; Wechsler, 1981). Moreover, reliabilities of Corsi's test and its relationships with sociodemographic variables were investigated.

Method

Subjects

The Italian edition of the WAIS–R and the Corsi's block-tapping test were administered to two Italian samples of 200 volunteer normal, healthy older adults (65–74 years and 75–100 years). The mean age of the sample ages 65–74 years ($n=200$) was 68.9 yr. ($SD=2.7$). The mean age for the women ($n=105$) was 68.9 yr. ($SD=2.6$); for the men ($n=95$) the mean age was 68.8 yr. ($SD=2.7$). The mean years of education for this sample was 5.8 yr. ($SD=3.1$). The mean years of education was 5.0 yr. ($SD=3.1$) for the women and 6.7 yr. ($SD=2.8$) for the men.

The mean age of the sample over 74 years ($n=200$) was 78.4 yr. ($SD=4.5$). The mean age was 78.0 yr. ($SD=4.2$) for the women ($n=114$) and 78.8 yr. ($SD=5.0$) for the men ($n=86$). The mean years of education for this sample was 5.9 yr. ($SD=3.7$). It was 5.5 yr. ($SD=3.4$) for the women and 6.4 yr. ($SD=4.0$) for the men.

The two samples consisted of pensioners and housewives and part of the data ($n=200$) was utilized in a previous paper to study the psychometric aspects of the WAIS–R in older age groups (Saggino, Balsamo, & Grieco, 1999). All subjects were free of neurological, psychiatric, or sensory disabilities. Information was requested on current or past illnesses with the aim of excluding people with neurological disorders, psychiatric histories, and alcohol or drug use.

Procedure

Subjects were administered the 11 subtests of the WAIS–R and immediately afterwards Corsi's block-tapping test. Some of them (104 for the sample 65–74 years of age and 99 for the sample over 74 years of age) were given a retest of WAIS–R Digit Span and Digit Symbol subtests and Corsi's block-tapping task within 15 days to study their reliabilities. Other tests not considered in the present paper were also administered. Some of the data regarding the WAIS–R scale were discussed in Saggino, *et al.* (1999). Other data, relating the WAIS–R to the NEO Personality Inventory Revised (NEO-PI–R; Costa & McCrae, 1992) were discussed by Saggino and Balsamo (2003).

The Corsi's test measures visuospatial short-term memory. In this task, nine identical small white cubes (side 4 cm) are arranged irregularly over a wooden board (26 × 32 cm). The sides of the cubes facing the examiner are numbered from 1 to 9 to ease administering the task and recording performance. The examiner taps some of the blocks (digits) in a particular sequence; the subject is required to tap out exactly the same pattern immediately afterwards. The examiner taps the blocks one at a time using the index finger at the rate of 1 block per 2 sec. The test begins with a sequence of two units and, if the subject succeeds, increasingly long sequences are presented. Each time a maximum of five equal-unit sequences is tapped out. The test ends when a subject reproduces five sequences of the same length incorrectly. The sequences used are from 2 to 9 digits for a total of 40 items (Orsini, *et al.*, 1987). Corsi's test score is the number of items correctly reproduced. The test scoring, the display procedures, and the administration of the test are the same as those used by Orsini (1994). These administration and scoring procedures were selected because they are more similar and comparable to those used with the Digit Span WAIS–R subtest.

The sum of the raw scores of the corresponding WAIS–R subtests was used as an estimate of the Verbal, Performance, and Full Scale IQs because there is at the moment no Italian standardization of the WAIS–R for subjects over 65 years of age. Therefore, we used the sum of the six verbal subtests' raw scores to obtain the Verbal Intelligence score, the sum of the five performance subtests' raw scores to obtain the Performance Intelligence score, and the sum of all the 11 subtests' raw scores to obtain the Full Scale Intelligence score. For purpose of comparisons, we calculated the correlations between these three scores and the corresponding three sums of the WAIS–R scaled scores based on the age group of 19–34 years in a subgroup of 100 subjects over 74 years old (Saggino & Balsamo, 2003). We obtained correlations higher than .90, indicating that the two scores can be considered substantially equivalent.

Results and Discussion

The mean for raw scores on Corsi's test was 15.7 ($SD=3.9$) for the sample of age 65–74 years, with a mean of 14.3 ($SD=3.5$) for the female sample and 17.3 ($SD=3.7$) for the male sample. The mean of raw scores for Corsi's test is 14.1 ($SD=3.3$) for the sample over 74 years of age, with a mean of 13.5 ($SD=3.5$) for the female sample and 14.9 ($SD=3.0$) for the male sample. The standard error of measurement corresponds to 4.6 for the sample 65–74 years of age (4.2 for the women and 4.5 for the men) and to 4.4 for the sample over 74 years of age (4.7 for the women and 4.0 for the men). All statistical analyses of the present paper were computed on raw scores.

Multiple regression analyses were calculated using sex, age, and years of education as predictors of Corsi's block-tapping test scores. In the group 65–74 years of age, all three variables collectively accounted for 18% of the score variance (adjusted $R^2=.18$; $F_{3,196}=15.52$, $p<.0005$). Only years of education (beta=.216, $t=3.21$, $p<.005$) and sex (beta=.324, $t=4.85$, $p<.0005$) accounted for a significant amount of unique explained variance in Corsi's block-tapping test scores. In the sample over 74 years of age, the three variables collectively accounted for 19% of the score variance (adjusted $R^2=.19$; $F_{3,196}=16.37$, $p<.0005$). All three predictors accounted for a significant amount of unique explained variance in the block-tapping test scores: years of education (beta=.339, $t=5.27$, $p<.0005$), age (beta=$-.201$, $t=-3.13$, $p<.005$), and sex (beta=.185, $t=2.86$, $p<.01$). Therefore, sex and education (and, to a lesser extent, age) represent important predictors of the Corsi test scores, as they are in general for all the variables of the cognitive domain (Orsini, *et al.*, 1986, 1987; Jensen, 1998).

Reliability of Corsi's test was calculated using both the split-half method (with correction by the Spearman-Brown formula) and the test-retest method. Split-half reliability was .86, and test-retest reliability was .85 for the sample 65–74 years of age. Split-half reliability was .85 and test-retest reliability was .75 for the sample 74 years and over. Therefore, Corsi's block-tapping test shows for normal older adults a good reliability (both internal consistency and temporal stability). The corresponding reliabilities for the WAIS–R subtests can be found in Saggino, *et al.* (1999).

Table 1 shows the conversion of raw scores for Corsi's test to scaled standard scores ($M=10$, $SD=3$) to allow comparison between scores obtained by subjects given Corsi's test and WAIS–R subtests. In fact, unlike raw scores, scaled scores allow comparison of results obtained on different tests. It facilitates the possible use of Corsi's test as a twelfth WAIS–R subtest.

Table 2 shows correlations for Corsi's test scores with those on the WAIS–R subtests and the three WAIS–R total scores (Verbal, Performance, and Full Scale). We present both the zero-order correlations and the partial correlation coefficients to control sex, age, and years of education because

TABLE 1
SCALED STANDARD SCORES FOR CORSI'S TEST EQUIVALENT TO RAW SCORES ($ns = 200$)

Scaled Standard Score	Raw Score Equivalent 65–74 yr.	Raw Score Equivalent 75–100 yr.	Scaled Standard Score
1	3	2	1
2			2
3	4	3–4	3
4	7–8	5–6	4
5	9–10	7–8	5
6	11	9–10	6
7	12	11–12	7
8	13	13	8
9	14		9
10	15–16	14	10
11	17	15	11
12	18–19	16	12
13	20	17	13
14	21	18	14
15	22	19	15
16	23–24	20	16
17	25	21	17
18			18
19	27		19

these three variables notoriously influence scores on cognitive tests, as we have already demonstrated (see also Orsini, *et al.*, 1986, 1987).

For the group 65–74 years of age, salient partial correlation coefficients

TABLE 2
ZERO-ORDER CORRELATIONS AND PARTIAL CORRELATIONS OF CORSI'S TEST SCORES WITH WAIS–R SUBTEST AND TOTAL SCORES ($ns = 200$)

WAIS–R Subscale and Total Scale	65–74 Years r	65–74 Years Partial r*	75–100 Years r	75–100 Years Partial r*
Information	.40	.23	.38	.15
Digit Span	.40	.28	.47	.36
Vocabulary	.34	.21	.41	.21
Arithmetic	.44	.29	.44	.27
Comprehension	.38	.24	.36	.15
Similarities	.31	.20	.30	.10
Picture Completion	.38	.22	.32	.12
Picture Arrangement	.27	.18	.35	.21
Block Design	.42	.32	.26	.07
Object Assembly	.39	.28	.18	.00
Digit Symbol	.40	.26	.36	.16
Verbal Scale Score	.42	.30	.47	.26
Performance Scale Score	.47	.36	.35	.12
Full Scale Score	.47	.37	.45	.22

*Partial correlations with sex, age, and education controlled.

for Corsi's test scores (that is, all the absolute correlations equal to or greater than .30) were with WAIS–R Full Scale (.37), Performance (.36), and Verbal scale scores (.30) and for WAIS–R Block Design (.32). For the sample over 74 years of age, the only salient partial correlation coefficient for Corsi's test was with the WAIS–R Digit Span (.36). All the zero-order correlations were greater than .30, with the only exception of Picture Arrangement (.27) in the sample 65–74 years of age; in the sample over 74 years of age, Block Design (.26) and Object Assembly (.18) were the only exceptions.

To obtain more precise information on Corsi's test validity for older adults, we located the Corsi's block-tapping task in cognitive factor space as represented by the 11 WAIS–R subtests. Thus, the intercorrelations of these 12 variables for each age group were subjected in an initial run, following Kaufman (1975) and Orsini (1994), to a principal components analysis to estimate the number of factors. Two criteria were used to obtain the number of factors to extract: the scree plot (Cattell, 1966) and the Kaiser's roots >1.00 criterion. Then a principal factor analysis was performed. We preferred the principal factor analysis method because it is considered more adequate in research on the g factor and cognitive abilities (Jensen, 1998).

A one-factor solution emerges by the Scree test for the sample 65–74 years of age. Furthermore, the initial eigenvalue of the first principal component is 6.72, while the initial eigenvalue of the second principal component is .998. Therefore, a one-factor principal axis solution was selected. The principal axis factoring solution explains 52.3% of the total variance. All the 12 variables present loadings higher than .50, as shown in Table 3. The Corsi's test has a loading of .51. Therefore, this factor represents the g factor, or general intelligence. In this sample Corsi's test seems to be a good measure of the g factor.

TABLE 3
Unrotated First Principal Factor Loadings For the Sample 65–74 Years of Age ($n = 200$)

Subscale	Loading
WAIS–R	
Information	.82
Digit Span	.60
Vocabulary	.84
Arithmetic	.66
Comprehension	.73
Similarities	.77
Picture Completion	.75
Picture Arrangement	.67
Block Design	.70
Object Assembly	.69
Digit Symbol	.86
Corsi's Test	.51

For the sample over 74 years of age, a three-factor solution emerges by the scree test. The initial eigenvalues of the principal components solution correspond to 6.01 for the first component, 1.13 for the second component, and 1.01 for the third component. The fourth component has an eigenvalue corresponding to .72. For this reason, only three factors were selected by the principal axis factoring method and rotated by the oblique direct oblimin method, which represents a choice better than the varimax when the factors are correlated (correlations range from .48 to .65). This solution explains 58.4% of the total variance after extraction. After this initial run we preferred a Schmid and Leiman hierarchical factor analysis as the definitive choice because it divides the variance of the variables into that due to unique variance (primary factors) and that due to the common variance (secondary factors). The hierarchical factor analysis is considered particularly useful when one is interested in studying the variables at different hierarchical levels because the interpretation of the second-order factors are based on the original variables and not on the interpretations of the first-order factors, as happens when we perform a first-order factor analysis followed by a second-order factor analysis. We obtained three primary and one secondary factor, as shown in Table 4. The first primary factor represents mainly the Verbal Comprehension factor. In fact, four out of the six verbal subtests (Compre-

TABLE 4
Schmid and Leiman Hierarchical Factor Analysis Loadings of WAIS–R Eleven Subtests and Corsi's Test For the Sample Over 74 Years of Age ($n = 200$)

Subscale	Secondary Factor 1	Primary Factor 1	Primary Factor 2	Primary Factor 3
WAIS—R				
Information	.65	.52	−.11	.04
Digit Span	.64	−.06	.07	.55
Vocabulary	.73	.45	−.02	.11
Arithmetic	.67	.06	.08	.43
Comprehension	.66	.53	−.09	.01
Similarities	.60	.57	−.06	−.11
Picture Completion	.66	.36	.22	−.06
Picture Arrangement	.56	.30	.19	−.04
Block Design	.63	.00	.62	−.02
Object Assembly	.56	−.06	.68	−.06
Digit Symbol	.71	.30	.25	.02
Corsi's Test	.54	.02	−.18	.59

hension, Similarities, Information, and Vocabulary) have their salient loadings (that is, absolute loadings equal to or higher than .30) on the primary Factor 1. Also, two performance subtests (Picture Completion and Digit-Symbol) have their salient loadings on this factor. Therefore, it does not seem to be a pure Verbal Comprehension factor. Factor 2 has its salient loadings on two performance subtests (Block Design and Object Assembly). Therefore, it appears to correspond to the Perceptual Organization factor, even if only two subtests from the Performance scale have their salient loadings on this factor. Factor 3 has its highest loadings on Digit Span, Arithmetic, and Corsi's block-tapping test so it seems to be the usual Freedom from Distractibility factor. In this sample, Corsi's test has its lowest loading on the Verbal Comprehension factor and its highest loading on the Freedom from Distractibility factor, as was found for children ages 11 to 16 years by Orsini (1994). As regards the secondary factor, both the 11 WAIS–R subtests and the Corsi's test have loadings greater than .50 on this factor. Therefore, it seems to be the usual g factor.

In conclusion, Corsi's test seems to be reliable for use with older normal Italian adults. As regards its validity, it loaded substantially on the WAIS–R g factor for adults 65–74 years old. In older subjects (over 74 years) it seems to measure particularly the Freedom from Distractibility factor together with the Digit Span and Arithmetic WAIS–R subtests at a primary level. At the secondary level, it loads on the general intelligence factor together with all the 11 WAIS–R subtests. Therefore, in the older sample, the Corsi's block-tapping test is largely a measure of short-term memory, loading on the same primary factor as the Digit Span subtest. Our results seem to confirm the recent view that verbal and spatial short-term memory are not independent (Jones, Farrand, Stuart, & Morris, 1995, cit. by Berch, et al., 1998). However, these preliminary findings still need to be confirmed in independent and, preferably, larger and more varied samples. In particular, the differences in the factor structure we have found in the two different age groups should be studied further.

REFERENCES

BERCH, D. B., KRIKORIAN, R., & HUHA, E. M. (1998) The Corsi Block-tapping Task: methodological and theoretical considerations. *Brain and Cognition*, 38, 317-338.

CAPITANI, E., LAIACONA, M., CICERI, E., & GRUPPO ITALIANO PER LO STUDIO NEUROPSICOLOGICO DELL'INVECCHIAMENTO. (1991) Sex differences in spatial memory: a reanalysis of block tapping long-term memory according to the short-term memory level. *The Italian Journal of Neurological Sciences*, 12, 461-466.

CATTELL, R. B. (1966) The scree test for the number of factors. *Multivariate Behavioural Research*, 1, 141-161.

CORSI, P. M. (1972) Human memory and the medial temporal region of the brain. *Dissertation Abstracts International*, 34, 891B.

COSTA, P. T., JR., & MCCRAE, R. R. (1992) *Revised NEO Personality Inventory (NEO-PI–R) and NEO Five-Factor (NEO-FFI) professional manual.* Odessa, FL: Psychological Assessment Resources.

DE RENZI, E., FAGLIONI, P., & PREVIDI, P. (1977) Spatial memory and hemispheric locus of lesion. *Cortex*, 13, 424-433.

JENSEN, A. R. (1998) *The g factor: the science of mental ability.* Westport, CT: Praeger.

JONES, D., FARRAND, P., STUART, G., & MORRIS, N. (1995) Functional equivalence of verbal and spatial information in serial short-term memory. *Journal of Experimental Psychology: Learning, Memory, and Cognition*, 21, 1008-1018.

KAUFMAN, A. S. (1975) Factor analysis of the WISC–R at 11 age levels between $6^{1}/_{2}$ and $16^{1}/_{2}$ years. *Journal of Consulting and Clinical Psychology*, 43, 135-147.

ORSINI, A. (1994) Corsi's Block-tapping Test: standardization and concurrent validity with WISC–R for children aged 11 to 16. *Perceptual and Motor Skills*, 79, 1547-1554.

ORSINI, A., CHIACCHIO, I., CINQUE, M., COCCHIARO, C., SCHIAPPA, O., & GROSSI, D. (1986) Effects of age, education and sex on two tests of immediate memory: a study of normal subjects from 20 to 99 years of age. *Perceptual and Motor Skills*, 63, 727-732.

ORSINI, A., GROSSI, D., CAPITANI, E., LAIACONA, M., PAPAGNO, C., & VALLAR, G. (1987) Verbal and spatial immediate memory span: normative data from 1355 adults and 1112 children. *Italian Journal of Neurological Sciences*, 8, 539-548.

SAGGINO, A., & BALSAMO, M. (2003) Relationship between WAIS–R intelligence and the five-factor model of personality in a normal elderly sample. *Psychological Reports*, 92, 1151-1161.

SAGGINO, A., BALSAMO, M., & GRIECO, A. (1999) Proprietà psicometriche della Wechsler Adult Intelligence Scale–Edizione Riveduta nella terza età: primi riscontri [Psychometric aspects of the Wechsler Adult Intelligence Scale Revised in old age: a preliminary report]. *Rassegna di Psicologia*, 16, 155-162.

WECHSLER, D. (1981) *Manual for the Adult Intelligence Scale–Revised.* San Antonio, TX: Psychological Corp.

Accepted February 27, 2004.

EFFECTIVENESS OF VIDEO OF CONSPECIFICS AS A REWARD FOR SOCIALLY HOUSED BONNET MACAQUES (*MACACA RADIATA*)[1]

ELIZABETH M. BRANNON

Duke University

MICHAEL W. ANDREWS

Southern Oregon University

LEONARD A. ROSENBLUM

SUNY Health Science Center

Summary.—Two experiments were conducted to examine the effectiveness of presenting brief video of conspecifics to socially housed bonnet macaques as a reward for performing a joystick task. Using a joystick, subjects tracked a moving target with the cursor on a computer monitor. In Exp. 1, subjects completed significantly more joystick trials for food reward than for video reward or no reward. Subjects also preferred viewing video of another group (Other Group Video) to receiving no reward or to viewing video of their own group (Own Group Video). In Exp. 2, subjects were given two reward conditions, video of a familiar social group or video of a new social group. Two monkeys contributed the vast majority of trials, and both responded more frequently when the reward was video of the new social group. Results of these two experiments suggest that viewing video of conspecifics may serve as an effective reward for at least some socially housed primates and suggests that novelty of the individuals depicted in the video is an important factor contributing to the reward value of video.

The opportunity to view video of a social group of conspecifics is an effective reward for individually housed bonnet macaques (Andrews & Rosenblum, 1993, 2001; Andrews, Bhat, & Rosenblum, 1995). An open question is whether video of conspecifics is effective as a reward for socially housed macaques. Although previous studies have examined the effects of viewing video of conspecifics for socially housed monkeys (e.g., Plimpton, Rosenblum, & Swartz, 1981; Capitanio, Boccia, & Colaiannia, 1985), the effectiveness of video of conspecifics as a reward for socially housed animals has not been systematically examined. There are multiple reasons that video of conspecifics might be rewarding for individually housed animals, but not for socially housed animals. First, individually housed monkeys are more likely to experience social deprivation, so viewing video of conspecifics might serve as a surrogate for live social interaction. Second, socially housed monkeys have more activities that compete for their attention than do individually

---

[1]This research was supported by an NIH grant to the second and third authors (2 R01 RR05321-05). The authors thank Marina Cords and Michael L. Platt for valuable comments on an earlier version of the manuscript. Address correspondence to Michael W. Andrews, Department of Psychology, Southern Oregon University, 1250 Siskiyou Blvd., Ashland, OR 97520 or e-mail (andrews@sou.edu).

housed animals, e.g., grooming group mates, or partaking in aggressive interactions. Nevertheless, if video of conspecifics is an effective reward for socially housed animals, this would allow investigators to use video reward without the necessity of putting subjects into social isolation.

Here we report two experiments with bonnet macaques in which video of conspecific groups was used as a reward for performing a joystick task. Exp. 1 examined the effectiveness of video as a reward by comparing response levels for video of conspecifics to response levels for a well-established food reward and no reward. A secondary purpose of Exp. 1 was to test further the view that the effectiveness of video of conspecifics derives to an important extent from the social stimulation it provides. Given previous findings suggesting that individually housed monkeys prefer to view video of conspecifics that contain novel individuals (Andrews & Rosenblum, 2001), we predicted that socially housed monkeys would show the same preference of viewing novel rather than familiar individuals in video rewards. Exp. 2 further tested the importance of novelty in the effectiveness of video of conspecifics as a reward for socially housed monkeys.

Method

Subjects

The subjects were a stable group of four male and three female 3.5-yr.-old bonnet macaques (*Macaca radiata*). Subjects had unique identification microchips (AVID; Norco, CA) implanted in both forearms (see Andrews, 1994).

Apparatus

The experiment was conducted in the group's indoor enclosure, a 2.0-m wide × 2.1-m high × 4.0-m long pen with opaque tile walls and floor. Two one-way mirror windows were located in the front wall of the pen. Two perches extended across the back of the pen, 74 and 154 cm above the pen floor. Lab chow and water were available *ad libitum*.

Two identical joystick-task systems were located side by side on the pen floor, facing opposite sides of the pen. Each system was contained within a clear Plexiglas box (74 × 63 × 74 cm). The joystick-task systems were identical to those described by Andrews, *et al.* (1995), with the exception that it was necessary to encase the monitors used for the current study in black wire mesh (openings .625 cm by .625 cm) to reduce interference with microchip radio frequencies.

Procedure

Task for Exps. 1 and 2.—More than one year prior to the onset of the experiments conducted for this report, the group members were shaped to perform a joystick task for food reward. Throughout shaping subjects received a food reward for contacting the green target area with the cursor. In the first phase of shaping the target consisted of a green border around the entire perimeter of the monitor screen. In the second phase of shaping one edge of the border (top, bottom, right or left) was randomly eliminated from the target area on each trial. In the third and fourth phases two and then three edges, respectively, were eliminated as target areas such that in stage four only one edge of the border was randomly available as a target. In the fifth phase the target was reduced in size in small increments. Finally, the small, rectangular target was set in motion. The target moved at 6 cm/sec. in a clockwise circle 7.5 cm from the center of the screen. A brief auditory signal followed completion of the task and preceded a reward. To grasp a joystick, subjects had to reach through the ring antenna of a microchip reader, thereby positioning the implanted microchip within the field of the microchip reader. The computer automatically recorded the subjects' identification numbers and the time and date for each trial. This task was used in both Exps. 1 and 2.

Experiment 1.—The critical manipulation in Exp. 1 was the nature of the reward. If the subject contacted the moving target with the cursor using the joystick, this was considered a successfully completed trial and rewarded. There were four reward conditions, and each condition occurred one day per week. Condition order was counterbalanced across weeks. The color of the target in the joystick task also varied across conditions to provide the subjects with a cue as to the reward that would be received on a given day. The task and rewards were available 10 hours (0900–1900) per day. Eight replications of each condition took place over an 8-wk. period. Data from Week 5, however, were lost due to equipment failure. Subjects received food and water *ad libitum* and were not food-deprived.

The four reward conditions were as follows: (1) In the Food Reward condition, completion of the task yielded a 190-mg banana-flavored food pellet followed by a 10-sec. intertrial interval; (2) in the Other Group Video condition, completion of the task resulted in a 10-sec. video segment of a 6-member social group of bonnet macaques with which the subject group had had no visual contact prior to the beginning of the experiment; (3) in the Own Group Video condition, a 10-sec. video segment of the subjects' own social group, excluding the task area, i.e., the subject could not view itself, was presented upon successful task completion; in both video-reward conditions, since the reward stimulus lasted for 10 sec., no additional intertrial interval was imposed; (4) in the No Reward condition, neither food nor any type of video was presented, but as in the food condition, a 10-sec. intertrial interval was imposed after trial completion. Note, that both video conditions used a live feed from a closed-circuit video camera. This meant that the video presented in the Own Group Video condition captured events that the subjects could view simply by turning away from the task system.

The physical features of the pen viewed in the Own Group Video condition were virtually identical to those of the pen viewed in the Other Group Video, and the two cameras were similarly positioned such that the field of view was also virtually identical in the two conditions. The novel group used in the Other Group Video condition contained six individuals: an adult male (7 years), 3 adult females (13–19 years), 1 subadult male (3 years), and an infant. A 6-member group was chosen for the Other Group Video to make the number of individuals viewed in the two video conditions comparable. Although the subjects' own group contained seven individuals, a maximum of only six individuals could be viewed in the video inasmuch as the task area with the seventh group member performing the task was always omitted from the field of view.

Post hoc analyses assessed whether the Own and Other Group Video segments differed in the number of individuals they displayed. The video segments observed by subjects between the hours of 0900 and 1300 in the sixth and seventh weeks of the study were sampled for both video conditions. To compare the average number of individuals visible in the segments used as rewards in the two conditions, the number of individuals visible in the last second of each 10-sec. video reward was recorded.

Informal observations suggested that more than one individual might be observing the video segments. This could contribute to differences in responding for food and video rewards by group members inasmuch as multiple individuals could observe each video, but only one individual could consume each pellet. To assess this possibility formally, direct behavioral observations were made to specify the number of individuals potentially able to view the video monitor in the 10 sec. immediately following task completion. During the fifth and sixth weeks, the focal group was observed by the first author between 0900 and 1030 hours for each condition. The maximum number of individuals in one of three possible viewing positions during the 10-sec. video presentations (Conditions 2 and 3) or the 10-sec. intertrial interval (Conditions 1 and 4) was recorded. A possible viewer of a video display was defined as any individual (a) directly in front of a system with its body positioned toward the monitor, (b) sitting on top of a system hanging its head upside down in front of the monitor, or (c) crouching on the corner of the lower perch with its head in line with the monitor.

Experiment 2.—The joystick systems and task were identical to those used in Exp. 1. Subjects were tested in an A-B-B-A design where blocks varied in the nature of the reward given for successful completion of a trial. The reward in Block A was video of the previously unfamiliar social group used in Exp. 1 (now called Familiar Group Video) and reward in B block was video of a new social group (New Group Video). All video rewards were again 10-sec. clips of live feed from a closed circuit camera. Each block was of 1 wk. duration, and four blocks were conducted. Subjects were given 24-hr.-per-day access, and data were not recorded on Sundays. The novel group consisted of five individuals: one adult male (6 years), and four adult females (7–19 years). A 5-member group was chosen because there was no 6-member group available, and a smaller novel group ensured that possible bias based on group size would be against the hypothesis that video of a novel group would elicit more responding. The stimulus groups were moved as necessary so that the same pen (described under Exp. 1) was used in both experimental conditions.

RESULTS

Experiment 1

Fig. 1a shows that subjects completed more trials per day in the Food Reward condition, the fewest number of trials per day in the No Reward condition, and an intermediate number of trials per day for the video-reward conditions. The average daily number of trials per subject for each condition across the seven weeks were as follows: Food Reward ($M = 292$ trials, $SE = 20.2$), Other Group Video ($M = 62$, $SE = 10.1$), Own Group Video ($M = 27$, $SE = 5.9$), No Reward ($M = 4$, $SE = .48$). A repeated-measures analysis of variance showed a main effect of condition ($F_{3,18} = 24.97, p < .01$) and a significant interaction between condition and week ($F_{18,108} = 10.2, p < .01$). The interaction is illustrated in Fig. 1a, which shows that the total number of trials completed per day remained approximately constant across the seven weeks for the Food Reward condition but decreased across the seven weeks

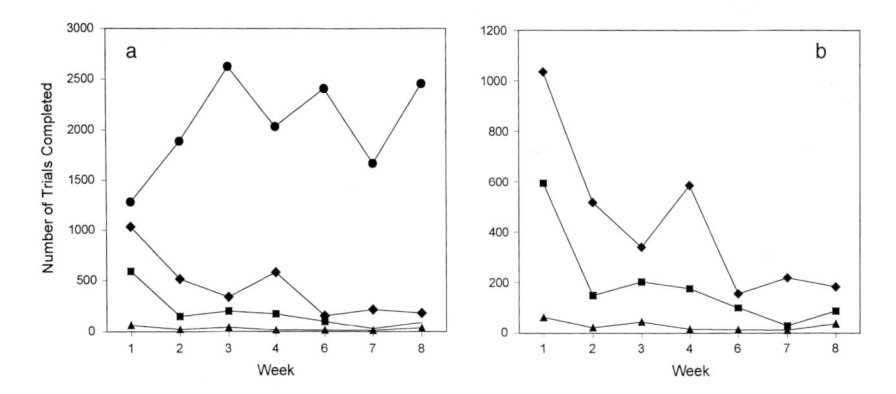

FIG. 1. (a) The total number of trials completed each day in each condition across the seven weeks. (b) The total number of trials completed across the seven weeks for the No Reward and two Video conditions. Note the difference in scale between Figs. 1a and 1b. (Food Reward ●, No Reward ▲, Other Group Video ♦, Own Group Video ■)

for video conditions. Scheffé *post hoc* tests indicated that the Food Reward condition differed from all others ($p < .05$), with no other significant differences.

Although the effectiveness of the Food Reward condition is indisputable, subjects completed more trials per day in the two video conditions than in the No Reward condition. Fig. 1b shows the same data as Fig. 1a without the Food Reward condition and illustrates that both video conditions elicited more trials per day than the No Reward condition. The comparatively high responding in the food-reward condition compared to all other conditions may have obscured statistical differences among the video conditions and the No Reward condition. To test this possibility, a second repeated-measures analysis of variance excluding the Food Reward condition was conducted. A significant main effect of condition was found ($F_{2,12} = 10.45$, $p < .01$). Scheffé *post hoc* tests indicated significantly higher responding to the Other Group Video condition compared to the No Reward condition ($p < .05$) and a weakly significant difference between the two video conditions ($p = .05$). The difference between the Own Group Video condition and the No Reward condition was not significant.

On average, subjects contributed approximately equal frequencies of total responding over the seven weeks (range 9 to 17% where an even distribution would predict 14%). However, individuals who ranked high on proportion of trials in the Food Reward condition tended to rank low on proportion of trials in both video conditions and vice versa. Whereas individual participation ranks were positively correlated for the two video reward conditions (Spearman $R = .92$, $p < .01$), these ranks for the Food Reward and both the Other Group and Own Group Video conditions were negatively correlated (Spearman $Rs = -.69$ and $-.53$, respectively), but these correlations were not significant as the sample was small.

To ensure that the two social video conditions did not differ in the number of individuals displayed, two 4-hr. samples of video rewards for each of the two video-reward conditions were analyzed. The mean number of individuals visible in the Own Group and Other Group Video conditions was 3.7 ($SE = .14$) and 4 ($SE = .12$), respectively. A paired t test indicated no significant difference between the two video conditions ($t_{78} = -1.60$, ns). Thus differences in task activity associated with these two conditions probably do not reflect a difference in the number of individuals present in the video segments.

To assess whether video rewards were being viewed only by the animal that directly obtained the reward or were being viewed by one or more additional individuals, the number of possible viewers was recorded during a subset of the 10-sec. video rewards (for the Own Group and Other Group Video conditions) and the 10-sec. intertrial intervals (for the Food and No

Reward conditions). The main effect of reward condition was significant ($F_{3,92} = 7.34$, $p < .01$). The mean number of viewers in the four conditions were for Food Reward = 1.5, Other Group Video = 2.4, Own Group Video = 2.8, and No Reward = 2.0. Fisher *post hoc* tests indicated significantly more viewers for both the Other Group Video and Own Group Video conditions than for the Food Reward condition ($p < .05$).

Experiment 2

In Exp. 2, two of the seven monkeys accounted for the vast majority of trials, 85%, 91%, 83%, and 92% in the four trial blocks, respectively. These two male monkeys did not dominate responding in Exp. 1; they earned 28% of the social video rewards and 10% of the food rewards where 29% would be predicted by an equal distribution among all group members. An analysis of variance for Exp. 2 showed a main effect of subject ($F_6 = 8.56$, $p < .001$), suggesting that subjects did not contribute equally to task activity. Scheffé's *post hoc* tests indicated that one individual contributed significantly more trials than 5 of the 6 other subjects ($p < .01$). That individual was responsible for 42%, 74%, 73%, and 62% of the trials in the four trial blocks, respectively, and it is of interest to note that he was the highest-ranking individual in the group (rank was based on informal observation of priority of access to food). Further analyses were restricted to the performance of the two high-responding individuals.

The main result of Exp. 2 was that the introduction of a new stimulus group in the second block of the ABBA design produced a dramatic in

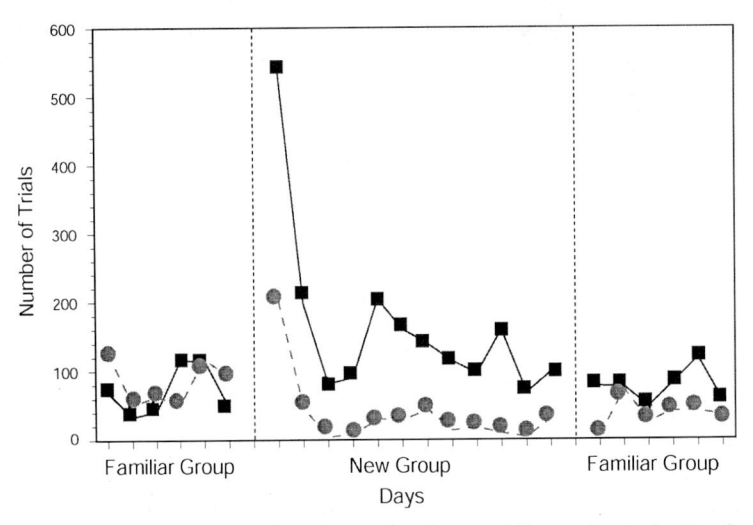

FIG. 2. The number of joystick trials completed successfully per day in the Familiar and New Group Video conditions of Exp. 2 for the two monkeys (Monkey 618 ■, Monkey 889 ●) that completed the vast majority of trials

crease in the number of trials performed by the two focal monkeys. Fig. 2 shows that, for those two monkeys, responding increased on the first day of the New Group Video condition and then rapidly decreased to the same level displayed for the Familiar Group Video condition. When the familiar group was reintroduced, an equivalent increment in activity was not observed.

Discussion

Exp. 1 suggested that food reward was more effective than either video reward condition in eliciting socially housed bonnet macaques to complete a joystick task. However, Exp. 1 also provided some evidence that video of conspecifics was an effective reward for these group-living monkeys. When the effect of the Food Reward condition was removed, the subjects engaged in significantly more trials per day to view video of a novel social group (Other Group Video condition) than to obtain no reward. It should be noted, however, that individual frequencies of responding for video reward conditions may underestimate the effectiveness of video reward in group-housed subjects. In contrast to an indivisible food-pellet reward that could be consumed by only a single individual, multiple individuals could consume, i.e., observe, each video reward. Indeed, it was found that, on average, 2.6 individuals tended to look toward the screen when a video was being presented. Thus, the recorded number of trials per subject for each condition may underestimate the efficacy of video reward for socially housed monkeys because individuals viewed rewards that they did not obtain themselves. In fact, the group generated over 400 video presentations per day in the Other Group Video condition, which is consistent with an average of 400 daily responses when video of conspecifics was a reward for individually housed monkeys (Andrews & Rosenblum, 1993).

This study provides some qualified support for the view that the reward value of video derives, at least in part, from the social content of the video. In Exp. 1, the hypothesis that Other Group Video would be a more effective reward for socially housed bonnet macaques compared to Own Group Video was supported. One strong possibility for these results is that Other Group Video elicited more responding because of its new social content. The Other Group Video condition displayed events and individuals that could be seen only through the task apparatus. In contrast, the Own Group Video displayed familiar individuals and events that were on-going activities in the subjects' enclosures and could consequently be viewed without the test apparatus.

However, there are other possible explanations for the results of Exp. 1. For example, it could be argued that the difference in the effectiveness of Own Group and Other Group Video rewards in eliciting task activity was due to differences in age or sex composition of the groups. However, such an explanation still would support the view that social stimulation is critical. Alternatively, it could be proposed that the videos differed in physical features of the images such as size, shape, or motion. This explanation cannot be completely dismissed, but it should be noted that the pens portrayed in the two video conditions were identical, and a video analysis indicated that Own Group and Other Group Video conditions were comparable in the average number of individuals observed. Indeed, because both Own Group and Other Group Videos were displaying the ongoing activities of natural organisms, and consequently both videos would be characterized as exhibiting a wide range of variation over time in the content of the images presented, e.g., individuals moving in and out of the field of the video camera, it would be difficult to propose a meaningful difference between the videos based upon physical properties alone.

In Exp. 2, the New Group Video elicited higher response rates than the Familiar Group Video, further supporting the hypothesis that video of conspecifics is an effective reward for socially housed bonnet macaques and again indicating that novelty of individuals featured in the videos was the main factor influencing the effectiveness of the videos. The findings of Exp. 2 also suggested that individual differences are likely to be an important consideration in long-term applications of this paradigm. Two monkeys were responsible for a vast majority of the trials in the social-video conditions (88%). Furthermore, the dominant monkey was responsible for the greatest number of trials (65%). Although this relationship may be coincidental, informal observations suggested that the dominant monkey's behavior was most affected by viewing rewards in the Other Group Video condition. This study was not designed to examine the role of dominance; therefore, dominance was not formally assessed but was inferred from informal observations of priority of access. Further work will be necessary to clarify the possible relationship between dominance and efficacy of video of conspecifics as a reward.

The conclusions must be tempered by several facts. First, despite producing response rates that were more than 15 times that of no reward, the effectiveness of social-video reward became statistically significant only after removing the effect of the food-reward condition from the analysis of Exp. 1. Second, difference in preference for the Own Group and Other Group Videos was of only marginal statistical significance despite more than a two-fold difference in the response rates for the two types of rewards (power was low). Third, individual differences were exhibited in Exp. 2, and two monkeys were responsible for the vast majority of trials. In addition, research should involve comparison of the effectiveness of video of conspecifics as a reward with other types of video of animate and inanimate footage. Nevertheless, our results do suggest that at least some socially housed monkeys will perform a complex task to view video of conspecifics. Furthermore, the two experiments reported support the hypothesis that a video of conspecifics can be an effective reward for socially housed monkeys and that the novelty of the individuals in the video is the main factor controlling efficacy of the video for reward.

REFERENCES

ANDREWS, M. W. (1994) An automated identification system for use with computer controlled tasks. *Behavior Research Methods, Instruments, & Computers*, 26, 32-34.

ANDREWS, M. W., BHAT, M. C., & ROSENBLUM, L. A. (1995) Acquisition and long term patterning of joystick selection of food-pellet vs. social video reward by bonnet macaques. *Learning & Motivation*, 26, 370-379.

ANDREWS, M. W., & ROSENBLUM, L. A. (1993) Live-social-video reward maintains joystick task performance in bonnet macaques. *Perceptual and Motor Skills*, 77, 755-763.

ANDREWS, M. W., & ROSENBLUM, L. A. (2001) Effects of change in social content of video rewards on response patterns of bonnet macaques. *Learning & Motivation*, 32, 401-408.

CAPITANIO, J. P., BOCCIA, M. L., & COLAIANNIA, D. J. (1985) The influence of rank on affect perception by pigtailed macaques (*Macaca nemestrina*). *American Journal of Primatology*, 8, 53-59.

PLIMPTON, E. H., ROSENBLUM, L. A., & SWARTZ, K. B. (1981) Response of juvenile bonnet macaques to social stimuli presented through color videotapes. *Developmental Psychobiology*, 14, 109-115.

Accepted March 2, 2004.

"THE SOUND MUST SEEM AN ECHO TO THE SENSE": POPE'S USE OF SOUND TO CONVEY MEANING IN HIS TRANSLATION OF HOMER'S ILIAD[1]

CYNTHIA WHISSELL

Laurentian University

Summary.—In his Essay on Criticism, Pope suggested that sound both could and should be used to convey meaning in poetry. To test his practice of this principle, the 52,000 sounds or phonemes in the first two Books of Pope's translation of the Iliad were scored with the help of Whissell's 2000 classification of sounds in terms of emotional meaning. A chi-squared contingency analysis indicated that there was a preferential and face valid use of Passive sounds in some passages and of Active sounds in others. There was also a significant difference between Books (Book I was more Active) and a distinct pattern of rise and then fall within each of them in the preferential use of Active phonemes.

Alexander Pope, an English poet of the Augustan period, was well aware of the manner in which sounds in poetry can be used to convey meaning. In his Essay on Criticism, written around 1709 (Audra & Williams, 1961, pp. 233-326), Pope affirmed that:

... The *Sound* must seem an *Eccho* to the *Sense*. *Soft* is the Strain when *Zephyr* gently blows, And the *smooth Stream* in *smoother Numbers* flows; But when loud Surges lash the sounding Shore, The *hoarse, rough Verse* shou'd like the *Torrent* roar (lines 365-369).

Pope was familiar with Plato's dialogue *Cratylus* which contrasted the naturalistic and conventional views of the role of sounds in language (Jones, 2002). In the extreme naturalistic view, sounds in the pure language of the gods conveyed information about the true nature of objects. A somewhat muted version of the naturalistic view is currently espoused by sound symbolists (e.g., Whissell, 2000, and to some extent Tsur, 1992), who contended that sounds in words can provide information about objects, actions, or dimensions of sensation and feeling. For sound symbolists, the nature of the sound itself is meaningful and symbolic. According to the extreme conventional view, which is echoed by de Saussure's doctrine of arbitrary relationships between sign and signified (de Saussure, 1983), sounds are arbitrarily employed in the description of objects and are meaningless in and of themselves.

Both extreme positions on the nature of sounds are ridiculed by Socrates in *Cratylus*, and the reader of the dialogue is encouraged to infer that

---

[1]Address enquiries to C. Whissell, Psychology Department, Laurentian University, Sudbury, ON P3E 2C6 Canada.

the sounds in the names of things are *sometimes* meaningful and *sometimes* arbitrary. Students of the use of sound in literature can be placed at different points along a continuum stretched between the two extremes described in *Cratylus*. Whissell (2000) maintained a position closer to the pole of natural meaning than many other students of poetry (e.g., Tsur, 1992). In this position, not every sound is assumed to represent an emotion every time it is used, but sound symbolism is seen as a stratum of meaning that underlies both poetry and the most banal use of language.

In the research described in this article, the first two Books of Pope's Iliad were analyzed specifically in terms of the sounds in them, to assess Pope's practice of his principle that "the sound must seem an echo to the sense." The main hypothesis of the research was that Pope should use sounds differently in different passages to enhance their varying emotional tone, which is not to suggest that sound was the only weapon in Pope's poetic arsenal. Jones (2002) suggested that Pope was sensitive not only to the role of sound but also to the role of rhythm and stress in establishing poetic effect.

Whissell (2000) classified sounds or phonemes in terms of their natural emotional meanings by investigating the proportional frequency of their occurrence in English words of known emotional character. Certain sounds were labelled as Active because they appeared relatively more often in Active words, while others were characterized as Passive because they appeared relatively more often in Passive words ("relatively more often" in this context implies that the null hypothesis of equal distribution of sounds in all types of words was rejected). Examples of Active sounds are those produced by the consonants **g**, **t**, **r**, and by the **er** in the word "murder." Examples of Passive sounds are those produced by the consonants **l** and **m**, the **ah** sound in the word "but" and the **eh** vowel in the word "get." .The relative use of **m** versus **r** and **t** in the third and fifth lines quoted above points to a relative Passivity in the third line (more **m**s) and a relative Activation in the fifth (more **r**s and **t**s). The "smooth stream" was more Passive in sound-tone than the "roaring torrent" which was more Active.

The meaning attached to sounds in Whissell's model (2000) was related to the muscular movements and facial expressions associated with the enunciation of each sound and to the characteristics of the various sound signals produced. Passive sounds were generally those produced by softer mouth positions, e.g., **l**, **ah**, and **eh**, while Active sounds were generally those produced by more rigid mouth positions, e.g., **r**, **er**. Active sounds were often plosives (sounds caused by a mini-explosion of air through the vocal apparatus, e.g., **t**, **g**). Whissell's assignment of meaning to sounds, which was purely statistical, is validated by the existence of systematic relationships between muscle use and sound meaning, and further by the fact that her statistical findings closely match those deduced by other methods and from the study of other languages (as delineated in Whissell, 1999, 2000). A note of caution should be struck, however, in connection with the fact that not all sounds are perceived in the same way in all contexts or in all combinations and patterns. Tsur (1992) mentioned the differing interpretations that attend sibilants in different situations ("hissing" versus "hushing" pp. 3, 43-44). Whissell's assignment of meaning to sound does not allow for such variability in meaning and therefore produces only a rough approximation to sound meaning that is most informative when averaged over a large number of cases. Interestingly enough, Whissell's method assigns no emotional meaning at all to the sibilant s (perhaps it was not possible to identify one particular kind of meaning because the sound was associated with several).

Books I and II of Pope's Iliad were downloaded from www.geocities.com/~bblair/iliad1.htm on 22/02/2003. The sounds or phonemes in them were scored with the help of two computer programs. One program transcribed the English text into phonetic text and a second tabulated the proportional occurrence of Active and Passive phonemes in various passages. Before analysis, the Books were divided into 31 passages according to content. Each passage is briefly described in Fig. 1. The comparisons in this paper were focused on the occurrence of Active and Passive sounds because these seem to be the ones most clearly referred to in Pope's Essay and also because Jones (2002) noted the important role that such sounds played in Pope's translations of the Iliad and Odyssey.

According to a contingency chi-squared analysis, there was a significant relationship ($\chi^2_{60} = 114.54$, $p = .00003$) between the nature of sounds (Active, Neutral, Passive) and passage. Fig. 1 portrays this relationship in terms of a single measure—the percent of average Active sounds in each passage minus the percent of average Passive sounds, where averages were established for the total sample of two Books or 52,000 phonemes. In Fig. 1, the horizontal axis represents passages (1–16 from Book I, 17–31 from Book II) while the vertical axis depicts the relative proportion of Active versus Passive sounds in each passage. For this axis, the zero point indicates that Active and Passive phonemes were both used at average rates for the passage. Positive numbers indicate higher-than-average Activation and negative ones a lower-than-average Activation or Passivity.

The highest proportion of Active sounds in comparison to Passive sounds occurred in the passage describing Achilles' withdrawal from the Greek camp after an argument with Agamemnon (passage 6). Two other Active points of Book I were Achilles' rant against Agamemnon (passage 8) and Thetis's response to Achilles' request for vengeance (passage 12). A relatively high use of Passive sounds in relation to Active sounds was found in the last section of Book I (passage 16), where Vulcan acted as mediator in a

862   C. WHISSELL

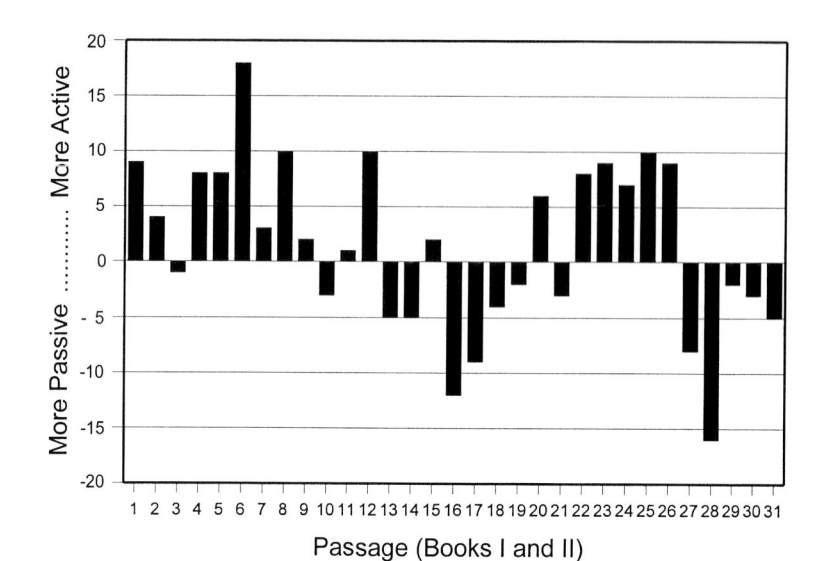

BRIEF OVERVIEW OF PASSAGES

Book I
1 Chryses asks to ransom his daughter Chryseis
2 Agamemnon refuses
3 Chryses calls on Apollo who sends a plague
4 The Greeks call a council
5 Agamemnon demands Briseis: Agamemnon and Achilles argue
6 Achilles withdraws from the Greek camp
7 Minerva stays Achilles' hand
8 Achilles rants against Agamemnon
9 Nestor mediates between Achilles and Agamemnon
10 Agamemnon takes Achilles' Briseis
11 Achilles calls on his Goddess-mother for help
12 Thetis answers
13 Chryseis is returned to Apollo's priest
14 Thesis obtains Jove's aid against Agamemnon
15 Juno argues with Jove about his interference
16 Vulcan mediates among the gods

Book II
17 Jove sends a vision to confuse and scare Agamemnon
18 Agamemnon responds with a stratagem
19 The Greeks prepare for flight
20 Juno and Minerva intervene to stop them
21 Ulysses detains the Greeks from flight
22 Thersites argues with Ulysses
23 Ulysses replies
24 Pallas advises submission to fate
25 Nestor advises a mustering of the troops
26 Agamemnon agrees
27 A propitiatory sacrifice is offered
28 The Greek forces are called out
29 The Greek forces are described in array
30 Achilles is still not with the Greeks
31 The forces ready for battle

FIG. 1. Changes in the use of Active sounds relative to the use of Passive sounds in 31 passages from Books I and II of Pope's translation of Homer's Iliad

conflict among the Greek gods. In Book II, several sequential passages made relatively high use of Active phonemes in describing the Greeks' preparation for flight from the battlefield, and the human and Olympian interventions that forestalled this flight (passages 22–26). The offering of a propitiatory sacrifice ("t'avert the dangers of the doubtful day"), and the calling out of the Greek forces for battle (passages 27, 28), which were both solemn rather than active passages, were characterized by the relative predominance of Passive phonemes. It is evident from Fig. 1 that each Book of Pope's Iliad had a central Activation peak, with scores rising from a quiet beginning to a peak of action and conflict, and then falling again towards the close of the Book. Overall, the second Book was relatively more Passive than the first ($\chi_2^2 = 20.42$, $p = .00004$), likely because it did not include the verbal pyrotechnics associated with the direct conflict between Achilles and Agamemnon.

The coefficient of relationship between passage and the employment of Active and Passive sounds was weak (Cramer $V = .05$). V is interpreted in much the same way as a Pearson product-moment correlation, and .05 would be an extremely weak correlation. Given enough power, however (and in this experiment power comes from the large number of phonemes studied), even such weak relationships may be statistically significant. The weakness of the relationship suggests that the differences encapsulated in Fig. 1 are differences of tone or flavouring, and that there was a considerable overlap between passages in the use of both types of sounds. Although certain kinds of sounds may predominate in certain groups of words, sounds such as **t** and **r** (which are very common in English) occur in both Active and Passive groups. This is evident in a comparison of the third and fifth lines of the quote discussed above, where **t** and **r** appear in both the relatively Passive and the relative Active lines, but more often in the latter. In his translation of the Iliad, Pope did not use one set of sounds for one type of emotion and a totally different set for another: rather he used all the common sounds of the English language, favouring those of an Active nature in some passages and those of a Passive nature in others.

On the basis of the data discussed above, it is possible to conclude that Pope used sounds differentially to convey the emotions associated with various passages, and that he did so in a manner that was face valid. Whissell (1999, 2000) reported many differences in sound use that can be assumed to have been unconscious, i.e., produced without intent, but in the case of Pope the use of sound to establish emotion was likely both conscious and purposeful. Pope's contention that "True Ease in Writing comes from Art, not Chance" (line 362 of the Essay) immediately precedes the material quoted above and confirms that Pope insisted upon a conscious and crafted application of the acknowledged principles of poetics. For him, one such principle was the importance of sound to meaning.

The relationship between sound and meaning is probabilistic and a rigid application of it to individual cases (for example, the insistence that two words including the same sounds must have similar meanings, or that two words with similar meanings must include the same sounds) will lead to some incredible conclusions. Only with large enough samples of language (the size of the sample ensures statistical power and also allows for probabilistic relationships to be discovered) can the "diagnosis" of language in terms of sound have meaning. Sound colours meaning and is part of meaning, but not the whole of meaning. By the same logic, sound colours poetry and is part of poetry, but not the whole of poetry (or even, for some poets, a very large part of poetry). Metaphorically speaking, sound symbolism is like the spice in an award-winning culinary masterpiece: spice forms a very small part of the whole—by weight or by volume—yet it is important enough to change the entire flavour of the whole.

REFERENCES

Audra, E., & Williams, A. (Eds.) (1961) *Alexander Pope: pastoral poetry and an essay on criticism*. London, UK: Methuen.

de Saussure, F. (1983) *Course in general linguistics*. (R. Harris, Transl.) London: Duckworth.

Jones, T. E. (2002) Plato's Cratylus, Dionysius of Halicarnassus, and the correctness of names in Pope's Homer. *The Review of English Studies*, 53, 484-499.

Tsur, R. (1992) *What makes sound patterns expressive? The poetic mode of speech perception*. Durham, NC: Duke Univer. Press.

Whissell, C. (1999) Phonosymbolism and the emotional nature of sounds: evidence of preferential use of particular phonemes in texts of differing emotional tone. *Perceptual and Motor Skills*, 89, 19-48.

Whissell, C. (2000) Phonoemotional profiling: a description of the emotional flavour of English texts on the basis of the phonemes employed in them. *Perceptual and Motor Skills*, 91, 617-648.

Accepted March 8, 2004.

SPATIAL VISUALIZATION OF UNDERGRADUATE EDUCATION MAJORS CLASSIFIED BY THINKING STYLES [1]

HAITHAM M. ALKHATEEB

University of Indianapolis

Summary.—180 undergraduate education majors studying mathematics were administered the Human Information Processing Survey and classified as showing Left ($n = 34$), Right ($n = 38$), Integrated ($n = 28$), or Mixed ($n = 80$) thinking styles. Rotation scores on the Purdue Spatial Visualization Test did not statistically differ among the four groups.

Although the brain functions as a composite whole, research has indicated that specialized cognitive functions can be more closely associated with different parts of the brain (Ornstein, 1997; Gazzaniga, 1998). Some researchers, for instance, indicated that the right hemisphere seems to show greater activation primarily with responses to nonverbal, concrete, spatial, analogic, emotional, and aesthetic materials, while the left hemisphere seems more activated by verbal, analytical, temporal, and digital materials (Torrance, 1982; Gazzaniga, 1985; Fountain & Fillmer, 1987; Springer & Deutsch, 1989). Such differences in the brain functions of each side have been inferred to underlie individuals' different styles of learning and information processing (Albaili, 1996), as individuals tend to endorse items for one thinking style over the other when processing information (Fountain & Fillmer, 1987; Gadzella & Kneipp, 1990; Albaili, 1993). The differences in preferences for information processing have been referred to as thinking styles (Albaili, 1993; Huang & Sisco, 1994; Chao & Huang, 2002) and as hemisphericity (Houtz & Frankel, 1988; Gadzella & Kneipp, 1990; Hassan & Abed, 1999). Style of thinking (hemisphericity) is the influence that an individual relies more on one than the other cerebral hemisphere for information processing (Torrance, 1982). Thinking styles are neither good nor bad, right nor wrong, and tend to remain constant, but they do change (Herrmann, 1995).

Studies have provided evidence for the association of spatial ability with the right hemisphere of the brain (Annett, 1985; Springer & Deutsch, 1989), although Hassan and Abed (1999) examined differences in spatial visualization scores between groups of mathematics teachers from the United Arab Emirates and found no significant differences in spatial visualization be-

---

[1]This work was completed during employment at the Department of Mathematics and Statistics, Miami University, Oxford, OH. Please address correspondence to Dr. Haitham Alkhateeb, Department of Mathematics and Computer Science, University of Indianapolis, Indianapolis, IN 46227 or e-mail (halkhateeb@uindy.edu).

tween subjects classified into Left, Right, and Integrated thinking style groups. Also, research shows that spatial scores are related to mathematical learning (Guay & McDaniel, 1977). Spatial scores, for instance, were related to solving problems in geometry (Battista, 1990). Gazzaniga (1985) and Springer and Deutsch (1989) found that students classified as preferring Right-hemispheric style tend to use spatial ways of dealing with information while those classified as preferring Left style tend to use verbal and analytic approaches to a problem. According to Kitchens, Barber, and Barber (1991), mathematics students who preferred a thinking style related to Right thinking style tended to prefer trigonometry, conics, vectors, and complex numbers. They also reported that most students classified as Left thinking style found it hard to do well in calculus courses. Conflicting evidence shows that college students majoring in mathematics preferred tasks associated with Left Hemisphericity (Monfort, Martin, & Frederickson, 1990). Few assessments have been made of differences in spatial visualization scores in relation to preferred thinking style scores of undergraduate education majors studying mathematics. In this study, differences in scores on spatial visualization between groups classified by scores on the Human Information Survey as showing Left, Right, Integrated, and Mixed styles of thinking were examined. No significant difference among students so classified were expected.

Method

The 180 participants (46% freshmen, 41% sophomores, and 13% juniors) were undergraduates enrolled in five classes of mathematics for education majors. There were 24 men and 156 women whose ages ranged from 18 to 28 years ($M = 18.9$).

Subjects were classified by their scores on the Human Information Processing Survey (Torrance, Taggart, & Taggart, 1984) into one of three groups: Left, Integrated, or Right thinking style. The survey is a self-report on 40 multiple-choice items. The three choices were designed to represent preference for Left, Right, or Integrated thinking style, e.g., "(A) no preference between algebra and geometry, (B) prefer algebra, (C) prefer geometry." A subject selects the alternative that is most descriptive of self. Thirty-four subjects were classified as preferring Left thinking style, 28 as Integrated, and 38 as Right. As 80 subjects did not meet the criterion for any style, they were categorized into a category of Mixed preference (Torrance, et al., 1984). The content validity of the test was described in the manual (Torrance, et al., 1984). Test-retest reliabilities also for graduate students in a class of Creative Thinking were provided by Torrance, et al. (1984).

The Purdue Spatial Visualization Test: Rotations, group-administered test, measured judged mental rotation of three-dimensional objects in drawings (Guay, 1977). Battista, Wheatley, and Talsma (1982) reported the test to be a valid measure of spatial ability. Cronbach alpha was .81 for the present sample.

RESULTS AND DISCUSSION

Table 1 presents the means and standard deviations of the Spatial Visualization scores by groups classified by preferences for Right, Left, Integrated, or Mixed thinking styles. Analysis of variance of scores for these groups showed no significant mean differences among these groups on Spatial Visualization ($F_{3,176} = 2.5$, ns).

TABLE 1
MEANS AND STANDARD DEVIATIONS FOR PURDUE SPATIAL
VISUALIZATION TEST BY INFERRED THINKING STYLE

Thinking Style	n	M	SD
Left	34	13.9	4.1
Integrated	28	15.3	4.5
Right	38	16.7	4.3
Mixed	80	15.8	4.8
Total	180	15.6	4.6

Since the present subjects were enrolled in the second semester of an elementary mathematics content course, it was expected that they would have higher spatial ability (Guay & McDaniel, 1977; Battista, 1980; Springer & Deutsch, 1989). However, the extent to which they reported using various styles depended on the type and complexity of the task employed. For example, complicated tasks would require the function of both the right and left hemispheres, as reported by Nishizawa (1994).

It is necessary to note that the proportion of women who participated in the current study is large. Since Springer and Deutsch (1989) maintained that the relationship between spatial abilities and thinking style may vary by sex, care must be taken in interpretation of this result. Further investigation with larger groups of both sexes is required to explore the association between thinking styles and mental rotation of undergraduate students majoring in education and to identify variables that may allow meaningful interpretation.

REFERENCES

ALBAILI, M. A. (1993) Inferred hemispheric thinking style, gender, and academic major among United Arab Emirates college students. *Perceptual and Motor Skills*, 76, 971-977.

ALBAILI, M. A. (1996) Inferred hemispheric style and problem-solving performance. *Perceptual and Motor Skills*, 83, 427-434.

ANNETT, M. (1985) *Left, right hand brain: the right shift theory*. London: Erlbaum.

BATTISTA, M. (1980) Interrelationships between problem solving ability, right hemisphere processing facility and mathematics learning. *Focus on Learning Problems in Mathematics*, 2, 53-60.

BATTISTA, M. T. (1990) Spatial visualization and gender differences in high school geometry. *Journal for Research in Mathematics Education*, 21, 47-60.

BATTISTA, M. T., WHEATLEY, G. H., & TALSMA, G. (1982) The importance of spatial visualization and cognitive development for geometry learning in preservice elementary teachers. *Journal for Research in Mathematics Education*, 13, 332-340.

CHAO, L., & HUANG, J. (2002) Thinking styles of school teachers and university students in mathematics. *Psychological Reports*, 91, 931-934.

FOUNTAIN, J. C., & FILLMER, H. T. (1987) Hemispheric brain preferences: what are the educational implications? *Reading Improvement*, 24, 252-255.

GADZELLA, B. M., & KNEIPP, L. B. (1990) Differences in comprehension process as a function of hemisphericity. *Perceptual and Motor Skills*, 70, 783-786.

GAZZANIGA, M. S. (1985) *The social brain*. New York: Basic Books.

GAZZANIGA, M. S. (1998) The split brain revisited. *Scientific American*, 279, 35-39.

GUAY, R. B. (1977) *Purdue Spatial Visualization Test: Rotations*. West Lafayette, IN: Purdue Research Foundation.

GUAY, R. B., & MCDANIEL, E. D. (1977) The relationship between mathematics achievement and spatial abilities among elementary school children. *Journal for Research in Mathematics Education*, 8, 211-215.

HASSAN, M. M., & ABED, A. S. (1999) Differences in spatial visualization as a function of scores on hemisphericity of mathematics teachers. *Perceptual and Motor Skills*, 88, 387-390.

HERRMANN, N. (1995) *The creative brain*. (2nd ed.) Quebec, Canada: Quebecor Printing Book Group.

HOUTZ, J. C., & FRANKEL, A. D. (1988) Hemisphericity and problem-solving ability. *Perceptual and Motor Skills*, 66, 771-774.

HUANG, J., & SISCO, B. R. (1994) Thinking styles of Chinese and American adult students in higher education: a comparative study. *Psychological Reports*, 74, 475-480.

KITCHENS, A., BARBER, W. D., & BARBER, D. B. (1991) Left brain/right brain theory: implications for developmental math instruction. *Review of Research in Developmental Education*, 8, 1-6. (ERIC No. ED 354963)

MONFORT, M., MARTIN, S. A., & FREDERICKSON, W. (1990) Information-processing differences and laterality of students from different college disciplines. *Perceptual and Motor Skills*, 70, 163-172.

NISHIZAWA, S. (1994) Cross-cultural effects on hemispheric specialization reflected on a task requiring spatial discrimination of the thumb by Japanese and American students. *Perceptual and Motor Skills*, 78, 771-776.

ORNSTEIN, R. (1997) *The right mind: making sense of the hemispheres*. New York: Harcourt Brace.

SPRINGER, S. P., & DEUTSCH, G. (1989) *Left brain, right brain*. (3rd ed.) New York: Freeman.

TORRANCE, E. P. (1982) Hemisphericity and creative functioning. *Journal of Research and Development in Education*, 15, 29-37.

TORRANCE, E. P., TAGGART, B., & TAGGART, W. (1984) *Human Information Processing Survey*. Bensenville, IL: Scholastic Testing Service.

Accepted March 5, 2004.

HANDEDNESS AND HOBBY PREFERENCE[1]

ORESTIS GIOTAKOS

Tripolis Army Hospital, Greece

Summary.—The objective of this study was to investigate the relationship between handedness and hobby preference in healthy individuals. For this reason, the Annett handedness questionnaire and a standard questionnaire on preference for hobbies were administered to 879 healthy young men (age, $M=22.3$, $SD=4.8$ yr.). Analysis showed more cultured individuals were much less likely to be strongly right-handed. Especially, pure right-handedness highly overrepresented among those who mainly preferred doing sports, pure left-handedness among those who preferred reading books, collecting, or going to the cinema/theater, and mixed-handedness among those who preferred arts, like playing music, drawing, or handicraft. The findings support evidence that handedness is associated with hobby preference.

It has been suggested that left-hemisphere dominant individuals approach the world more analytically, whereas the right-hemisphere dominant individuals tend to approach situations from a more holistic perspective (Bogen, 1997). In addition, right-hemisphere dominance is considered to be associated with superior visuospatial and mathematical ability (Smith, Meyers, & Kline, 1989), as well as with talent in arts like architecture, sculpture, and music (Peterson, 1974, 1979, 1980; Mebert & Michel, 1980).

In the current study the relationship between handedness and hobby preference was investigated, i.e., studying the handedness in a group of young men, in relation to their hobby preference, and hypothesizing that the more cultured individuals will be less likely to be strongly right-handed. Although nonright-handedness is generally not considered pathological, the belief that at least some deviations from normal right-handedness is traceable to disease or brain damage remains widespread (Previc, 1996; Giotakos, 2001, 2002). For this reason, the relationship between handedness and hobby preference was investigated in healthy individuals.

Method

Eight hundred seventy-nine men (age, $M=22.3$, $SD=4.8$ yr.), who were recruits following the basic training in the Greek army, consented to participate. They were all healthy because all recruits are screened for mental and physical diseases, and anyone with severe symptoms was excluded. All subjects were asked for their hobby preference, and they were classified according to their main preference of (1) reading books, collecting, and going

---

[1]Please address correspondence to O. Giotakos, M.D., 2 Erifilis str, Athens 11634, Greece or e-mail (giotakos@tri.forthnet.gr).

to the cinema/theater, (2) doing sport, and (3) doing art, like playing music, drawing, and handicraft. All were administered the Annett Hand Preference Questionnaire (1970, 1985; see McMeekan & Lishman, 1975; for additional psychometric data) which assesses hand preference according to the stated and demonstrated preference for 12 discrete actions. Subjects stated and demonstrated "right," "left," or "either" for each action. Based on his response pattern, the subject was assigned to one of eight categories outlined by Annett. According to the "broad" definition of mixed-handedness (cf. discussion by Malesu, Cannon, Jones, McKenzie, Gilvary, Rifkin, Toone, & Murray 1996), subjects were considered to be mixed-handers, if they were not totally right or left-handed (Annett classes 2 to 7). Pure right- and pure left-handers were considered to be the Annett groups 1 and 8, respectively. After an overall 3 × 3 table of chi square, data were analyzed with Mantel-Haenszel odds-ratio and 2 × 2 chi-squared analysis using Fisher's two-tailed probability tests.

RESULTS

The overall 3 × 3 table of chi square was statistically significant ($p < .009$). There were 508 (58%) pure right-handers (Annett class 1), 31 (3%) pure left-handers (Annett class 8), and 340 (39%) mixed-handers (Annett classes 2 to 7) among 879 individuals. Table 1 shows the proportion of subjects classified according their hobby preferences. The frequency of pure right-handedness among subjects who preferred sports was significantly higher than the frequency of pure right-handedness of subjects who did not prefer sports (61.6% vs 51.4%, Odds Ratio: 1.51, 95% CI: 1.1–2.0, $p < .002$). The frequency of pure left-handedness in the subjects who preferred read-

TABLE 1
HOBBY PREFERENCE IN RELATION TO HANDEDNESS IN 879 HEALTHY MEN

Hobbies	Pure Right-handedness f	Pure Right-handedness %	Mixed-handedness f	Mixed-handedness %	Pure Left-handedness f	Pure Left-handedness %
Reading books, collecting, going to cinema/theater	74	52	59	41	10	7
Sports	340	61	197	36	15	3
Arts: playing music, drawing, handicraft	94	51	84	46	6	3
Total	508	58	340	39	31	3

*3 × 3 chi-square test value: 13.4, df: 4, $p < .009$.

ing, collecting, and going to the cinema/theater, was significantly higher than the frequency of pure left-handedness of subjects who did not prefer these hobbies (7.0% vs 2.9%, Odds Ratio: 2.56, 96% CI: 1.1–5.5, $p < .02$). Finally, the frequency of mixed-handedness of subjects who preferred art, such as playing music, drawing, and handicraft, was higher than that of mixed-handedness for subjects who did not prefer art (45.7% vs 36.8%, Odds Ratio: 1.44, 95% CI: 1.0–2.0, $p < .02$).

Discussion

The main limitation of this study was the lack of a female comparison group; however, the present young males were fairly representative of the general population because military service is compulsory for all males in Greece, while individuals suffering from serious physical and mental disorders are exempted. It should be noted also that during last years Greek parents do not discourage left-handedness.

Right-handedness was highly represented or more like the general population among the present subjects who preferred sports. Previous studies showed a high proportion of left-handers among top sportsmen (Grouios, Tsorbatzoudis, Alexandris, & Barkoukis, 2000; Holtzen, 2000), but this superiority of the left-handers in many sports may reflect the nature of the specific sports and not an innate neurological advantage (Wood & Aggleton, 1989). In addition, Grouios, et al. (2000) found the excess of left handers among sporting competitors applies only to competitors in interactive or confrontational sports, i.e., basketball or boxing, and not to competitors in noninteractive or nonconfrontational sports, i.e., cycling, running, or swimming in which left-handers occur about as frequently as they do in the nonsporting population.

Pure left-handedness was highly represented among the subjects who preferred reading books, collecting, and going to the cinema/theater, while mixed-handedness was highly represented among the subjects who preferred art, such as playing music, drawing, and handicraft. Although the educational achievement was not assessed, we can suggest that as a whole, the more cultured conscripts were much less likely to be strongly right-handed. These findings can be discussed in parallel with previous findings which suggested that right-hemisphere dominance may be associated with talent in architecture, sculpture, mathematics, and music (Peterson, 1974, 1979, 1980; Mebert & Michel, 1980; Smith, et al., 1989). Recent studies suggest that left hemisphere-dominant individuals tend to be self-controlled, introverted, and with strong leadership qualities, while right hemisphere-dominant individuals have been described as extroverted, independent, intuitive, and as tending to approach situations from a holistic perspective (Power & Lundsten, 1997; Gadzella, 1999). In most of these studies such remarks have been inferences rather than hard or direct measurement of cerebral function by fMRI, for example. The present findings are consistent with an association between handedness and preference for hobbies or self-amusements. This might provide useful suggestions to the educational system, which, although it uses methods associating learning process with pleasure or playing, is mainly based on a linear model of thinking, characterized by learning piece by piece (Vitale, 1982).

REFERENCES

ANNETT, M. (1970) A classification of hand preference by association analysis. *British Journal of Psychiatry*, 61, 303-321.
ANNETT, M. (1985) *Left, right, hand and brain: the right shift theory.* London: Erlbaum.
BOGEN, J. E. (1997) Some educational implications of hemisphere specialization. In M. C. Wittrock (Ed.), *The human brain.* Englewood Cliffs, NJ: Prentice Hall. Pp. 8-76.
GADZELLA, B. M. (1999) Differences among cognitive processing styles groups on personality traits. *Journal of Instructional Psychology*, 26, 161-166.
GIOTAKOS, O. (2001) Narrow and broad definition of mixed handedness in male psychiatric patients. *Perceptual and Motor Skills*, 93, 631-638.
GIOTAKOS, O. (2002) Crossed hand-eye dominance in male psychiatric patients. *Perceptual and Motor Skills*, 95, 728-732.
GROUIOS, G., TSORBATZOUDIS, H., ALEXANDRIS, K., & BARKOUKIS, V. (2000) Do left-handed competitors have an innate superiority in sports. *Perceptual and Motor Skills*, 90, 1273-1282.
HOLTZEN, D. W. (2000) Handedness and professional tennis. *International Journal of Neuroscience*, 105, 101-119.
MALESU, R. R., CANNON, M., JONES, P. B., MCKENZIE, K., GILVARY, K., RIFKIN, L., TOONE, B. K., & MURRAY, R. M. (1996) Mixed handedness in patients with functional psychosis. *British Journal of Psychiatry*, 168, 234-236.
MCMEEKAN, E. R. I., & LISHMAN, W. A. (1975) Retest reliabilities and interrelationships of the Annett Hand Preference Questionnaire and the Edinburg Handedness Inventory. *British Journal of Psychology*, 66, 53-59.
MEBERT, C. J., & MICHEL, G. E. (1980) Handedness in artists. In J. H. Herron (Ed.), *Neuropsychology of left-handedness.* New York: Academic Press. Pp. 273-278.
PETERSON, J. M. (1974) Left handedness among architects: some facts and speculation. *Perceptual and Motor Skills*, 38, 547-550.
PETERSON, J. M. (1979) Left-handedness: differences between student artists and scientists. *Perceptual and Motor Skills*, 48, 961-962.
PETERSON, J. M. (1980) Success in architecture: handedness and visual thinking. *Perceptual and Motor Skills*, 50, 1139-1143.
POWER, S. J., & LUNDSTEN, L. L. (1997) Studies that compare type theory and left-brain/right-brain theory. *Journal of Psychological Type*, 43, 22-28.
PREVIC, F. H. (1996) Nonright-handedness, central nervous system and related pathology, and its lateralization: a reformulation and synthesis. *Developmental Neuropsychology*, 12, 443-515.
SMITH, B. D., MEYERS, M. B., & KLINE, R. (1989) For better or worse: left handedness, pathology, and talent. *Journal of Clinical and Experimental Neuropsychology*, 11, 944-958.
VITALE, B. (1982) *Unicorns are real: a right brain approach to learning.* New York: Jalmar Press.
WOOD, C. J., & AGGLETON, J. P. (1989) Handedness in "fast ball" sports: do left handers have an innate advantage? *British Journal of Psychology*, 80, 227-240.

Accepted March 12, 2004.

INFLUENCE OF ALCOHOL INTAKE ON THE PARAMETERS EVALUATING THE BODY CENTER OF FOOT PRESSURE IN A STATIC UPRIGHT POSTURE [1]

MASAHIRO NODA	SHINICHI DEMURA
Jin-ai University	*Department of Physical Education Kanazawa University*
SHUNSUKE YAMAJI	TAMOTSU KITABAYASHI
Fukui National College of Technology	*Graduate School of Natural Science and Technology Kanazawa University*

Summary.—To examine the influence of alcohol intake on various parameters evaluating the change in body center of foot pressure during a static upright posture, 11 healthy young males and females gave measures of blood pressure, heart rate, whole body reaction time, standing on one leg with eyes closed, and body stability for 60 sec. in the Romberg posture (open eyes, closed feet) before and after the alcohol intake. The measurement was made with an Anima's stabilometer G5500. Data sampling frequency was 20 Hz. The subjects drank alcohol (Japanese sake 540 ml) within 10 min. After 10, 20, and 30 min. of alcohol intake, the same measurements were carried out. 24 parameters with higher trial-to-trial reliability were selected from the following 7 domains: distance, mean center of foot pressure, distribution of amplitude, area, velocity, frequency (power spectrum), and direction (vector) of body-sway and velocity. Parameters for distance, velocity, and area of body-sway significantly changed after alcohol intake, but the mean center of foot pressure and frequency of body-sway were unchanged. It was inferred that the mean center of foot pressure and frequency for body-sway did not change even if a nervous function decreased by the alcohol intake, and an upright posture was maintained by increasing the distance, area, and velocity of body-sway. Further, body-sway tends to increase in the medial/lateral direction as compared with the anterior/posterior direction.

Static upright posture of human beings is controlled by integrating afferent signals from vestibular and semicircular ducts, visuosensory, propriospinal reflex, and somatosensory systems in the cerebellum and brainstem (Markham, 1987; Baker, Newstead, Mossberg, & Nicodemus, 1998). It has been clarified that the people with disequilibrium cannot integrate these afferent signals (labyrinthine vertigo, Parkinsonism, etc.), show a unique sway type around the body center of foot pressure (CFP) during static upright posture (Kanter, Rubin, Armstrong, & Cummins, 1991). The center of foot pressure test is used as a useful test to screen disequilibrium in clinical set-

---

[1]Address correspondence to Shunsuke Yamaji, Fukui National College of Technology, Geshi, Sabae, Fukui 916-8507, Japan or e-mail (yamaji@fukui-nct.ac.jp).

tings (Goldie, Bach, & Evans, 1989; Dickstein & Dvir, 1993). That is, it is possible to assess the state of standing posture control observed at the center of foot pressure. However, because center of foot pressure is a conclusive output that includes various physiological mechanisms for posture control, it is difficult to assess the physical and physiological function using center of foot pressure. On the other hand, many researchers have examined the possibility of the center of foot pressure test during static upright posture as a balance test for healthy people (Kapteyn, Bles, Njiokiktjien, Kodde, Massen, & Mol, 1983; Ekdahl, Jarnlo, & Andersson, 1989; Goldie, et al., 1989; Geurts, Nienhuis, & Mulder, 1993; Nakagawa, Ohashi, Watanabe, & Mizukoshi, 1993; Woolley, Rubin, Kanter, & Armstrong, 1993; Baker, et al., 1998). Although they proposed many parameters from time-series center of foot pressure data moving on a two-dimensional coordinate plane, parameters regarding distance or area of body-sway have not been sufficiently examined to evaluate balancing by healthy people. Static upright posture of human beings is controlled by integrating afferent signals as stated above, and, in addition, lower and trunk muscle strength significantly affects postural control. Previous studies have shown body-sway in a static upright posture is larger with aging. Since muscle strength and nervous function decrease with aging, it is not clear that the contribution for the increase of body-sway with aging is as large in either function as the physiological mechanism. Therefore, we hypothesized that, when the nervous function transiently declines, the relationship between center of foot pressure parameters and postural control can clarify by dividing into the parameters which are influenced by decline of nervous function. Stimulation of visual perception, alcohol intake, or physical fatigue are considered stimulation disturbances in the decline of nervous function.

Alcohol intake causes a nervous function decline, leads to an inhibition of the central nervous system, and dilatation of blood vessels, and brings decreases in perception, concentration, judgment, coordination, balance, and memory. Moreover, an effect on autokinesia and reflex movement systems has been recorded. Many researchers have examined the relationship between alcohol intake and postural control or balance. However, few studies have examined the relationship between alcohol intake and center of foot pressure parameters. Mangold, Laubli, and Krueger (1996) examined the influence of alcohol intake on bipedal and monopedal balance, fine motor activity, and mental performance. They reported that, although fine motor activity and mental performance were not significantly declined, the distance parameter of center of foot pressure was significantly larger. In fact, it is suggested that the distance parameter of center of foot pressure is affected immediately by alcohol intake. Kubo, Sakata, Matsunaga, Koshimune, Sakai, Ameno, and Ijiri (1989) reported that blood alcohol concentration (BAC) correlated moderately with the distance, area, and velocity of center of foot pressure parameters. Moreover, Uimonen, Laitakari, Bloigu, Reinila, and Sorri (1994) and Nieschalk, Ortmann, West, Schmal, Stoll, and Fechner (1999) also reported that these center of foot pressure parameters were larger with alcohol intake. Most previous studies have examined the influence of alcohol intake by focusing on the change of the distance, area, and velocity of center of foot pressure parameters, but few studies have focused on change in the period, direction, or center of body-sway. These parameters possibly assess the qualitative aspects of body-sway differently from the quantitative aspects such as the distance, area, and velocity of center of foot pressure parameters. Although alcohol intake makes the body-sway increase, it is not clear whether it affects the body-sway pattern or upright posture during static upright postural control. The relationship between the physiological mechanism of postural control and body-sway evaluated by center of foot pressure parameters may clarify this viewpoint.

The purpose of this study was to clarify the influence of a decline in nervous functions by alcohol intake on various body-sway parameters during static upright posture.

Method

Subjects

Five healthy young men (ages: 20.4 yr. ± 0.55, height: 175.2 ± 6.45 cm, weight: 69.9 ± 7.94 kg) and six women (ages 21.5 yr. ± 2.03, height: 160.5 ± 5.72 cm, weight: 60.1 ± 7.92 kg) participated. Subjects were enrolled in a university and participated as volunteers. The subjects had no evidence or known history of a gait, postural, or skeletal disorder. Their physical characteristics approximated the standard values of the same age cohort in Japan (Laboratory of Physical Education in Tokyo Metropolitan University, 2000). Informed consent was obtained from each subject after a full explanation of the experimental project and its procedures.

Experimental Equipment

Postural static was evaluated using a stabilometer (G5500, Anima Inc., Japan) to measure the time-series of the subject's center of foot pressure. The center of foot pressure of vertical load with this instrument was calculated from values of three sensors on the peak of the isosceles triangle of a level surface. The sampling frequency was 20 Hz.

Evaluation Parameters

Twenty-four body-sway parameters (Demura, Yamaji, Noda, Kitabayashi, & Nagasawa, 2001; Yamaji, Demura, Noda, Nagasawa, Nakada, & Kitabayashi, 2001) were selected from the following seven domains (Table 1): distance (2 parameters), area (2 parameters), mean center of foot pres-

TABLE 1
CENTER OF FOOT PRESSURE (CFP) PARAMETERS

Parameter	Property
Distance	
1 Mean path length, cm/sec.	M length of center of foot pressure (CFP) path
2 Root mean square, cm	Equation: $\sqrt{[(\sum X_i - \bar{X})^2 + (\sum Y_i - \bar{Y})^2]/N}$ Dispersion from CFP
Displacement	
3 Mean CFP of X-axis, cm	M displacement of CFP for X- and Y-axis
4 Mean CFP of Y-axis, cm	
Amplitude	
5 SD of X-axis sway, cm	Equation: $S_X = \sqrt{\Sigma(X_i - \bar{X})^2/N}$
6 SD of Y-axis sway, cm	Equation: $S_Y = \sqrt{\Sigma(Y_i - \bar{Y})^2/N}$
Area	
7 Area surrounding maximal amplitude rectangle, cm^2	Area surrounding maximal amplitude rectangular for each axis
8 Area surrounding SD ellipse, cm^2	Ellipse area with the radius of body-sway for X, Y-axis
Velocity	
9 M velocity of X-axis sway, cm/sec.	M velocity of X-, Y-axis for body-sway
10 M velocity of Y-axis sway, cm/sec.	
Frequency of sway (power spectrum)	
11 Ratio of A domain for power spectrum of R-axis sway, %	Power spectrum area by the furier translate for the body-sway value (X-, Y-, R-direction) divided A, B, C, domain. A domain: 0–0.2 Hz, B domain: 0.2–2 Hz, C domain: above 2 Hz
12 Ratio of B domain for power spectrum of R-axis sway, %	
13 Ratio of C domain for power spectrum of R-axis sway, %	
Frequency of velocity (power spectrum)	
14 Ratio of A domain for power spectrum of R-axis velocity, %	Power spectrum area by the furier translate for the body-sway velocity (X-, Y-, R-direction) divided A, B, C, domain. A domain: 0–0.2 Hz, B domain: 0.2–2 Hz, C domain: above 2 Hz
15 Ratio of B domain for power spectrum of R-axis velocity, %	
16 Ratio of C domain for power spectrum of R-axis velocity, %	

(continued on next page)

Parameter	Property
Direction of sway	M distance of body-sway in 4 directions (A to H)
17 M vector length of A direction sway, cm	
18 M vector length of C direction sway, cm	
19 M vector length of E direction sway, cm	
20 M vector length of G direction sway, cm	
Direction of velocity	M distance of body-sway velocity in 4 directions (A to H)
21 M vector length of A direction velocity, cm/sec.	
22 M vector length of C direction velocity, cm/sec.	
23 M vector length of E direction velocity, cm/sec.	
24 M vector length of G direction velocity, cm/sec.	

sure (2 parameters), amplitude (2 parameters), velocity (2 parameters), frequency of sway and velocity (power spectrum)(6 parameters), and direction of sway and body-sway velocity (vector) (8 parameters). These parameters were developed based on logical validity and had high trial-to-trial and day-to-day reliability parameters in previous studies (Demura, et al., 2001; Yamaji, et al., 2001).

Blood pressure and heart rate were measured with an auto-hemodynamometer to check the subject's body condition before and after the alcohol intake. The nervous function tests for whole body reaction time and standing time on one leg with eyes closed were done before and after the alcohol intake to confirm the decline of the global coordination system. The former (whole body reaction) test measured the reaction time from light stimulation from the measurement instrument to jumping from the plate (Takei Co., Ltd., whole body reaction type II). The measurement was carried out five times, and the mean value of data for three trials, except the maximal and minimal data, was used for further analysis. The latter (standing time on one leg with eyes closed) test measured the continuous time with one leg standing and eyes closed. Both hands set on the waist, and another with the leg raised up and forward were measured twice, and the mean value of the two trials was used for further analysis.

Experimental Procedure

Fig. 1 shows the experimental procedure in this study. The subject's physical and mental conditions and fatigue feeling were noted on a 5-point scale (condition: 1 = very good and 5 = very poor, fatigue: 1 = not at all and 5 = very tired) during a rest for 30 min. before measurement. The measurement was called off if subject's rating was above 3 points. Platform stabilometry during 60 sec. in an upright Romberg posture (open eyes and feet together) was done twice with 1 min. rest after the measurement of blood pressure and heart rate. The measurement procedure for platform stabilometry followed the test standard by Kapteyn, et al. (1983). The subjects were asked to hold their upper extremities at their sides while looking straight ahead to the center of an eye-level target and to stand in a quiet stance with eyes open on a stable platform. The subjects drank 540 ml of alcohol (Japanese sake) during 10 min. after the nervous function tests. Thus, they drank 1.00–1.37 ml/kg alcohol standardized by body mass. Blood alcohol concentration (BAC) for each subject was calculated using the equation for estimation. The average euhydration volume in young adults is approximately two-thirds of body mass. Since the specific gravity of ethyl alcohol is 0.794, the gravity of alcohol intake volume (540 ml, 15%) is 64.314 g (540 × 0.15 × 0.794 = 64.314). Therefore, BAC was indicated from the gravity ratio between alcohol intake and average euhydration volume {64.314/[2 × body mass (g)]}/

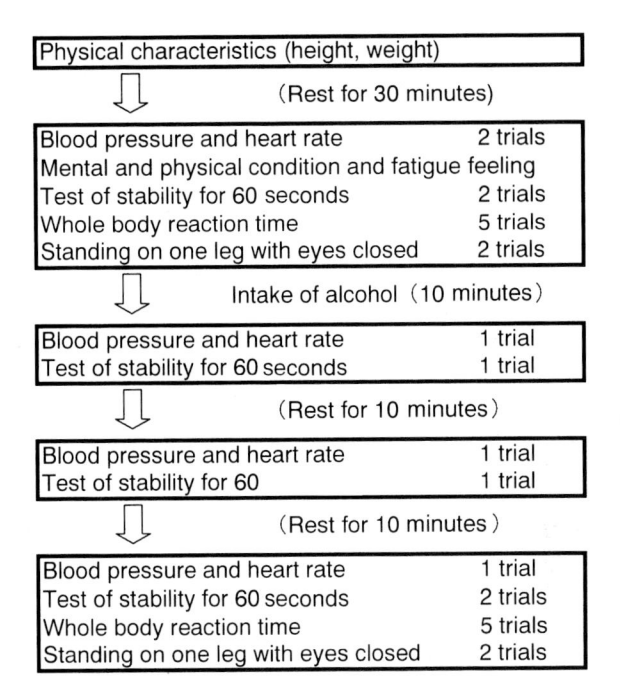

Physical characteristics (height, weight)	
⇩ (Rest for 30 minutes)	
Blood pressure and heart rate	2 trials
Mental and physical condition and fatigue feeling	
Test of stability for 60 seconds	2 trials
Whole body reaction time	5 trials
Standing on one leg with eyes closed	2 trials
⇩ Intake of alcohol (10 minutes)	
Blood pressure and heart rate	1 trial
Test of stability for 60 seconds	1 trial
⇩ (Rest for 10 minutes)	
Blood pressure and heart rate	1 trial
Test of stability for 60	1 trial
⇩ (Rest for 10 minutes)	
Blood pressure and heart rate	1 trial
Test of stability for 60 seconds	2 trials
Whole body reaction time	5 trials
Standing on one leg with eyes closed	2 trials

FIG. 1. Experimental procedure

3}. BAC for each subject was in the range of 0.11–0.18%. It is inferred that the subject was in a state of alcoholic drunkenness. The blood pressure, heart rate, and platform stabilometry were measured at 10, 20, and 30 min. after alcohol intake. The nervous function tests were performed at 30 min. after alcohol intake. All measurements were done from 10:00–12:00 a.m. The subjects were instructed not to eat, drink, or exercise for 2 hr. before the measurement. We confirmed in the pilot experiments that the parameters (stability performance, blood pressure, and heart rate) in the experimental protocol did not influence the bias (fatigue or subject's concentration).

Data Analysis

A repeated-measures one-way analysis of variance was used to examine the mean difference in body-sway parameters before and after alcohol intake. Tukey *HSD* method was used for multiple comparison tests. The probability level of .05 was considered as indicative of statistical significance.

RESULTS AND DISCUSSION

Physical and Mental Conditions and Nervous Function Tests

Fig. 2 shows the test results of one-way analysis of variance of selected parameters. Although the diastolic and systolic blood pressures were significantly unchanged after alcohol intake, the heart rate significantly increased (10, 20, 30 min.). Nervous function tests showed a significant change. Namely, the whole body reaction time became longer and the standing time on one leg with eyes closed became shorter (Fig. 2).

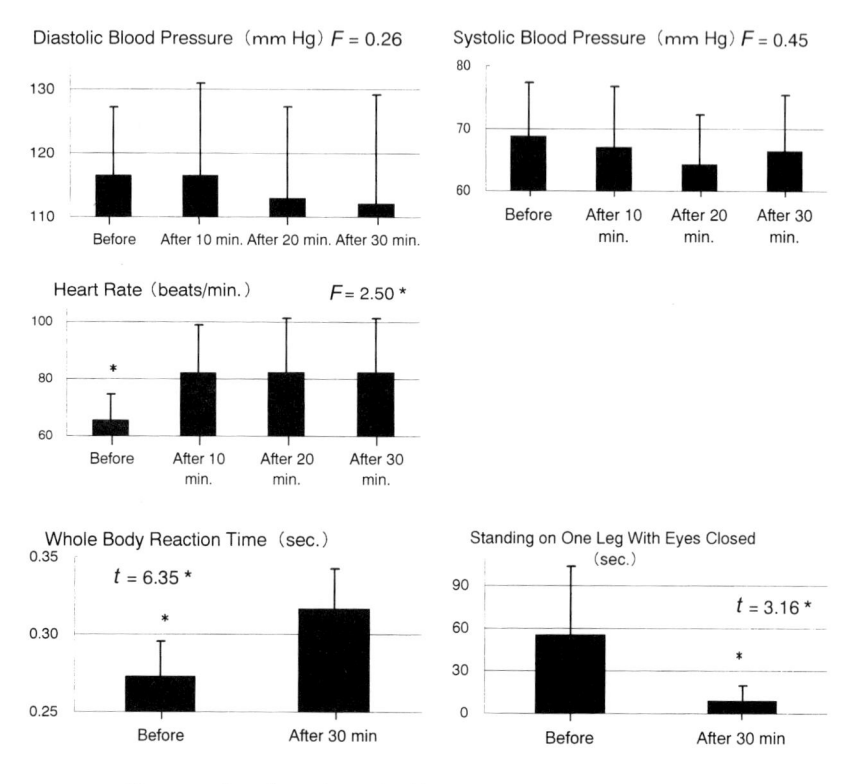

FIG. 2. Change in diastolic and systolic blood pressure, pulse, whole body reaction time, and standing time on one leg with eyes closed before and after the intake of alcohol. *Significant difference before and after the intake of alcohol ($p < .05$).

Comparison of Parameters Regarding Body-sway Before and After Alcohol Intake

Fig. 3 shows the typical pattern of the center of foot pressure change before and after alcohol intake in a subject. All subjects tended to increase the center of foot pressure change. There were significant differences in all parameters except for mean center of foot pressure for the X and Y directions, and the total area ratio of the power spectrum for body-sway (cf. Table 2). There were significant differences for all parameters except for mean center

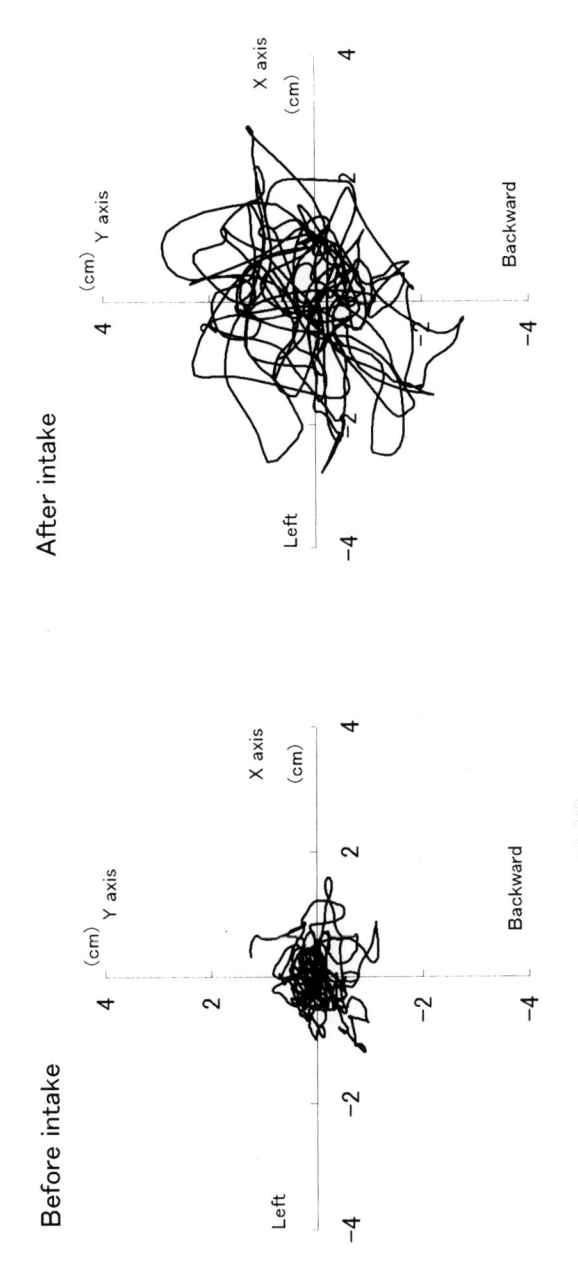

Fig. 3. The typical pattern of the CFP change before and after alcohol intake by a subject

TABLE 2
RESULTS OF ONE-WAY ANALYSES OF VARIANCE ON PARAMETERS OF BODY-SWAY

Parameter	Before Intake M	Before Intake SD	After Intake 10 min. M	10 min. SD	20 min. M	20 min. SD	30 min. M	30 min. SD	F	Post hoc Tukey HSD
Distance										
M path length, cm/sec.	0.88	0.16	1.76	0.66	2.05	0.88	2.15	1.45	8.60*	A3, A2, A1 > B
Root mean square, cm	0.65	0.17	1.35	0.59	1.39	0.56	1.46	0.72	9.59*	A3, A2, A1 > B
Displacement (M CFP), cm										
X-axis	0.34	0.64	0.07	0.62	0.01	0.82	0.11	0.57	0.81	
Y-axis	−1.70	1.62	−1.94	1.71	−2.09	1.62	−1.77	1.36	0.31	
Amplitude, (SD), cm										
X-axis sway	0.43	0.14	0.81	0.35	0.86	0.32	0.87	0.34	9.10*	A3, A2, A1 > B
Y-axis sway	0.47	0.17	1.07	0.50	1.08	0.48	1.16	0.65	8.74*	A3, A2, A1 > B
Area, cm²										
Maximal amplitude rectangle	5.80	3.21	29.06	21.77	32.13	22.36	35.71	32.28	6.79*	A3, A2, A1 > B
SD ellipse	0.63	0.29	3.19	2.38	3.36	2.50	3.79	3.78	6.08*	A3, A2, A1 > B
Velocity (M), cm/sec.										
X-axis sway	0.55	0.12	1.01	0.31	1.22	0.48	1.20	0.62	12.53*	A3, A2, A1 > B
Y-axis sway	0.47	0.09	1.07	0.50	1.24	0.59	1.35	1.12	6.49*	A3, A2, A1 > B
Frequency of sway (power spectrum), %										
Ratio of A domain	28.30	4.83	24.96	6.49	22.99	4.79	24.46	7.56	1.66	
Ratio of B domain	58.60	5.84	62.61	4.78	64.34	5.38	61.06	7.31	2.21	
Ratio of C domain	13.11	2.96	12.43	4.08	12.67	3.30	14.48	4.26	0.59	
Frequency of velocity (power spectrum), %										
Ratio of A domain	9.04	1.81	9.80	1.28	11.28	3.07	9.92	1.48	3.17*	A2 > B
Ratio of B domain	49.67	3.72	54.20	4.84	54.78	3.43	54.19	3.77	5.55*	A3, A2, A1 > B
Ratio of C domain	41.29	4.94	35.99	5.03	33.93	3.77	35.89	3.46	768*	B1 > A1, A2, A3

(continued on next page)

TABLE 2 (CONT'D)
RESULTS OF ONE-WAY ANALYSES OF VARIANCE ON PARAMETERS OF BODY-SWAY

Parameter	Before Intake M	Before Intake SD	After Intake 10 min. M	10 min. SD	20 min. M	20 min. SD	30 min. M	30 min. SD	F	Post hoc Tukey HSD
Direction of sway (M vector length), cm										
A direction sway	0.57	0.28	1.46	0.73	1.51	0.76	1.54	0.90	7.91*	A3, A2, A1 > B
C direction sway	0.52	0.15	1.08	0.45	1.08	0.46	1.08	0.39	9.87*	A3, A2, A1 > B
E direction sway	0.57	0.17	1.15	0.56	1.21	0.48	1.26	0.56	9.30*	A3, A2, A1 > B
G direction sway	0.53	0.19	1.00	0.60	1.06	0.44	1.04	0.38	5.27*	A3, A2, A1 > B
Direction of velocity (M vector length), cm										
A direction velocity	0.72	0.16	1.80	0.82	1.98	0.87	2.15	1.63	7.23*	A3, A2, A1 > B
C direction velocity	0.84	0.17	1.71	0.62	1.87	0.71	1.85	0.87	13.66*	A3, A2, A1 > B
E direction velocity	0.77	0.16	1.78	0.98	1.99	1.05	2.15	1.85	6.09*	A3, A2, A1 > B
G direction velocity	0.90	0.20	1.58	0.50	1.94	0.74	2.05	1.12	11.14*	A3, A2, A1 > B

of foot pressure for the X and Y directions, and the total ratio of the power spectrum for body-sway. The values of these parameters became larger after alcohol intake, except the C area ratio of the power spectrum of body-sway velocity. There were no significant differences among 10, 20, and 30 min. on all parameters.

Comments

It has been reported that alcohol intake inhibits the central nervous function, dilates blood vessels, and decreases performance related to global nervous functions such as reaction time, hand-eye coordination, and balance (Franks, Hensley, Hensley, Starmer, & Teo, 1976; Roebuck, Simmons, Mattson, & Riley, 1998; Nieschalk, *et al.*, 1999). The performance on nervous function tests in this study changed significantly after alcohol intake. Persons with a nervous function abnormality showed a body-sway distinct from disequilibrium cases such as labyrinthine vertigo and Parkinsonism (Kanter, *et al.*, 1991). Alcohol intake causes a temporary nervous function decline and influences the center of foot pressure sway. It is interesting to note which parameters widely used by many researchers strongly influence body-sway with a nervous function decline. Previous studies (Franks, *et al.*, 1976; Kubo, *et al.*, 1989; Unimonen, *et al.*, 1994; Roebuck, *et al.*, 1998; Nieschalk, *et al.*, 1999) examined the influence of alcohol intake on the body-sway parameters, mainly distance, area, and velocity, reporting that all parameters increased after alcohol intake. Their results agree with those of this study. The values for their parameters for all subjects in this study increased even after alcohol intake. Kubo, *et al.* (1989) stated that the sway area was the most sensitive parameter relating to the body-sway change after alcohol intake. Unimonen, *et al.* (1994) reported that the body-sway velocity was more effective than area in evaluating body-sway change after alcohol intake. Alcohol intake causes a decrease in the cerebral cortex function and physiological changes to neurocyte matter and then inhibits synapse transmission. Namely, alcohol intake affects the global nervous system related to body-sway. Therefore, the influence appears remarkable for parameters regarding the magnitude of body-sway. The nervous function decline with alcohol intake may need a larger range of body-sway to keep a stable upright posture.

This study examined the influence of alcohol intake for 24 body-sway parameters including the amplitude, frequency (power spectrum), and direction (vector) in the center of foot pressure sway and body-sway velocity, which have not been examined to date. The mean center of foot pressure for X and Y directions, total area ratios of the power spectrum for body-sway did not largely change. Taguchi and Yoda (1976) reported that the time-varying parameters for mean center of foot pressure are influenced by each individual's posture and skeleton. Kitabayashi, Demura, Yamaji, Nakada, Noda, and Imaoka (2002) reported that the distance and velocity parameters related to the height and length of lower limbs, and the parameters for mean center of foot pressure and body-sway frequency related to body composition. Therefore, it is inferred that the parameters regarding the magnitude of body-sway are influenced by both factors of body linearity and nervous function, whereas the parameters regarding mean center of foot pressure and body-sway frequency are influenced more strongly by body physique and body composition than by nervous function. Moreover, it is assumed that there was a postural control attempt to maintain a similar frequency of body-sway by making sway-size greater because the frequency of body-sway hardly changed after alcohol intake in spite of producing a greater distance and velocity. In the Romberg posture for closed feet, the medial/lateral axis as a support basis (foot length × foot width) is shorter (narrower) than for the anterior/posterior axis. This can be explained as one of the causes for the distance, area, and velocity after alcohol intake on the medial/lateral axis, changing remarkably as compared with the anterior/posterior axis. Further, because the ankle and knee joints can move easily in an anterior/posterior direction during the Romberg posture, control of anterior/posterior directions is easier than that of the medial/lateral directions. Body-sway of the distance, area, and velocity become large by the alcohol intake because perception of the body-sway delay as compared with a normal state. However, even if nervous function declines with alcohol intake during keeping the static standing posture, when the body-sway appears for the same direction, the postural control system attempts to back the former position on the same speed disordering the balance. Therefore the mean center of foot pressure and frequency for body-sway (X and Y axis) did not change. In other words, the decline of the stability function to the stable position of the center of gravity may be small as compared with that to hold the body-sway.

Franks, et al. (1976) suggested that the influence of alcohol intake on body-sway change differs with the amount, giving an alcohol amount as a ratio of body weight for each subject. However, all subjects took the same volume (540 ml) of alcohol in this study. The intake volume converted to a ratio of the subject's weight was equal to or over that in previous studies (Franks, et al., 1976). Moreover, the effect of alcohol intake in the nervous function tests was confirmed for all subjects. Therefore, the intake volume in this study is considered to be enough to decrease the nervous functions. Examining the influence of alcohol intake by considering the intake volume by each subject on body-sway must be undertaken.

In conclusion, we examined the influence of alcohol intake on 24 parameters regarding the change of center of foot pressure (CFP) in a static upright posture. Parameters regarding the magnitude of body-sway, such as distance, velocity, and direction, remarkably increased after alcohol intake, whereas the parameters regarding mean center of foot pressure and frequency of body-sway changed very little. The former parameters are considered to be strongly influenced by nervous function. Further, postural stability is maintained by making the distance and velocity of body-sway greater without changing body-sway frequency after alcohol intake.

REFERENCES

BAKER, C. P., NEWSTEAD, A. H., MOSSBERG, K. A., & NICODEMUS, C. L. (1998) Reliability of static standing balance in nondisabled children: comparison of two methods of measurement. *Pediatric Rehabilitation*, 2, 15-20.

DEMURA, S., YAMAJI, S., NODA, M., KITABAYASHI, T., & NAGASAWA, Y. (2001) Examination of parameters evaluating the center of foot pressure in static standing posture from the viewpoints of trial-to-trial reliability and interrelationships among parameters. *Equilibrium Research*, 60, 44-55.

DICKSTEIN, R., & DVIR, Z. (1993) Quantitative evaluation of stance balance performance in the clinic using a novel measurement device. *Physiotherapy Canada*, 45, 102-108.

EKDAHL, C., JARNLO, G. B., & ANDERSSON, S. I. (1989) Standing balance in healthy subjects. *Scandinavian Journal of Rehabilitation and Medicine*, 21, 187-195.

FRANKS, H. M., HENSLEY, V. R., HENSLEY, W. J., STARMER, G. A., & TEO, R. K. C. (1976) The relationship between alcohol dosage and performance decrement in humans. *Journal of Studies on Alcohol*, 37, 284-297.

GEURTS, A. C. H., NIENHUIS, B., & MULDER, T. W. (1993) Intrasubject variability of selected force-platform parameters in the quantification of postural control. *Archives of Physical Medicine and Rehabilitation*, 74, 1144-1150.

GOLDIE, P. A., BACH, T. M., & EVANS, O. M. (1989) Force platform measures for evaluating postural control: reliability and validity. *Archives of Physical Medicine and Rehabilitation*, 70, 510-517.

KANTER, R. M., RUBIN, A. M., ARMSTRONG, C. W., & CUMMINS, V. (1991) Stabilometry in balance assessment of dizzy and normal subjects. *American Journal of Otolaryngology*, 12, 196-204.

KAPTEYN, T. S., BLES, W., NJIOKIKTJIEN, C. J., KODDE, L., MASSEN, C. H., & MOL, J. M. F. (1983) Standardization in platform stabilometry being part of posturography. *Agressologie*, 24, 321-326.

KITABAYASHI, T., DEMURA, S., YAMAJI, S., NAKADA, M., NODA, M., & IMAOKA, K. (2002) Gender differences and relationships between physique and parameters evaluating the body center of pressure in static standing posture. *Equilibrium Research*, 61, 56-62.

KUBO, T., SAKATA, Y., MATSUNAGA, T., KOSHIMUNE, A., SAKAI, S., AMENO, K., & IJIRI, I. (1989) Analysis of body-sway pattern after alcohol ingestion in human subjects. *Acta Otolaryngologica, Suppl.*, 468, 247-252.

LABORATORY OF PHYSICAL EDUCATION IN TOKYO METROPOLITAN UNIVERSITY. (Eds.) (2000) *New physical fitness standards of Japanese people*. Tokyo: Fumaido.

MANGOLD, S., LAUBLI, T., & KRUEGER, H. (1976) Effects of a low alcohol dose on static balance, fine motor activity, and mental performance. *Neurotoxicology and Teratology*, 18, 547-554.

MARKHAM, C. H. (1987) Vestibular control of muscular tone and posture. *Canadian Journal of Neurological Science*, 14, 493-496.

NAKAGAWA, H., OHASHI, N., WATANABE, Y., & MIZUKOSHI, K. (1993) The contribution of proprioception to posture control in normal subjects. *Acta Oto Laryngologica, Suppl.*, 504, 112-116.

NIESCHALK, M., ORTMANN, C., WEST, A., SCHMAL, F., STOLL, W., & FECHNER, G. (1999) Effects of alcohol on body-sway patterns in human subjects. *International Journal of Legal Medicine*, 112, 253-260.

ROEBUCK, T. M., SIMMONS, R. W., MATTSON, S. N., & RILEY, E. P. (1998) Prenatal exposure to alcohol affects the ability to maintain postural balance. *Alcoholism—Clinical and Experimental Research*, 22, 252-258.

TAGUCHI, K., & YODA, M. (1976) [Analysing techniques of the center of gravity-area occupied and length of lucus followed by the center of gravity]. [*Japanese Journal of Otolaryngology*], 79, 1576-1589.

UNIMONEN, S., LAITAKARI, K., BLOIGU, R., REINILA, M., & SORRI, M. (1994) Static posturography and intravenous alcohol. *Journal of Vestibular Research*, 4, 277-283.

WOOLLEY, S. M., RUBIN, A., KANTER, R. M., & ARMSTRONG, C. W. (1993) Differentiation of balance deficits through examination of selected components of static stabilometry. *The Journal of Otolaryngology*, 22, 368-375.

YAMAJI, S., DEMURA, S., NODA, M., NAGASAWA, Y., NAKADA, M., & KITABAYASHI, T. (2001) The day-to-day reliability of parameters evaluating the body center of pressure in static standing posture. *Equilibrium Research*, 60, 217-226.

Accepted January 30, 2004.

INFLUENCE OF MUSIC AND DISTRACTION ON VISUAL SEARCH PERFORMANCE OF PARTICIPANTS WITH HIGH AND LOW AFFECT INTENSITY[1]

LEE CRUST

Sports Department
Lincoln College

PETER J. CLOUGH

Department of Psychology
Hull University

COLIN ROBERTSON

Department of Psychology
University of Lincoln

Summary.—This study examined the role of music and distraction on the performance of a visual search task (grid test) for 57 volunteer sports science undergraduates ($M = 21.6$ yr., $SD = 3.0$), comprising 39 men and 18 women who were subsequently classified as either high or low in Affect Intensity (responsiveness to emotional stimuli). Participants were instructed to identify as many numbers in sequence from an 8 × 8 concentration grid while being randomly exposed to four conditions: silence (Control), distraction (Talking), Instrumental Music, and Lyrical Music. Each trial lasted 120 sec., with 180-sec. rest periods between trials. A one-way repeated-measures analysis of variance and Newman-Keuls *post hoc* analysis for the entire sample ($N = 57$) indicated that significantly higher scores on the grid test were attained with Lyrical Music than with Instrumental Music ($p < .05$), Talking ($p < .01$), or Control conditions ($p < .01$). The Instrumental Music condition had significantly better performance than either the Talking or Control condition ($p < .01$). When the 20 highest and lowest Affect Intensity scores were analysed, no significant between-group mean differences in performance were evident. Results suggest that music may facilitate a simple visual search task.

Many investigators have observed performance alterations when participants exercise with musical accompaniment; one of the supposed mechanisms responsible is improved attentional processing (Anshel & Marisi, 1978; Copeland & Franks, 1991; Szabo, Small, & Leigh, 1999). Despite this, little consideration has been given to examining experimentally the effects of music on the attentional processes of sports performers. Szabo, *et al.* (1999) suggested that increases in work output during stationary cycling were achieved by careful selection of musical accompaniment, which potentially diverted attention from unpleasant, fatigue-related cues and promoted a switch from internal to external processing. This finding offered support to Rejeski's Parallel Information Processing Model (Rejeski, 1985) that proposed an explanation of 'dissociation' strategies based on attentional flooding due to limited channel capacity. Szabo, *et al.* (1999) proposed that whether music altered attentional processing was likely to be dependent on the arousing qualities of given selections.

---

[1]Address enquiries to Lee Crust, Sports Department, Lincoln College, Monks Road, Lincoln, LN2 5HQ, United Kingdom or e-mail (lcrust@lincolncollege.ac.uk).

In a task requiring high attention (a motor-racing computer game), the presence of arousing music has interfered with the task, yielding performance decrements (North & Hargreaves, 1999). Participants performed better when completing simple tasks in the presence of less arousing music. This further supports the claim that arousing music occupies attentional space, with an evident interaction between music and task characteristics.

Other researchers (Copeland & Franks, 1991; Szmedra & Bacharach, 1998) have provided evidence that music can promote a relaxation response during exercise trials. It is highly plausible that the effects of music on exercise performance are a result of the interrelationship between arousal and attention (Szabo, et al., 1999). Easterbrook's cue-utilisation hypothesis (1959) could explain how changes in arousal promote a more optimal focus on a task by either increasing or decreasing the performer's perceptual field. Presumably promotion of optimal arousal could be achieved through either relaxation or stimulation.

Outside of sports and exercise, North and Hargreaves (1997b, p. 275) suggested music research provides some support for Mehrabian and Russell's model of environmental psychology (1974). This model predicts increasing approach or avoidance type behaviors in response to environmental conditions. More pleasurable environments are predicted to influence the desire to stay, explore, and be satisfied with task performance in a given environment (North & Hargreaves, 1997a). Music may not just divert attentional processes but may indirectly influence performance by promoting pleasant feelings such as enjoyment (Boutcher & Trenske, 1990) that could induce a more optimal focus for a task.

Although the emphasis for researchers in the sports and exercise domain has been on manipulating music characteristics, Karageorghis, Terry, and Lane (1999) also acknowledged the role of personal factors. Past equivocal findings may in part reflect individual differences in the responses of exercise participants, although this has received little experimental consideration. Music has consistently elicited changes in mood and affective states (Richards, 1981; Hayakawa, Miki, Takada, & Tanaka, 2000), and individuals have reliably differed in intensity of responses to emotionally provoking stimuli (Larsen, Diener, & Emmons, 1986; Larsen, Diener, & Cropanzano, 1987). There appears to be a need to examine whether some individuals are more likely to respond to such stimulation in work-related contexts. Larsen's construct of Affect Intensity—a stable trait-like difference in emotional arousability, similar to the augmenter/reducer construct but related to emotional rather than sensory stimuli—has been operationalized via the Affect Intensity Measure (Larsen, et al., 1986).

Affect Intensity appears to apply to both positive and negative emotions, with those scoring higher values on the Affect Intensity Measure reporting more extreme reactions than those scoring low to objectively rated emotional stimuli. It appears that participants with high Affect Intensity can also be distinguished by different cognitive operations such as selectively attending to the emotion-provoking aspects of events, generalising and focussing on personalising meanings (Larsen, et al., 1987).

The objectives of this research were to examine how music and distraction influence responses to a visual search task. If music operates by occupying cognitive processing space, it might be predicted that lower visual search performance should be associated with exposure to music. If music promotes a more pleasant environment, one might predict performance increments due to increased arousal. Secondly, the role of individual differences was explored to evaluate whether some participants are more likely to be influenced by music stimuli than others. It was hypothesised that participants with higher Affect Intensity would respond more intensely to motivational music.

Method

Participants

Participants were 57 sports science undergraduates (M age = 21.6 yr., $SD = 3.0$), 38 men and 19 women who volunteered to participate. They were solicited from penultimate and final year sports and exercise psychology classes. All were briefed on experimental requirements and signed informed consent forms prior to testing.

Tests

A 5-page booklet incorporating a front-page of instructions with a small 3×3 practice grid, and four 8×8 randomised concentration grids (printed on A5 sized paper) was given to each participant, with the scores on the four grids used to assess visual search skills. Concentration grids have been extensively used prior to competition to give a sense of what it means to be totally focussed (Weinberg & Gould, 2003, p. 375). The 8×8 grid contained 64 cells, with a two-digit number in each cell. The numbers were randomly positioned in cells with the objective to search the grid and to identify and cross-out numbers in the correct sequence, e.g., 01, 02, 03, etc. A Philips (Model No. AZ2030) portable stereo system was used to deliver the music. Sound intensity was set at 70 decibels using a Castle GA202 Sound Level Meter.

The Affect Intensity Measure (Larsen, et al., 1986), a 40-item inventory, designed to assess the characteristic strength of intensity with which an individual typically experiences emotions, was completed by each participant. Each item was rated on a 6-point scale with scoring achieved by averaging the responses across the 40 items. Larsen, et al. (1986) used a sample of 62 participants from a population of 280 introductory psychology students to represent extremes of Affect Intensity. Participants with High and Low Affect Intensity had mean scores of 4.3 and 3.5 using the Affect Intensity Measure. Construct validity has been provided, with Larsen (1984) reporting a significant correlation of .50 ($p < .01$) between Affect Intensity and reports of typical affect response intensity by the participants' parents. Retest correlations after 1, 2, and 3 mo. were .80, .81, and .81, respectively. Coefficients alpha in the range of .90 to .94 were also noted across four samples (Larsen, 1984). Larsen, et al. (1986) found the Affect Intensity Measure was significantly correlated with scores on the Arousability Scale (Mehrabian, 1979) and on the Reactivity subscale of the Mood Survey (Underwood & Froming, 1980). Negative correlations between Affect Intensity and peripheral physiological arousal were also noted which suggests participants with high Affect Intensity are underaroused in quiet, stimulus-reduced environments.

Selection of Interventions

Careful consideration was given to the selection of interventions in this study. The two chosen musical selections were both from popular music, with similar high tempi (between 120 and 130 beats per minute^{-1}) and both were previous Top Twenty songs on the Official British Music Chart. One of the selections was instrumental[2] (Instrumental Music Condition) while the other contained positive, stimulating lyrics[3] (Lyrical Music Condition).

Pilot work included the Brunel Music Rating Inventory (Karageorghis, et al., 1999) to assess the motivational qualities of the music and employed 12 participants from the same population as the study participants. The 13-item inventory has recently been shown to be an appropriate measurement device in the selection of motivational music for sports and exercise (Szabo & Griffiths, 2003). An overall motivational quotient is calculated between 3.33 and 33.3, with scores higher than the *Mdn* of 18.33 regarded as motivational. The mean motivational quotients of Instrumental ($M = 19.4$, $SD = 2.2$) and Lyrical Music ($M = 20.8$, $SD = 3.6$) conditions were above the minimum requirements to be classified as motivational music (cf. Karageorghis, et al., 1999). A *t* test showed that the two music conditions did not differ significantly ($p > .05$) from each other in overall motivational properties. A 120-sec. edited portion of each selection accompanied trials.

The Talking condition was taken from the National Coaching Foundation's Mental Training Programme for Concentration Training (Hardy & Fazey, 1990). The audiocassette tape featured a 120-sec. sequence including ver-

---

[2]'Children—Dream Version' performed by Robert Miles, Courtesy of Deconstruction, Ltd. (1996).
[3]'Music Gets The Best Of Me' performed by Sophie Ellis Bexter, Courtesy of Polydor, Ltd. (2002).

bal conversations and calling-out of random numbers which was used in an attempt to interfere with the attentional focus of the participants. A 120-sec. period of silence was used for the Control Condition.

Procedure

The experiment took place in a quiet room while participants sat at desks. Participants performed the task in groups of 11 to 16. Each participant was provided a pen and an A5 sized 5-page booklet containing four (64 items—8 × 8) grids. Strict instructions were given not to turn the pages until told to do so. Standardised instructions were given, and participants completed a small 3 × 3 practice grid by searching for the numbers in sequence from 01 to 09, contained in the random grid, and crossing out the identified target numbers as quickly as possible before searching for the next target.

After successful completion of the practice grid, participants attempted to search visually four 8 × 8 grids, identifying and crossing out as many numbers in the correct sequence starting with 01 and working up towards 64. The participants were not instructed to follow a particular search strategy, i.e., left to right, top to bottom. Trials began with the participant turning over a page to a new grid. Each trial lasted for 120 sec. with 180-sec. rest intervals between trials. Four testing sessions were completed, with up to a maximum of 16 participants at a time, who were exposed to the four conditions in a random order. These conditions were Control (silence), Talking (interference), Instrumental Music, and Lyrical Music. Following the fourth and final trial, all participants completed the Affect Intensity Measure (Larsen, *et al.*, 1986) before leaving the room.

Results

Initial analysis of the entire data set ($N=57$) was completed using a one-way repeated-measures analysis of variance. In line with Larsen, *et al.* (1986), the data set was subsequently placed into rank order on the basis of Affect Intensity scores, with the 20 highest and lowest scores selected to represent High and Low Affect Intensities. The mean scores of High ($M=4.2$, $SD=0.2$) and Low ($M=3.4$, $SD=0.2$) Affect Intensity groups were consistent with data reported by Larsen, *et al.* (1986). These data were analysed using a two-way mixed-model (2 groups × 4 conditions) analysis of variance. *Post hoc* analysis was conducted using Newman-Keuls tests.

A one-way repeated-measures analysis of variance for the entire sample yielded significant differences for conditions ($F_{3,165}=18.74$, $p<.01$). *Post hoc* Newman-Keuls comparisons showed significantly better visual search performance in the Lyrical Music condition, compared to Instrumental Music ($p<.05$), Talking ($p<.01$), and Control ($p<.01$). Further, performance in the Instrumental Music condition was significantly greater than for those exposed to Talking or Control ($p < .01$). In comparison to the Control condition, the effect sizes for Lyrical and Instrumental Music were moderate (ES = 0.5) and small (ES = .03), respectively. Table 1 shows the mean performance for each condition in relation to the total sample and High and Low Affect Intensity subgroups.

TABLE 1
Mean Grid Test Scores by Groups and Conditions

Group	n	Control[a] M	SD	Talking[b] M	SD	Music Instrumental[c] M	SD	Lyrical[d] M	SD
Total Sample	57	42.1[cd]	10.9	41.4[cd]	9.7	45.3[abd]	10.6	47.1[abc]	7.7
Low AIM	20	43.5[cd]	8.6	44.1[cd]	9.0	49.3[ab]	8.8	49.5[ab]	9.4
High AIM	20	42.8[d]	12.4	40.9[cd]	10.2	44.4[b]	11.1	46.3[ab]	10.9

Note.—Different superscripts indicate differences between conditions ($p < .05$).

To assess potential effects pertaining to sex or order of treatments a two-way (sex × order of treatments) mixed-model analysis of variance was applied. There were no significant main effects for sex ($F_{1,55} = 2.51$, $p > .1$), order of treatments ($F_{3,165} = 0.31$, $p > .1$), and no interactions ($F_{3,165} = 0.72$).

To examine whether responses differed as a function of Affect Intensity when exposed to conditions, a two-way (2 groups × 4 conditions) mixed-model analysis of variance showed a significant main effect for conditions ($F_{3,114} = 12.55$, $p < .01$) but not for their interaction ($F_{3,114} = 1.26$, $p > .1$) or between groups ($F_{1,38} = 1.07$, $p > .1$). Table 1 shows the mean grid scores for both the High and Low AIM groups.

To examine the significant main effects for conditions, Newman-Keuls comparisons were applied. Consistent with data collected for the total sample, both Lyrical and Instrumental Music were associated with significantly better visual search performance than either Talking ($p < .01$) or the Control ($p < .01$). No further differences were noted.

Discussion

These results show that music played during a visual search task can facilitate or increase performance. This finding appears consistent with Mehrabian and Russell's model of environmental psychology (1974), which predicts increased approach type behaviours in more pleasurable environments. Music might have provided a more pleasurable environment that increased enthusiasm for the task. The exact mechanism by which music increased performance remains unclear although the relationship between arousal and attention proposed by Easterbrook (1959) could offer a plausible explanation. The Cue Utilisation Hypothesis suggests arousal that is either too high or too low yields suboptimal attentional processing and consequently lower task performance. With a resultant perceptual field that is either too wide or too narrow, important targets may be missed while visually searching.

Past research suggests that music can promote alterations in arousal resulting in either stimulation or relaxation, depending upon musical characteristics (Hohler, 1989; Karageorghis & Terry, 1997; Szabo, et al., 1999). It is likely that the motivational music elicited a motivational response that altered arousal and consequently attentional processes, resulting in a more optimal focus on the task. The highest mean performance was found in the Lyrical Music condition which may reflect the importance of lyrics and meaning to the individual. Given that the Lyrical Music condition promoted significantly better visual search performance than Instrumental Music, while both possessed a similar tempo, suggests that more subtle musical characteristics were responsible for such differences. Research both within and outside of sports and exercise contexts has shown fast music was related to increased speed of behavioural responding (Anshel & Marisi, 1978; Milliman, 1986; McElrea & Standing, 1992), but the present research suggests tempo alone is an inadequate explanation for results. Both Snyder (1993) and Karageorghis (1998) have emphasised the importance of lyrics that convey meaning to the individual.

Unlike North and Hargreaves (1999), who found arousing music interfered with performance on an attentional demanding task, present results do not suggest that motivational music takes up cognitive space to the detriment of visual search performance. In part, this difference could be due to task complexity since North and Hargreaves (1999) reported tasks of lower complexity were not negatively affected by music.

Although it was hypothesised that those participants who rate experienced emotions more intensely (affectively intense) and were inferred to be physiologically underaroused in stimulus-reduced conditions would respond more positively to a music stimulus, in this study no significant differences were evident. Larsen, et al. (1986) proposed that, given the same level of emotion-provoking stimuli, more affectively intense participants would characteristically respond more strongly regardless of whether stimulation was mild, moderate, or extreme. Larsen's work was, however, essentially based upon self-report measures and cognitive operations. Present results, which employed objectively rated motivational music (as assessed by a subset of the experimental population), do not support the transposition of Larsen's findings from self-report measures and cognitive operations (Larsen, et al., 1986, 1987) to responses during a visual search task. No between-group differences were found for visual search performance in this study, suggesting affect intensity did not influence responses. With regards to individual differences, Davidson (2000) warned against assuming symmetry across emotional response systems. Thus an individual with a low threshold for elicitation of the subjective experience (measured by self-report) may actually have a much higher threshold for the elicitation of physiological or behavioural responses.

The objectives of this study were to identify performance changes, but it is clear that any firmer explanations will require future researchers to devote attention to concurrent physiological parameters of arousal. Physiological measures of arousal would allow the identification of any changes due to treatments and potentially enable researchers to determine if the effects of music in a given situation involve either a relaxation response, arousal increments, or simply enable participants to function optimally. If transposed to exercise settings, this research could suggest that rather than simply operating as a distraction from feelings of fatigue that music may promote a more optimal task focus.

REFERENCES

ANSHEL, M. H., & MARISI, D. Q. (1978) Effect of music and rhythm on physical performance. *Research Quarterly*, 49, 109-113.

BOUTCHER, S. H., & TRENSKE, M. (1990) The effects of sensory distraction and music on perceived exertion and affect during exercise. *Journal of Sport and Exercise Psychology*, 12, 167-176.

COPELAND, B. L., & FRANKS, B. D. (1991) Effects of types and intensities of background music on treadmill endurance. *The Journal of Sports Medicine and Physical Fitness*, 15, 100-103.

DAVIDSON, R. J. (2000) The functional neuroanatomy of affective style. In R. D. Lane & L. Nadel (Eds.), *Neuroscience of emotion*. Oxford, Eng.: Oxford Univer. Press. Pp. 371-379.

EASTERBROOK, J. A. (1959) The effect of emotion on cue utilisation and the organisation of behaviour. *Psychological Review*, 66, 183-201.

HARDY, L., & FAZEY, J. (1990) *Concentration training*. [Audio cassette tape] Leeds, Eng.: National Coaching Foundation.

HAYAKAWA, Y., MIKI, H., TAKADA, K., & TANAKA, K. (2000) Effects of music on mood during bench stepping exercise. *Perceptual and Motor Skills*, 90, 307-314.

HOHLER, V. (1989) Sport and music. *Sport Science Review*, 12, 41-44.

KARAGEORGHIS, C. I. (1998) Music for sport and exercise. *Ultra-fit*, 8(6), 30-32.

KARAGEORGHIS, C. I., & TERRY, P. C. (1997) The psychophysical effects of music in sport and exercise: a review. *Journal of Sport Behavior*, 20, 54-68.

KARAGEORGHIS, C. I., TERRY, P. C., & LANE, A. M. (1999) Development and initial validation of an instrument to assess the motivational qualities of music in exercise and sport: the Brunel Music Rating Inventory. *Journal of Sport Sciences*, 17, 713-724.

LARSEN, R. J. (1984) Theory and measurement of affect intensity as an individual difference characteristic. *Dissertation Abstracts International*, 5, 2297B. (University microfilms No. 84-22112)

LARSEN, R. J., DIENER, E., & CROPANZANO, R. (1987) Cognitive operations associated with individual differences in affect intensity. *Journal of Personality and Social Psychology*, 53, 767-774.

LARSEN, R. J., DIENER, E., & EMMONS, R. A. (1986) Affect intensity and reactions to daily life events. *Journal of Personality and Social Psychology*, 51, 803-814.

MCELREA, H., & STANDING, L. (1992) Fast music causes fast drinking. *Perceptual and Motor Skills*, 75, 362.

MEHRABIAN, A. (1979) *Manual for the questionnaire measure of stimulus screening and arousability*. Los Angeles, CA: Univer. of California, Los Angeles.

MEHRABIAN, A., & RUSSELL, J. A. (1974) *An approach to environmental psychology*. Cambridge, MA: MIT Press.

MILLIMAN, R. E. (1986) The influence of background music on the behavior of restaurant patrons. *Journal of Consumer Research*, 13, 286-289.

NORTH, A. C., & HARGREAVES, D. J. (1997a) Experimental aesthetics and everyday music listening. In D. J. Hargreaves & A. C. North (Eds.), *The social psychology of music*. Oxford, Eng.: Oxford Univer. Press. Pp. 84-103.

NORTH, A. C., & HARGREAVES, D. J. (1997b) Music and consumer behaviour. In D. J. Hargreaves & A. C. North (Eds.), *The social psychology of music*. Oxford, Eng.: Oxford Univer. Press. Pp. 268-289.

NORTH, A. C., & HARGREAVES, D. J. (1999) Music and driving game performance. *Scandinavian Journal of Psychology*, 40, 285-292.

REJESKI, W. J. (1985) Perceived exertion: an active or passive process? *Journal of Sport Psychology*, 7, 371-378.

RICHARDS, C. (1981) The use of music to induce mood. (Unpublished manuscript, Oxford, Eng., Univer. of Oxford)

SNYDER, E. E. (1993) Responses to musical selections and sport: an auditory elicitation approach. *Sociology of Sport Journal*, 10, 168-182.

SZABO, A., & GRIFFITHS, L. (2003) Evaluation of the motivational quality of music played during exercise at two fitness centres using the Brunel Music Rating Inventory. *Journal of Sport Sciences*, 21, 360.

SZABO, A., SMALL, A., & LEIGH, M. (1999) The effects of slow- and fast-rhythm classical music on progressive cycling to voluntary physical exhaustion. *The Journal of Sports Medicine and Physical Fitness*, 39, 220-225.

SZMEDRA, L., & BACHARACH, D. W. (1998) Effect of music on perceived exertion, plasma lactate, norepinephrine and cardiovascular hemodynamics during treadmill running. *Physiological Biochemistry*, 19, 32-37.

UNDERWOOD, B., & FROMING, W. J. (1980) The Mood Survey: a personality measure of happy and sad moods. *Journal of Personality Assessment*, 44, 404-414.

WEINBERG, R. S., & GOULD, D. (2003) *Foundations of sport and exercise psychology*. (3rd ed.) Champaign, IL: Human Kinetics.

Accepted March 8, 2004.

RETENTION OF PRACTICE EFFECTS ON SIMPLE REACTION TIME FOR PERIPHERAL AND CENTRAL VISUAL FIELDS [1]

SOICHI ANDO, NORIYUKI KIDA, AND SHINGO ODA

Kyoto University

Summary.—Previous researchers reported that EMG Reaction Time (RT) for a key press in peripheral and central visual fields decreases with practice. The practice effects on the RT for peripheral visual field transferred to the RT for the central visual field, and vice versa. The present study investigated whether practice effects on the RT for peripheral and central visual fields and the corresponding transfer effects lasted 3 wk. or not. 16 male subjects were divided into two groups, one practicing using peripheral vision, the other practicing using central vision. Each group practiced RT tasks for 3 wk. 3 wk. after practice terminated, the practice effects and the transfer effects were maintained as a significant decrease in RT was found over the 3-wk. retention interval, suggesting that once the neural correlates of responding quickly are improved, the improved performances are remarkably stable for at least 3 wk.

With practice people can improve responding quickly. Recently, we have reported that reaction time (RT) for both peripheral visual field and central visual field decreases with practice (Ando, Kida, & Oda, 2002). The practice effects established on the RT for peripheral visual field transferred to the RT for central visual field, and vice versa. The transfer effects suggest that the decrease in the RT resulted from a decrease in the central nervous system's processing time common to the two RT tasks.

Proctor, Reeve, Weeks, Dornier, and Van Zandt (1991) investigated whether practice effects on choice RT using spatial precuing and symbolic cuing tasks were retained after a 1-wk. interval. They indicated that the response-selection procedures acquired with practice were retained fairly well for at least 1 wk. Compared to literatures about the practice effects on simple and choice RT (see references in Ando, *et al.*, 2002), few studies have addressed how long lasting the practice effects on RT are, i.e., how well the effects are retained. No study of the retention of practice effects on simple RT for peripheral visual field was located so the present study was designed to examine retention of practice effects on simple RT for both peripheral and central visual fields. Behavioral evaluation of retention of these practice effects is important since retention suggests changes in neural correlates with practice are lasting after retention interval.

---

[1]Address enquiries to Shingo Oda, Laboratory of Human Motor Control, Graduate School of Human and Environmental Studies, Kyoto University, Sakyo-ku, Kyoto 606-8501 Japan or e-mail (m54899@sakura.kudpc.kyoto-u.ac.jp).

Method

Subjects

Sixteen male university students (M age = 22.3 yr., SD = 1.4) volunteered to participate. They were randomly divided into two groups of the same age (ns = 8); one practiced using peripheral vision and the other practiced using central vision. All subjects reported normal visual acuity either unaided or while wearing their own corrective lenses. The subjects all wrote with the right hand.

Apparatus

A computer (NEC PC9821) was used to control visual stimulus presentation and record the RT for a key press throughout the experiments. All visual conditions were conducted using binocular vision. The subject's head rested on a head and chin rest placed 30 cm from the computer screen (3 cd/m^2) so the eyes were directly in front of and at the same level as the position of the fixation point. The exposure duration of the visual stimulus was 50 msec. Four intertrial intervals (2, 3, 4, and 5 sec.) were randomly used. They also served as the foreperiods. The stimulus 8-mm diameter (1.52° in central vision) in all conditions was in the shape of a ring (14 cd/m^2). The contrast ratio was 0.65, and the sign of the contrast was bright (white on black background). Subjects responded to the onset of each stimulus by pressing the space key of the computer as fast as possible. The response key was manipulated using the index finger of the right hand.

Electromyograms (EMG) were measured from the flexor digitorum superficialis muscle of responding forearm. EMG-RT is the time from stimulus onset to the appearance of the electromyogram (EMG). Morris (1977) and Ando, *et al.* (2002) reported that decrease in the RT with practice reflected changes in the premotor components. Therefore, EMG-RT was used as the index to assess the practice effects.

Testing Procedure

Before practice, after the date of practice, and three weeks after practice, RT for the key press and EMG-RT were measured in the following three retinal positions: (I) Central condition, (II) Near Peripheral condition, and (III) Far Peripheral condition. In the Central condition, the stimulus was presented at the fixation point and in the Near Peripheral condition was presented at an angle of 10° to the right from the midpoint of the subject's eyes. The stimulus in the Far Peripheral condition was presented at an angle of 30° to the right from the midpoint of the subject's eyes. In the Peripheral conditions, the fixation point remained illuminated throughout the experiments. The subjects were instructed to keep their eyes on the fixation point. One experimental block consisted of a series of 25 trials. Before each block, the subjects were visually familiarized with the stimuli and given 10 practice trials. Experimental conditions of (I), (II), and (III) were tested in a randomized order. The condition was constant during each block. Horizontal components of eye movement were measured by an infrared reflection system (T.K.K. 2930a Takei Scientific Instruments Co., Ltd., Japan) and showed that subjects could hold their eyes on a fixation point throughout each response.

Practice Procedure

During the practice period, the group practicing using peripheral vision practiced RT tasks in the Far Peripheral condition. The group practicing using central vision practiced RT tasks in the Central condition. Each group practiced three blocks five days a week for three weeks for a total of 1,125 trials. During the practice period, RT for the key press was recorded for each group. The RT for the key press before practice, during the practice period, and after practice was analyzed to confirm that subjects' performance had peaked with practice. The RT for the key press during the practice period was averaged by week for each group.

RESULTS AND DISCUSSION

Table 1 shows the means and standard deviations of the RT for the key press before practice, during the practice period, and after practice for each group. Friedman's nonparametric one-way analysis of variance was performed on the RT between times of measurement for each group, indicating that mean RT significantly differed between times of measurement for the group using peripheral vision $[\chi_4^2(N=8) = 18.66, p<.05]$ and for the group practicing using central vision $[\chi_4^2(N=8) = 21.70, p<.05]$.

TABLE 1
RT (MSEC.) FOR A KEY PRESS BEFORE, DURING, AND AFTER PRACTICE FOR EACH GROUP

Measure	Before Practice	Week 1	Week 2	Week 3	After Practice
The Group Practicing Using Peripheral Vision (n = 8)					
Far Peripheral Condition					
M	265	249*	239*†	243*	243*
SD	14	13	11	17	16
The Group Practicing Using Central Vision (n = 8)					
Central Condition					
M	245	238*	227*†	229*†	232*
SD	14	14	12	13	16

Note.—Mean RT during the practice period was averaged by week. *Significant difference with RT before practice for each condition ($p<.05$). †Significant difference with RT at the first week during the practice period for each condition ($p<.05$).

A Wilcoxon paired signed-rank test showed that the RT before practice was significantly larger than the other times of measurement for each group ($p<.05$, respectively). Mean RT at the first week during the practice period was significantly larger than that at the second week during the practice period for the group using peripheral vision ($p<.05$). Mean RT at the first week during the practice period was significantly larger than that at the second and third weeks during the practice period in the group using central vision ($p<.05$, respectively). There were no significant differences in the RT between after practice and at each week during the practice period. It was suggested that the majority of practice effects for both groups occurred during the first block, which was defined before practice in the present study, and the first week of the practice period. Afterward, mean RT leveled off and almost unchanged. Therefore, we can assume that subjects' performance had peaked after the practice period had elapsed.

Three-way analysis of variance was performed on the EMG-RT with condition and time of measurement as the within factors and group as the between factor. A main effect of group was not significant ($F_{1,14}=0.99$), indicating that there were no differences in mean RT between groups. The interaction of time of measurement by condition was significant ($F_{4,56}=3.39, p<$

.05). One-way analysis of variance was performed for each condition. There were significant main effects of time of measurement for the Central, the Near Peripheral, and the Far Peripheral conditions ($F_{2,30}=24.39$, $p<.001$; $F_{2,30}=10.17$, $p<.001$; $F_{2,30}=26.83$, $p<.001$, respectively).

EMG-RT for both groups was summarized for further analysis as there were no differences between groups and no interactions related to group (Table 2). The multiple comparisons by the Tukey HSD showed that mean EMG-RT after practice was shorter than the EMG-RT before practice for the Central, the Near Peripheral, and the Far Peripheral conditions ($p<.001$, $p<.01$, and $p<.001$, respectively).

TABLE 2
EMG-RT (msec.) For All Subjects by Condition and Time of Measurement

Measure	Time of Measurement		
	Before Practice	After Practice	3 Wk. After Practice
Central Condition			
M	175	165‡	161‡
SD	11	15	13
Near Peripheral Condition			
M	179	167†	167†
SD	12	15	14
Far Peripheral Condition			
M	194	177‡	182‡
SD	13	15	18

Note.—Significant difference with the EMG-RT before practice for each condition.
†$p<.01$. ‡$p<.001$.

The multiple comparisons also indicated that the EMG-RT three weeks after practice was shorter than the EMG-RT before practice for the Central, the Near Peripheral, and the Far Peripheral conditions ($p<.001$, $p<.01$, and $p<.001$, respectively). No differences were observed between the EMG-RT after practice and the EMG-RT three weeks after practice for each condition. These results indicated that the practice effects and the transfer effects were maintained over the retention interval, suggesting that once simple RT for peripheral and central visual fields decreases with practice, the improved performances are stable and retained for at least three weeks. Visual information is processed in various ways until eventually it is output as observable motor activity. It appears that once the neural correlates of responding quickly are improved, the improved performances are retained for at least three weeks. Further investigation would be needed to ascertain whether the practice effects on simple RT are retained for longer periods than this.

REFERENCES

ANDO, S., KIDA, N., & ODA, S. (2002) Practice effects on reaction time for peripheral and central visual fields. *Perceptual and Motor Skills*, 95, 747-751.
MORRIS, H. H. (1977) Effects of practice and set upon reaction time and its fractionated components. In D. M. Landers & R. W. Christina (Eds.), *Psychology of motor behavior and sport*. Champaign, IL: Human Kinetics. Pp. 259-268.
PROCTOR, R. W., REEVE, T. G., WEEKS, D. J., DORNIER, L., & VAN ZANDT, T. (1991) Acquisition, retention, and transfer of response selection skill in choice reaction tasks. *Journal of Experimental Psychology: Learning, Memory, and Cognition*, 17, 497-506.

Accepted March 15, 2004.

DIFFERENTIAL EFFECTS OF LAUGHTER ON ALLERGEN-SPECIFIC IMMUNOGLOBULIN AND NEUROTROPHIN LEVELS IN TEARS [1]

HAJIME KIMATA

Department of Allergy
Ujitakeda Hospital

Summary.—Laughter after viewing a humorous video "Modern Times" decreased Japanese cedar pollen-specific immunoglobulin E (IgE) and IgG4 levels, while it enhanced Japanese cedar pollen-specific IgA levels in tears of patients with atopic keratoconjunctivitis, while viewing a nonhumorous weather information video did not do so. Laughter after viewing "Modern Times" also decreased nerve growth factor levels without affecting neurotrophin-3 levels in tears of those patients, while viewing a weather information video did not. These results indicate that laughter decreased allergen-specific IgE and IgG4 production and increased allergen-specific IgA production with concomitant decrease in nerve growth factor. These results indicate that laughter may have some implications for study and treatment of allergic diseases.

It has been reported that allergen-specific immunoglobulin E (IgE), IgG4, and IgA levels are elevated in blood and tears of patients with allergic conjunctivitis (Aghayan-Ugurluouglu, Ball, Vrtala, Schweiger, Kraf, & Valenta, 2000; Somos, Schneider, & Farkas, 2001). In addition, nerve growth factor (NGF) levels in blood have been elevated in patients with vernal keratoconjunctivitis (Lambiase, Bonini, Micera, Magrini, Bracci-Laudiero, & Aloe, 1995), atopic dermatitis (Kimata, 2003a), and bronchial asthma (Noga, Hanf, Schaper, O'Conner, & Kunkel, 2001). In contrast, the blood levels of another neurotrophin, neurotrophin-3 (NT-3) were not elevated in patients with bronchial asthma (Noga, *et al.*, 2001). These results indicate that neurotrophin may be involved in allergic responses. Patients with atopic dermatitis report physiological and psychological stress, and stress increases IgE levels in blood of patients with atopic dermatitis (Buske-Kirschbaum, Geiben, Hollig, Morschhauser, & Hellhammer, 2002). In contrast, it has been previously reported that laughter induced by viewing humorous videos, Charlie Chaplin's "Modern Times" and Rowan Atkinson's "The Best Bits of Mr. Beans," was associated with reduced allergen-induced skin wheal responses in 25 and 8 patients with atopic dermatitis, respectively, while viewing nonhumorous video did not do so (Kimata, 2001a, 2001b). Since the levels of NGF and NT-3 in tears of allergic patients have not been reported but might be expected to have similar associations, the possible effect of laughter on allergen-specific

---

[1]Address correspondence to Dr. Hajime Kimata, Department of Allergy, Ujitakeda Hospital, 24-1, Umonji, Uji, Uji-City, Kyoto Prefecture, 611-0021, Japan or e-mail (h-kimata@takedahp.or.jp).

IgE, IgG4, and IgA, and NGF and NT-3 levels in tears of patients with atopic dermatitis having atopic keratoconjunctivitis were investigated. It was expected that laughter could modulate allergic responses and neurotrophins simultaneously in allergic patients, which would directly prove the involvement of neurotrophin in allergy.

Method

After obtaining informed consent, 24 normal subjects (12 women and 12 men, M age 26 yr., range 20–41) and 24 patients with atopic dermatitis having atopic keratoconjunctivitis (12 women and 12 men, M age 27 yr., range 22–43) were studied. The patients had moderate to severe atopic dermatitis (SCORAD index: $M=40$, range 33–51) (Kunz, Oranje, Labreze, Stalder, Ring, & Taieb, 1997), and all were allergic to Japanese cedar pollen as shown by positive serum Japanese cedar pollen-specific IgE levels (M 82.5 IU/ml). All of the patients were treated with oral anti-allergic medication, oxatomide (60 mg/day) (Kyowa, Hakkou Industries, Ltd., Osaka, Japan) and skin care, including washing with povidone iodine and application of the nonsteroidal anti-inflammatory ointment azulen, and tranilast eyedrops (Kissei Pharmaceutical, Co. Ltd., Tokyo, Japan) (Kimata, 2001c). The half-lives of oxatomide and tranilast were 5 hr. and 4 hr., respectively. The patients did not use oxatomide and tranilast eye drops for 2 days prior to the study.

Study 1 was conducted in the conference room of the Ujitakeda Hospital. A cross-over design was used. Twelve of 24 normal subjects or patients with atopic keratoconjunctivitis were randomly assigned to view an 87-min. video, "Modern Times" once. After 1 mo., they viewed an 87-min. nonhumorous weather information video (the control condition) once. The other 12 normal subjects or patients with atopic keratoconjunctivitis first viewed the control video once, and after 1 mo. they viewed "Modern Times" once. Medical staff ascertained that all of the subjects laughed when they viewed "Modern Times," while they did not laugh at all when they viewed the control video. Just before and immediately after viewing the control video or "Modern Times," they rated their stress using a one-item overall stress rating scale. The item asked them to rate their overall stress on a scale using anchors of 0: no stress and 10: extremely stressed (Kang & Fox, 2001). Moreover, just before, immediately after, 2 hr. after, and 4 hr. after viewing the video, tears were collected with a micropipette (Drummond Scientific, Broomall, PA) (Yamada, Ogata, Kawai, Mashima, & Nishida, 2002) by medical staff who were blind to the purpose of the study. Japanese cedar pollen-specific IgE, IgG4, and IgA levels in tears were measured by Enzyme-linked immunosorbent assay (ELISA) by staff who were blind to the purpose of the study (Kimata, Fujimoto, Ishioka, & Yoshida, 1996; Kimata, 2003b). Briefly, ELISA plates were coated with Japanese cedar-pollen allergen (0.5 μg/well) and incubated with tears. Biotinylated anti-IgE, anti-IgG4, and anti-IgA antibodies and peroxidase-labeled ExtrAvidine were used to develop allergen-specific IgE, IgG4, and IgA. Sensitivity of the assay was 0.3 ng/ml. NGF and NT-3 levels in tears were measured by commercial ELISA (Promega Corp., Madison, WI) (Noga, et al., 2001).

The effect of laughter was also studied by viewing another humorous video in Study 2 in which seven patients with atopic keratoconjunctivitis were randomly assigned to view a 73-min. humorous video, "The Best Bits of Mr. Beans" once, and 1 mo. after the study they viewed the control video once. The other eight patients with atopic keratoconjunctivitis first viewed the control video, and 1 mo. after the study they viewed "The Best Bits of Mr. Beans" once. All of the patients laughed when they viewed "The Best Bits of Mr. Beans" but not the control video. Just before and immediately after viewing a video, tears were collected as above, and Japanese cedar pollen-specific IgE, IgG4, and IgA, and NGF were measured. "Modern Times" and "The Best Bits of Mr. Beans" were dubbed in English, but a Japanese translation was added on the screen. This study was approved by the Ethics Committee at our hospital. Since parameters were paired and nonparametric, statistical analysis was performed using a Wilcoxon signed-ranks test to calculate probability (p) levels. Also, effect sizes (ES) were calculated.

Results

Effect of Viewing "Modern Times" (Study 1)

Stress ratings.—As shown in Table 1, the mean stress rating did not change significantly in normal subjects before and after viewing the control video (ns, ES = –0.12), while after viewing the humorous video, it was slightly, but significantly ($p = .03$, ES = .30), decreased. In contrast, the baseline stress rating was significantly ($p = .0001$, ES = –.75) elevated in patients with

TABLE 1
Effect of Viewing Humorous Video on Stress Ratings: Means and 95% Confidence Intervals (CI) ($N = 24$)

	Stress Rating			
	Viewing Control Video		Viewing Humorous Video	
	Before	Immediately After	Before	Immediately After
Normal Subjects				
M	1.1[a]	1.3[a]	1.2[b]	0.7[c]
95% CI	0.7, 1.5	0.9, 1.7	0.9, 1.6	0.3, 1.1
Patients With Atopic Keratoconjunctivitis				
M	4.7[d]	4.9[d]	4.8[e]	1.4[f]
95% CI	4.3, 5.1	4.1, 5.7	4.6, 5.6	1.2, 1.6

Note.—Means in rows with differing superscripts are different at the p levels by Wilcoxon signed-ranks test and by effect sizes (ES). [b vs c]$p = .03$ and ES = .30. [e vs f]$p = .0001$ and ES = .73.

atopic keratoconjunctivitis compared to those in normal subjects, and it was not significantly different when they viewed the control video ($p = 0.66$, ES = −.05). However, immediately after viewing the humorous video, the mean stress rating significantly decreased ($p = .0001$, ES = .73). From these results one infers patients with atopic keratoconjunctivitis report stress and viewing a humorous video significantly reduces their self-reported stress.

Immunological Results

As shown in Table 2, assays of Japanese cedar pollen-specific IgE, IgG4, or IgA indicated that none of these were detected in the tears of normal subjects. No significant changes in these levels occurred after the normal subjects viewed the control video or the humorous video. In contrast, significantly elevated levels of Japanese cedar pollen-specific IgE ($p = .00001$, ES =

TABLE 2
Effect of Viewing Humorous Video on Immunoglobulin Levels in Tears: Means and 95% Confidence Intervals For Japanese Cedar Pollen-specific IgE, IgG4, IgA (ng/ml) ($N = 24$)

Tear	Before	Time After Viewing		
		Immediately	2 Hours	4 Hours
Viewing Control Video				
Normal Subjects				
IgE	<0.3	<0.3	<0.3	<0.3
IgG4	<0.3	<0.3	<0.3	<0.3
IgA	<0.3	<0.3	<0.3	<0.3
Patients With Atopic Keratoconjunctivitis				
IgE	10.6[a]	10.9[a]	10.7[a]	10.4[a]
	8.4, 12.8	8.5, 13.4	8.7, 13.8	8.1, 12.0
IgG4	13.7[b]	14.4[b]	14.1[b]	13.9[b]
	11.2, 16.3	11.5, 17.3	11.3, 16.6	11.4, 16.6
IgA	3.3[c]	3.7[c]	3.5[c]	3.2[c]
	2.9, 3.7	3.1, 4.3	3.0, 4.1	2.7, 3.6
Viewing Humorous Video				
Normal Subjects				
IgE	<0.3	<0.3	<0.3	<0.3
IgG4	<0.3	<0.3	<0.3	<0.3
IgA	<0.3	<0.3	<0.3	<0.3
Patients With Atopic Keratoconjunctivitis				
IgE	10.3[d]	6.1[e]	8.1[f]	10.1[d]
	8.3, 12.4	5.3, 6.9	6.7, 9.5	7.7, 12.5
IgG4	14.7[g]	9.3[h]	11.2[i]	14.3[g]
	11.2, 18.2	7.3, 11.3	8.7, 13.7	11.0, 17.6
IgA	3.6[j]	5.8[k]	4.9[l]	3.9[j]
	3.0, 4.3	5.0, 6.6	4.3, 5.5	3.3, 4.5

Note.—Means in rows with differing superscripts are different at the p levels by Wilcoxon signed-ranks test and by effect sizes (ES). [d vs e]$p = .0002$ and ES = .50; [d vs f]$p = .003$ and ES = .15; [g vs h]$p = .0004$ and ES = .35; [g vs i]$p = .003$ and ES = .17; [j vs k]$p = .0005$ and ES = −.53; [j vs l]$p = .001$ and ES = −.25.

.88), IgG4 ($p = .00001$, ES = 0.85), and IgA ($p = .0001$, ES = 0.76) were detected in the tears of patients with atopic keratoconjunctivitis. There were no significant differences in the levels after the patients viewed the control video. However, immediately after viewing the humorous video, the levels for Japanese cedar pollen-specific IgE and IgG4 significantly decreased, while Japanese cedar pollen-specific IgA levels significantly increased.

Time-course study showed that there was a still significant decrease in Japanese cedar pollen-specific IgE and IgG4 levels, and increase in Japanese cedar pollen-specific IgA levels after 2 hr. of viewing the humorous video (Table 1). However, after 4 hr. of viewing, there was no significant change of Japanese cedar pollen-specific IgE ($p = .06$, ES = –.09), IgG4 (ns, ES = .04), or IgA (ns, ES = –.03) compared to baseline levels.

Neurogenic Results

NGF and NT-3 were detectable in tears of normal subjects, but neither viewing the control video nor the humorous video significantly affected the levels of these neurotrophins in normal subjects (Table 3). In contrast, NGF levels were significantly elevated compared to those in normal subjects ($p = .0001$, ES = –.95), while NT-3 levels were not significantly elevated (ns, ES = –.09) in tears of patients with atopic keratoconjunctivitis. Immediately after viewing the control video, NGF or NT-3 levels were not significantly changed. However, immediately after viewing the humorous video, NGF levels were significantly decreased, while NT-3 levels were not significantly changed.

Time-course study showed that there was a still significant decrease in NGF levels after 2 hr. of viewing the humorous video (Table 3). However, 4 hr. after viewing the humorous video, there was no significant change of NGF levels compared to baseline levels ($p = .09$, ES = –.24).

Effect of Viewing "The Best Bits of Mr. Beans" (Study 2)

The effect of viewing another humorous video "The Best Bits of Mr. Beans" was studied. Immediately after viewing this video, there was also a significant decrease in tear levels of Japanese cedar pollen-specific IgE (M [95% CI] ng/ml, 9.2 [7.4–11.0] before vs 6.3 [5.7–6.9] after; $p = .0001$, ES = .52), Japanese cedar pollen-specific IgG4 (13.6 [11.8–15.4] before vs 9.5 [6.6–12.4] after; $p = .0002$, ES = 0.38), and NGF (M[95% CI] pg/ml, 214 [170–265] before vs 139 [125–153] after; $p = .0006$, ES = .71), while there was a significant increase in Japanese cedar pollen-specific IgA (M[95% CI] ng/ml, 4.0 [3.0–5.0] before vs 7.3 [6.1–8.5] after; $p = .0001$, ES = –.60). In contrast, immediately after viewing the control video, these parameters were not significantly modulated (data not shown).

TABLE 3
Effect of Viewing Humorous Video on Immunoglobulin Levels in Tears: Means and 95% Confidence Intervals For NGF, NT-3 (pg/ml) (N = 24)

Tear	Before	Time After Viewing		
		Immediately	2 Hours	4 Hours

Viewing Control Video

Normal Subjects				
NGF	45.6[a]	48.1[a]	44.7[a]	47.5[a]
	39.7, 51.9	40.5, 55.7	38.9, 50.4	40.1, 56.4
NT-3	24.3[b]	27.2[b]	26.6[b]	25.3[b]
	21.0, 27.6	23.7, 30.7	22.5, 30.1	21.7, 29.4
Patients With Atopic Keratoconjunctivitis				
NGF	238[c]	256[c]	247[c]	251[c]
	213, 264	227, 285	224, 271	230, 282
NT-3	26.3[d]	29.7[d]	27.5[d]	28.1[d]
	22.4, 30.2	25.4, 34.0	23.0, 31.8	24.3, 33.5

Viewing Humorous Video

Normal Subjects				
NGF	47.0[e]	46.3[e]	47.4[e]	45.9[e]
	40.1, 53.9	39.0, 53.6	40.5, 54.3	38.5, 52.4
NT-3	28.1[f]	26.5[f]	27.6[f]	28.9[f]
	24.4, 31.8	23.0, 30.0	24.0, 31.5	24.7, 31.9
Patients With Atopic Keratoconjunctivitis				
NGF	245[g]	136[h]	186[i]	242[g]
	218, 273	118, 154	164, 208	215, 277
NT-3	25.5[j]	28.9[j]	25.1[j]	27.6[j]
	22.2, 28.8	24.8, 32.9	22.0, 28.5	23.9, 31.5

Note.—Means in rows with differing superscripts are different at the p levels by Wilcoxon signed-ranks test and by effect sizes (ES). [g vs h] $p = .0001$ and ES = .69; [g vs i] $p = .0009$ and ES = .59.

Discussion

These results indicated that laughter after viewing a humorous video was associated with decreased levels of Japanese cedar pollen-specific IgE and IgG4, and NGF levels in tears. This was not due to nonspecific decrease of flow in tears, since Japanese cedar pollen-specific IgA or NT-3 levels did not decrease. This is consistent with previous report that these chemicals were produced locally in the eyes but not inflow from blood (Nomura & Takemura, 1998). Collectively, measurement of these parameters in tears may be suitable for the study of production of immunoglobulins and neurotrophins.

There is precedence that laughter modulates various parameters *in vivo*. Laughter caused by viewing a humorous video elevated natural kill cell activity and serum IgA levels in normal subjects (Berk, Felten, Tan, Bittman, & Westengard, 2001). Exposure to rakugo, a traditional Japanese comic story, decreased levels of interleukin 6 in the blood of patients with rheumatoid arthritis (Yoshino, Fujimori, & Kohda, 1996). Similarly, laughter significantly decreased stress-induced high levels of growth hormone in blood (Berk, Tan, Fry, Napier, Lee, Hubbard, Lewis, & Eby, 1989). Laughter while attending MANZAI, one form of Japanese comedy performance, which is carried out by two people, was associated with significantly less increase in postprandial blood glucose in patients with diabetes (Hayashi, Hayashi, Iwanaga, Kawai, Ishii, Shoji, & Murakami, 2003). These results suggest that laughter may enhance basal immune responses or counteract abnormal parameters. Japanese cedar pollen-specific IgA levels were elevated in patients with atopic keratoconjunctivitis, which was further increased by laughter. Since it has been reported that IgA may counteract allergic responses (Aghayan-Ugurluouglu, *et al.*, 2000), laughter-induced increase in Japanese cedar pollen-specific IgA levels may act as a blocking antibody in patients with atopic keratoconjunctivitis.

The magnitude of change of these parameters may be clinically relevant since laughter alleviates pain in patients with rheumatoid arthritis (Yoshino, *et al.*, 1996) or reduces itching in patients with atopic dermatitis (Kimata, 2001b). However, detailed study is necessary to elucidate the clinical effect of laughter on various diseases.

The mechanisms of laughter on differential effects on Ig production are currently under investigation. Kimata (2001a) previously reported that laughter decreased IgE-mediated allergen-induced skin wheal response, while stress increased IgE levels in the blood of patients with atopic dermatitis (Buske-Kirschbaum, *et al.*, 2002). NGF levels were increased by stress (Aloe, Bracci-Laudiero, Alleva, Lambiase, Micera, & Tirassa, 1994). In a preliminary *in vitro* experiment, NGF increased Japanese cedar pollen-specific IgE and IgG4 production, while it decreased Japanese cedar pollen-specific IgA production (manuscript in preparation). Therefore, one can speculate that stress may elevate NGF levels, which in turn may augment Japanese cedar pollen-specific IgE and IgG4 production, while it may decrease Japanese cedar pollen-specific IgA production in patients with atopic keratoconjunctivitis. In contrast, laughter decreases NGF levels, which in turn may decrease Japanese cedar pollen-specific IgE and IgG4 levels and may increase Japanese cedar pollen-specific IgA levels. Moreover, the dissociation of allergen-specific IgE, IgG4, and IgA responses has been reported (Aghayan-Ugurluouglu, *et al.*, 2000). It has also been reported that relaxation increases salivary IgA (Green & Green, 1987), in accordance with the present results.

It has been reported that the levels of NGF in blood are elevated in patients with atopic dermatitis, bronchial asthma, or vernal keratoconjunctivitis (De Simmone, Alleva, Tirassa, & Aloe, 1990; Lambiase, *et al.*, 1995; Noga, *et al.*, 2001; Kimata, 2003a). Moreover, neurogenic inflammation has increased NGF levels in tears (Vesaluoma, Muller, Gallar, Lambiase, Moilanen, Hack, Belmonte, & Tervo, 2000). Collectively, these results indicate that NGF may play some role in allergic responses in tears. In contrast, the levels of NT-3 in the blood of patients with bronchial asthma were not elevated (Noga, *et al.*, 2001). These reports suggest that NT-3 may not be involved in allergic responses in tears. Since NT-3 levels in tears were not elevated in patients with atopic keratoconjunctivitis, it is not surprising that NT-3 levels were not decreased by viewing humorous video.

Taken together, laughter may be useful at least temporally in the study of neuroimmunology and treatment of allergic diseases.

REFERENCES

AGHAYAN-UGURLUOUGLU, R., BALL, T., VRTALA, S., SCHWEIGER, C., KRAF, D., & VALENTA, R. (2000) Dissociation of allergen-specific IgE and IgA responses in sera and tears of pollen-allergic patients: a study performed with purified recombinant pollen allergens. *Journal of Allergy and Clinical Immunology*, 105, 803-813.

ALOE, L., BRACCI-LAUDIERO, L., ALLEVA, E., LAMBIASE, A., MICERA, A., & TIRASSA, P. (1994) Emotional stress induced by parachute jumping enhances blood nerve growth factor and the distribution of nerve growth factor receptors in lymphocytes. *Proceedings of the National Academy of Sciences USA*, 91, 10440-10444.

BERK, L. S., FELTEN, D. L., TAN, S. A., BITTMAN, B. B., & WESTENGARD, J. (2001) Modulation of neuroimmune parameters during the eustress of humor-associated mirthful laughter. *Alternative Therapies in Health and Medicine*, 7, 62-76.

BERK, L. S., TAN, S. A., FRY, W. F., NAPIER, B. J., LEE, J. W., HUBBARD, R. W., LEWIS, J. E., & EBY, W. C. (1989) Neurogenic and stress hormone changes during mirthful laughter. *American Journal of Medical Science*, 298, 390-396.

BUSKE-KIRSCHBAUM, A., GEIBEN, A., HOLLIG, H., MORSCHHAUSER, E., & HELLHAMMER, D. (2002)

Altered responsiveness of the hypothalamus-pituitary-adrenal axis and the sympathetic adrenomedullary system to stress in patients with atopic dermatitis. *Journal of Clinical Endocrinology & Metabolism*, 87, 4245-4251.

DE SIMMONE, R., ALLEVA, E., TIRASSA, P., & ALOE, L. (1990) Nerve growth factor released into the bloodstream following intraspecific fighting indices mast cell degranulation in adult male mice. *Brain, Behavior and Immunity*, 4, 74-81.

GREEN, R. G., & GREEN, M. L. (1987) Relaxation increases salivary immunoglobulin A. *Psychological Reports*, 61, 623-629.

HAYASHI, K., HAYASHI, T., IWANAGA, S., KAWAI, K., ISHII, H., SHOJI, S., & MURAKAMI, K. (2003) Laughter lowered the increase in postprandial blood glucose. *Diabetes Care*, 26, 1651-1652.

KANG, D-H., & FOX, C. (2001) Th1 and Th2 cytokine response to academic stress. *Research in Nursing & Health*, 24, 245-257.

KIMATA, H. (2001a) Effect of humor on allergen-induced wheal reactions. *Journal of the American Medical Association*, 285, 738.

KIMATA, H. (2001b) [The effect of laughter on atopic dermatitis]. *Stress and Clinics*, 10, 33-37. [in Japanese]

KIMATA, H. (2001c) In vitro induction of IgE antibody to latex. *Allergy*, 56, 914.

KIMATA, H. (2003a) Enhancement of allergic skin wheal responses in patients with atopic eczema/dermatitis syndrome by playing video games or by a frequent ringing mobile phone. *European Journal of Clinical Investigation*, 33, 513-517.

KIMATA, H. (2003b) Enhancement of allergic skin wheal responses and in vitro allergen-specific IgE production by computer-induced stress in patients with atopic dermatitis. *Brain, Behavior and Immunity*, 17, 134-138.

KIMATA, H., FUJIMOTO, M., ISHIOKA, C., & YOSHIDA, A. (1996) Histamine selectively enhances human immunoglobulin E (IgE) and IgG4 production induced by anti-CD58 monoclonal antibody. *Journal of Experimental Medicine*, 184, 357-364.

KUNZ, B., ORANJE, A. P., LABREZE, L., STALDER, J-F., RING, J., & TAIEB, A. (1997) Clinical validation and guidelines for the SCORAD index: consensus report of the European Task Force on Atopic Dermatitis. *Dermatology*, 195, 10-19.

LAMBIASE, A., BONINI, S., MICERA, A., MAGRINI, L., BRACCI-LAUDIERO, L., & ALOE, L. (1995) Increased plasma levels of nerve growth factor in vernal keratoconjunctivitis and relationship to conjunctival mast cells. *Investigative Ophthalmology & Visual Science*, 36, 2127-2132.

NOGA, O., HANF, G., SCHAPER, C., O'CONNER, A., & KUNKEL, G. (2001) The influence of inhalative corticosteroids on circulating nerve growth factor, brain-derived neurotrophic factor and neurotrophin-3 in allergic asthmatics. *Clinical and Experimental Allergy*, 31, 1906-1912.

NOMURA, K., & TAKEMURA, E. (1998) Tear IgE concentrations in allergic conjunctivitis. *Eye*, 12, 296-298.

SOMOS, S., SCHNEIDER, I., & FARKAS, B. (2001) Immunoglobulins in tears and sera in patients with atopic dermatitis. *Allergy and Asthma Proceeding*, 22, 81-86.

VESALUOMA, M., MULLER, L., GALLAR, J., LAMBIASE, A., MOILANEN, J., HACK, T., BELMONTE, C., & TERVO, T. (2000) Effects of olroresin capsicum pepper spray on human corneal morphology and sensitivity. *Investigative Ophthalmology and Visual Science*, 41, 2238-2147.

YAMADA, M., OGATA, M., KAWAI, M., MASHIMA, Y., & NISHIDA, T. (2002) Substance P and its metabolites in normal human tears. *Investigative Ophthalmology and Visual Science*, 43, 2622-2625.

YOSHINO, S., FUJIMORI, J., & KOHDA, M. (1996) Effects of mirthful laughter on neuroendocrine and immune system in patients with rheumatoid arthritis. *Journal of Rheumatology*, 23, 793-794.

Accepted March 11, 2004.

EXACT GOODNESS-OF-FIT TESTS FOR UNORDERED EQUIPROBABLE CATEGORIES [1,2]

KENNETH J. BERRY, JANIS E. JOHNSTON, AND PAUL W. MIELKE, JR.

Colorado State University

Summary.—An algorithm and computer program to calculate exact goodness-of-fit tests for unordered categories with equal probabilities under the null hypothesis are presented. FORTRAN program EBGF utilizes partitions and multinomial weights to reduce computation times for Fisher's exact, exact chi-square, exact likelihood-ratio, exact Freeman-Tukey, and exact Cressie-Read goodness-of-fit tests.

The assessment of goodness-of-fit for unordered equiprobable categories is common in psychological research; for example, log-linear analyses (Mielke, Berry, & Johnston, 2004). This paper presents a fast recursion algorithm for Fisher's exact, exact chi-square, exact likelihood-ratio, exact Freeman-Tukey, and exact Cressie-Read goodness-of-fit tests for k unordered categories with equal probabilities under the null hypothesis. Exact tests are free from any asymptotic assumptions; consequently, they are ideal for sparse tables where expected values may be small.

STATISTICS

Consider the random assignment of n objects to k unordered, mutually-exclusive, exhaustive, equiprobable categories, i.e., the probability for each of the k categories is $p_i = 1/k$ for $i = 1, \ldots, k$, under the null hypothesis. Then, the probability that o_i objects occur in the ith of k categories is the multinomial probability given by

$$P(o_i \mid n, p_i) = P(o_1, \ldots, o_k \mid n, p_1, \ldots, p_k) = \left(n! \bigg/ \prod_{i=1}^{k} o_i! \right) \prod_{i=1}^{k} p_i^{o_i}, \quad [1]$$

where

$$\sum_{i=1}^{k} p_i = 1$$

and

$$\sum_{i=1}^{k} o_i = n.$$

Fisher's exact goodness-of-fit test is the sum of all distinct $P(o_i \mid n, p_i)$ values that are less than or equal to the observed value of $P(o_i \mid n, p_i)$ associated

---

[1]Address correspondence to K. J. Berry, Department of Sociology, Colorado State University, Fort Collins, CO 80523-1784 or e-mail (berry@lamar.colostate.edu).
[2]The program has been filed in Document APD2004-011. Remit $15.00 for photocopy to the Archive for Psychological Data, P.O. Box 7922, Missoula, MT 59807-7922.

with a set of observations $o_1, \ldots, o_k$ (Mielke & Berry, 1993, 2001, pp. 239-240).

The Pearson (1900) chi-square goodness-of-fit test statistic for n objects in k unordered categories is given by

$$\chi^2 = \sum_{i=1}^{k} \frac{(o_i - e_i)^2}{e_i} \qquad [2]$$

and the Wilks (1935, 1938) likelihood-ratio test statistic is given by

$$G^2 = 2 \sum_{i=1}^{k} o_i \ln\left(\frac{o_i}{e_i}\right), \qquad [3]$$

where the expected frequency of the ith category under the null hypothesis of equal category probabilities is $e_i = n/k$ for $i = 1, \ldots, k$.

Two other tests which have received attention are the Freeman-Tukey (1950) goodness-of-fit test statistic given by

$$T^2 = \sum_{i=1}^{k} \left[\sqrt{o_i} + \sqrt{o_i + 1} - \sqrt{4n/k + 1} \right]^2, \qquad [4]$$

and the Cressie-Read (1984) goodness-of-fit test statistic given by

$$I(\lambda) = \frac{2}{\lambda(\lambda+1)} \sum_{i=1}^{k} o_i \left[\left(\frac{o_i}{n/k}\right)^\lambda - 1 \right]. \qquad [5]$$

Cressie and Read (1984) showed that the statistic with λ set to 2/3 is considered to be best both in terms of attained significance level and small sample power properties.

Under the null hypothesis, the χ^2, G^2, T^2, and $I(2/3)$ goodness-of-fit test statistics are asymptotically distributed as chi-squared with $k-1$ degrees-of-freedom. However, when n is small or k is large, the expected frequencies are often small, and the chi-squared approximation to these tests is suspect. Based on early work by Bartlett (1937, 1953a, 1953b, 1954, 1955), Box (1949), and Lawley (1956), Williams (1976) introduced a correction to G^2 given by

$$q = 1 + \frac{1}{6n(k-1)} \sum_{i=1}^{k} \frac{1-p_i}{p_i}. \qquad [6]$$

An additional correction to G^2 by Smith, Rae, Manderscheid, and Silbergeld (1981) is given by

$$q' = 1 + \frac{1}{6n^2(k-1)} \sum_{i=1}^{k} \frac{(1-p_i)(1+np_i)}{p_i^2}. \qquad [7]$$

Under the null hypothesis of equal category probabilities, i.e., $p_i = 1/k$ for $i = 1, \ldots, k$, Equation 6 reduces to

$$q = 1 + \frac{k+1}{6n}, \qquad [8]$$

and Equation 7 reduces to

$$q' = 1 + \frac{k+1}{6n} + \frac{k^2}{6n^2}. \qquad [9]$$

Both the Williams (1976) $G_W^2 = G^2/q$ and the Smith, et al. (1981) $G_S^2 = G^2/q'$ test statistics are asymptotically distributed as chi-squared with $k-1$ degrees-of-freedom.

Algorithm

In general, for an exact goodness-of-fit test with n events in k categories there are

$$M = \binom{n+k-1}{k-1} \qquad [10]$$

distinct ordered configurations to be examined. Under the null hypothesis that the probability of each of k categories is equal, a vastly reduced number of distinct partitions of the data can be considered using a further condensation of the M ordered configurations. However, if the probabilities are not equal, then the total number of distinct ordered configurations cannot be condensed. In such cases, programs exist for the general case (Mielke & Berry, 1993, 2001, p. 322). This further condensation is based on a 1748 result by Euler which provides a generating function for the number of decompositions of n into integer summands without regard to order using the recurrence relation

$$p(n) = \sum_{j=1}^{} (-1)^{j-1} p[n - (3j^2 \pm j)/2] \qquad [11]$$

where $p(0) = 1$ and j is a positive integer satisfying $2 \leq 3j^2 \pm j \leq 2n$ (Euler, 1988, pp. 256-282). Note that if $n = 1$, then $j = 1$ with only the $-$ sign allowed; if $2 \leq n \leq 4$, then $j = 1$ with both the $+$ and $-$ signs allowed; if $5 \leq n \leq 6$, then $j = 1$ with both the $+$ and $-$ signs allowed and $j = 2$ with only the $-$ sign allowed; and so forth. In order to maintain consistency with the mathematical notation first employed by Euler, $p(n)$ denotes the number of partitions of n into distinct parts and should not be confused with the common statistical use of p which usually indicates a probability value. Hardy and Ramanujan (1918, p. 79) provided the asymptotic formula for $p(n)$, as n approaches ∞, given by

$$p(n) \sim \frac{1}{4n\sqrt{3}} \exp\left(\pi \sqrt{2n/3}\right). \qquad [12]$$

Given the observed categorical frequencies, $o_1, \ldots, o_k$, the algorithm generates all $p(n)$ partitions, computes the exact probability for each partition, calculates the observed χ^2, G^2, G_W^2, G_S^2, T^2, and $I(2/3)$ test statistics, and the number of ways each partition can occur, i.e., the partition weights. The partition weights are multinomial and are given by

$$W = k! \Big/ \prod_{i=1}^{m} f_i! \qquad [13]$$

where f_i is the frequency for each of m distinct numbers comprising a partition. For example, if the observed partition is {3 2 2 1 0 0} where $n = 8$, $k = 6$, and $m = 4$, then $f_1 = 1$, $f_2 = 2$, $f_3 = 1$, $f_4 = 2$, and $W = 180$. If $k \geq n$, then the number of distinct partitions is $p(n)$. If $k < n$, the number of distinct partitions is reduced to eliminate those partitions where the number of partition values exceeds k. For example, if $k = 3$ and $n = 5$, then the two partitions {2 1 1 1} and {1 1 1 1 1} cannot be considered as the respective number of partitions, four and five, both exceed $k = 3$. The sum of the values of W for the included distinct partitions is equal to M.

The exact probability values for the Fisher exact, χ^2, G^2, T^2, and $I(2/3)$ goodness-of-fit tests are obtained by comparing observed values to partition probabilities. In the case of Fisher's exact test, partition probabilities equal to or less than the observed partition probability are weighted and summed. For the exact χ^2, G^2, T^2, and $I(2/3)$ goodness-of-fit tests, partition probabilities associated with partition test statistics equal to or greater than the observed test statistic values are weighted and summed. Under the null hypothesis, G_W^2 and G_S^2 are simple scalar functions of G^2; consequently, the exact probability values for G_W^2 and G_S^2 are identical to the probability value for G^2.

Examples

Three examples illustrate the application of the goodness-of-fit tests. The first example is based on $n = 8$ events in $k = 8$ categories, i.e., $n = k$; the second example is based on $n = 45$ events in $k = 20$ categories, i.e., $n > k$; and the third example is based on $n = 10$ events in $k = 50$ categories, i.e., $n < k$.

Example 1

Consider an example application where $n = 8$ learning-disabled elementary school children are classified into $k = 8$ categories of learning disability with eight categorical frequencies $o_1 = o_2 = 3$, $o_3 = 2$, and $o_4 = o_5 = o_6 = o_7 = o_8 = 0$. The null hypothesis specifies that the k expected category probabilities are equally likely, i.e., $p_i = 1/k = .125$ for $i = 1, \ldots, 8$. Table 1 lists the $p(8) = 22$ distinct partitions of the $n = 8$ events into the $k = 8$ categories, the partition probabilities, the multinomial weight for each partition, and the weight-

TABLE 1
Partitions, Exact Partition Probabilities, Multinomial Weights, and Exact Weighted Probabilities For $n = 8$ and $k = 8$

Number	Partition	Partition Probability	Multinomial Weight	Weighted Probability
1	1 1 1 1 1 1 1 1	$.2403 \times 10^{-2}$	1	$.2403 \times 10^{-2}$
2	2 1 1 1 1 1 1 0	$.1202 \times 10^{-2}$	56	$.6729 \times 10^{-1}$
3	2 2 1 1 1 1 0 0	$.6008 \times 10^{-3}$	420	$.2523$
4	2 2 2 1 1 0 0 0	$.3004 \times 10^{-3}$	560	$.1682$
5	2 2 2 2 0 0 0 0	$.1502 \times 10^{-3}$	70	$.1051 \times 10^{-1}$
6	3 1 1 1 1 1 0 0	$.4005 \times 10^{-3}$	168	$.6729 \times 10^{-1}$
7	3 2 1 1 1 0 0 0	$.2003 \times 10^{-3}$	1120	$.2243$
8	3 2 2 1 0 0 0 0	$.1001 \times 10^{-3}$	840	$.8411 \times 10^{-1}$
9	3 3 1 1 0 0 0 0	$.6676 \times 10^{-4}$	420	$.2804 \times 10^{-1}$
10*	3 3 2 0 0 0 0 0	$.3338 \times 10^{-4}$	168	$.5608 \times 10^{-2}$
11	4 1 1 1 1 0 0 0	$.1001 \times 10^{-3}$	280	$.2804 \times 10^{-1}$
12	4 2 1 1 0 0 0 0	$.5007 \times 10^{-4}$	840	$.4206 \times 10^{-1}$
13	4 2 2 0 0 0 0 0	$.2503 \times 10^{-4}$	168	$.4206 \times 10^{-2}$
14	4 3 1 0 0 0 0 0	$.1669 \times 10^{-4}$	336	$.5608 \times 10^{-2}$
15	4 4 0 0 0 0 0 0	$.4172 \times 10^{-5}$	28	$.1168 \times 10^{-3}$
16	5 1 1 1 0 0 0 0	$.2003 \times 10^{-4}$	280	$.5608 \times 10^{-2}$
17	5 2 1 0 0 0 0 0	$.1001 \times 10^{-4}$	336	$.3365 \times 10^{-2}$
18	5 3 0 0 0 0 0 0	$.3338 \times 10^{-5}$	56	$.1869 \times 10^{-3}$
19	6 1 1 0 0 0 0 0	$.3338 \times 10^{-5}$	168	$.5608 \times 10^{-3}$
20	6 2 0 0 0 0 0 0	$.1669 \times 10^{-5}$	56	$.9346 \times 10^{-4}$
21	7 1 0 0 0 0 0 0	$.4768 \times 10^{-6}$	56	$.2670 \times 10^{-4}$
22	8 0 0 0 0 0 0 0	$.5960 \times 10^{-7}$	8	$.4768 \times 10^{-6}$

*Observed categorical frequencies for Example 1 are identified with an asterisk.

ed partition probabilities. Partition number 10 in Table 1 corresponds to the observed categorical frequencies. Table 2 illustrates the calculation of exact cumulative partition probabilities for Fisher's exact, χ^2, and G^2 goodness-of-fit tests. The partition probabilities for Fisher's exact test are accumulated according to the magnitudes of the partition probabilities. The P value for Fisher's exact goodness-of-fit test is the sum of the partition probabilities equal to or less than the observed partition probability value. The χ^2 (G^2) partition probabilities are accumulated according to the magnitudes of the associated χ^2 (G^2) test statistics. The P value for the χ^2 (G^2) goodness-of-fit test is the sum of the partition probabilities associated with χ^2 (G^2) test statistics equal to or greater than the observed χ^2 (G^2) test statistic value. The T^2 and $I(2/3)$ partition probabilities are accumulated in like manner to the χ^2 and G^2 tests. The P values for Fisher's exact, χ^2, and G^2 goodness-of-fit tests are indicated by asterisks in Table 2.

Under the null hypothesis of no difference between the observed and expected frequencies, Fisher's exact goodness-of-fit P value is .02538. The observed χ^2 test statistic is 14.00 with an exact P value of .06744 and an

TABLE 2
Exact P Values For Fisher's Exact, Chi-square, and Likelihood-Ratio Tests

Fisher's Exact P Value	Chi-square Statistic	P Value	Likelihood-Ratio Statistic	P Value
$.4768 \times 10^{-6}$	56.00	$.4768 \times 10^{-6}$	33.27	$.4768 \times 10^{-6}$
$.2718 \times 10^{-4}$	42.00	$.2718 \times 10^{-4}$	27.24	$.2718 \times 10^{-4}$
$.1206 \times 10^{-3}$	32.00	$.1206 \times 10^{-3}$	24.27	$.1206 \times 10^{-3}$
$.3076 \times 10^{-3}$	30.00	$.6814 \times 10^{-3}$	22.69	$.3076 \times 10^{-3}$
$.8683 \times 10^{-3}$	26.00	$.8683 \times 10^{-3}$	22.18	$.4244 \times 10^{-3}$
$.9851 \times 10^{-3}$	24.00	$.9851 \times 10^{-3}$	21.50	$.9851 \times 10^{-3}$
$.4350 \times 10^{-2}$	22.00	$.4350 \times 10^{-2}$	18.87	$.4350 \times 10^{-2}$
$.9957 \times 10^{-2}$	20.00	$.9957 \times 10^{-2}$	17.68	$.9957 \times 10^{-2}$
$.1556 \times 10^{-1}$	18.00	$.1556 \times 10^{-1}$	16.64	$.1416 \times 10^{-1}$
$.1977 \times 10^{-1}$	16.00	$.1977 \times 10^{-1}$	16.09	$.1977 \times 10^{-1}$
$.2538 \times 10^{-1}$*	14.00	$.2538 \times 10^{-1}$	15.96	$.2538 \times 10^{-1}$*
$.6744 \times 10^{-1}$	14.00	$.6744 \times 10^{-1}$*	13.86	$.6744 \times 10^{-1}$
$.9547 \times 10^{-1}$	12.00	$.9547 \times 10^{-1}$	13.18	$.9547 \times 10^{-1}$
.1796	12.00	.1235	12.14	.1796
.2076	10.00	.2076	11.09	.2076
.2181	8.00	.2181	11.09	.2181
.4424	8.00	.4424	9.36	.4424
.6107	6.00	.6107	8.32	.6107
.6780	6.00	.6780	6.59	.6780
.9303	4.00	.9303	5.55	.9303
.9976	2.00	.9976	2.77	.9976
1.0000	0.00	1.0000	0.00	1.0000

*Observed P values are identified with an asterisk.

asymptotic P value of .05118. The observed G^2 test statistic is 15.96 with an exact P value of .02538 and an asymptotic P value of .02552. The observed G_W^2 test statistic is 13.44 with an asymptotic P value of .06216. The observed G_S^2 test statistic is 11.78 with an asymptotic P value of .10793. Recall that as scalar functions of G^2, the exact probabilities for G_W^2 and G_S^2 are identical to the exact probability of G^2. The observed T^2 test statistic is 12.94 with an exact P value of .01977 and an asymptotic P value of .07349. The observed $I(2/3)$ test statistic is 13.78 with an exact P value of .02538 and an asymptotic P value of .05524.

Given the different criteria used to determine the Fisher, χ^2, and G^2 probabilities in Table 2, the exact P values for Fisher's test, χ^2, and G^2 will sometimes differ, e.g., Fisher's test and χ^2 on the one hand and χ^2 and G^2 on the other hand, and sometimes agree, e.g., Fisher's test and G^2. Note that although the P values for Fisher's test and G^2 are both .02538 in this case, the cumulative distributions differ. It is also interesting to note that the Fisher and G^2 P values of .02538 lie on the rejection side of a nominal significance level of $\alpha = .05$, while the χ^2 P value of .06744 lies on the other side of $\alpha = .05$ in this example.

Example 2

Consider $n=45$ patients with a history of substance abuse classified into $k=20$ substance types, with categorical frequencies $o_1=o_2=o_3=6$, $o_4=5$, $o_5=4$, $o_6=3$, $o_7=2$, and $o_8=\cdots=o_{20}=1$. For this example, only 81,801 of the $p(45)=89,134$ partitions are relevant to the analysis, i.e., it is not possible to distribute all $n=45$ events into the $k=20$ categories and have all categories contain two or fewer observations. The null hypothesis specifies that the k expected category probabilities are equally likely, i.e., $p_i=1/k=.05$, for $i=1,\ldots,20$. Under the null hypothesis of no difference between the observed and expected frequencies, Fisher's exact goodness-of-fit P value is .06927. The observed χ^2 test statistic is 32.78 with an exact P value of .02864 and an asymptotic P value of .02550. The observed G^2 test statistic is 28.07 with an exact P value of .16668 and an asymptotic P value of .08212. The observed G_W^2 test statistic is 26.04 with an asymptotic P value of .12899. The observed G_S^2 test statistic is 25.27 with an asymptotic P value of .15181. The exact probabilities for G_W^2 and G_S^2 are identical to the exact probability of G^2. The observed T^2 test statistic is 22.28 with an exact P value of .35793 and an asymptotic P value of .27044. The observed $I(2/3)$ test statistic is 30.70 with an exact P value of .03701 and an asymptotic P value of .04359.

Example 3

For this example, consider that a patient is asked to check any of $k=50$ symptoms experienced in the past six months, resulting in $n=10$ selections for categorical frequencies of $o_1=4$, $o_2=3$, $o_3=2$, $o_4=1$, and $o_5=\ldots=o_{50}=0$. In this example, all of the $p(10)=42$ partitions are relevant to the analysis, given that $n<k$. The null hypothesis specifies that the k expected category probabilities are equally likely, i.e., $p_i=1/k=.02$ for $i=1,\cdots,50$. Under the null hypothesis of no difference between the observed and expected frequencies, Fisher's exact goodness-of-fit P value is $.17950 \times 10^{-5}$. The observed χ^2 test statistic is 140.00 with an exact P value of $.37880 \times 10^{-4}$ and an asymptotic P value of $.10766 \times 10^{-9}$. The observed G^2 test statistic is 52.64 with an exact P value of $.17950 \times 10^{-5}$ and an asymptotic P value of .33495. The observed G_W^2 test statistic is 28.46 with an asymptotic P value of .99173. The observed G_S^2 test statistic is 8.75 with an asymptotic P value of 1.00. Again, the exact probabilities for G_W^2 and G_S^2 are equal to the exact probability value for G^2. The observed T^2 test statistic is 23.87 with an exact P value of $.17950 \times 10^{-5}$ and an asymptotic P value of .99906. The observed $I(2/3)$ test statistic is 89.87 with an exact P value of $.83559 \times 10^{-5}$ and an asymptotic P value of $.33388 \times 10^{-3}$.

Discussion

Goodness-of-fit tests for unordered equiprobable categories are important tools in log-linear analyses and other psychological research applications. Recent exact multinomial model tests for log-linear analyses of r-way contingency tables depended on the present partitioning technique (Mielke, et al., 2004). Because small samples are prevalent in psychology (Holmes, 1979, 1990, pp. 41-42), sparse goodness-of-fit tables are common, for which asymptotic tests are notoriously poor choices, as shown here and elsewhere (Mielke & Berry, 2001, pp. 239-246). Exact tests are widely recognized to be preferred over asymptotic tests when feasible. In this paper, a fast recursion algorithm is presented that computes exact probability values for seven well-known goodness-of-fit tests. The algorithm is very fast when n is small because it computes only a maximum of $p(n)$ partition probability values instead of the M configuration probability values required by other exact algorithms. For example, in Example 3 with $n = 10$ and $k = 50$, there are $M = 62,828,356,305$ possible configurations to be examined, but only $p(10) = 42$ partitions.

Example 1 illustrates the algorithm with $n = 8$ observations in $k = 8$ unordered equiprobable categories. Thus, the expected value for each category is $e_i = 1.00$ for $i = 1, \ldots, 8$. Fisher's exact, G^2, G_W^2, G_S^2, and $I(2/3)$ goodness-of-fit tests yield identical exact P values of .02538, which is less than the nominal significance level of $\alpha = .05$, while χ^2 yields an exact P value of .06744, which is greater than $\alpha = .05$. The exact P value for T^2 is .01977. In comparison, the asymptotic P values for χ^2 and G^2 are good approximations to the corresponding exact P values, while the asymptotic P values for G_W^2 and G_S^2 provide increasingly conservative estimates of the corresponding exact P values. The asymptotic P values for both T^2 and $I(2/3)$ are much too conservative with asymptotic P values of .07349 and .05524, respectively.

Example 2 analyzes the data with $n = 45$ observations in $k = 20$ unordered equiprobable categories. The expected value for each category is $e_i = 2.25$ for $i = 1, \ldots, 20$. Unlike Example 1 where Fisher's exact, G^2, G_W^2, G_S^2, and $I(2/3)$ goodness-of-fit tests yielded exact P values less than $\alpha = .05$ and χ^2 yielded an exact P value greater than $\alpha = .05$, in Example 2 χ^2 and $I(2/3)$ yield exact P values less than $\alpha = .05$, while G^2, G_W^2, G_S^2, and T^2 all yield very conservative exact P values greater than $\alpha = .05$. In comparison, the asymptotic P values for χ^2 and $I(2/3)$ are good approximations to the corresponding exact P values, while the asymptotic P values for G^2, G_W^2, and T^2 provide poor approximations to the corresponding exact P values. On the other hand, the asymptotic P value for G_S^2 of .15181 is a good approximation to the exact G_S^2 P value of .16668. As in Example 1, the asymptotic P values for G_W^2 and G_S^2 result in pronounced increases over the value for G^2 with the added corrections of Williams (1976) and Smith, et al. (1981).

Example 3 analyzes very sparse data with $n = 10$ observations in $k = 50$ unordered equiprobable categories. In this example analysis, the expected value for each category is only $e_i = .2$ for $i = 1, \ldots, 50$. Fisher's exact test, G^2,

G_W^2, G_S^2, and T^2 yield identical exact P values of $.17950 \times 10^{-5}$ and the exact P values for χ^2 and $I(2/3)$ are not far removed at $.37880 \times 10^{-4}$ and $.83559 \times 10^{-5}$, respectively. On the other hand, the asymptotic P values range from $.10766 \times 10^{-9}$ for χ^2 to 1.00 for G_S^2. The asymptotic P value of $.33388 \times 10^{-3}$ for $I(2/3)$ is the only asymptotic P value that even remotely approximates the corresponding exact P value.

In general, asymptotic goodness-of-fit P values are heavily influenced by small sample sizes leading to sparse tables with low expected values. As is evident in Example 3, asymptotic P values are of little use for very sparse tables. Moreover, asymptotic P values provide conservative estimates of the corresponding exact P values in some cases, and in other cases, liberal estimates. As asymptotic goodness-of-fit P values are neither dependable nor reliable for sparse tables, exact P values are recommended. Other things being equal, Fisher's exact test is probably the best of the exact tests since the P value is based solely on the underlying exact probability structure, rather than an artificial test statistic.

Program

Program EBGF computes exact P values for Fisher's exact, χ^2, G^2, T^2, and $I(2/3)$ goodness-of-fit tests. When the null hypothesis specifies equal probabilities for all categories, Program EBGF employs the further condensation of the M ordered configurations which provides substantial computational improvement over exact programs that compute test statistic values for all M configurations. Table 3 compares the $p(n)$ partitions analyzed by Program EBGF with the M possible configurations for $1 \leq n = k \leq 20$. For example, with $n = 15$ observations in $k = 15$ categories, there are only $p(15) = 176$ partitions, but $M = 77{,}558{,}760$ total configurations to be analyzed. This indicates why such a gain in program speed is attained under the null hypothesis that the probability of each of k categories is equal. When k is very much larger than n, the efficiency of Program EBGF is increased, and exact programs utilizing M configurations are useless.

Program EBGF is written in FORTRAN-77 in double precision. Comment lines provide input/output specification, documentation, and an example analysis. Input into Program EBGF is interactive and consists of a problem heading, the number of categories (k), and the number of observed events in each of the categories, $o_1, \ldots, o_k$. Output of Program EBGF consists of

(1) the exact probability of the observed partition
(2) the exact Fisher P value,
(3) the observed Pearson (1900) χ^2 test statistic,
(4) the exact Pearson χ^2 P value,
(5) the asymptotic Pearson χ^2 P value,

TABLE 3
COMPARISON OF $p(n)$ AND M WHEN $1 \leq n = k \leq 20$

n	$p(n)$	M
1	1	1
2	2	3
3	3	10
4	5	35
5	7	126
6	11	462
7	15	1,716
8	22	6,435
9	30	24,310
10	42	92,378
11	56	352,716
12	77	1,352,078
13	101	5,200,300
14	135	20,058,300
15	176	77,558,760
16	231	300,540,195
17	297	1,166,803,110
18	385	4,537,567,650
19	490	17,672,631,900
20	627	68,923,264,410

(6) the observed Wilks (1935, 1938) G^2 test statistic,
(7) the exact Wilks G^2 P value,
(8) the asymptotic Wilks G^2 P value,
(9) the Williams (1976) observed G_W^2 test statistic,
(10) the Williams asymptotic G_W^2 P value,
(11) the Smith, et al. (1981) observed G_S^2 test statistic,
(12) the Smith, et al. asymptotic G_S^2 P value,
(13) the Freeman-Tukey (1950) observed T^2 test statistic,
(14) the Freeman-Tukey exact T^2 P value,
(15) the Freeman-Tukey asymptotic T^2 P value,
(16) the Cressie-Read (1984) observed $I(2/3)$ test statistic,
(17) the Cressie-Read exact $I(2/3)$ P value, and
(18) the Cressie-Read asymptotic $I(2/3)$ P value.

In addition, a number of checks on calculations are provided in the output. Program EBGF is dimensioned for $k = 50$ categories and $n = 120$ observed events and accommodates $k \geq n$ and $k < n$. The dimensions of Program EBGF can be changed by the user. Copies of Program EBGF are available at www.stat.colostate.edu/permute and also from the Archive for Psychological Data.[2]

REFERENCES

BARTLETT, M. S. (1937) Properties of sufficiency and statistical tests. *Proceedings of the Royal Society of London, Series A*, 160, 268-282.

BARTLETT, M. S. (1953a) Approximate confidence intervals. *Biometrika*, 40, 12-19.

BARTLETT, M. S. (1953b) Approximate confidence intervals: II. More than one unknown parameter. *Biometrika*, 40, 306-317.

BARTLETT, M. S. (1954) A note on the multiplying factors for various χ^2 approximations. *Journal of Royal Statistical Society, Series B*, 16, 296-298.

BARTLETT, M. S. (1955) Approximate confidence intervals: III. A bias correction. *Biometrika*, 42, 201-204.

BOX, G. E. P. (1949) A general distribution theory for a class of likelihood criteria. *Biometrika*, 36, 317-346.

CRESSIE, N., & READ, T. R. C. (1984) Multinomial goodness-of-fit tests. *Journal of the Royal Statistical Society, Series B*, 46, 440-464.

EULER, L. (1748/1988) *Introduction to analysis of the infinite, Book 1.* (J. D. Blanton, Transl.) New York: Springer-Verlag.

FREEMAN, M. F., & TUKEY, J. W. (1950) Transformations related to the angular and the square root. *The Annals of Mathematical Statistics*, 21, 607-611.

HARDY, G. H., & RAMANUJAN, S. (1918) Asymptotic formulae in combinatory analysis. *Proceedings of the London Mathematical Society*, 17, 75-115.

HOLMES, C. B. (1979) Sample size in psychological research. *Perceptual and Motor Skills*, 49, 283-288.

HOLMES, C. B. (1990) *The honest truth about lying with statistics.* Springfield, IL: Thomas.

LAWLEY, D. N. (1956) A general method for approximating to the distribution of likelihood ratio criteria. *Biometrika*, 43, 295-303.

MIELKE, P. W., JR., & BERRY, K. J. (1993) Exact goodness-of-fit probability tests for analyzing categorical data. *Educational and Psychological Measurement*, 53, 707-710.

MIELKE, P. W., JR., & BERRY, K. J. (2001) *Permutation methods: a distance function approach.* New York: Springer-Verlag.

MIELKE, P. W., JR., BERRY, K. J., & JOHNSTON, J. E. (2004) Asymptotic log-linear analysis: some cautions concerning sparse frequency tables. *Psychological Reports*, 94, 19-32.

PEARSON, K. (1900) On a criterion that a given system of deviations from the probable in the case of a correlated system of variables is such that it can reasonably be supposed to have arisen in random sampling. *Philosophical Magazine*, 50, 157-175.

SMITH, P. J., RAE, D. S., MANDERSCHEID, R. W., & SILBERGELD, S. (1981) Approximating the moments and distribution of the likelihood ratio statistic for multinomial goodness of fit. *Journal of the American Statistical Association*, 76, 737-740.

WILKS, S. S. (1935) The likelihood test of independence in contingency tables. *The Annals of Mathematical Statistics*, 6, 190-196.

WILKS, S. S. (1938) The large-sample distribution of the likelihood ratio for testing composite hypotheses. *The Annals of Mathematical Statistics*, 9, 60-62.

WILLIAMS, D. A. (1976) Improved likelihood-ratio tests for complete contingency tables. *Biometrika*, 63, 33-37.

Accepted March 8, 2004.

OPTIMAL HANDLE ANGLE OF THE FENCING FOIL FOR IMPROVED PERFORMANCE[1,2]

FANG-TSAN LIN

National Taiwan College of Physical Education

Summary.—Improperly designed hand tools and sports equipment contribute to undesired injuries and accidents. The idea of bending the tool, not the wrist, has been applied to sports equipment. According to Bennett's idea, the design of an ideal handle angle should be in the range of 14° to 24°. Thus design of the handle angle in the sport of fencing is also important. A well-designed handle angle could not only reduce ulnar deviation to avoid wrist injury but also enhance performance. An experiment with several different handle angles was conducted to analyze the effect on performance. Analysis showed an angle of 18° to 21° provided best overall performance in fencing.

Aghazadeh and Mital (1987) indicated there were over 260,000 hand tool-related injuries in the United States each year and that the associated medical costs alone come to some 400 million dollars. Mirka, Shivers, Smith, and Taylor (2002) suggested that hand tools should be redesigned to reduce risk of wrist and upper extremity injury of workers and athletes. Read and Wade (1999, pp. 8-9) indicated that use of a little thought and effort can go a long way in preventing injuries and improving performance. For example, the idea of bending the tool, not the wrist, has been applied to other things by Bennett (cf. Sanders & McCormick, 1993, p. 388), who patented the idea of bent handles (19° ± 5°) for tools and sports equipment.

Many sports tools are not designed for their efficient and safe operation by humans especially in repetitive activity. Improperly designed tools and devices have many undesired consequences, including accidents and injuries (Sanders & McCormick, 1993, pp. 383-409). For example, Lephart, Abt, and Ferris (2002) indicated that extrinsic factors associated with ligament injury during exercise are related to the conditioning of the athlete, equipment used, type of sport, and environmental conditions. Playing a sport without stretching or adequate training and awkward postures were also recognized as key ergonomic risk factors for cumulative trauma disorders and sport injuries in the literature (Armstrong & Radwin, 1986; Putz-Anderson, 1988; Muggleton, Allen, & Chappell, 1999). Dane, Can, and Karsan (1999) investigated the incidences of sport injuries in right- and left-handed subjects;

---

[1]This study was supported by National Science Council of Taiwan, under operating Grant No. NSC90-2218-E-028-001. The author gratefully acknowledges Mr. Chang, Chih-Lin in Hsiuping Institute of Technology for his assistance in experimental procedure and data collecting.
[2]Please address correspondence to Fang-Tsan Lin, National Taiwan College of Physical Education, No. 16, Section 1, Shuan-Shih Road, Taichung, Taiwan 402 or e-mail (ftlin@mars.ntcpe.edu.tw).

they found 83.0% of left-handed athletes and 68.0% of right-handed athletes had sports injuries. Ridenour (1998) indicated that different accident patterns for golf equipment were noted for adults and children. Previous publications investigating accidents involving golf clubs and over 2,000 incidents involving emergency room treatment of children injured by golf clubs were reviewed. Most injuries occurred when unsupervised children played with golf clubs at home. Kingma and ten Duis (1998) investigated about the incidence rate of sports injuries in five different types of sports and found that the most frequent type of sports injury was sprain. For all five types of sports, about 90% of the injuries were observed on either the lower or upper extremities. The possible health problems associated with intensive handling activity include localized muscle pain of the lower back and cardiovascular problems (Heppel, Fhawley, & Channer, 1991; Degani, Asfour, Waly, & Koshy, 1993; Hung & Paquet, 2002).

Huthon (1996, pp. 60-77) also indicated that almost any type of hand and wrist injury could occur during sport. For example, the hand might be pierced by a flying javelin or crushed by the collapse of a heavy stand. An opponent's racquet, foil, blade, stick, club, bat, etc. may strike the player accidentally. However, an athlete's own implement may do the damage, especially if it suddenly strikes a hard object in mid-swing, as when a golfer's club hits the ground. The upper end of the handle is driven forcibly against the front of the wrist, and this is actually the commonest cause of a rare but important injury—fracture of the hook of the hamates. The combination of maturation changes, and increased competitiveness of sports activity may also increase the likelihood of sport injury (Hass, Schick, Chow, Tillman, Brunt, & Cauraugh, 2003). But in practice sports injuries to the hand and wrist are almost always closed injuries, usually to bone or joint, such as the tennis wrist and carpal tunnel syndromes which have been associated with activity in a variety of fencing exercises.

The sport of fencing is an excellent form of exercise; it is still a popular sport in Taiwan. There are four attack tactics including active attacks, simultaneous attacks, parry riposte, and timing attacks in fencing. Chang and Lin (2001b) indicated that offensive defense tactics include parry riposte and timing attacks. The parry riposte is the basis of defense tactics, so there is no difference in hit performance between winner and loser. Chang and Lin (2001a) also found that the key point for winning the game is use of timing attack tactics properly, and practice could improve athletes' overall tactics. Strict training is necessary to accomplish successful use of these tactics. The main requirement for training includes muscular strength, movement velocity, durability, body softness, and sensitivity, especially with arms, legs, and wrists (Beijing College of Physical Education, 1996). Since tactics are the key factor in victory and practiced skill is the basis for performance of the tactics, coaches frequently modify skills training to develop correct use of tactics. If coaches ignore the athlete's physiological characteristics, exercise excessively, or adopt incorrect equipment and training methods which are non-ergonomically appropriate during the training period, athletes may suffer serious injuries (Nigg, Denoth, & Neukomm, 1981). The main regions in which a fencer frequently suffers injuries are the joints of the ankles, knees, hips, and wrist. Injuries affect training so that the athlete cannot make continuous progress in skill (Fink, 1993). Thus design of the handle angle in the sport of fencing is also important. A well-designed handle angle could not only reduce ulna deviation to avoid wrist injury but could also enhance performance in fencing (Lin & Chang, 2001a, pp. 351-354).

Today, various tools are often crafted for many specific applications as well as for general-purpose activities (Sanders & McCormick, 1993, pp. 383). So the design of fencing foils is also very important and should be considered (Shi, 1991). Ergonomic design of the handle angle is necessary to prevent injuries and to enhance performance. For example, Lin and Chang (2001a, 2001b) found that a suitable downward handle angle could contribute to the accomplishment of effective hit, accuracy, and the users' rating of subjective satisfaction. Read and Wade (1999, pp. 8-9) also indicated that using the right equipment and technique could prevent sport injuries. Athletes' bodies are different in shape and size so the design of the handle angle or a running shoe, the weight of a racquet head, the position of a car seat or computer keyboard must suit individual athletes. Technique is just as important. If faulty, technique can even produce an injury, whether paddling a kayak or lifting a box of groceries. In sports, using the right equipment and training a certain way may suit one person's body shape and lead to a gold medal, but if those methods produce injuries, other techniques would be needed or equipment redesigned.

Li (2002) found that unnatural posture and repetitive forceful exertion have been risk factors for hand or wrist injury. Such effects may be reduced via redesign of handles. A suitable downward angle of the fencing foil's handle could also reduce ulnar deviation and prevent wrist injury. Lin and Chang (2001b) conducted an experiment with handle angles from 3° to 15° (including 3°, 6°, 9°, 12°, 15°). They found that 9° and 15° downward handle angle were associated with highest performance on the effective hit and accuracy hit, but the 15° handle had the highest subjective satisfaction rating. The larger the handle angle, the more comfortable on use of the wrist, and fewer injuries may occur. According to Bennett, the design of an ideal handle angle of sports equipment should be in the range of 14° to 24° (Sanders & McCormick, 1993). The main purpose of the study was to assess fencing performance with different handle angles in the range of 14° to 24°. The study used the fencing foil as an experimental sword.

Method

Subjects

Of eight participants, all reported having normal vision. All subjects, right-handed fencers, were members of the university fencing team.

Experimental Design

A fencing experiment using several different handle angles was conducted to analyze their effects on fencing performance. The independent variable was downward handle angle, specifically, 9°, 15°, 18°, 21°, and 24°. The angle of 12° was eliminated in this experiment because performance was not sensitive to that angle in Lin and Chang (2001a). The dependent variables were the hit rate, hit accuracy, and a users' rating of subjective satisfaction. The one-way analysis of variance was adopted for inferential statistics.

Equipment

There were eight France Lames swords for international competition, a 5-point target for accuracy hitting, a fencing outfit with a 20-cm × 16-cm copper plate for attack hitting, and a list for users' rating of subjective satisfaction (1 = very comfortable, 5 = very uncomfortable).

Procedure

For measurement of attack hits, all attack actions were the same as those in Chang and Lin's experiment (2001a). The distance between the coach and subject was kept constant. The coach was always in the initiative position. The subject had to follow the coach's instructions for required actions, such as simultaneous attack, parry riposte, or active attack. The subjects always kept the same distance to the coach by an advancing or retreating step. The attack hit might use lunges or retreating steps, depending on the distance from the coach. Each subject performed 10 attack hits for each handle angle, for a total of 50 hits per subject in this experiment.

To measure hit accuracy this study used 5-point targets to range scores from 5 to 1 point. The target circle diameters were 3 cm, 5 cm, 7 cm, 9 cm, and 11 cm. Any hit outside the area or nontouch hitting was assigned 0 point. The distance from the starting line to the target was the length of a straight-arm with a blade plus the length of two steps in retreat. Each subject had 10 trials for a lunge with each handle angle, for a total of 50 hits per subject in this experiment.

Results and Discussion

Analysis of Hit Rate

Five types of handle angles, for each of which 10 attack-hit trials were performed. The measure of total attack-hits for each subject was 50. Means and standard deviations are presented in Table 1. A one-way analysis of variance with angles as the independent variable and hit rates as the dependent variable indicated that hit rates were significantly affected by using different handle angles ($F_{4,35} = 11.7$, $p \leq .001$, see Table 1). Post hoc testing by the Scheffé test ($p \leq .05$) indicated that the angles 18°, 21°, and 24° downward had the highest mean hit rate (see Table 1), but there was no significant difference on mean rating of users' subjective satisfaction.

TABLE 1
MEANS, STANDARD DEVIATIONS, AND ONE-WAY ANALYSIS OF VARIANCE
FOR HIT RATE AND HIT ACCURACY (%)

	Handle Angle	M	SD	$F_{4,7}$	p	Post hoc Test
Hit Rate				11.7	<.001	c=d=e>b>a
a	9°	58.80	17.27			
b	15°	76.30	5.18			
c	18°	77.55	12.82			
d	21°	93.80	7.44			
e	24°	85.00	5.35			
Hit Accuracy				6.50	<.001	c=d=b>e>a
a	9°	53.50	8.99			
b	15°	67.00	6.85			
c	18°	72.50	5.32			
d	21°	69.30	10.58			
e	24°	56.00	13.05			

Analysis of Hit Accuracy

The five handle angles were the same as those for the attack hit. Ten lunge trials were performed with each angle for a total of 50 lunge hits for each subject. Means and standard deviations are presented in Table 1. A one-way analysis of variance with angles as the independent variable and hit accuracy as the dependent variable indicated that hit accuracy was significantly affected by using different handle angles ($F_{4,35} = 6.5$, $p \leq .001$, see Table 1). Post hoc testing by the Scheffé test ($p \leq .05$) indicated that the angles 15°, 18°, and 21° downward had the highest mean hit accuracy (see Table 1). There was also no significant difference for mean ratings of subjective satisfaction.

The important finding is that 18° to 21° (19.5° ± 1.5°) downward angle was associated with the best overall fencing performance. Both downward angles had the highest effective hits and accuracy scores with the same rating of subjective satisfaction. This finding is almost the same as Bennett's idea (cf. Sanders & McCormick, 1993, pp. 388) of bending handles in the range 14° to 24° (19° ± 5°) for all tools and sports equipment. But the range here is more restricted and smaller than in the earlier finding. The reason may be that fencing requires highly dynamic movements (Cavanagh & Lafortune, 1980) and requires extreme accuracy, so such an optimal angle range should be restricted or smaller than for other hand tools.

Finally, this study suggests that the handle angle design of all sport equipment should be considered within ergonomics theory because suitable design of hand tools could not only reduce ulnar deviation to avoid wrist injuries but could also enhance sports performance, including accuracy and effective hits.

REFERENCES

AGHAZADEH, F., & MITAL, A. (1987) Injuries due to hand tools. *Applied Ergonomics*, 18, 273-278.

ARMSTRONG, T. J., & RADWIN, R. D. (1986) Repetitive trauma disorders: job evaluation. *Journal of Occupational Medicine*, 21, 481-486.

BEIJING COLLEGE OF PHYSICAL EDUCATION. (1996) *Fencing in Beijing College of Physical Education*. Beijing: Beijing College of Physical Education.

CAVANAGH, P., & LAFORTUNE, M. (1980) Ground reaction forces in distance running. *Journal of Biomechanics*, 13, 397-406.

CHANG, C. L., & LIN, F. T. (2001a) Effects of foil downward angle on attack hit. *Journal of National Taiwan College of Physical Education*, 9, 591-607.

CHANG, C. L., & LIN, F. T. (2001b) Statistical analysis of the influence on fencing tactics in competition. *Journal of National Taiwan College of Physical Education*, 8, 239-251.

DANE, E., CAN, S., & KARSAN, O. (1999) Sport injuries in right- and left-handers. *Perceptual and Motor Skills*, 89, 846-848.

DEGANI, A., ASFOUR, S., WALY, S. M., & KOSHY, J. G. (1993) A comparative study of two shovel designs. *Applied Ergonomics*, 24, 306-312.

FINK, P. (1993) Force in the forward leg during a fencing lunge. Unpublished doctoral dissertation of Purdue Univer.

HASS, C. J., SCHICK, E. A., CHOW, J. W., TILLMAN, M. D., BRUNT, D., & CAURAUGH, J. H. (2003) Lower extremity biomechanics differ in prepubescent and postpubescent female athletes during stride jump landings. *Journal of Applied Biomechanics*, 19, 139-152.

HEPPEL, R., FHAWLEY, S. K., & CHANNER, K. S. (1991) Shoveller's infarction. *British Medical Journal*, 302, 469-470.

HUNG, C. T., & PAQUET, V. (2002) Kinematic evaluation of two snow-shovel designs. *International Journal of Industrial Ergonomics*, 29, 319-330.

HUTHON, M. A. (1996) *Sports injuries—recognition and management*. New York: Oxford Univer. Press.

KINGMA, J., & TEN DUIS, H. J. (1998) Sports members' participation in assessment of incidence rate of injuries in five sports from records of hospital-based clinical treatment. *Perceptual and Motor Skills*, 86, 675-686.

LEPHART, S. M., ABT, J. P., & FERRIS, P. (2002) Neuromuscular contributions to anterior cruciate ligament injuries in females. *Current Opinion in Rheumatology*, 14, 168-173.

LI, K. W. (2002) Ergonomics design and evaluation of wire-typing hand tools. *International Journal of Industrial Ergonomics*, 30, 149-161.

LIN, F. T., & CHANG, C. L. (2001a) An application research of human factors on foil blade angle. In W. Sheng & Z. Kan (Eds.), *Occupational ergonomics*. Beijing: Tianjin Science and Technology Press. Pp. 351-354.

LIN, F. T., & CHANG, C. L. (2001b) Human factors design and application of foil blade angle. *Proceeding of 21st FISU Congress in Beijing*. Pp. 211-212.

MIRKA, G. A., SHIVERS, C., SMITH, C., & TAYLOR, J. (2002) Ergonomic interventions for the furniture manufacturing industry: Part II. Hand tools. *International Journal of Industrial Ergonomics*, 29, 275-287.

MUGGLETON, J. M., ALLEN, R., & CHAPPELL, P. H. (1999) Hand and arm injuries associated with repetitive manual work in industry: a review of disorders, risk factors and preventive measures. *Ergonomics*, 42, 714-739.

NIGG, B. M., DENOTH, J., & NEUKOMM, P. A. (1981) Quantifying the load on the human body: problems and some possible solutions. In R. C. Nelson (Ed.), *Biomechanics VIB*. Baltimore, MD: University Park Press. Pp. 88-99.

PUTZ-ANDERSON, V. (1988) *Cumulative trauma disorders: a manual for musculoskeletal diseases of upper limbs*. London: Taylor & Francis.

READ, M., & WADE, P. (1999) *Sports injuries*. Oxford, UK: Butterworth Heinemann.

RIDENOUR, M. V. (1998) Golf clubs: hidden home hazard for children. *Perceptual and Motor Skills*, 86, 747-753.

SANDERS, M. S., & MCCORMICK, E. J. (1993) *Human factors in engineering and design*. New York: McGraw-Hill.

SHI, S. K. (1991) Human factors and sports. *Journal of Culture and Physical Education, Taipei*, 18, 48-51.

Accepted March 16, 2004.

PREVALENCE OF UNIVERSITY STUDENTS' SUFFICIENT PHYSICAL ACTIVITY: A SYSTEMATIC REVIEW[1]

JENNIFER D. IRWIN

The University of Western Ontario

Summary.—This study reviewed and analyzed the prevalence of university students' participation in physical activity at the level necessary to acquire health benefits. 19 primary studies (published 1985–2001) representing a total of 35,747 students (20,179 women and 15,568 men) from a total of 27 countries (Australia, Canada, China, Germany, Nigeria, United States, and 21 European countries) are described and the amount of activity identified within each study is analyzed in accordance with the American College of Sports Medicine (ACSM) guidelines for physical activity. With respect to these guidelines, more than one-half of university students in the United States and Canada are not active enough to gain health benefits. Internationally, the same is true, although Australian students appear to have the highest level of sufficient activity (at 60%). Women, and especially African-American women, are among the least active students, and students living off-campus are more active than those on-campus. Insufficient activity is a serious health concern among university students. Appropriate interventions and tools to measure ACSM-recommended physical activity are needed.

Long-term, insufficient physical activity is a prevalent and a preventable leading risk factor for chronic disease and death (McGinnis, 1992, p. S197). University students, given their numbers and future societal roles, "are a group worthy of study, especially [because] little is known about their physical activity patterns and other health-related attributes" (Leslie, Owen, Salmon, Bauman, Sallis, & Kai Lo, 1999 p. 21). Although inactivity-related morbidities tend to be expressed later in life, the associated behavioral patterns tend to be formed during childhood to early adulthood (McGinnis, 1992; Bungum & Vincent, 1997). Therefore, it is critical to establish active lifestyles during youth (Bungum & Vincent, 1997). The purpose of this paper was to review the current literature pertaining to the prevalence of physical activity participation among university students and analyze findings against the American College of Sports Medicine (ACSM, 2000) guidelines for moderate activity, i.e., the level of physical activity necessary for health benefits. This review is unique because it analyzes the literature in accordance with standards for health. The resulting information is particularly valuable for determining the actual level of sufficient physical activity among this population and, therefore, identifying the strength of the need for early physical (in)activity interventions.

---

[1]Address enquiries to J. D. Irwin, Ph.D., Room 2319, Somerville House, Faculty of Health Sciences, University of Western Ontario, London, ON, Canada N6A 4K7 or e-mail (jenirwin@uwo.ca).

Regular physical activity reduces the risk of many diseases including coronary heart disease, stroke, and hypertension (Salonen, Puska, & Tuomelehto, 1982); noninsulin-dependent diabetes mellitus (Sothern Loftin, Suskind, Udall, & Blecker, 1999; ACSM, 2000); osteoporosis (Ebeling, 1998; Damilakis, Perisinakis, Kontakis, Vagios, & Gourtsoyiannis, 1999; Rubin, Hawker, Peltekova, Fielding, Ridout, & Cole, 1999); some kinds of cancer (Powell, Caspersen, Koplan, & Ford, 1998; Rockhill, Willett, Hunter, Manson, Hankinson, & Colditz, 1999; Wyrwich & Wolinsky, 2000; Freidenreich, Bryant, & Courneya, 2001); mental health ailments, such as stress and mood disturbances (Barabasz, 1991; Brevard & Ricketts, 1996; DiLorenzo, Bargman, Stucky-Ropp, Brassington, Frensch, & LaFontaine, 1999; McGuigan, 1999; Moore, Babyak, Wood, Napolitano, Khatri, Craighead, Herman, Krishman, & Blumenthal, 1999; Sothern, *et al.*, 1999; ACSM, 2000); back injuries; and development of gallstones (Sothern, *et al.*, 1999). Physical activity, however, does not just provide long-term protection from disease; physical activity also reduces stress and therefore provides immediate benefits. Furthermore, there is a dose-response relationship between physical activity and longevity (Pekkanen, Marti, Nissinen, Tuomelehto, Punsar, & Karvonen, 1987; Ferrucci, Izmirlian, Leveille, Phillips, Corti, Brock, & Guralnik, 1998), and the protective health effect of physical activity may persist for some time after activity is discontinued (Rubin, *et al.*, 1999; Wyrwich & Wolinsky, 2000). In light of this evidence, it seems logical that more people are exercising on a regular basis now than ever before (Cash, Novy, & Grant, 1994; Chen, 1998). However, participation in exercise decreases significantly between adolescence and adulthood, the age range of most university students (Stephens, Jacobs, & White, 1985; Caspersen, Christensen, & Pollard, 1986; Statistics Canada, 1998).

It is important to understand patterns of regular physical activity during the formative stage when young people are entering adulthood and laying a foundation for the adult life patterns. There may be opportunities to encourage the development of regular physical activity during these years. Since 9.4 million young adults in the United States (Martinez & Curry, 1998) and nearly 25% of Canadians ages 18–24 years attend university (Statistics Canada, 2000, 2001), there may be specific opportunities to influence the physical activity patterns of this subpopulation. Further, this group may be important because those who attend university may play an important role in establishing social and cultural norms as they move into roles as decision-makers and opinion leaders within the population (Leslie, Owen, & Sallis, 1999; Leslie, Owen, Salmon, Bauman, Sallis, & Kai Lo, 1999). For these reasons, it is important to gauge the physical activity patterns of this population and find effective ways to increase their exercise participation.

The recommendation to "accumulate 30 minutes or more of moderate-intensity physical activity on most, preferably all, days of the week" was published in 1995 by the American College of Sports Medicine in conjunction with the Centers for Disease Control and Prevention [hereafter referred to as the ACSM prescription/guidelines]. This recommendation was born from a workshop in which 20 researchers specializing in physical activity and health examined "pertinent scientific evidence and... develop[ed] a clear, concise 'public health message' regarding physical activity" (Pate, Pratt, Blair, Haskell, Macera, Bouchard, Buchner, Ettinger, Heath, King, Kriska, Leon, Marcus, Morris, Paffenbarger, Patrick, Pollock, Rippe, Sallis, & Wilmore, 1995, p. 402). The recommendation underscored the health benefits of physical activity of moderate intensity and promoted the acceptability of achieving the 30-min. duration in shorter bouts throughout the day. The recommendations are supported by physical activity and health research and are consistent with the panel's goal to create a message that can readily be integrated into behavioral interventions (Pate, *et al.*, 1995). Since their publication, the guidelines have received widespread acceptance. For example, the guidelines are prominent within the United States government's "Healthy People 2010" publication (U.S. Department of Health and Human Services, 2000), Health Canada's Physical Activity Guide to Healthy Active Living (Health Canada and the Canadian Society for Exercise Physiology, 1998), and Sports Medicine New Zealand's physical activity recommendations for the population (Sports Medicine New Zealand, 1998). The guidelines are intended to enhance, rather than replace, previous ACSM guidelines which promoted higher intensity activities for maximal benefits. It should be noted that ACSM has recommendations for other forms of physical activity such as resistance training, which may be a common form for physical activity among university students. Resistance training is engaged in most commonly by men, ages 17–29 years. Of those who regularly lift weights, 82% also engage in other forms of physical activity at least five times per week (Galuska, Earle, & Fulton, 2002). However, for the purpose of this study, the ACSM guidelines of accumulating 30 min. or more of moderate-intensity physical activity on most, preferably all, days of the week was the standard used.

Method

To obtain relevant literature for this systematic review, five databases were searched: Medline 1997–2003 and 1993–1996; HealthSTAR 1996–1998; 'Current Contents' all weeks; CINAHL 1982–2003; and PsycINFO 1984–2003. The search terms used to identify the chosen articles were university students, college students, physical activity, and exercise. The reference pages of articles identified by the database searches were also examined, and additional literature was discovered and retrieved. More than 35 articles were identified as potentially appropriate and acquired. The abstracts, introductions, and methodologies of each study were reviewed to assess its purpose, method, and sample. Consequently, a total of 19 studies, summarized in Table 1, were identified as appropriate, given that they met the criterion of being primary studies in which the prevalence of physical activity for university or college students was assessed.

RESULTS

Prevalence of Insufficient Physical Activity Among University Students in Canada and the United States

From the 19 studies (published 1985–2001), representing a total of 35,747 students (20,179 females and 15,568 males) from a total of 27 countries (Australia, Canada, China, Germany, Nigeria, United States, and 21 European countries), approximately one-half (or more) of Canadian and American university students studied did not engage in sufficient levels of physical activity. For instance, Troyer and colleagues (Troyer, Ullrich, Yeater, & Hopewell, 1990) found that fewer than 50% of their 69 medical school subjects engaged in 'hard' (e.g., dancing, basketball, scrubbing floors) or 'very hard', e.g., running, racquetball, tennis singles, physical activities according to their 7-day recall questionnaire. In short, similar to the 607 Canadian students who completed the Makrides, Veinot, Richard, McKee, and Gallivan (1998) version of the Physical Activity Behavioral Scale, more than 50% of respondents did not meet minimum physical activity recommendations utilized by the researchers. Similarly, 46% of the 59 students living on-campus and 56% of the 55 students living off-campus in the study by Brevard and Ricketts (1996) and 46% of the 800 first-year students studied by Pinto and Marcus (1995) led an insufficiently active lifestyle (with active lifestyle defined by Pinto and Marcus as engaging in physical activity 3 to 4 times/week; Brevard and Ricketts did not provide an operational definition). Leslie, Owen, Salmon, Bauman, Sallis, & Kai Lo's (1999, p. 23) definition of "sufficiently active" required students to meet the ACSM prescription, and nearly 40% of respondents were categorized as insufficiently active.

Sex Differences

Sex differences in activity levels were identified by Leslie, Owen, Salmon, Bauman, Sallis, and Kai Lo (1999) who found that males were more likely than females to be both moderately active and highly active at 42% versus 38% and 26% versus 16%, respectively. Dinger and Waigandt's (1997) investigation of 2,772 students who completed the Youth Risk Behavior Survey for College Students and Lowry, Galuska, Fulton, Wechsler, Kann, and Collins' (2000) assessment of 4,838 students from the National

College Health Risk Behavior Survey also found female students to be less likely than their male counterparts to engage in vigorous activities, i.e., activities that evoked sweating and/or breathing hard during a 20-min. period, 3 times/week) at 33% and 43.7%, respectively (Lowry, *et al.*'s results). Also, Dinger and Waigandt did not describe the specific percentage differences across sex. Additionally, Lowry, *et al.* found that males were more likely than females to engage in strength training activities, at 33.9% and 26.8%, respectively. However, female and male students were equally likely (19.5%) to engage in moderate physical activities, i.e., walking or cycling to or from class or work for 30 or more minutes per session, 5 days/week. For each of the three questionnaires used by Sarkin, Nichols, Sallis, and Calfas (1998) in their study of 575 students, men were identified consistently as more active than women. Likewise, Pinto and Marcus (1995) found statistically significant differences in the activity patterns of males and females, with 42% of males compared to 50% of females being inactive. The recent study by Pinto, Cherico, Szymanski, and Marcus (1998), a follow-up to the 1995 study by Pinto and Marcus (1995), found that, when the exercise classifications were adjusted to reflect the current ACSM guidelines, 58% of their original sample of first-year students ($n=332$) were considered sufficiently active, and 42% were considered inactive. During their second year of university, the sufficiently active student population rose to 64%, and the inactive population decreased to 36%, with fewer women being sufficiently active than men.

Highest Inactivity Rates

The highest inactivity rates were found by Douglas, Collins, Warren, Kann, Gold, Clayton, Ross, and Kolbe (1997), Haberman and Luffey (1998), Ford and Goode (1994), Page (1987), and Sarkin, *et al.* (1998) each of whom found students' inactivity levels at 60% or greater. Douglas and colleagues, who analysed physical activity data from 4,838 students who completed the National College Health Risk Behavior Survey, and Haberman and Luffey, who studied 302 students' physical activity levels from the Survey of Selected Nutritional Health Practices of College Students, found that 62% and 61% of their respondents, respectively, did not meet the study's criteria for a physically active lifestyle, i.e., only 37.6% and 39%, respectively, engaged in physical activity three or more times each week. Haberman and Luffey found no difference between male and female students; however, Douglas, *et al.* found a significant difference in favour of males. Likewise, Page found that nearly 65% of 274 students reported not to have a "regular schedule" of physical activity according to "a health attitudes and practices survey," with males being more likely than females to have such a schedule, at 40.4% and 32.3%, respectively. Using three different question-

TABLE 1
Prevalence of Insufficient Physical Activity Among University Students, 1985–2001

Author	Study Population	Test	Definition of Sufficient Physical Activity [and unique contribution of the study to this body of literature]	Prevalence of Insufficient Activity
Brevard & Ricketts (1966)	114 university students enrolled in introductory nutrition class; 18–41 yr.; M age = 20 years; 81% female; 54% of women and 47% of men lived on campus	2-page questionnaire	"Physical activity was analyzed for intensity, duration, and mode.... Exercise mode was analysed by placing subjects into four groups: aerobic, anaerobic, combination of aerobic and anaerobic, or no exercise. Subjects rated their activity level as sedentary, lightly active, active, or very active" (p. 36). [Revealed potentially important influence of living quarters on university students' physical activity levels.]	51% (46% on-campus, 56% off-campus.
Chen (1998)	289 Chinese students (155 males, 134 females) in Beijing and 180 students from the United States (93 males, 87 females) at the University of Alabama	Motives for Activity Participation questionnaire	"... the subjects were presented a list of sports and physical activities and asked to report in which sport or physical activity they were engaged. Then the subjects reported how often (frequency) and how long (duration) they had been participating in those activities from a list of forced choices of frequencies and durations. Frequency and duration were multiplied together for the activities so that the total number represented an individual's current level of participation" (p. 1464). [Revealed physical activity differences between Chinese and American university students.]	Chinese men and women exercised for 204 and 93 min./wk., respectively; American men and women for 273 and 206.4 min./wk., respectively
Dinger & Waigandt (1997)	2,772 students at a midwestern university; 62% female, 38% male; 90% Caucasian, 4% Asian, 3% African American, 3% other; 90% of sample were 22 years or younger	Youth Risk Behavior Survey for College Students	"... participating in vigorous exercise at least 3 days the previous week" (p. 361).	55%
Douglas, et al. (1997)	U.S. nationally representative sample of 4,838 undergraduate university students	National College Health Risk Behavior Survey	"...vigorous physical activity (that made you sweat and breathe hard) for at least 20 minutes on 3 or more of the 7 days preceding the survey ... walking or bicycling (moderate physical activity) for at least	62.4% (67% female, 56.3% male)

TABLE 1 (CONT'D)
PREVALENCE OF INSUFFICIENT PHYSICAL ACTIVITY AMONG UNIVERSITY STUDENTS, 1985–2001

Author	Study Population	Test	Definition of Sufficient Physical Activity [and unique contribution of the study to this body of literature]	Prevalence of Insufficient Activity
Ford & Goode (1994)	244 American undergraduate university students enrolled in health education classes at one urban school setting in the U.S.; ages ranged from 18–33 years with 81% between ages of 18 and 21 years; 76% women, 24% men	a health needs assessment questionnaire	30 minutes at a time on 5 or more of the 7 days preceding the survey" (p. 63). [Representativeness of sample; findings based on a nationally representative sample of U.S. university students.]	50% (40% male, 60% female)
Haberman & Luffey (1998)	302 college undergraduate students at the University of Pittsburgh	Survey of Selected Nutritional Health Practices of College Students	No definition given. [Revealed physical activity data specific to African American students.]	61%
Kelley & Kelley (1994)	253 African-American freshmen at a historically African-American university in the South, 90 males, 163 females; M age for males 18.5 yr., for females 18.2 yr.	Lipid Research Clinics Physical Activity Questionnaire and Physical Activity History Questionnaire	"... exercise vigorously for at least 20 minutes" (described on SSNHPCS) 3 or more times per week. "... frequent participation ... 2 to 5 hours per week for 9 months or longer" (p. 209). [The survey tools were previously deemed highly reliable (88% and 84% test-retest) and were validated using VO_2 max and BMI (research physical activity) and a cardiovascular fitness test (history). Both tests were used within this study to assess physical activity prevalence, thus enabling researchers to place greater confidence in their results.]	54% (42% male, 65% female)

(continued on next page)

TABLE 1 (CONT'D)
PREVALENCE OF INSUFFICIENT PHYSICAL ACTIVITY AMONG UNIVERSITY STUDENTS, 1985–2001

Author	Study Population	Test	Definition of Sufficient Physical Activity [and unique contribution of the study to this body of literature]	Prevalence of Insufficient Activity
Kelley, Lowing, & Kelley (1998)	212 (79 male, 133 female) Black, first-year university students enrolled in a historically Black university in the South; average age of men 18.7 yr., of women 18.7 yr.	Physician-based Assessment and Counseling for Exercise	"Students were categorized as 'active' if they reported engaging in moderate activity, i.e., brisk walking, for 30 min. at a time, or vigorous activity, i.e., running, for 20 min. at a time, 3 or more times per week" (p. 86). [This was one of the very few studies that was theoretically grounded (a modified Stages of Change Approach).]	56% (43% male, 68% female)
Leslie, et al. (1999a, 1999b)	905 males, 1,243 females (total=2,148) of two metropolitan university campuses and two rural campuses in Australia	self-completed survey	"... 30 min. of moderate physical activity on most, preferably all, days of the week; this equates to 3.5 hr. per week or 800 to 1000 Kcal per week" (p. 198). [A previously validated measure was used in this study; physical activity was operationally defined using the ACSM guidlines.]	39% (32% male, 46% female)
Lowry, et al. (2000)	4,838 college students over the age of 18 years were sampled via a 2-stage cluster sample design for the survey	used data from the 1995 National College Health Risk Behavior Survey	"... vigorous physical activity ≥ 3 days/week ... muscle strengthening exercises ≥ 3 days/week ... 30 min. of moderate physical activity such as walking or bicycling ≥ 5 days/week ..." [A previously validated measured was used in this study.]	62.4% (67% female, 56.3% male)
Makrides, et al. (1998)	607 university students living in residence (male and female) at Dalhousie University in Halifax, Nova Scotia	a closed ended questionnaire	"exercising ... three times per week" (p. 172) [This was a Canadian study; and a focus group was used to ensure that survey items were clear to potential respondents.]	51%

TABLE 1 (CONT'D)
PREVALENCE OF INSUFFICIENT PHYSICAL ACTIVITY AMONG UNIVERSITY STUDENTS, 1985–2001

Author	Study Population	Test	Definition of Sufficient Physical Activity [and unique contribution of the study to this body of literature]	Prevalence of Insufficient Activity
Onifade (1985)	350 (217 men, 133 women) Nigerian students (enrolled in universities in the U.S.)	*modified version* of the Physical Activity Behaviour Scale	"Subjects indicated the frequency of participation in physical activity for each of the six domains of Kenyon's conceptual model for charactering physical activity, thus revealing the frequency of: twice or more per week, once per week, twice per month, once per month, and *less often or never*" (p. 185). [Revealed information specific to the physical activity habits of Nigerian students, which was rare in the literature.]	*very high* (active only 1-2 times/mo.)
Page (1987)	274 students enrolled in a health course at a northeastern university in the U.S.; 63.3% were female; 50.4% freshmen, 23.2% sophomores, 13.6% juniors, 11% seniors, 1.8% graduate students; 85.3% of sample white, 9.1% black, 5.6% Asian, Hispanic, and other social groups	a health attitudes and practices survey	"... a regular schedule of physical activity" (p. 28). "... exercising hard enough to significantly increase heart rate for 20 continuous minutes or more" (p. 28). [The author examined both attitudes and corresponding practices pertaining to students' physical activity behaviours.]	65% (59.6% male, 67.7% female)
Pinto, *et al.* (1998)	332 first-year students at a private university in the Northeast; average age 18.6 yr., 60% women	4-page questionnaire	The ACSM guidelines for moderate physical activity were used to define physically active. [A longitudinal study was utilized to assess physical activity changes from year 1 to year 2 of university.]	42% (while in 1st-yr. university); 36% (while in 2nd-yr. university)
Pinto & Marcus (1995)	800 university students from a private school in Rhode Island (500 undergraduate students, 300 graduate students)	7-page questionnaire assessing satisfaction with health services	"... exercising for 20 minutes or longer three or more times a week" (p. 28).	46% (50% female, 42% male)

(continued on next page)

TABLE 1 (CONT'D)
PREVALENCE OF INSUFFICIENT PHYSICAL ACTIVITY AMONG UNIVERSITY STUDENTS, 1985–2001

Author	Study Population	Test	Definition of Sufficient Physical Activity [and unique contribution of the study to this body of literature]	Prevalence of Insufficient Activity
Sarkin, et al. (1998)	575 university students in southern California; 256 men, 319 women; 46% non-European-American	Seven-Day Physical Activity Recall Interview, Youth Risk Behavior Survey, National Health Interview Survey 1991	[This was one of the very few studies that was theoretically grounded (an altered Stages of Change Approach).] "A MET value ... was assigned to each of the physical activities reported.... Moderate intensity was defined as 3-5.9 MET and vigorous intensity was defined as 6 MET or greater"; "To determine the prevalence of meeting the health-related guidelines ... the protocols included one that considered a frequency of five times per week and another that considered an accumulation of 150 min.week^{-1} instead of frequency" (p. 151). [Triangulation (3 different questionnaires) was used to assess prevalence rates; this method demonstrated the impact that the questionnaire/tool itself can have on a study's physical activity prevalence findings.]	62.8% (ACSM guideline) 60% 67.8%
Steptoe, et al. (1997)	16,483 (7,302 male, 9,181 female) university students from among 21 countries *recruited from nonhealth-related courses	The European Health and Behaviour Survey	"Physical exercise was assessed by responses to the question 'over the past two weeks have you taken any exercise (e.g. sport, physically active pastime)?' Those who responded positively were asked what activity they had carried out and how many times they had exercised. In subsequent analyses, participants were divided into those who exercised one to four times and those who had exercised five or more times in the past two weeks" (p. 846-847). [Study findings pertain to a large sample of European university students.]	67% (64% male, 70% female)
Stock, et al. (2001)	650 freshmen students from the University of Bielefeld,	a self-administered questionnaire as-	The physical activity measure asked for the number of self-reported hours of exercise per week, with	66.3% (59.2% male, 72% female)

TABLE 1 (Cont'd)
PREVALENCE OF INSUFFICIENT PHYSICAL ACTIVITY AMONG UNIVERSITY STUDENTS, 1985–2001

Author	Study Population	Test	Definition of Sufficient Physical Activity [and unique contribution of the study to this body of literature]	Prevalence of Insufficient Activity
	Germany (288 men, 362 women)	sessing health behaviors	highly active being defined as four or more hours per week. [The operational definition of physical activity may lend itself to a higher standard than the ACSM guidelines.]	
Troyer, et al. (1990)	69 second-year medical students at West Virginia University in Morgantown, U.S. (50 men, 19 women)	modified form of a 7-day recall questionnaire developed by Sallis, et al. in 1985	"Moderate activity included activities such as sweeping, mowing the lawn, walking, golfing, or calisthenic exercises. Examples of hard activity were scrubbing floors, dancing, or half-court basketball; very hard activity illustrations were running, playing racquetball, or tennis singles" (p. 304). [Triangulation (laboratory fitness tests) was used to validate questionnaire.]	51%

naires, Sarkin, *et al.* (1998) found that each questionnaire indicated a different, yet high, rate of insufficient activity, ranging between 60-68% when using the ACSM guidelines. The overall insufficient activity rate of the African-American students studied by Ford and Goode (1994), Kelley and Kelley (1994), and Kelley, Lowing, and Kelley (1998) were not atypical at 50%, 54%, and 56%, respectively, However, the sex differences were large; 40% of men and 60% of women (Ford & Goode, 1994, $n=244$), 42% of men and 65% of women (Kelley & Kelley, 1994, $n=290$), and 43% of men and 68% of women (Kelley, *et al.*, 1998, $n=212$) were insufficiently active.

International Comparisons

Physical activity levels of European, Australian, German, Nigerian, and Chinese university students are comparable to the aforementioned physical activity prevalence information, which pertains to university students within Canada and the United States. For example, Steptoe, Wardle, Fuller, Holte, Justo, Sanderman, and Wichstrom (1997) studied 16,483 university students from 21 European countries using the European Health and Behaviour Survey and found that less than 36% of men and 30% of women engaged in physical activity five or more times over a 14-day period (the sex difference was statistically significant in Belgium, Iceland, Greece, Portugal, Spain, and Italy). In Finland, women were significantly more likely to be physically active than men, at 52.7% and 35.7%, respectively.

In his study on 289 Chinese and 180 American students' participation in physical activities using the Motives for Activity Participation questionnaire, Chen (1998) found that Chinese students spent significantly less time participating in physical exercise. Specifically, both American men and women exercised for longer durations than Chinese men and women; Chinese men and women exercised for a total of 204 and 93 min./week, respectively, while American men and women exercised for 273 and 206 min./week, respectively. Chen's findings are inconsistent with Xuming's inference (1992) that female Chinese students placed a higher value on physical activity than their male peers.

Stock, Wille, and Krämer (2001) found particularly high inactivity rates similar to the highest inactivity rates within Canada and the United States. Of the 650 freshmen studied at a German university (56% female), over 66% of students were not 'highly active'. More specifically, 72% of female students engaged in less than 4 hr. of exercise per week, compared with 59% of their male counterparts. However, the operational definition of 'very active' at four or more hours per week is unique, and may provide an elevated standard, e.g., a total four hours per week could result in more than 30 min. each day.

To identify the physical activity preferences of Australian university students, Leslie, Owen, and Sallis (1999) differentiated those who were insufficiently active from those who were sufficiently active using the ACSM guidelines. Responses from the 864 subjects showed that 39% of Australian students were inactive, with women being significantly more likely than men to be inactive, 46% to 32%, respectively.

While using a modified version of the Physical Activity Behaviour Scale to study the relationship among physical activity behavior, attitude, and beliefs among 450 Nigerian university students, Onifade (1985) found the highest insufficient activity rates of the studies in this review. After tabulating all of the subdomains of physical activity, it was clear that both Nigerian men and women engaged in any type of physical activity only once or twice per month.

From the foregoing discussion it is clear that this set of studies indicates Australian students have the highest prevalence of regular physical activity participation. Yet, within that population, 40% remain insufficiently active. Therefore, it is evident that insufficient physical activity is a problem all across the student samples studied.

Conclusion

Approximately half or more of university students in the United States, Canada, and China were categorized as insufficiently active. In Australia, 40% of students were insufficiently physically active; in Europe, 67% were inactive; and in Nigeria virtually no students engaged in any physical activity. Sarkin, *et al.* (1998) demonstrated the challenge of comparing physical activity prevalence rates across studies using dissimilar measurement tools. Nonetheless, Sarkin, *et al.*'s findings from each of the questionnaires used, together with all of the other studies' findings, indicated that regardless of the measure, university students were not sufficiently active to achieve health benefits. University women, and especially African Americans, have been identified as more likely to be insufficiently active than university men. Students living on-campus were at greater risk for inactivity than those living off-campus. Results from all of the aforementioned studies indicated a low prevalence of sufficient physical activity relative to the ACSM prescription; at best, 60% of students were sufficiently active, falling short by at least 40% when compared to the goal of having 100% active.

It is important to note that only four sets of researchers used the ACSM operational definition for physical activity (Pinto, *et al.*, 1998; Sarkin, *et al.*, 1998; Leslie, Owen, & Sallis, 1999; Lowry, *et al.*, 2000). Therefore, "sufficiently active" and "insufficiently active" statuses were often compared and contrasted using different definitions. Because the ACSM prescription requires more frequent participation than most of the guidelines utilized in the studies, subjects categorized as sufficiently active in a number of studies may be considered insufficiently active using the ACSM guidelines. The inverse is also possible; because the ACSM prescription accepts lower intensity activity than many of the studies reviewed, subjects categorized as insufficiently active may be sufficiently active using the ACSM guidelines. Further, because the vast majority of measuring procedures in these studies were not published, it is unclear which domains the tests encompassed, e.g., leisure activity, transportation, occupation, etc. Since many of the tests were unpublished self-report measures, and their psychometric characteristics (such as reliability) were not reported, it is possible that subjects over-reported their actual amount of exercise. The lack of a standardized instrument to measure the prevalence of physical activity according to the ACSM guidelines posed limitations when requiring comparative inferences across the different samples. Consequently, from the preceding literature review, two conclusions can be drawn. First, to track better and compare students' physical activity patterns at the level necessary for health gains, the construction of a standardized tool using the ACSM prescription is needed. For further studies, the International Physical Activity Questionnaire should be considered as a potential measure of physical activity. This questionnaire produces cross-national monitoring and has reasonable measurement properties for monitoring population levels of physical activity among 18- to 65-yr.-olds (Craig, Marshall, Sjostrom, Bauman, Booth, Ainsworth, Pratt, Ekelund, Yngve, Sallis, & Oja, 2003). Second, insufficient activity is a serious health problem among university students, and the creation and implementation of early intervention activities are warranted. Physical activity reduces stress and therefore provides immediate benefits, not just long-term protection (McGuigan, 1999; Haugland, Wold, & Torsheim, 2003). Regular activity also promotes healthy weight, and weight is an immediate concern to many students (Page, 1987; Brevard & Ricketts, 1996; Haberman & Luffey, 1998; Makrides, et al., 1998). Although physical activity can help students to maintain a healthy body composition and to manage stress, it is during stressful periods, e.g., examinations, that students tend to exercise even less than their usual amount (Steptoe, Wardle, Pollard, Canaan, & Davies, 1996). University students may be receptive to adopting regular physical activity; they have to deal with such stressful events in their lives as moving away from home, separating from friends and family, living in residence, and beginning university (Makrides, et al., 1998; Pinto, et al., 1998; Leslie, Owen, Salmon Baumen, Sallis, & Kai Lo, 1999). All of the evidence points in one direction; university students are in need of efficacious programs for physical activity that are tailored to provide health gains. Those attempting to develop and evaluate structured university courses aimed at promoting physical activity may find this information particularly useful; although some universities require their students to pass physical activity courses, there have been only a limited number of studies with conclusive results regarding their impact (Cardinal, Jacques, & Levy, 2002). Thus, it may be critical to include students' activity and scheduling preferences in the creation of such programs and ensure that these programs have the potential for self-sustaining behavioural patterns. Then, programmers will have a strong chance of truly facilitating a positive health change in the lives of young people today, and for their years to come.

REFERENCES

AMERICAN COLLEGE OF SPORTS MEDICINE. (2000) *ACSM's Guidelines for exercise testing and prescription.* (6th ed.) Philadelphia, PA: Lippincott, Williams & Wilkins.

BARABASZ, M. (1991) Effects of aerobic exercise on transient mood state. *Perceptual and Motor Skills,* 73, 657-658.

BREVARD, P. B., & RICKETTS, C. D. (1996) Residence of college students affects dietary intake, physical activity, and serum lipid levels. *Journal of the American Dietetic Association,* 96, 35-38.

BUNGUM, T. J., & VINCENT, M. L. (1997) Determinants of physical activity among female adolescents. *American Journal of Preventive Medicine,* 13(2), 115-122.

CARDINAL, B. J., JACQUES, K. M., & LEVY, S. S. (2002) Evaluation of a university course aimed at promoting exercise behaviour. *Journal of Sports Medicine and Physical Fitness,* 42, 113-122.

CASH, T. F., NOVY, P. L., & GRANT, J. R. (1994) Why do women exercise? Factor analysis and further validation of the reasons for exercise inventory. *Perceptual and Motor Skills,* 78, 539-544.

CASPERSEN, C. J., CHRISTENSEN, C. M., & POLLARD, R. A. (1986) Status of the 1990 physical fitness and exercise objectives—evidence from NHIS (1985). *Public Health Report,* 101, 587-592.

CHEN, W. (1998) Chinese and American college students' motives for participation in physical activities. *Perceptual and Motor Skills,* 87, 1463-1470.

CRAIG, C. L., MARSHALL, A. L., SJOSTROM, M., BAUMAN, A. E., BOOTH, M. L., AINSWORTH, B. E., PRATT, M., EKELUND, U., YNGVE, A., SALLIS, J. F., & OJA, P. (2003) International Physical Activity Questionnaire: 12-country reliability and validity. *Medicine & Science in Sports & Exercise,* 35, 1381-1395.

DAMILAKIS, J., PERISINAKIS, K., KONTAKIS, G., VAGIOS, E., & GOURTSOYIANNIS, N. (1999) Effect of lifetime occupational physical activity on indices of bone mineral status in healthy postmenopausal women. *Calcified Tissue International,* 64, 112-116.

DILORENZO, T. M., BARGMAN, E. P., STUCKY-ROPP, R., BRASSINGTON, G. S., FRENSCH, P. A., & LAFONTAINE, T. (1999) Long-term effects of aerobic exercise on psychological outcomes. *Preventive Medicine,* 28, 75-85.

DINGER, M. K., & WAIGANDT, A. (1997) Dietary intake and physical activity behaviors of male and female college students. *American Journal of Health Promotion,* 1, 360-362.

DOUGLAS, K. A., COLLINS, J. L., WARREN, C., KANN, L., GOLD, R., CLAYTON, S., ROSS, J. G., & KOLBE, L. J. (1997) Results from the 1995 National College Health Risk Behavior Survey. *Journal of American College Health,* 46, 55-66.

EBELING, P. R. (1998) Osteoporosis in men: new insights into aetiology, pathogenesis, prevention and management. *Drugs & Aging,* 13, 421-434.

FERRUCCI, L., IZMIRLIAN, G., LEVEILLE, S., PHILLIPS, L. L., CORTI, M. C., BROCK, D. B., & GURALNIK, J. M. (1998) Smoking, physical activity, and active life expectancy. *American Journal of Epidemiology,* 149, 645-653.

FORD, D. S., & GOODE, C. R. (1994) African American college students' health behaviors and perceptions of related health issues. *Journal of American College Health,* 42, 207-210.

FREIDENREICH, C. M., BRYANT, H. G., & COURNEYA, K. S. (2001) Case-control study of lifetime physical activity and breast cancer risk. *American Journal of Epidemiology,* 154, 336-347.

GALUSKA, D., EARLE, D., & FULTON, J. (2002) The epidemiology of U.S. adults who regularly engage in resistance training. *Research Quarterly for Exercise and Sport,* 73, 330-334.

HABERMAN, S., & LUFFEY, D. (1998) Weighing in college students' diet and exercise behaviors. *Journal of American College Health*, 46, 189-191.

HAUGLAND, S., WOLD, B., & TORSHEIM, T. (2003) Relieving the pressure? The role of physical activity in the relationship between school-related stress and adolescent health complaints. *Research Quarterly for Exercise and Sport*, 74, 127-135.

HEALTH CANADA AND THE CANADIAN SOCIETY FOR EXERCISE PHYSIOLOGY. (1998) *Canada's physical activity guide to healthy active living*. Ottawa, ON: Minister of Supply and Services Canada. (Catalogue No. H39-429/1998-1E. ISBN 0-662-86627-7)

KELLEY, G. A., & KELLEY, K. S. (1994) Physical activity habits of African-American college students. *Research Quarterly for Exercise and Sport*, 65, 207-212.

KELLEY, G. A., LOWING, L., & KELLEY, K. (1998) Psychological readiness of black college students to be physically active. *Journal of American College Health*, 47, 83-87.

LESLIE, E., OWEN, N., & SALLIS, J. (1999) Inactive Australian college students preferred activities, sources of assistance, and motivators. *American Journal of Health Promotion*, 13, 197-199.

LESLIE, E., OWEN, N., SALMON, J., BAUMAN, A., SALLIS, J. F., & KAI LO, S. (1999) Insufficiently active Australian college students: perceived personal, social, and environmental influences. *Preventive Medicine*, 28, 20-27.

LOWRY, R., GALUSKA, D. A., FULTON, J. E., WECHSLER, H., KANN, L., & COLLINS, J. L. (2000) Physical activity, food choice, and weight management goals and practices among U.S. college students. *American Journal of Preventive Medicine*, 18, 18-26.

MAKRIDES, L., VEINOT, P., RICHARD, J., MCKEE, R., & GALLIVAN, T. (1998) A cardiovascular health needs assessment of university students living in residence. *Canadian Journal of Public Health*, 89, 175-181.

MARTINEZ, G. M., & CURRY, A. (1998) *School enrollment—social and economic characteristics of students (update)*. Washington, DC: U.S. Department of Commerce Economics and Statistics Administration, U.S. Bureau of the Census.

MCGINNIS, J. M. (1992) The public health burden of a sedentary lifestyle. *Medicine and Science in Sports and Exercise*, 24(Suppl.) S196-S200.

MCGUIGAN, F. J. (1999) *Encyclopedia of stress*. London: Allyn & Bacon.

MOORE, K. A., BABYAK, M. A., WOOD, C. E., NAPOLITANO, M. A., KHATRI, P., CRAIGHEAD, W. E., HERMAN, S., KRISHNAN, R., & BLUMENTHAL, J. A. (1999) The association between physical activity and depression in older depressed adults. *Journal of Aging and Physical Activity*, 7, 55-61.

ONIFADE, S. A. (1985) Relationship among attitude, physical activity behavior and physical activity belief of Nigerian students toward physical activity. *International Journal of Sport Psychology*, 16, 183-192.

PAGE, R. M. (1987) Assessing college students' personal choices about health. *College Student Journal*, 1, 26-30.

PATE, R. R., PRATT, M., BLAIR, S. N., HASKELL, W. L., MACERA, C. A., BOUCHARD, C., BUCHNER, D., ETTINGER, W., HEATH, G. W., KING, A. C., KRISKA, A., LEON, A. S., MARCUS, B. H., MORRIS J., PAFFENBARGER, R. S., PATRICK, K., POLLOCK, M. L., RIPPE, J. M., SALLIS, J., & WILMORE, J. H. (1995) Physical activity and public health: a recommendation from the Centers for Disease Control and Prevention and the American College of Sports Medicine. *The Journal of the American Medical Association*, 273, 402-407.

PEKKANEN, J., MARTI, B., NISSINEN, A., TUOMELEHTO, J., PUNSAR, S., & KARVONEN, M. J. (1987) Reduction of premature mortality by high physical activity: a 20-year follow-up of middle-aged Finnish men. *Lancet*, 1(8548), 1473-1477.

PINTO, B. M., CHERICO, N. P., SZYMANSKI, L., & MARCUS, B. H. (1998) Longitudinal changes in college students' exercise participation. *Journal of American College Health*, 47, 23-27.

PINTO, B. M., & MARCUS, B. H. (1995) A stages of change approach to understanding college students' physical activity. *College Health*, 44, 27-31.

POWELL, K. E., CASPERSEN, C. J., KOPLAN, J. P., & FORD, E. S. (1998) Physical activity and chronic disease. *American Journal of Clinical Nutrition*, 49, 999-1006.

ROCKHILL, B., WILLETT, W. C., HUNTER, D. J., MANSON, J. E., HANKINSON, S. E., & COLDITZ, G. A. (1999) A prospective study of recreational physical activity and breast cancer risk. *Archives of Internal Medicine*, 159, 2290-2296.

Rubin, L. A., Hawker, G. A., Peltekova, V. D., Fielding, L. J., Ridout, R., & Cole, D. E. C. (1999) Determinants of peak bone mass: clinical and genetic analyses in a young female Canadian cohort. *Journal of Bone Mineral Research*, 14, 633-643.
Salonen, J. T., Puska, P., & Tuomelehto, J. (1982) Physical activity and risk of myocardial infarction, cerebral stroke and death: a longitudinal study in Eastern Finland. *American Journal of Epidemiology*, 115, 526-537.
Sarkin, J. A., Nichols, J. F., Sallis, J. F., & Calfas, K. J. (1998) Self-report measures and scoring protocols affect prevalence estimates of meeting physical activity guidelines. *Medicine & Science in Sports & Exercise*, 32, 149-156.
Sothern, M. S., Loftin, M., Suskind, R. M., Udall, J. N., & Blecker, U. (1999) The health benefits of physical activity in children and adolescents: implications for chronic disease prevention. *European Journal of Pediatrics*, 158, 271-274.
Sports Medicine New Zealand. (1998) *Policy statement: physical activity and health*. Sidney, New Zealand: Author.
Statistics Canada. (1998) *How active are Canadians?* Ottawa, ON: Canadian Fitness and Lifestyle Research Institute. (Bulletin No. 1. 1995. Catalogue No. 82-221-XDE)
Statistics Canada. (2000) CANSIM, *Cross-classified tables 00580701, 00580702, Matrix 6367*. Ottawa, ON: Author.
Statistics Canada. (2001) CANSIM II, Table 051-0001-*Estimates of population, by age group and sex*. Ottawa, ON: Author.
Stephens, T., Jacobs, D. R., & White, C. C. (1985) A descriptive epidemiology of leisure-time physical activity. *Public Health Report*, 100, 147-158.
Steptoe, A., Wardle, J., Fuller, R., Holte, A., Justo, J., Sanderman, R., & Wichstrom, L. (1997) Leisure-time physical exercise: prevalence, attitudinal correlates, and behavioural correlates among young Europeans from 21 countries. *Preventive Medicine*, 26, 845-854.
Steptoe, A., Wardle, J., Pollard, T. M., Canaan, L., & Davies, J. (1996) Stress, social support, and health-related behavior: a study of smoking, alcohol consumption and physical exercise. *Journal of Psychosomatic Research*, 41, 171-180.
Stock, C., Wille, L., & Krämer, A. (2001) Gender-specific health behaviors of German university students predict the interest in campus health promotion. *Health Promotion International*, 16, 145-154.
Troyer, D., Ullrich, I. H., Yeater, R. A., & Hopewell, R. (1990) Physical activity and condition, dietary habits, and serum lipids in second-year medical students. *Journal of American College Nutrition*, 9, 303-307.
U.S. Department of Health and Human Services. (2000) *Healthy People 2010: understanding and improving health*. (2nd ed.) Washington, DC: U.S. Government Printing Office.
Wyrwich, K. W., & Wolinsky, F. D. (2000) Physical activity, disability, and the risk of hospitalization for breast cancer among older women. *Journal of Gerontology: Series A, Biological Sciences and Medical Sciences*, 55, M418-M421.
Xuming, C. (1992) Chinese college students' perceived values of physical activity. *Dissertation Abstracts International*, 53(10), 147.

Accepted March 10, 2004.

INFLUENCE OF COLOR ON NUMBER PERSEVERATION IN A SERIAL ADDITION TASK[1]

HARIKLIA PROIOS

Technological Institute Patras

AND

PETER BRUGGER

University Hospital Zürich

Summary.—The present study examined the influence of coloring the repeated number in a serial addition task that elicits perseveration in normal subjects. 110 undergraduates were administered the original, black-and-white version of the task, 112 other undergraduates the new, colored version. The task required adding the following numbers: 1000 + 40 + 1000 + 30 + 1000 + 20 + 1000 + 10. We predicted that, in the colored version, the enhanced saliency of the repeated number 1000 would reduce the incidence of perseverative errors. Results with the black-and-white version replicated our 1994 findings, i.e., the majority of subjects produced the perseverative response 5000 rather than the correct answer of 4100. Contrary to our expectation, color did not improve performance but rather *increased* both perseverative and nonperseverative errors. We speculate that the enhanced saliency of the 4 repeated 4-digit terms may have further distracted subjects from discovering the critical lure, namely, the repetitive digit changes in the partial sums at irrelevant positions, i.e., in the thousands and tens but never in the hundreds.

The American Heritage Dictionary of English Language (Pickett, 2000) defines "perseveration" as an "uncontrollable repetition of a particular response despite the absence or cessation of a stimulus, or the tendency to continue or repeat an act or activity after the cessation of the original stimulus". Although mainly described in the behavioral neurology literature (e.g., Sandson & Albert, 1987), perseveration can also be found in normal subjects if appropriate task demands are chosen. For instance, a fairly high number of perseverative responses can be obtained from healthy subjects attempting to solve an apparently trivial calculation task (Brugger & Gardner, 1994). In this task, participants sequentially add a series of Arabic numbers, presented one by one: 1000 + 40 + 1000 + 30 + 1000 + 20 + 1000 + 10. The partial sums of this serial addition have nonexplicit repetitive changes in digits at the thousands (first from left) or tens position (third from left). For example, in 1000 + 40 = 1040 it is the position of the tens (third from the left) that changes, whereas in 1040 + 1000 = 2040 it is the thousands position (first from the left). At the last step, however, the final result changes at the *hundreds* position, i.e., the 1 in 4100, which is the *second* digit from the left. Thus, at this critical step significantly more participants respond with the wrong answer 5000 rather than the correct one, 4100.

---

[1]The authors gratefully acknowledge the support of Swiss National Science Foundation grant SNF-PIOIA-103089. Address correspondence to Professor Hariklia Proios, Mitropoleos 52, Thessaloniki 54621, Greece or e-mail (hproios@npsy.unizh.ch).

The goal of the present experiment was to examine the influence of enhancing the saliency of the repeated number 1000. In the learning literature, a well-documented finding is that coloring an item primes attention to a target (Dwyer, 1978, for a review). Therefore, we constructed two versions of the calculation task. In one version, all digits were printed black on a white background, whereas in the other version, the numbers "1000" were printed in bright red (also on white background). We predicted an improved calculation accuracy with the colored compared to the original black-and-white version of the serial addition task.

Method

The participants were 222 undergraduate students of both sexes with a mean age of 24 yr. (range 18 to 36), recruited from several institutions, Swiss Federal Institute of Technology (Zurich), Columbia University (New York), Montclair State University (New Jersey), and Hofstra University (New York). Test procedure was adopted from Brugger and Gardner (1994); in a classroom setting, single numbers were presented as a vertical array on an overhead projector at a rate of approximately 2 seconds per number, in the sequence indicated above. A window was used to mask all other numbers as each of the numbers was displayed one at a time down the column. Subjects were required to add up consecutive numbers mentally and, on appearance of a question mark after the last number, to write down the final sum. There were eight test sessions, four of which used the regular black-and-white version of the task, and four a colored version. Classes were randomly assigned to the two test versions. In the colored version the four digits "1000" were colored in bright red; all other digits and the question mark remained black.

Results and Discussion

Overall, 33.3% of the subjects produced the correct result, i.e., "4100," replicating our previous finding (Brugger & Gardner, 1994), whereas 49.6% produced the perseverative error 5000, and 17.1% another incorrect response. These percentages as well as the respective percentages for the two experimental groups separately are displayed in Table 1. The subjects administered the colored version produced more incorrect responses (perseverative and nonperseverative combined) than the subjects who received the black-and-white version ($\chi^2 = 4.4$, $p = .04$). Although numerically, the increase in nonperseverative errors was higher than that for perseverative errors, the incidence of the two error types was statistically comparable among those subjects of the two experimental groups who produced incorrect responses ($n = 148$; $\chi^2 = 1.2$, $p = .26$).

Thus, contrary to our prediction, coloring the repeated number 1000 did not improve performance but rather *increased* the number of errors. Obviously, enhancing the saliency of each "1000" did not help participants monitor how many of them had been presented. One interpretation is that the critical lure for committing a perseverative error is solely the repeated changes at irrelevant digit positions; the four red "1000s" did not reduce the pervasiveness of this lure, but, if anything, further distracted subjects from consciously detecting it.

TABLE 1
Percentages of Different Types of Responses in Serial Addition Task For Groups Administered the Black-and-White (Traditional) and Colored (All "1000s" Colored Red) Versions of the Task and Two Groups Combined

Test	n	Correct ("4100")	Perseverative ("5000")	Nonperseverative
Black-and-White	110	40.0	47.3	12.7
Colored	112	26.8	51.8	21.4
All Subjects	222	33.3	49.6	17.1

The original, black-and-white version of the serial addition task was recently employed to measure perseveration tendencies in healthy subjects as a function of preferred cognitive styles (Tranum & Grasha, 2002). Field dependence was the only dimension found to be associated with a differential inclination to commit perseverative errors. Interestingly, field dependence was also a relevant predictor of subjects' susceptibility to color coding in a variety of psychological tests (Dwyer & Moore, 1992). It remains unclear whether the color manipulation introduced in the present experiment will interact with subjects' cognitive styles, resulting in an increased perseveration tendency in some subjects, but a decreased one in others.

REFERENCES

Brugger, P., & Gardner, M. (1994) Perseveration in healthy subjects: an impressive classroom demonstration for educational purposes. *Perceptual and Motor Skills*, 78, 777-778.

Dwyer, F. M. (1978) *Strategies for improving visual learning.* State College, PA: Learning Services.

Dwyer, F. M., & Moore, D. M. (1992) Effect of color coding on visually and verbally oriented tests with students of different field dependence levels. *Journal of Educational Technology Systems*, 20, 311-320.

Pickett, J. (Ed.) (2000) *The American Heritage Dictionary of English language.* (4th ed.) Boston, MA: Houghton Mifflin.

Sandson, J., & Albert, M. L. (1987) Perseveration in behavioral neurology. *Neurology*, 37, 1736-1741.

Tranum, D., & Grasha, A. F. (2002) Susceptibility to illusions and cognitive style: implications for pharmacy dispensing. *Perceptual and Motor Skills*, 95, 1063-1086.

Accepted March 25, 2004.

RESISTANCE TRAINING IS ASSOCIATED WITH IMPROVED MOOD IN HEALTHY OLDER ADULTS [1,2]

CHARLES L. McLAFFERTY, JR., CARLA J. WETZSTEIN, AND GARY R. HUNTER

Department of Human Studies
University of Alabama at Birmingham

Summary.—This study examined the effects of 24 wk. of resistance training on mood in healthy but sedentary older adults. 28 participants performed resistance training 3 times per week for 24 weeks. No significant differences were found in mood scores between high and variable resistance groups, and there were no significant interactions between resistance and sex or intervention, or among all three factors. For pooled data, significant improvement was found on measures of Confusion, Tension, Anger, and Total Mood Scores, although not for scores for Fatigue, Vigor, and Depression. Sex differences were found on some subscales, but no significant interactions between sex and resistance training. These findings support the effectiveness of resistance training in improving mood in healthy older adults, although further study is needed to control for effect size, as well as cohort, social, and attentional effects.

As individuals approach late adulthood, declines are expected in health, physical strength, and cognitive abilities. Exercise has been shown to attenuate declines in physiological processes (Fiatarone, Marks, Ryan, Meredith, Lipsitz, & Evans, 1990; Hurley & Hagberg, 1998). Resistance training has also been shown to improve the ability of older adults to carry out everyday activities, such as walking, standing up, carrying groceries, and climbing stairs (Hunter, Treuth, Weinsier, Kekes-Szabo, Kell, Roth, & Nicholson, 1995).

It is generally accepted that exercise is associated with improvement in mood, depression, and anxiety. Studies have shown positive effects of resistance training and aerobic exercise on measures of mood and depression (North, McCullagh, & Tran, 1990; Stewart & King, 1991). These effects have been shown to be associated with short-term exercise interventions (McGowan, Pierce, & Jordan, 1991; Maroulakis & Zervas, 1993) and long-term (Doyne, Ossip-Klein, Bowman, Osborn, McDougall-Wilson, & Neimeyer, 1987; Martinsen, Hoffart, & Solberg, 1989; Emery & Gatz, 1990; Norvell &

---

[1] This research was supported by The Ralph L. Smith Foundation, Kansas City. Special thanks are extended to the participants, whose commitment and persistence made this study possible. The authors also thank Marcas Bamman, who helped design the resistance training protocol and assisted with training, as well as Amanda Brown, Paul Zuckerman, and Kathlene Landers for their tireless assistance with the training of these participants. Portions of this article were presented at the 2000 annual meeting of the American College of Sports Medicine.
[2] Direct correspondence to Charles L. McLafferty, Jr., Ph.D., University of Alabama at Birmingham, Room 202 Education Building, 1530 3rd Avenue South, Birmingham, AL 35294-1250 or e-mail (clm@uab.edu).

Belles, 1993). The majority of studies have focused on mood changes in college- and middle-aged populations, using aerobic exercise (Maroulakis & Zervas, 1993; McGowan, Talton, & Thompson, 1996), resistance training (Norvell, Martin, & Salamon, 1991), or resistance training and aerobic training (Doyne, et al., 1987; Martinsen, et al., 1989). Several studies have associated resistance training with a reduction in state anxiety, primarily in college-age individuals (O'Connor, Bryant, Veltri, & Gebhardt, 1993; Koltyn, Raglin, O'Connor, & Morgan, 1995; Bartholomew & Linder, 1998).

Although aerobic exercise is generally associated with changes in mood and depression in adults over 60 years of age, the results have been more ambiguous than in younger populations. The failure to find a consistent association between mood and exercise in older adults has been well documented (Emery & Blumenthal, 1991). It is likely that older adults have more variability in their health status and ability to exercise, thus causing a narrowing of effect size and lessening of consistency of exercise studies, as noted in Rossi (1990, 1997). Even so, more recent studies have provided a more coherent set of findings regarding exercise and mood, particularly regarding depressed older adults.

It is possible that resistance training does not affect mood in the same manner as aerobic exercise. In a meta-analysis of 66 exercise studies in young and middle-aged adults, North, et al. (1990) found that resistance training had an effect size on depression indices three times greater than aerobic exercise. However, the meta-analysis included only two studies of resistance training. In contrast, at least one controlled study did not find a significant difference between resistance training and aerobic exercise in depressed patients trained for 8 wk.; similar improvement was observed in both groups (Martinsen, et al., 1989).

Several studies explore mood changes in depressed older adults who engage in resistance training. In a randomized, controlled study Singh, Clements, and Fiatarone (1997) found that 10 wk. of resistance training in 16 depressed older adults resulted in a significant reduction in measures of depression compared to 16 similar participants in an attention-control group. Intensity of resistance training (defined as a ratio of strength gain) significantly correlated with the amount of improvement.

Another controlled study randomized clinically depressed older adults into 10 wk. of education ($n=16$) or resistance training ($n=16$), after which the exercise group was given 10 wk. of unsupervised weight training. Depression scores were significantly reduced in exercisers at 20 wk. and at 26-mo. follow-up (Singh, Clements, & Fiatarone Singh, 2001).

Depressed older adults with knee osteoarthritis showed improvements in depression scores with aerobic exercise ($n=144$) but not resistance training ($n=146$), when compared with controls ($n=144$) over 18 mo. in one large-scale, controlled study (Penninx, Rejeski, Pandya, Miller, Di Bari, Applegate, & Pahor, 2002). However, compliance rates in this study average 63%. Participants in the resistance training group whose compliance was in the top tertile (≥ 79%) demonstrated greater improvement in depression than all compliance tertiles of aerobic exercisers, although whether this effect was significant was not reported. The lack of a significant effect of resistance training may be accounted for by those in the lowest compliance tertile (≤ 50%), whose depression scores *increased* 28%, a significant amount compared to controls ($p < .03$). Further investigation is needed to determine if resistance exercise may be injurious in some arthritic patients, resulting in further inflammation and a sense of failure in those participating, thus confounding such studies.

To our knowledge, only one study has examined effects on mood of resistance training in healthy older adults. Tsutsumi, Don, Zaichkowsky, Takenaka, Oka, and Ohno (1998) studied mood changes in healthy women who performed resistance training three times per week for 12 weeks using two intensity levels and a control group ($n = 12$ in each group). The researchers found increased scores on Vigor and decreased scores on Tension for both intensity groups but did not find significant changes in Depression on the Profile of Mood States.

Clearly, there was a wide difference in protocols and populations being studied. Specifically, factors involved in the studies mentioned above were healthy vs depressed or arthritic, length of intervention, compliance, and number of participants (power). When compliance was considered in the Penninx, *et al.* study (2002), consistently resistance exercise had a significant effect on mood.

The meta-analysis by North, *et al.* (1990) also found a relationship between length of intervention and effect size in young and middle-aged adults: exercise programs of 21 to 24 wk. had an effect size more than *nine times* greater than programs of 9 to 12 wk. Interventions longer than 24 wk. demonstrated a significantly smaller effect size than those of 21 to 24 wk. This finding implies that length of intervention may also account for part of the effect of exercise on mood, as the studies cited in older adults varied from 10 wk. to 18 mo.

The present study was intended to explore the effects of an extended regimen of resistance training on measures of mood in a sample of healthy, older men and women. Previous studies have used shorter (or much longer) interventions, generally in depressed populations. It was hypothesized that 24 wk. of resistance training would be associated with an improvement of mood in a healthy, older population. Intensity was considered as a possible mediator of mood change.

Method

Sample

Thirty healthy and mostly sedentary older adults between 60 and 77 years of age ($M = 66.9$, $SD = 4.3$) were recruited through newspaper advertisements, word of mouth, and flyers in local community centers. Participants were screened to be free of cardiovascular, metabolic, or physical disorders. All were nonsmokers and of normal body mass index. None of the participants had participated in resistance training, and all except one were sedentary (defined as exercising less than once per week for the past year). One male participant was a runner and ran about 7 miles per week in three to four exercise sessions. He continued running at the same level throughout the course of the study. All female participants were postmenopausal. Participants were instructed not to make changes in their diet, eating habits, or weight during the study. Institutional Review Board-approved written consent was obtained prior to participation in compliance with the Department of Health and Human Services Regulations for Protection of Human Research Subjects.

Two of the participants were excluded from the findings of this study. One did not accurately complete the psychological measures, and the other did not participate regularly in the exercise sessions. Of the 28 remaining participants, 15 men and 13 women, 27 were Euro-American and one African American. Participants began to enter into the study in May, and the last participant finished in March the following year. Detailed descriptive information is in Table 1 below.

Procedure

Body composition.—Body composition was measured at the beginning and end of the study by air displacement plethysmography conducted in a BOD POD Version 1.69 (Body Composition System; Life Measurement Instruments, Concord, CA) as described by Fields, Hunter, and Goran (2000).

Strength training program.—Participants trained 3 times per week for 24 weeks at a local fitness center using the following protocol. Stretching and warm-up was performed for 5 min. on a bike or treadmill. Training consisted of two sets of 10 repetitions using eight resistance training exercises: shoulder press, seated row, back extension, elbow flexion (Cybex), knee flexion, knee extension, bench press (Keiser), and either Smith rack squat or Cybex leg press. Situps were also performed. Random assignment was made to one of two resistance groups. High resistance was based on 80% of one-repetition maximum for 8 to 10 repetitions. Variable resistance was based on 80, 50, or 65% of maximum for 8 to 10 repetitions, with sessions arranged so that no more than three exercises were at each resistance level. Sessions were supervised by exercise physiologists. Participants were encouraged to rest no more than 2 min. between sets and could socialize with each other during exercise sessions. Average adherence rate of the participants was over 90% and was not significantly different between exercise groups.

Strength testing.—After three initial familiarization sessions, strength was assessed using a one-repetition maximum protocol on seven exercises (all but the seated row and back extension). Strength testing was repeated every nine sessions and used to adjust workout protocols. Target weights were increased between strength testing sessions whenever the participant reached 10 repetitions of a given exercise. Further details of the exercise protocol and physiological testing is reported by Hunter, Wetzstein, McLafferty, Zuckerman, Landers, and Bamman (2001).

Psychological testing.—The Profile of Mood States (McNair, Lorr, & Droppleman, 1992) was administered to assess mood "over the past week, including today" prior to the strength testing sessions at the beginning and end of the study. The Profile of Mood States uses 65 adjectives that are rated on a scale with anchors of 0: Not at all and 4: Extremely to measure Tension, Depression, Anger, Vigor, Fatigue, and Confusion. A Total Mood Disturbance score was derived by adding the negative mood scores, subtracting Vigor, and adding 100.

The Profile of Mood States is a well-tested, clinically validated test. It was originally developed for use on a psychiatric outpatient population, with guarded recommendations for its use in research on healthy populations such as college students (McNair, *et al.*, 1992). However, it has been used in hundreds of exercise-related studies (LeUnes & Burger, 1998) and is considered a valid measure in exercise studies.

Statistics.—Two (pre vs post) × 2 (high vs variable resistance) × 2 (male vs female) analysis of variance with repeated measures on time was run to assess differences for POMS mood scores at the beginning and end of the study. Paired two-tailed t tests were conducted to compare pre- and posttest measures on body fat, weight, Body Mass Index, and one-repetition maximum values for squat, arm curl, leg extension, leg curl, shoulder press, chest press, and leg press. A correlation was also calculated for overall strength gain with each of the POMS mood scores to estimate association between mood and intensity, as defined by Singh, *et al.* (1997). SPSS (for Windows Versions 10 and 11.5) was used for all analyses. A two-tailed p value <.05 was adopted for significance.

Interviews.—Twenty-three of the original 30 participants were interviewed in a semistructured, open-ended format. Participants were asked to tell what, if anything, had changed for them as a consequence of participating in the study. Complete examination of the qualitative data is in preparation for later presentation.

Results

Body Composition and Strength

There were no significant changes in weight or Body Mass Index following 24 wk. of resistance training (see Table 1). However, there was a significant decrease in body fat % (2.5%, $p < .001$) as well as a significant increase in fat-free mass (1.8 kg, $p < .001$). On measures of strength testing, all changes were significant ($p < .01$). Strength increased, on average, 41.9% across the tested exercises for these participants. Further details of physiological changes are reported by Hunter, *et al.* (2001).

TABLE 1
AGE, BODY COMPOSITION, AND STRENGTH VARIABLES BEFORE
AND AFTER 24 WEEKS OF RESISTANCE TRAINING

Measure	Pretest M	Pretest SD	Posttest M	Posttest SD	n
Age, yr.	66.93	4.34			28
Weight, kg	72.66	11.92	72.69	12.39	28
Body Mass Index, kg · m^{-2}	24.79	3.18	24.55	3.15	28
% body fat, ADP	31.4	10.6	28.9	10.9†	28
Fat-free mass, kg	49.9	11.2	51.7	12.0†	28
Fat mass, kg	22.8	8.9	21.0	8.9†	28
Squat, lb.	121.30	37.36	192.83	57.40†	23
Curl, lb.	38.06	18.96	56.67	25.68†	27
Leg Extension, lb.	72.59	29.75	118.15	52.39†	27
Leg Curl, lb.	54.36	19.05	75.65	27.82†	27
Shoulder Press, lb.	41.67	15.24	55.96	21.59†	27
Chest Press, lb.	92.41	28.50	116.11	38.29†	27
Leg Press, lb.	115.00	39.81	151.85	47.07†	27

†$p < .01$.

Mood Scores

No significant differences were found between variable and high resistance groups. Furthermore, there were no significant interactions between intensity and time or sex, or all three factors combined. Therefore data were pooled to increase statistical power, and the statistical analysis run as a 2 (pre vs post) × 2 (male vs female) analysis of variance with repeated measures on the first measure (see Table 2) to assess whether there were any significant differences in mood before and after training. On the POMS scales, significant improvement in raw scores was found on measures of Confusion, Tension, Anger, and Total Mood Scores. Scores for Fatigue, Vigor, and Depression did not change significantly.

There were significant differences between men and women for raw scores on the subscales of Depression, Anger, Confusion, and Total Mood. However, there were no statistically significant interactions between sex and resistance training.

TABLE 2
Effects of Resistance Training on Profile of Mood States Scores in Healthy Older Adults by Sex

Mood State	Women (n = 13) Pretest M	SD	Posttest M	SD	Men (n = 15) Pretest M	SD	Posttest M	SD	Main Effects p	d	Sex Effects p	d
Tension	6.8	4.7	4.4	3.7	4.8	3.1	2.7	3.0	.02	.61	ns	.48
Depression	3.5	4.1	2.6	2.3	0.9	1.4	0.7	1.6	ns	.17	.001	.68
Anger	3.1	3.0	1.5	1.9	1.5	1.7	0.1	0.3	.02	.78	.002	.59
Vigor	19.5	4.9	20.2	7.3	21.9	4.6	23.3	4.8	ns	.20	ns	.44
Fatigue	6.7	5.8	5.2	5.9	4.3	4.0	2.2	2.8	ns	.38	.03	.46
Confusion	6.3	3.4	4.9	3.2	3.1	2.7	1.5	1.0	.01	.50	.001	.99
Total Mood	6.8	16.2	−1.8	20.0	−7.3	10.6	−16.1	9.5	.03	.54	.001	.78

Note.—No significant interactions between sex and time.

Interview Data

Sixteen of the 23 participants interviewed after the study noted at least some improvement in mood as a result of the study; this indicates that the Profile of Mood States may underreport meaningful changes in healthy adults. Interviewees made comments such as "it changed my life" and "I thought we were going over the hill [before the study]; we're still going up it." One participant called the study "exhilarating," adding "I feel great!"

Discussion

As previously reported in a nearly identical subgroup (Hunter, *et al.*, 2001), participants in this study showed a significant increase in strength and fat-free mass, and a significant reduction in body fat, regardless of resistance intensity. These changes are consistent with other studies of resistance training in older adults (Fiatarone Singh, 2002).

The study of women conducted by Tsutsumi, *et al.* (1998) showed improvement in POMS scores on the Tension and Vigor scales for both resistance intensities. The present study yielded significant improvement in Tension though not for Vigor. We also found significant improvement on Confusion and Anger scales. Unfortunately, Tsutsumi, *et al.* did not report results for these scales.

No significant training differences were found for Vigor, Depression, and Fatigue in this study. However, the sample size and power for detecting a training effect for these variables were small, and all means showed a trend for improvement following training. Rossi (1990, 1997) advocated for nonsignificant results that projections be made for sample sizes in such research. In the use of the Profile of Mood States, such sample sizes needs to be reported for each scale, as the effect size is different for each one. Based on the present study, projected sample sizes for the Vigor, Depression, and Fatigue scales are 208, 266, and 57, respectively, based on an unpublished 2000 account of a power calculator provided by the UCLA Department of Statistics[3] for a projected power of .80 using a two-sided test at $p < .05$. These projections should be considered conservative, as the use of a separate control group would lower effect sizes.

Several factors may explain any differences between the present study and those of Tsutsumi, et al. (1998). First, in the previous study, the data were not pooled when no significant differences were found between intensities. Second, Tsutsumi, et al. used a different protocol for the intensities, which varied both percentage of 1RM (75–80% vs 55–65%) and number of repetitions (8 to 10 vs 14 to 16) used for the high and low groups, respectively.

Finally, length of the intervention may have been a factor (12 vs 24 wk.). As mentioned, North, et al. (1990) reported in their meta-analytic review that length of intervention has a dramatic influence on effect size. This meta-analysis, however, did not show how much of this increased effect size is related to the length of the exercise protocol as opposed to the natural tendency of depressive episodes to be self-limiting. Most episodes of major depression last six months or less (Maxmen & Ward, 1995).

That depression scores did not improve significantly was unexpected. However, the average depression score was not high to begin with, and further decrease was unlikely. This is congruent with Gitlin, Lawton, Windsor Landsberg, and Kleban (1992) and Penninx, et al. (2002), who did not find significant improvement in depression scores in nondepressed samples.

Although the changes on some of the POMS scales are significant, it is also important to ask if they are clinically relevant. The scales themselves are centered mainly on pathology, e.g., Confusion, Depression, Fatigue, and the healthy sample in this study had raw scores near scale extremes. In this study, 11 out of 28 participants scored a "0" on the prestudy scale of depression. Their scores could not improve; they could change only in the direction of more depression. Also, the Profile of Mood States was administered before strength-testing sessions, when short-term changes in mood as a result of exercise are minimized. Even so, 16 of the 23 participants interviewed noted a change in their mood as a result of resistance training. For some individuals, the perceived effects were dramatic.

---

[3]The 2002 power calculator can be obtained from the Department of Statistics, University of California at Los Angeles as of April 8, 2004 from http://calculators.stat.ucla.edu/powercalc/. It is based on an unpublished computer program written by Brown, B. W., Brauner, C., Chan, A., Gutierrez, D., Herson, J., Lovato, J., Polsley, J., and Venier, J. (2000), Calculations for sample sizes and related problems. The University of Texas M. D. Anderson Cancer Center, Houston. Last accessed April 8, 2004 at http://odin.mdacc.tmc.edu/anonftp/. Source code for the PC is available (as of April 8, 2004) by file transfer protocol from ftp://odin.mdacc.tmc.edu/pub/win32/dstplan_4.2_se.exe or e-mail: bwb@mdanderson.org.

The interview data indicate that most interviewees reported improvement, although the Profile of Mood States data indicate a far more subtle effect. Studies have not readily clarified the extent to which resistance training improves mood in healthy older adults. Part of the problem may lie in the lack of standardization of intensity. Studies of aerobic exercise tend to use an age-based formula to derive prescribed target heart rate, while resistance training studies have used an exercise prescription based on a percentage of maximum ability, as in the current study (Hunter, *et al.*, 1995; Tsutsumi, *et al.*, 1998), self-reports of intensity (Bartholomew & Linder, 1998), or an after-study measure of intensity based on attained increases in strength (Singh, *et al.*, 1997).

Limitations

The lack of a control group who engaged in a parallel social, attentional, or interactional activity may limit these experimental conclusions. In addition, participants were recruited for an exercise study, and their motivation to exercise may not be generalizable to the population. Such individuals may have positive expectations of exercise, resulting in a kind of "Pygmalion effect" from participation. These design limitations have been previously noted (Folkins & Sime, 1981; Morgan, 1985). A control group might also help to account for the inevitable effects of aging on older adults in a study of this length. However, randomly assigned control groups in long-term exercise studies such as this one suffer from high dropout rates that hinder their effective use. Participants unable to exercise who do not withdraw may experience loss of morale, which might confound any attempt to serve as a control.

Another limitation has to do with the small to moderate effect sizes inherent in these phenomena. Part of the problem lies in the arbitrary use of significance levels as absolute cutoff points (Rossi, 1997). Rossi also noted that studies of phenomena which have small to moderate effect sizes have a greater chance of Type II error, which results when a given intervention has a small effect but the null hypothesis is retained because the measured value is not "significant".

In summary, resistance training in healthy older adults may be related to small but significant changes on Confusion, Tension, Anger, and Overall Mood scores; the small amounts of improvement noted on scales of Depression, Vigor, and Fatigue were not sufficient to meet significance levels. Power estimates of sample sizes were conducted for further study of these scales. Although scores on the Depression subscale do not appear to improve with resistance training in these healthy older adults, our sample was not depressed initially. Interview data from participants indicated that 16 of the 23 interviewees reported at least some improvement in mood. Further study is needed to control for cohort, social, and attentional effects of resistance training.

REFERENCES

BARTHOLOMEW, J. B., & LINDER, D. E. (1998) State anxiety following resistance exercise: the role of gender and exercise intensity. *Journal of Behavioral Medicine*, 21, 205-219.

DOYNE, E. J., OSSIP-KLEIN, D. J., BOWMAN, E. D., OSBORN, K. M., McDOUGALL-WILSON, I. B., & NEIMEYER, R. A. (1987) Running versus weight lifting in the treatment of depression. *Journal of Consulting and Clinical Psychology*, 55, 748-754.

EMERY, C. F., & BLUMENTHAL, J. A. (1991) Effects of physical exercise on psychological and cognitive functioning of older adults. *Annals of Behavioral Medicine*, 13, 99-107.

EMERY, C. F., & GATZ, M. (1990) Psychological and cognitive effects of an exercise program for community-residing older adults. *Gerontologist*, 30, 184-188.

FIATARONE, M. A., MARKS, E. C., RYAN, N. D., MEREDITH, C. N., LIPSITZ, L. A., & EVANS, W. J. (1990) High-intensity strength training in nonagenarians: effects on skeletal muscle. *Journal of the American Medical Association*, 263, 3029-3034.

FIATARONE SINGH, M. A. (2002) Exercise comes of age: rationale and recommendations for a geriatric exercise prescription. *Journals of Gerontology Series A–Biological Sciences & Medical Sciences*, 57, M262-M282.

FIELDS, D. A., HUNTER, G. R., & GORAN, M. I. (2000) Validation of the BOD POD with hydrostatic weighing: influence of body clothing. *Medicine and Science in Sports and Exercise*, 24, 200-205.

FOLKINS, C. H., & SIME, W. E. (1981) Physical fitness training and mental health. *American Psychologist*, 36, 373-389.

GITLIN, L. N., LAWTON, M. P., WINDSOR LANDSBERG, L. A., & KLEBAN, M. H. (1992) In search of psychological benefits: exercise in healthy older adults. *Journal of Aging and Health*, 4, 174-192.

HUNTER, G. R., TREUTH, M. S., WEINSIER, R. L., KEKES-SZABO, T., KELL, S. H., ROTH, D. L., & NICHOLSON, C. (1995) The effects of strength conditioning on older women's ability to perform daily tasks. *Journal of the American Geriatrics Society*, 43, 756-760.

HUNTER, G. R., WETZSTEIN, C. J., McLAFFERTY, C. L., JR., ZUCKERMAN, P. A., LANDERS, K., & BAMMAN, M. M. (2001) High resistance versus variable resistance training in older adults. *Medicine and Science in Sports and Exercise*, 33, 1759-1764.

HURLEY, B. F., & HAGBERG, J. M. (1998) Optimizing health in older persons: aerobic or strength training? *Exercise and Sport Sciences Reviews*, 26, 61-89.

KOLTYN, K. F., RAGLIN, J. S., O'CONNOR, P. J., & MORGAN, W. P. (1995) Influence of weight training on state anxiety, body awareness and blood pressure. *International Journal of Sports Medicine*, 16, 266-269.

LEUNES, A., & BURGER, J. (1998) Bibliography on the Profile of Mood States in sport and exercise psychology research, 1971-1998. *Journal of Sport Behavior*, 21, 53-70.

MAROULAKIS, E., & ZERVAS, Y. (1993) Effects of aerobic exercise on mood of adult women. *Perceptual and Motor Skills*, 76, 795-801.

MARTINSEN, E. W., HOFFART, A., & SOLBERG, O. (1989) Comparing aerobic with nonaerobic forms of exercise in the treatment of clinical depression: a randomized trial. *Comprehensive Psychiatry*, 30, 324-331.

MAXMEN, J. S., & WARD, N. G. (1995) *Essential psychopathology and its treatment.* (2nd ed.) New York: Norton.

McGOWAN, R. W., PIERCE, E. F., & JORDAN, D. (1991) Mood alterations with a single bout of physical activity. *Perceptual and Motor Skills*, 72, 1203-1209.

McGOWAN, R. W., TALTON, B. J., & THOMPSON, M. (1996) Changes in scores on the Profile of Mood States following a single bout of physical activity: heart rate and changes in affect. *Perceptual and Motor Skills*, 83, 859-866.

McNAIR, D. M., LORR, M., & DROPPLEMAN, L. F. (1992) *EdITS manual for the Profile of Mood States.* San Diego, CA: Educational and Industrial Testing Service.

MORGAN, W. P. (1985) Affective beneficence of vigorous physical activity. *Medicine and Science in Sports and Exercise*, 17, 94-100.

North, T. C., McCullagh, P., & Tran, Z. V. (1990) Effect of exercise on depression. *Exercise and Sport Sciences Reviews*, 18, 379-415.

Norvell, N., & Belles, D. (1993) Psychological and physical benefits of circuit weight training in law enforcement personnel. *Journal of Consulting and Clinical Psychology*, 61, 520-527.

Norvell, N., Martin, D., & Salamon, A. (1991) Psychological and physiological benefits of passive and aerobic exercise in sedentary middle-aged women. *Journal of Nervous and Mental Disease*, 179, 573-574.

O'Connor, P. J., Bryant, C. X., Veltri, J. P., & Gebhardt, S. M. (1993) State anxiety and ambulatory blood pressure following resistance exercise in females. *Medicine and Science in Sports and Exercise*, 25, 516-521.

Penninx, B., Rejeski, W., Pandya, J., Miller, M., Di Bari, M., Applegate, W., & Pahor, M. (2002) Exercise and depressive symptoms: a comparison of aerobic and resistance exercise effects on emotional and physical function in older persons with high and low depressive symptomatology. *Journal of Gerontology Series B–Psychological Sciences & Social Sciences*, 57, P124-P132.

Rossi, J. S. (1990) Statistical power of psychological research: what have we gained in 20 years? *Journal of Consulting and Clinical Psychology*, 58, 646-656.

Rossi, J. S. (1997) A case study in the failure of psychology as a cumulative science: the spontaneous recovery of verbal learning. In L. L. Harlow, S. A. Mulaik, & J. H. Steiger (Eds.), *What if there were no significance tests?* Mahwah, NJ: Erlbaum. Pp. 175-197.

Singh, N. A., Clements, K. M., & Fiatarone, M. A. (1997) A randomized controlled trial of progressive resistance training in depressed elders. *Journals of Gerontology Series A–Biological Sciences & Medical Sciences*, 52A, M27-M35.

Singh, N. A., Clements, K. M., & Fiatarone Singh, M. A. (2001) The efficacy of exercise as a long-term antidepressant in elderly subjects: a randomized, controlled trial. *Journal of Gerontology: Medical Sciences*, 56A, M497-M504.

Stewart, A. L., & King, A. C. (1991) Evaluating the efficacy of physical activity for influencing quality-of-life outcomes in older adults. *Annals of Behavioral Medicine*, 13, 108-116.

Tsutsumi, T., Don, B. M., Zaichkowsky, L. D., Takenaka, K., Oka, K., & Ohno, T. (1998) Comparison of high and moderate intensity of strength training on mood and anxiety in older adults. *Perceptual and Motor Skills*, 87, 1003-1011.

Accepted March 16, 2004.

GEOPHYSICAL VARIABLES AND BEHAVIOR: XCIX. REDUCTIONS IN NUMBERS OF NEURONS WITHIN THE PARASOLITARY NUCLEUS IN RATS EXPOSED PERINATALLY TO A MAGNETIC PATTERN DESIGNED TO IMITATE GEOMAGNETIC CONTINUOUS PULSATIONS: IMPLICATIONS FOR SUDDEN INFANT DEATH [1,2]

M. J. DUPONT, B. E. McKAY, G. PARKER, AND M. A. PERSINGER

Laurentian University

Summary.—Correlational analyses have shown a moderate strength association between the occurrence of continuous pulsations, a type of geomagnetic activity within the 0.2-Hz to 5-Hz range, and the occurrence of Sudden Infant Deaths. In the present study, rats were exposed continuously from two days before birth to seven days after birth to 0.5-Hz pulsed-square wave magnetic fields whose intensities were within either the nanoTesla or microTesla range. The magnetic fields were generated in either an east-west (E-W) or north-south (N-S) direction. At 21 days of age, the area of the parasolitary nucleus (but not the solitary nucleus) was significantly smaller, and the numbers of neurons were significantly less in rats that had been exposed to the nanoT fields generated in the east-west direction or to the microTesla fields generated within either E-W or N-S direction relative to those exposed to the N-S nanoTesla fields. These results suggest nanoTesla magnetic fields, when applied in a specific direction, might interact with the local geomagnetic field to affect cell migration in structures within the brain stem that modulate vestibular-related arousal and respiratory or cardiovascular stability.

The occurrence of Sudden Infant Death has been correlated with various increments of geomagnetic activity during the months in which the deaths occur. More specifically, O'Connor and Persinger (1997) found a strong correlation between the incidence of Sudden Infant Deaths in Canada and specific bands of intensity of geomagnetic activity. Their subsequent analyses (O'Connor & Persinger, 1999) suggested a role of protracted periods of weak (< 1 nT) symmetrical rhythmic activity, continuous geomagnetic pulsations (pc1), in the association between global geomagnetic activity and Sudden Infant Death.

Although there are many hypotheses concerning the cause of sudden death in infants, anomalies within the neuronal arrangement or electrical activity of specific structures in the brain stem have been considered the

---

[1]This research was supported by a grant from the Canadian Foundation for the Study of Infant Deaths (Sidney Segal Research Foundation) and by the Laurentian University Neuroscience Research Group. Thanks to Linda Vaillancourt for technical contributions.
[2]Address correspondence to Dr. M. A. Persinger, Department of Biology, Behavioral Neuroscience Laboratory, Laurentian University, Sudbury, ON Canada P3E 2C6 or e-mail (mpersinger @laurentian.ca).

most common predisposing factor. Transient anomalous dysfunctions that lead to recurrent intermittent episodes of hypoxia may contribute to sudden death. Waters, Meehan, Huang, Gravel, Michaud, and Cote (1999) found that most of the infants who died suddenly, compared to the reference group, displayed apoptosis of neurons within the brain stem. The resultant reduction of cell numbers would be compatible with the magnitude of the marginally significant cytometric changes in neuronal soma, specifically within medullary structures that modulate heart rate and respiration, in the brains of infants who died suddenly (Oehmichen, Linke, Zilles, & Saternus, 1989).

The present experiment was designed to imitate a temporal pattern of specific geomagnetic conditions, particularly the simulation of repeated rhythmic shapes of magnetic fields (similar to pc1 pulsations), that might contribute to Sudden Infant Death. Because the incidence of Sudden Infant Death is relatively low, it was suspected that it would be produced by a series of interacting variables. One of these would involve the activities of the medullary reticular nuclei that affect arousal. Recently, Barmack and Yakhnitsa (2000) showed that the parasolitary nucleus is the source of GABAnergic projections to two regions: the inferior olive and the nucleus reticularis gigantocellularis. They are involved with the level of physiological arousal.

If the occurrence of a specific geomagnetic pattern during a critical period of neurodevelopment affected cell numbers in the parasolitary nucleus, then subsequent exposure to these fields might produce an electrical anomaly that would produce cessation of respiration and heart beats (Eckert, 1992). For comparison and to help control for the role of "nonspecific effects," the solitary nucleus was selected for examination. It is adjacent to the parasolitary nucleus. Unlike the parasolitary nucleus, the solitary nucleus receives sensory fibers from the facial, glossopharyngeal, and vagus nerves. Whereas the cells within the rostral third of this nucleus are associated with gustation, those within the posterior two-thirds are involved with visceral afferents.

METHOD

In two separate blocks, a total of 16 pregnant, approximately 90-day-old Wistar albino rats housed singly in standard plastic cages (with aluminum tops containing food and a water bottle) were exposed to magnetic fields produced by one of two 112-cm by 125-cm aluminium racks that were separated by at least 2 m and arranged either in an east-west or north-south direction. Each rack was wrapped around its perimeter with 72 turns of 30-gauge (AWG) copper wire to form a band 13 cm wide.

In different blocks of the experiments, one coil served as the active coil while the other served as the reference coil. As a result, there were four litters for each of the four conditions. When a coil was activated a 0.5-Hz pulsed-square wave magnetic field was generated continuously through the coil and the cages by a custom-made device. When the current was delivered through the coil the magnetic field was generated in the perpendicular direction within the horizontal plane. The resulting fields, as measured by a MEDA FM-300 magnetometer, were a continuous rhythmic series of signals. The total duration of each complex square wave that composed the continuous rhythmic signals was about 600 msec. Its onset was associated with a transient spike with a rise time of between 1.5 and 3.5 microsec. that was about four times the amplitude of the major plateau. The offset was associated with a similar spike with opposite polarity with comparable amplitude.

The amplitudes of the continuously presented 0.5-Hz waves were changed every 30 min. These protracted changes in amplitude occurred in 4-hr. cycles with six cycles per day (McKay, Koren, & Persinger, 2003). The duration of 4 hr. was selected given its similarity to natural pulsations. The maximum intensities of the amplitude modulations according to the magnetometer (placed within the same plastic cage and lid involved with housing the mothers) during each 30-min. period were 0, 870 nT, 1040 nT (1.04 microT), 1300 nT (1.30 microT), 1770 nT (1.77 microT), 1330 nT, 1040 nT, and 870 nT within the active coil. Given induction effects, the maximum field strengths in the inactive coil per successive 30-min. period were 0, 4 nT, 8 nT, 11 nT, 13 nT, 11 nT, 8 nT, and 4 nT. These changes were superimposed upon the ambient geomagnetic activity (see McKay, et al., 2003 for sample figures). The rats were exposed from two days before birth to seven days after birth. This period was selected because it involved the perinatal period shown to be most sensitive to the effects of magnetic fields (Persinger, Lafreniere, & Ossenkopp, 1974). The litters were not culled so that potential postnatal deaths could be detected. Except to discern whether the pups were alive once per day, they were not touched.

At 21 days of age, one male and one female rat from each litter were randomly selected and decapitated. The 32 brains were fixed in ethanol-formalin acetic acid, processed, embedded in paraffin, and sectioned at 10 micrometers. The required sections were stained with toluidine blue O. The numbers of neurons and glial cells within the solitary nucleus and parasolitary nucleus were counted in a 6 × 6 grid at 400 X. The sections included the parasolitary nucleus in 28 of the rats and the solitary nucleus in 31 of the rats. However, the four treatments were more or less equally represented. Three-way analyses of variance as a function of sex, field (activated or reference), and orientation of the applied field (E–W vs N–S) were completed for the numbers of neurons, glial cells (oligodendroglia and astroglia), and neuronal/glial ratios by SPSS software on a VAX 2000 computer. Significance by Tukey *post hoc* tests was set at $p < .05$.

Results

The means and standard deviations for numbers of neurons and glial cells, neuronal/glia ratios, and areas for the two structures are shown in Table 1. There were significantly ($F_{1,19} = 4.79$, $p < .05$; $\eta^2 = .36$) fewer neurons within the parasolitary nuclei of rats that had been exposed to the activated field compared to the reference field. However, this main effect was confounded by the statistically significant interaction between the orientation of the applied field and its intensity ($F_{1,19} = 9.28$, $p < .01$). Post hoc analysis indicated that the rats exposed to the microT fields showed reduced numbers of neurons, regardless of field orientation. Those exposed to the nanoT field generated in the E–W direction also showed reduced numbers of neurons compared to those exposed to the nanoT field generated in the N–S direction. The areas of the parasolitary nuclei of the rats exposed to the microT field, regardless of coil orientation, were significantly smaller ($F_{1,19} = 4.25$, $p < .05$; $\eta^2 = .37$) relative to those exposed to the nanoT intensities.

TABLE 1
Means and Standard Deviations For Numbers of Neurons, Glial Cells, Neuronal/Glial Ratios and Area (um^2) of the Structure Per Section Within the Parasolitary and Solitary Nuclei in Rats Perinatally Exposed to Various Simulated "Geomagnetic" Conditions

	nanoTesla Field				microTesla Field			
	\multicolumn{8}{c}{Direction of Applied Field}
	N–S		E–W		N–S		E–W	
	M	SD	M	SD	M	SD	M	SD
Parasolitary Nucleus								
Area (um^2)	34720[a]	15190	26474	6553	19288[b]	5520	24159	7194
Neurons	152[a]	66	88[b]	11	75[b]	30	93[b]	20
Glial cells	47	28	44	19	40	19	42	17
Neuron/Glial cells	3.5	.8	2.3	.9	2.2	1.0	2.4	.8
Solitary Nucleus								
Neurons	4413	196	3462	620	3897	1019	3921	564
Glial cells	67[a]	14	88	15	104[b]	13	91	16
Neuron/Glial cells	2.6[a]	.3	1.9	.6	1.5[b]	.4	2.1[a]	.4

Note.—Fields are applied in a north–south (N–S) or east–west (E–W) direction.
[a] vs [b] $p < .05$.

Except for the significantly ($F_{1,22} = 7.26$, $p < .01$; $\eta^2 = .43$) fewer numbers of neurons within the solitary nucleus for the male brains ($M = 157$ neurons, $SD = 30$) compared to those for the female brains ($M = 180$ neurons, $SD = 24$), there were no statistically significant treatment effects or interactions between treatments and sex. However, there were significantly more glial cells ($F_{1,22} = 4.15$, $p < .05$; $\eta^2 = .32$) in the solitary nuclei of rats that had been exposed to the microT fields compared to the nanoT field. The interaction between the orientation and the activation of the fields was significant ($F_{1,22} = $

7.49, $p = .01$) and, due to the fact that the rats exposed to the microT fields generated in the N–S direction, had more glial cells than those exposed to the nanoT field while this discrepancy was not present for those exposed to the field generated in the E–W direction.

By far the most powerful treatment effect was for the ratios of neurons to glial cells within the solitary nucleus. Male rats displayed significantly ($F_{1,22} = 12.30$, $p < .001$; $\eta^2 = .43$) lower ratios than did the females. There was a significant interaction ($F_{1,22} = 15.63$, $p < .001$) between intensity of the field and its orientation. Post hoc analysis indicated that rats exposed to the microT field generated in the north–south direction showed lower ratios than those exposed to the nanoT field generated in the north–south direction while those exposed to the microT or nanoT fields generated in the east-west direction had comparable values.

Discussion

The results of this study suggest that the geomagnetic orientation of the source generating complex magnetic fields designed to simulate geomagnetic pulsations was a significant variable. The rats that had been exposed to the nanoTesla strength magnetic fields generated in an east–west direction displayed fewer cells within the parasolitary nucleus compared to the rats that had received the same-strength field generated in a north–south direction. Rats that had been exposed to the field strengths one-thousand times stronger than the nanoTesla ranges displayed comparable reduced numbers of cells, regardless of the fields' orientations.

The results of the study do not indicate whether the source of the diminished numbers of neurons was necrosis or apoptosis. Significant neuronal apoptosis was found in the brain stem for 96% of infants who had died suddenly (Waters, et al., 1999). The distribution of apoptosis was mostly in dorsal nuclei, including the spinal trigeminal tract and the vestibular nuclei. These structures are involved with sensation to the face and position of the head. Waters, et al. (1999) suggested that enhanced neuronal death by apoptosis and the involvement of these specific brain stem nuclei might be linked to the role of prone sleeping as a significant risk factor for Sudden Infant Death.

It was assumed that the values for the numbers of neurons within a cross-section of the parasolitary nucleus and its cross-sectional area in the rats that had been exposed perinatally to the nanoTesla 0.5-Hz fields generated in a north–south direction are typical of normal estimates. Consequently, the lower numbers of neurons seen in rats exposed to the nanoTesla fields generated in an east–west direction would reflect an effect from this treatment. If this assumption is valid then geomagnetic pulsations (pc1) or less symmetrical temporal variations of correlative geomagnetic activity generated along this spatial dimension could be important for affecting the development of neuronal conditions that might increase the organism's later sensitivity to specific patterns of weak magnetic fields.

Our daily magnetometer recordings (24-sec. samples) have clearly shown that on some days only the north–south, east–west, or vertical component may be the most affected component of the earth's magnetic field during a geomagnetic storm. Global values, such as the average antipodal index (aa), reflect the most "disturbed" magnetometric components. As a result days with similar quantitative values may have been dominated by qualitatively different types of disturbances. If the spatial vector of the geomagnetic disturbance is a critical variable, then gross correlations between numbers of Sudden Infant Deaths and aa values might underestimate the strength of the true association.

Cells within the parasolitary nucleus are the primary source of the inhibitor neurotransmitter GABA to portions of the inferior olive and giant reticular nucleus. Cells from components of the inferior olive project to the contralateral cerebellar uvula-nodulus (Barmack, 1996) that project back to the parasolitary nucleus. The average discharge rate for these cells in response to sinusoidal stimulation between 0.2 Hz and .4 Hz was about 10 Hz (Barmack & Yakhnitsa, 2000). The activities of these cells were also modulated by vestibular stimulation in either the pitch or roll planes (dynamic roll-tilt along the longitudinal plane) but not the horizontal plane. If during development these cells were affected by pc1-like geomagnetic patterns, then head movements within a particular plane could significantly affect the stability and frequency of the discharge rates of aggregates of these neurons.

Such responses to stimuli with specific orientation may explain the relationship between the developmental window associated with Sudden Infant Death and periods when head movements, particularly when the infant is placed on its stomach, are prominent (Stulbach, 2003). It is suggested that appropriate synchronization by periodic geomagnetic oscillations within the pc1 range (around 0.5 Hz) when presented with the optimal ratio of time-varying-to-static intensities produces a resonance within the parasolitary circuit. Because the parasolitary nucleus lacks a commissural projection, mutual or reciprocal inhibition does not occur, and the inhibitory discharges become markedly synchronized. A reduction in the number of neurons as seen in this study may encourage this synchronization if the neurons that have died or failed to develop determined primarily inhibitory intranuclear functions.

It may be of interest that the locus ceruleus, which processes sensory input and regulates the forebrain's functional state, exhibits intrinsic oscillations with periods in the .02-Hz to .5-Hz range (Filippov, Gladyshev, &

Williams, 2002). The presence of these "infraslow potentials" as well as their amplitudes can be exacerbated by the stress of physical restraint. In infants under six months of age, lying on the ventral surface (face down) may simulate this stress. Developmental abnormalities within the medullary reticular formation have been strongly implicated in at least a subset of Sudden Infant Deaths (Kinney, Filiano, & White, 2001). If our hypothesis is correct, the paucity of neurons within at least the parasolitary nucleus may reflect a network of developmental deficiencies that, given the specific combination of stimuli, result in sudden death.

That the results of our study were nonspecific artifacts was not likely in light of the absence of significant group differences for the numbers of neurons within the nearby solitary nucleus. However, there were significantly greater numbers of glial cells within the solitary nucleus of the rats that had been exposed to the east–west generated nanoTesla fields, compared to the rats that had been exposed to the north–south generated fields. If we assume that increased numbers of glial cells suggest reactive gliosis from an earlier period, then their evaluation in conjunction with the reduction of neurons might reflect the consequences of early deafferentiation. The present model would predict that infants who die suddenly must have been exposed several times to similar stimuli during their development to produce the deficit that would allow the precipitating stimulus within the geomagnetic field to produce sudden death.

This model would be similar to the predictions of Eckert (1992) who hypothesized two elements were required, a selection factor and a trigger factor, for the occurrence of Sudden Infant Death. The first involved disturbed geomagnetic fields within the residence or surroundings of a pregnant woman that interrupted the normal development of the central organ that controls respiration in the fetus. Were this infant then exposed to an electromagnetic pulsation similar to its own breathing frequency, but inverted in phase, value, or form (the trigger factor), the impulses from the "respiratory control organ" to the breathing organs would be disturbed. This would have a fatal effect.

There is one final implication of this reasoning. If vulnerable organisms do not die as infants, they may be vulnerable, perhaps as adults, to other physiological transients such as cardiac arrhythmias. Persinger and O'Connor (2001) found increased incidences of cardiac arrhythmias in adults and sudden deaths in infants occurred on the same days. In our first series of experiments of reintroducing adult rats to the 0.5-Hz, 5-nT to 10-nT field in which they were born, there was a sudden cardiac death in a healthy 4-mo.-old adult male rat within one hour of an abrupt and persistent decrease in the intensity of the north–south component of the geomagnetic field within the coils.

Although the vertical component remained relatively stable during this event, there was a decrease from 4,250 nT to 4,158 nT (102 nT) within the X-component (N–S direction) of the earth's magnetic field over a period of 1.8 hr. Superimposed on this gradual decline was a rapid (within a few minutes) decrease of 45 nT followed 28 min. later after no change by another rapid decrease of 36 nT. There were concomitant rapid increases of about 10 to 20 nT in the Y-component (E–W direction) during these periods. This same event in more northern latitudes, for example Finland (Sodankyla Geophysical Laboratory), was associated with a comparable temporal structure but a greater decrease of more than 500 nT in the X-component.

The rat had been placed in the exact cage position (and static geomagnetic configuration) and orientation (E–W) of the experimental magnetic field in which he had been born four months previously. There has never been a sudden death in this age range of normal rats in the population of approximately 4,000 rats we have studied over the last 20 years. However, we (Persinger, McKay, O'Donovan, & Koren, in revision) have found that nocturnal exposures for only 6 min. once per hour to experimental fields whose intensities decreased by about 50 nT in the north–south direction resulted in increased sudden death in male rats within 24 hr. after epileptic seizures had been induced.

REFERENCES

BARMACK, N. H. (1996) GABAergic pathways convey vestibular information to the beta nucleus and dorsomedial cell column of the inferior olive. *Annals of the New York Academy of Science*, 781, 541-552.

BARMACK, N. H., & YAKHNITSA, V. (2000) Vestibular signals in the parasolitary nucleus. *Journal of Neurophysiology*, 83, 3559-3569.

ECKERT, E. E. (1992) Magnetic influences on fetus and infant as reason for sudden infant death syndrome: a new testable hypothesis. *Medical Hypotheses*, 38, 66-69.

FILIPPOV, I. V., GLADYSHEV, A. V., & WILLIAMS, W. C. (2002) Role of infraslow (0-0.05 Hz) potential oscillations in the regulation of brain stress response by locus ceruleus system. *Neurocomputing*, 44-46, 795-798.

KINNEY, H. C., FILIANO, J. J., & WHITE, W. F. (2001) Medullary serotonergic network deficiency in the sudden infant death syndrome: a review of a 15-year study of a single data set. *Journal of Neuropathology and Experimental Neurology*, 60, 228-247.

MCKAY, B. E., KOREN, S. A., & PERSINGER, M. A. (2003) Behavioral effects of combined perinatal L-name and 0.5 Hz magnetic field treatments. *International Journal of Neuroscience*, 113, 119-139.

O'CONNOR, R. P., & PERSINGER, M. A. (1997) Geophysical variables and behavior: LXXXII. A strong association between sudden infant death (SIDs) and increments of global geomagnetic activity-possible support for the melatonin hypothesis. *Perceptual and Motor Skills*, 84, 1376-1378.

O'CONNOR, R. P., & PERSINGER, M. A. (1999) Sudden infant death, bands of geomagnetic activity, and pc1 (0.2 to 5 Hz) geomagnetic pulsations. *Perceptual and Motor Skills*, 88, 391-397.

OEHMICHEN, M., LINKE, P., ZILLES, K., & SATERNUS, K. S. (1989) Reactive astrocytes and macrophages in the brain stem of SIDS victims? Eleven age- and sex-matched SIDS and control cases. *Clinical Neuropathology*, 8, 276-283.

PERSINGER, M. A., LAFRENIERE, G. F., & OSSENKOPP, K-P. (1974) Behavioral, physiological, and histological changes in rats exposed during developmental stages to ELF magnetic fields.

In M. A. Persinger (Ed.), *ELF and VLF electromagnetic field effects*. New York: Plenum. Pp. 177-225.

PERSINGER, M. A., MCKAY, B. E., O'DONOVAN, C. A., & KOREN, S. A. (in revision) Sudden death in epileptic rats exposed to nocturnal magnetic fields that simulate the shape and the intensity of sudden changes in geomagnetic activity: an experiment in response to Schnabel, Beblo and May. *International Journal of Biometerology*.

PERSINGER, M. A., & O'CONNOR, R. P. (2001) Geophysical variables and behavior: CIII. Days with sudden infant deaths and cardiac arrhythmias in adults share a factor with pc1 geomagnetic pulsations: implications for pursuing mechanism. *Perceptual and Motor Skills*, 92, 653-654.

STULBACH, N. (2003) New biological approach and solution to SIDs. *Medical Hypothesis*, 61, 16-17.

WATERS, K. A., MEEHAN, B., HUANG, J. Q., GRAVEL, R. A., MICHAUD, J., & COTE, A. (1999) Neuronal apoptosis in Sudden Infant Death Syndrome. *Pediatric Research*, 45, 166-172.

Accepted March 22, 2004.

ON A GENERAL CLASS OF CHI-SQUARED GOODNESS-OF-FIT STATISTICS[1]

TARALD O. KVÅLSETH

University of Minnesota

Summary.—A class of chi-squared goodness-of-fit statistics is presented as being based on the so-called divergence of one probability distribution from another. A still more general class of goodness-of-fit statistics is then presented by eliminating some of the restrictions required of divergence-based statistics. This most general class of statistics includes, as particular cases, a variety of statistics used in the published literature.

The concept and measures of *divergence* (discrepancy, "distance," or cross-entropy) of one probability distribution from another have wide interest and applicability to various fields of study. Mutual or transmitted information, which is a frequently used measure of human performance in stimulus-response tasks (e.g., Wickens & Hollands, 2000, Ch. 2, 9), can be viewed as a divergence of the joint stimulus-response probabilities from those of the statistical independence condition (e.g., Kvålseth, 1991). Divergence minimization is used to estimate probability distributions (e.g., Kapur, 1994, Part B). In terms of testing statistical hypotheses, which is the main concern of this paper, the Cressie-Read statistic for goodness-of-fit tests is based on a family of divergence measures (e.g., Read & Cressie, 1988). In particular, what is presented here is a general class of chi-squared goodness-of-fit statistics based on divergences as well as a further generalization.

A Class of Divergence Statistics

Consider that P and Q, or $\{p_i\}$ and $\{q_i\}$, are two probability distributions, each having k elements, with $\sum_{i=1}^{k} p_i = \sum_{i=1}^{k} q_i = 1$. If, for $x = p/q$, $d(x)$ is a value of the *divergence function* d, with

$$D(P:Q) = \sum_{i=1}^{k} q_i d(p_i/q_i), \qquad [1]$$

then $D(P:Q)$ is defined as the (directed) *divergence* of P from Q if (a) d is convex for all x and strictly convex at $x=1$, (b) the first derivative of $d(x)$ with respect to x is zero at $x=1$, i.e., $d'(1)=0$, and (c) $d(1)=0$. This general divergence is known as Csiszár's class of divergencies, after Csiszár (1972), although the restriction $d(1)=0$ has been added as a reasonable requirement of any divergence function. See also discussions by Kapur (1994).

---

[1]Address correspondence to T. O. Kvålseth, Department of Mechanical Engineering, University of Minnesota, Minneapolis, MN 55455.

Consider next the categorical data case when, for $i = 1, \ldots, k$ categories, the $p_i = n_i/n$ are the observed proportions and $q_i = m_i/n$ are the expected probabilities under the null hypothesis (H_0), with $n = \sum_{i=1}^{k} n_i = \sum_{i=1}^{k} m_i$ being the sample size. Given the three restrictions imposed on d in Equation [1] and expanding it in a Taylor series about $x_i = p_i/q_i = n_i/m_i = 1$, the following result is obtained:

$$\frac{2n}{d''(1)} D(\{n_i\} : \{m_i\}) = \frac{2n}{d''(1)} \sum_{i=1}^{k} q_i [d(1) + d'(1)(x_i - 1) + \frac{d''(1)}{2!}(x_i - 1)^2$$

$$+ \frac{d'''(1)}{3!}(x_i - 1)^3 + \ldots] \qquad [2a]$$

$$= \sum_{i=1}^{k} \frac{(n_i - m_i)^2}{m_i} + \frac{2}{d''(1)} \sum_{i=1}^{k} m_i [\frac{d'''(1)}{3!}(x_i - 1)^3 + \ldots] \qquad [2b]$$

$$= X^2 + o_p(1) , \qquad [2c]$$

since $d(1) = d'(1) = 0$ and where $o_p(1)$ represents a stochastic term that converges to zero in probability (see, e.g., Read & Cressie, 1988, pp. 45-47). Consequently, the class of divergence statistics $2n[d''(1)]^{-1} D(\{n_i\} : \{m_i\})$ has the same asymptotic chi-squared distribution as the well-known Pearson's X^2 with the appropriate degrees of freedom.

This class of divergence statistics for goodness-of-fit tests has been used in some of this author's unpublished research for some time and has also independently been proposed by Menéndez and Pardo (2002). Of course, the best-known members of this class of statistics are Pearson's X^2, which corresponds to $d(x) = (x - 1)^2$ and the likelihood-ratio statistic G^2, which corresponds to $d(x) = x \log x - x + 1$, with $\log x$ being the natural (base $-e$) logarithm. The Cressie-Read one-parameter family of statistics also clearly belongs to this class (see, e.g., Read & Cressie, 1988, Ch. 7).

Further Generalization

The class of goodness-of-fit statistics defined by Equations [1] and [2] can be further generalized by replacing the divergence function d with a less restrictive (nondivergence) function f. What shall be required is that (1) $f''(1) \neq 0$, and (2) all derivatives $f^{(r)}(x)$ exist so that $f(x)$ can be expanded in a Taylor series about $x = 1$. Of course, some or all $f^{(r)}(x)$ may be 0 for $r > 2$ as, for example, with $f(x) = x^3$. Then, the following shall be proved:

$$K^2 = \frac{2}{f''(1)} \sum_{i=1}^{k} m_i \left[f\left(\frac{n_i}{m_i}\right) - f(1) \right] \qquad [3]$$

has the asymptotic chi-squared distribution with $k-1$ degrees of freedom under simple H_0 and $k-1-s$ degrees of freedom under composite H_0 when the estimated expected frequencies $\hat{m}_i = nq_i$ are functions of a set of s estimated parameters.

Due to the two requirements that (1) $f''(1) \neq 0$ and (2) $f(x)$ is Taylor-series expansible at $x=1$, the K^2 statistic in Equation [3] can be expressed as:

$$K^2 = \frac{2}{f''(1)} \sum_{i=1}^{k} m_i \left[f(1) + f'(1)(x_i - 1) + \frac{f''(1)}{2!}(x_i - 1)^2 + O_p(n^{-3/2}) - f(1) \right]. \quad [4a]$$

The $f(1)$ terms cancel out and $\sum_{i=1}^{k} m_i(x_i - 1) = 0$ so that

$$K^2 = \sum_{i=1}^{k} \frac{(n_i - m_i)^2}{m_i} + O_p(n^{-1/2}) = X^2 + o_p(1). \quad [4b]$$

That is, K^2 has the same asymptotic chi-squared distribution under the null hypothesis H_0 as Pearson's X^2. For the meaning of the probabilistic convergence notation O_p and o_p, see, for example, Agresti (2002, Ch. 14).

Particular members of this general class of statistics in Equation [3], besides the subclass in Equations [1] through [2], include the following: Pearson's X^2 with $f(x) = (x-1)^2$ or $f(x) = x^2$; the likelihood-ratio statistic G^2 with $f(x) = x \log x$, the modified likelihood-ratio statistic GM^2 (e.g., Read & Cressie, 1988, p. 11) with $f(x) = \log x$, the Neuman-modified X^2 statistic (e.g., Read & Cressie, 1988, p. 11) with $f(x) = 1/x$, the Freeman-Tukey statistic F^2 (e.g., Read & Cressie, 1988, p. 11) with $f(x) = x^{1/2}$, and the Cressie-Read statistics with $f(x) = x^\alpha$ for the real-valued parameter α. Any linear function of two or more of these functions $f(x)$, is also a member of the K^2 class in Equation [3].

Another interesting member of the K^2 class of goodness-of-fit statistics is obtained from $f(x) = \log(x+1)$, for which

$$f'(x) = (x+1)^{-1}, f''(x) = -(x+1)^{-2}, \text{ and } f''(1) = -1/4.$$

By denoting the statistic as K_1^2, it follows from Equation [3] that

$$K_1^2 = \frac{2}{-1/4} \sum_{i=1}^{k} m_i \left[\log\left(\frac{n_i}{m_i} + 1\right) - \log 2 \right] = 8 \sum_{i=1}^{k} m_i \log\left(\frac{2m_i}{n_i + m_i}\right). \quad [5]$$

As a numerical example involving this K_1^2 statistic, consider the four-category multinomial case with sample size $n=75$, observed frequencies (counts) $n_i = 40, 3, 25, 7$ for $i = 1, \ldots, 4$, and expected frequencies $m_i = 37.5, 7.5, 22.5, 7.5$ for $i = 1, \ldots, 4$ under the simple null hypothesis $H_0: q_i$ (or p_{oi} as usually denoted) $= .5, .1, .3, .1$. From Equation [5], $K_1^2 = 3.87$, as compared to Pearson's $X^2 = 3.18$ and the likelihood-ratio statistic $G^2 = 3.97$. Since the values of these three statistics are all less than the tabulated chi-squared value $\chi^2_{.05,3} = 7.81$ for $k - 1 = 3$ degrees of freedom and $\alpha = .05$, the H_0 cannot be rejected at the 5% level of significance.

REFERENCES

AGRESTI, A. (2002) *Categorical data analysis*. (2nd ed.) New York: Wiley.

CSISZÁR, I. (1972) A class of measures of informativy of observation channels. *Peridica Mathematica Hungarica*, 2, 191-213.

KAPUR, J. N. (1994) *Measures of information and their applications*. New York: Wiley.

KVÅLSETH, T. O. (1991) On generalized information measures of human performance. *Perceptual and Motor Skills*, 72, 1059-1063.

MENÉNDEZ, M. L., & PARDO, J. A. (2002) Tests of symmetry in three-dimensional contingency tables based on *phi*-divergence statistics. Paper presented at the 24th European Meeting of Statisticians and the 14th Prague Conference on Information Theory, Statistical Decision Functions and Random Processes, Prague, the Czech Republic, August 19-23.

READ, T. R. C., & CRESSIE, N. A. C. (1988) *Goodness-of-fit statistics for discrete multivariate data*. Berlin: Springer-Verlag.

WICKENS, C. D., & HOLLANDS, J. G. (2000) *Engineering psychology and human performance*. (3rd ed.) Upper Saddle River, NJ: Prentice Hall.

Accepted March 2, 2004.

PERCEPTUAL ENCODING OF FINGERSPELLED AND PRINTED ALPHABET BY DEAF SIGNERS: AN fMRI STUDY [1,2]

ANDRÉ DUFOUR

Centre d'Etudes de Physiologie Appliquée
CNRS - Université Louis Pasteur

RENAUD BROCHARD

Laboratoire d'Etudes des Acquisitions
et du Développement
Dijon, France

OLIVIER DESPRÉS

Centre d'Etudes de Physiologie Appliquée
CNRS - Université Louis Pasteur

CHRISTIAN SCHEIBER

Institut de Physique Biologique
CNRS, Strasbourg, France

CHRISTEL ROBERT

Laboratoire de Psychologie Expérimentale
Université Pierre Mendes France, Grenoble

Summary.—We measured brain activation during the perception of fingerspelled letters, printed letters, and abstract shapes (control condition) in six congenitally, profoundly deaf signers and six normal hearing subjects. Normal hearing subjects showed essentially extrastriate activation in the fingerspelled letters and printed letters conditions whereas deaf subjects showed activation of a broader network in printed letters and fingerspelled conditions, comprising supplementary frontal and posterior areas, and the supramarginal gyrus (Brodmann Area 6). These results suggest that, on one hand, different cerebral areas in deaf and hearing subjects mediate processing of printed letters and, on the other hand, common cerebral areas are activated in deaf signers when they are engaged in processing fingerspelled or printed letters.

Sign language is the primary visual-gestural language of the deaf community and is acquired as a native language by children of deaf parents. Those who use sign language as a primary means of communication also use fingerspelling for concepts that lack a sign. Fingerspelling a word involves the rapid execution of a sequence of hand configurations, one for each letter of the word being represented. In deaf families young deaf children are exposed at an early age to fingerspelling used by their parents and older siblings and begin to fingerspell themselves long before they are able to read and write, and even before they are aware of the correspondence between fingerspelling and print. Unlike sign language, a natural language historically and structurally unrelated to spoken or printed language, French fingerspell-

---

[1]We are grateful to all deaf and hearing subjects for their participation. Special thanks are extended to Albert Tabao, manager of the school of French Sign Language in Strasbourg, and to Christel Feig, sign language instructor.
[2]Address enquiries to A. Dufour, Centre d'Etudes de Physiologie Appliquée, CNRS–Université Louis Pasteur, 12 rue Goethe - 6700 Strasbourg, France or e-mail (andre.dufour@c-strasbourg.fr).

ing is composed of 26 distinct hand displays, one for each letter of the alphabet.

Fingerspelling is not a representation of spoken language. It does not encode phonological alternations found in language, e.g., vowel alternations; nor does it encode the various tiers that construct the spoken signal: tone, pitch, stress (word or phrase). Although fingerspelling has a one-to-one correspondence with each letter of the alphabet, it is not an identical representation of print, since the nature of the activity—executing the hand signals in sequence—disallows the scanning capacity of the reader of the printed page. Some of the system's internal features do not appear in print, e.g., the execution of certain clusters of fingerspelled hand configurations take on characteristic global movements so they are identifiable independently of the units composing the cluster. As opposed to printed letters, fingerspelling is a dynamic, i.e., a changing-state, representation of the graphic form of a spoken language (Wilcox, 1992).

Previous studies using imaging techniques have shown activation of language-specific areas in deaf signers while perceiving or producing signed language (Bavelier, Corina, Jezzard, Clark, Karni, Lalwani, Rauschecker, Braun, Turner, & Neville, 1998; Hickok, Bellugi, & Klima, 1998a, 1998b; Neville, Bavelier, Corina, Rauschecker, Karni, Lalwani, Braun, Clark, Jezzard, & Turner, 1998; Nishimura, Hashikawa, Doi, Iwaki, Watanabe, Kusuoka, & Kubo, 1999; Petitto, Zatorre, Gauna, Nikelski, Dostie, & Evans, 2000). However, neuronal circuits involved in fingerspelling processing cannot be predicted from cerebral activation observed while processing signed language. In terms of structure, fingerspelling differs from signing in a number of ways. Hence, to express a word, sign language uses one, or at most two, distinct hand configurations, but a fingerspelled word has as many separate configurations as there are letters in the word. Moreover, the space of articulation for a sign extends from the top of the head to the waist and well out from the sides of the body, but fingerspelling is strictly confined to a small region in front of the fingerspeller's body. In addition, while the orientation of the palm relative to the body in a sign can vary from facing upward, downward, to the sides, fingerspelling orientation is limited: the palm must face outward from the speller's body. Hsu (1979) cautioned that we should not think of fingerspelling as equivalent to speech; it is purely a representation of orthography and does not encode any more information than print. It is therefore a medium for transmitting linguistic information (Savage, Evans, & Savage, 1981; Quigley & Paul, 1984).

While movement is an important component of the processing of fingerspelling as well as signing, it has been shown that fingerspelling and signing can be differentially disrupted (Kegl, Gilmore, Lionard, Bowers, Fennell, Roper, Trowbridge, Poizner, & Heilman, 1996). These authors reported study of a deaf signer undergoing intraoperative cortical stimulation prior to brain surgery. They found separate localizations for the production of fingerspelling and signing. At a site wherein disruption of fingerspelling occurred, speech and signing might persist, while at another site signing could be interrupted, with sparing of speech and fingerspelling. Finally, although learning of individual fingerspelled letters may be acquired in less than one hour (Sutcliffe, 1981), this ease is misleading. Not only does their use in communication require considerable speed and fluency, but also observation of experienced users belies the description that they are spelling with their fingers. Rather their productions are continuous, the finger positions for words forming what Akamatsu (1985) described as 'visual envelopes'. In production, letters run together to create patterns, which signify letter sequences or words, and, in reception, it is these patterns that the proficient user must detect. The most striking demonstration of this 'whole word' approach is in cases where children use fingerspelling before acquiring the reading and spelling skills necessary to use the 'letter by letter' approach (Maxwell, 1998). These illustrate the nature of the proficient use of fingerspelling and suggest that its acquisition may be achieved without resort to a stage at which words are translated letter by letter into a finger position. As a consequence, it may be hypothesized that processes involved in reading of fingerspelled letters involve a different cerebral circuit than those involved in printed letters or sign language reading.

This study examined whether processing of fingerspelled or printed letters is mediated by the same cerebral organization in congenitally, profoundly deaf signers. Using high-field (2 Tesla) functional resonance imaging (fMRI), we measured brain activation during the presentation of fingerspelled letters, printed letters, and abstract shapes (control condition) in six congenitally, profoundly deaf French signers and six subjects with normal hearing. We assumed that normal hearing subjects would process fingerspelled letters like a series of representations of familiar objects (a hand under different meaningless configurations). Deaf subjects should process fingerspelled letters as visual items that can be decoded as meaningful components of language and can be given a similar status as that of letters in normal hearing people. So, we expected that fingerspelled letters would lead to the activation of different cerebral areas in deaf than in hearing subjects. According to previous imaging studies (Pugh, Shaywitz, Shaywitz, Constable, Skudlarski, Fulbright, Bronen, Shankweiler, Katz, Fletcher, & Gore, 1996; Binder, Frost, Hammeke, Cox, Rao, & Prieto, 1997; Sugio, Inui, Matsuo, Matsuzawa, Glover, & Nakai, 1999), areas generally associated with auditory or phonological processes are not activated when hearing people read single printed letters. So we did not expect to observe distinct patterns of cerebral activation in hearing and deaf subjects when they read printed letters.

Method

Subjects.—The subjects were six right-handed congenitally, profoundly deaf signers (three males and three females ages 22 to 38 years; $M=27$ yr.) and six normal-hearing right-handed volunteers (three males and three females ages 25 to 35 years; $M=29$). The mean hearing loss reported by deaf participants was 115 dB hearing loss (range 105–119 dB hearing loss). All deaf participants had hearing parents. All deaf signers were recruited from a local association in Strasbourg. All had participated in the same educational program, which ensured that they had similar language skills. All were native signers and were selected for their good French reading and writing. The hearing subjects were not familiar with the signed alphabet. All participants gave written informed consent in accordance with the Declaration of Helsinki.

Experimental design/stimulus material.—Before scanning, subjects were presented examples of the visual stimuli (fingerspelled letters from the French Sign Language alphabet, printed letters or abstract shapes, see Fig. 1 for examples) and were told to watch them carefully during the experiment to perform a recognition test at the end of the session. During scanning subjects passed four repetitions of one block of four experimental conditions in a fixed order (ON1, ON2, ON3, and OFF). Subjects were presented, respectively, with static fingerspelled letters in ON1 condition, printed letters in ON2 condition, abstract shapes in ON3 condition, and black screen (no stimulus) in the OFF condition. In this latter condition (rest), subjects were instructed to fixate the white fixation cross and to wait for the next se-

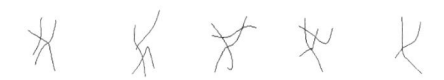

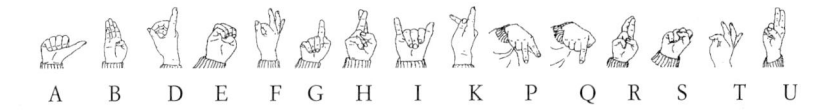

Abstract Shapes

Abstract Shapes

A B C D E F G I J K L P R S U

Abstract Shapes

A B D E F G H I K P Q R S T U

Fig. 1. Examples of abstract shapes, presented printed and fingerspelled letters during the scanning session

quence without doing anything. We chose to subtract the activation measured in each experimental condition (ON1, ON2, and ON3) from the rest condition (OFF) since the processing of printed or fingerspelled letters can not just be thought of as a mere addition of supplementary processing to abstract shape processing (Sartori & Umiltà, 2000). Each condition lasted 50 msec., resulting in the presentation of 100 stimuli per condition for the all-scanning session.

All three kinds of stimuli were presented through a fiber optic device (Avotec, Jensen Beach, Florida, USA) at a rate of 2 items/sec. which is the average production rate of deaf signers (Reed, Delhorne, & Durlach, 1990). See Fig. 1 for a list of presented fingerspelled and printed letters. Hearing subjects were not told that hand shapes corresponded to letters to avoid their guessing the corresponding letter.

MR Analysis

A Bruker (Karlsruhe, Germany) 2.0-T system equipped with a 30mT · m^{-1} gradient coil set for echo planar imaging (EPI) was used to perform the study. Ten image volumes were acquired for each condition presented in the following sequence: Fingerspelled Letters (ON1), Printed Letters (ON2), Abstract Shapes (ON3), and rest condition (OFF). Four successive blocks of these four conditions (ON1-ON2-ON3-OFF) were passed during the scanning session, resulting in 200 scans in total. At the end of each condition, the subject was instructed visually about the next sequence of stimuli that were to be presented (see behavioral tests, described below).

The paradigm was triggered by the MRI system that ran continuously during the experimental phase. The acquisition consisted of 32 transaxial gradient-echo planar (GE-EPI) 64 × 64 brain isotropic (4-mm) slices, so-called volume and was repeated each 5000 msec. (repetition time). Before statistical analysis, preprocessing of the images was performed (realignment, normalization, and smoothing) according to the procedures proposed by Friston, Ashburner, Frith, Poline, Heather, and Frackowiak (1995), Friston, Holmes, Worsley, Poline, Frith, and Frackowiak (1995), and as implemented in the Statistical Parametric Mapping (SPM99) software (Welcome Department of Cognitive Neurology) (Friston, Ashburner, Frith, Poline, Heather, & Frackowiak, 1995; Friston, Holmes, Worsley, Poline, Frith, & Frackowiak, 1995). Realignment of the fMRI series to the first image volume decreased the deleterious effect of head motion during the acquisition procedure on the massively parallel single voxel statistical data analysis. After correction, the center of mass coordinates were within ±0.6 mm for each of the experimental time series. Spatial transformation was computed between an EPI subject reference volume and an EPI template in a standard system coordinates (Montreal Neurological Institute template) and applied to the data series. During this procedure the data were interpolated to 128 × 128 (2-mm theoretical voxel size). The data were smoothed using a 4-mm full width at half maximum kernel to improve signal-to-noise ratio and to approximate normal distribution of the data.

Statistical analysis was performed. The single condition paradigm (two tasks) was modeled using delayed (5 sec.) boxcar hemodynamic model function in the context of the general linear model (Friston, Ashburner, Frith, Poline, Heather, & Frackowiak, 1995; Friston, Holmes, Worsley, Poline, Frith, & Frackowiak, 1995), resulting in a t statistic for each and every voxel. These t statistics were transformed to z statistics. Voxels that met the statistical criteria of significance ($p < .01$, one-tailed), corrected for multiple comparisons, constitute a statistical parametric map. These images were interpreted by referring to the probabilistic behavior of a Gaussian field. Data were analyzed, and reproducibility was confirmed for each subject individually. Anatomical identification of activated areas was performed individually by mapping areas onto the subject's own anatomical normalized (T1) images (T1 images on T1 template). Following individual anatomical identification of activated areas for each subject, the activated areas were mapped onto the best-fitted area of the normalized template T1 image in the Talairach reference coordinate system (Talairach & Tournoux, 1988).

Behavioral tests.—At the end of each session, subjects were asked recognition (yes/no) questions on the printed letters, fingerspelled letters, and the abstract shapes to ensure attention to the experimental stimuli (see Table 1). Subjects indicated to the experimenter whether those had appeared during the run or not. Half of the test stimuli had appeared before, and half were new.

Results

Behavioral Test

The behavioral data (reported in Table 1) indicated that subjects were attending to the stimuli. Both groups performed equally well in remembering abstract shapes (ns, $\delta = 0.32$, $1 - \beta = 0.04$ for $\alpha = .05$). In both groups performance is at chance. This indicates that abstract shapes were too complicated to be encoded as meaningful objects. Hearing subjects were signifi-

TABLE 1
Behavioral Data For Hearing and Deaf Subjects

Recognition Task	Hearing		Deaf	
	% Correct	Hits/False Alarms	% Correct	Hits/False Alarms
Fingerspelled letters	0.78	0.50/0.22	0.79	0.40/0.09
Printed letters	0.96	0.49/0.03	0.81	0.43/0.12
Abstract shapes	0.56	0.36/0.30	0.54	0.34/0.30

cantly better at recognizing printed letters than fingerspelled letters ($p < .05$, $\delta = 2.92$, $1 - \beta = 0.69$, Newman-Keuls *post hoc* comparison), deaf subjects performed equally well in remembering both the fingerspelled and the printed letters (ns, $\delta = 0.48$, $1 - \beta = 0.07$ for $\alpha = .05$). Both groups perform equally well in the fingerspelled condition when only considering percentage of correct responses (ns, $\delta = 0.24$, $1 - \beta = 0.045$ for $\alpha = .05$). However, results show that false alarm rate is significantly higher in hearing subjects than in deaf subjects ($p < .05$, $\delta = 2.45$, $1 - \beta = 0.58$, Newman-Keuls *post hoc* comparison). This suggests that deaf subjects were better than hearing subjects at rejecting the fingerspelled letters that were not shown during the experimental session. The opposite tendency can be observed with printed letters where hearing subjects show lower false alarm rates than deaf subjects (ns, $\delta = 1.47$, $1 - \beta = 0.30$ for $\alpha = .05$). These results suggest that the recall strategy consisted of trying to identify those stimuli subjects had not seen during the experimental session rather than trying to recognize those that they had actually seen.

NeuroImaging Data

Comparisons of the visual stimuli fingerspelled letters, printed letter, and abstract shapes with the rest condition produced significant increases in the blood oxygen level dependent (BOLD) signal. Cortical areas, which had statistically significant activations ($p < .01$) as contrasted against the rest condition, are described in Tables 2 through 4. To test differences between the presentation conditions for each group we conducted an additional conjunction analysis between subjects in a fixed effect model (Friston, Ashburner, Frith, Poline, Heather, & Frackowiak, 1995; Friston, Holmes, Worsley, Poline, Frith, & Frackowiak, 1995) using a significance threshold for active voxels of $p = .05$.

Abstract Shapes

While seeing abstract shapes, both hearing and deaf subjects displayed

TABLE 2
Significant Activation Foci Obtained in Individual Subject Analysis of Abstract Shapes Processing According to the Talairach and Tournoux Atlas

Cerebral Region	Right/Left	Brodmann Area	No. of Deaf Subjects ($n = 6$)	No. of Hearing Subjects ($n = 6$)
Inferior Occipital Gyrus	R/L	18	6	6
Middle Occipital Gyrus	R/L	18-19	6	6
Fusiform Gyrus	R/L	19-37	4	5
Lingual Gyrus	R/L	18	2	1
Precuneus	R/L	19	3	4
Cuneus	R/L	18	3	2

activation within visual extrastriate areas, including inferior and middle occipital gyri (BA 18, 19), the fusiform and lingual gyri (BA 18, 19, 37), the precuneus and cuneus (BA 18, 19) (see Table 2).

Fingerspelled Letters

When seeing fingerspelled letters, hearing subjects displayed activation of the same areas observed in the abstract shape condition. Additionally, the inferior temporal gyrus was active in four of the six hearing subjects. Given that our hearing subjects were not familiar with sign language, perception of fingerspelled letters could be considered as a mere object recognition task. For instance, the object to be recognized is a noncanonical view of a hand.

In addition to the activated areas observed in hearing subjects, deaf subjects displayed activation of the inferior and superior parietal lobule (BA 7, 40) and of the frontal cortex (inferior, middle, and superior gyri) on both hemispheres. Activation also involved the precentral gyrus (BA 4, 6) (see Table 3). These areas are generally activated when familiar or meaningful visual items are presented.

TABLE 3
SIGNIFICANT ACTIVATION FOCI OBTAINED IN INDIVIDUAL SUBJECT ANALYSIS OF FINGERSPELLED LETTERS PROCESSING ACCORDING TO TALAIRACH AND TOURNOUX ATLAS

Cerebral Region	Right/Left	Brodmann Area	No. of Deaf Subjects ($n=6$)	No. of Hearing Subjects ($n=6$)
Inferior Occipital Gyrus	R/L	18	6	6
Middle Occipital Gyrus	R/L	18-19	6	6
Fusiform Gyrus	R/L	19-37	2	3
Lingual Gyrus	R/L	18	3	2
Precuneus	R/L	19	4	3
Cuneus	R/L	18-19	3	3
Inferior Temporal Gyrus	R/L	19-37	6	3
Inferior Parietal Lobule	R/L	40	6	
Superior Parietal Lobule	L	7	6	
Precentral Gyrus	R/L	4-6	6	
Inferior Frontal Gyrus	R	44	4	
Middle Frontal Gyrus	R/L	9-10	5	
Superior Frontal Gyrus	R/L	9-10	4	

Printed Letters

In the printed letter condition hearing subjects displayed a similar pattern of activation as in the fingerspelling condition (see Table 4). Activation of the extrastriate cortex in hearing subjects is in agreement with recent studies, suggesting that these areas are involved in letter processing (Pugh, *et al.*, 1996; Polk & Farah, 1998; Pugh, Mencl, Jenner, Katz, Frost, Lee, Shaywitz, & Shaywitz, 2000). Involvement of the inferior temporal gyrus has

TABLE 4
SIGNIFICANT ACTIVATION FOCI OBTAINED IN INDIVIDUAL SUBJECT ANALYSIS OF PRINTED LETTERS PROCESSING ACCORDING TO TALAIRACH AND TOURNOUX ATLAS

Cerebral Region	Right/Left	Brodmann Area	No. of Deaf Subjects ($n=6$)	No. of Hearing Subjects ($n=6$)
Inferior Occipital Gyrus	R/L	18	6	6
Middle Occipital Gyrus	R	18-19	6	6
Lingual Gyrus	R	18	3	3
Fusiform Gyrus	L	19-37	3	2
Inferior Parietal Lobule	L	40	2	1
Precuneus	R	19-7	3	2
Inferior Temporal Gyrus	R/L	19-37	4	3
Inferior Frontal Gyrus	R	44	2	
Middle Frontal Gyrus	R	10	1	
Middle Frontal Gyrus	L	9-10-11	2	
Superior Frontal Gyrus	R/L	9-10	5	
Precentral Gyrus	R/L	4-6	6	

been observed in previous fMRI studies of language areas (Binder, et al., 1997).

Deaf subjects displayed a similar pattern of activation as in the fingerspelling condition. Most notable was the bilateral activation of the precentral gyrus (BA 4, 6) in all six subjects. However, activation of frontal areas, as described above, was less marked since they were observed in only two subjects. This was attested by statistical analysis which showed activation in the inferior and middle frontal gyrus only in the fingerspelled condition.

DISCUSSION

The main aim of this study was to investigate whether processing of fingerspelled or printed letters is mediated by the same cerebral organization in deaf signers. A second point of interest was to compare the brain structures activated when hearing and deaf readers were presented printed letters.

Analysis showed that processing of printed letters was associated with different patterns of cerebral activation in hearing and deaf subjects. Hearing subjects displayed activation of extrastriate areas. This pattern of activation was comparable to those observed in simple object- or letter-recognition tasks (Pugh, et al., 1996; Sugio, et al., 1999). In contrast, deaf subjects showed bilateral activation of frontal areas and, more intensively, of the precentral gyrus (BA 4, 6). These areas have already been reported to be involved in sign language processing in profoundly deaf signers (Bavelier, et al., 1998; Corina, McBurney, Dodrill, Hinshaw, Brinkley, & Ojemann, 1999). More interestingly, deaf subjects displayed a very similar pattern of activation in processing of fingerspelled and printed letters. Especially, deaf subjects displayed bilateral activation of the supramarginal gyrus (BA 4, 6) in both conditions. Additionally, a large cortical region activated by fingerspelled letters involved the inferior and superior parietal lobules. Activation of posterior frontal regions (BA 6, mouth and face premotor regions), in both the fingerspelled and printed letter conditions, is consistent with a recent fMRI study (Bavelier, et al., 1998). These authors evoked semantic-phonological errors when these regions were stimulated in a deaf signer. As suggested by the authors, the supramarginal gyrus may play a critical role in the selection of phonological feature information and in the association of such information with semantic representations in the service of language production. Although participants were explicitly asked not to talk during the scanning session, it is possible that they silently repeated each stimulus to facilitate its memorization. This could explain why these areas were activated since it is quite frequently observed in brain-imaging studies that imagining or producing activates the same areas.

Previous cerebral imaging and cortical mapping studies on sign language comprehension or production have essentially focused on sentence processing in both native and late signers (Bavelier, et al., 1998; Hickok, et al., 1998a, 1998b; Nishimura, et al., 1999; Petitto, et al., 2000). While classical language areas within the left hemisphere were activated by both in English and in American Sign Language, American Sign Language strongly activated right hemisphere structures. This was true irrespective of whether the native signers were deaf or hearing (Bavelier, et al., 1998; Corina, et al., 1999). In the present study, we found no predominance of either hemisphere in the activations when processing fingerspelled letters. Nor did we find in either groups differences in the areas activated in fingerspelled letters and printed letters. Two speculations emerge from this observation. On one hand, since no difference in activation is found at a sublexical level (as in our study), activation differences might be present at a lexical level. This argument is supported by magnetic transcortical stimulation in which fingerspelling could be interrupted with sparing speech or signing (Kegl, et al., 1996). On the other hand, it is important to note that the similar patterns of activation observed in deaf subjects do not ensure similar processes in the fingerspelled and printed letter conditions. The observed activation of common sites might simply reflect that deaf subjects automatically translated printed into fingerspelled letters.

Recent findings have shown that brains of deaf individuals are organized differently from those of hearing individuals. For instance, Bavelier, Brozinsky, Tomann, Mitchell, Neville, and Liu (2001) have shown that the lateralization of the medial and medial superior temporal areas was found to shift toward the left hemisphere in early signers, suggesting that early exposure to sign language leads to a greater reliance on the left medial and medial superior temporal areas. Deaf signers also showed enhanced activation of the medial and medial superior temporal areas compared to hearing subjects during peripheral attention, and they displayed increased activation of the posterior parietal cortex. Finally, in deaf signers attention to motion resulted in enhanced activation in the posterior superior temporal sulcus, establishing for the first time in humans that early sensory deprivation can result in different patterns of activation in this polymodal area. Another study carried out by Finney, Fine, and Dobkins (2001) found that deaf subjects, when processing visual stimuli, exhibit activation in a region of the right auditory cortex corresponding to Brodmann's Areas 42 and 22, as well as in Area 41, i.e., the primary auditory cortex. However, it seems unlikely that these differences in cerebral activation between deaf and hearing individuals have any implication in the differences we observed, since they mainly concern low-level and visual-motion processes.

Conclusion

Taken together, our results suggest that, on one hand, different cerebral areas in deaf and hearing subjects are activated when processing printed letters. On the other hand, common cerebral areas are activated in deaf subjects when they are engaged in processing fingerspelled or printed letters. Further evidence will be required to assess whether these common areas underlie similar functions. It has to be noted that we cannot affirm whether the obtained results were exclusively associated with differences in hearing status. Observed differences might also be explained by fingerspelling ability, since deaf signers were only compared with hearing nonsigners and with hearing signers. Studies including hearing signers should be conducted to clarify this point.

REFERENCES

AKAMATSU, C. (1985) Fingerspelling formulae: a word is more or less the sum of its letters. In W. Stokoe & V. Volterra (Eds.), *SLR '83: Proceedings of the 3rd International Symposium on Sign Language Research*. Silver Spring, MD: Linstock Press. Pp. 126-132.

BAVELIER, D., BROZINSKY, C., TOMANN, A., MITCHELL, T., NEVILLE, H., & LIU, G. (2001) Impact of early deafness and early exposure to sign language on the cerebral organization for motion processing. *Journal of Neuroscience*, 21, 8931-8942.

BAVELIER, D., CORINA, D., JEZZARD, P., CLARK, V., KARNI, A., LALWANI, A., RAUSCHECKER, J., BRAUN, A., TURNER, R., & NEVILLE, H. (1998) Hemispheric specialization for English and ASL: left invariance-right variability. *NeuroReport*, 9, 1537-1542.

BINDER, J., FROST, J., HAMMEKE, T., COX, R., RAO, S., & PRIETO, T. (1997) Human brain language areas identified by functional magnetic resonance imaging. *Journal of Neuroscience*, 17, 353-362.

CORINA, D., MCBURNEY, S., DODRILL, C., HINSHAW, K., BRINKLEY, J., & OJEMANN, G. (1999) Functional roles of Broca's area and SMG: evidence from cortical stimulation mapping in a deaf signer. *Neuroimage*, 10, 570-581.

FINNEY, E., FINE, I., & DOBKINS, K. (2001) Visual stimuli activate auditory cortex in the deaf. *Nature Neuroscience*, 4, 1171-1173.

FRISTON, K., ASHBURNER, J., FRITH, C., POLINE, J., HEATHER, J., & FRACKOWIAK, R. S. J. (1995) Spatial registration and normalization of images. *Human Brain Mapping*, 2, 165-189.

FRISTON, K., HOLMES, A., WORSLEY, K., POLINE, J., FRITH, C., & FRACKOWIAK, R. (1995) Statisti-

cal parametric maps in functional imaging: a general linear approach. *Human Brain Mapping*, 2, 189-210.
HICKOK, G., BELLUGI, U., & KLIMA, E. (1998a) The neuronal organization of language: evidence from sign language aphasia. *Trends in Cognitive Science*, 2, 129-136.
HICKOK, G., BELLUGI, U., & KLIMA, E. (1998b) What's right about the neural organization of sign language? A perspective on recent neuroimaging results. *Trends in Cognitive Science*, 2, 465-468.
HSU, C. (1979) Six years of observation of Visible English at Louisiana State School for the Deaf. *Teaching English to Deaf*, 6, 27-34.
KEGL, J., GILMORE, R., LIONARD, C., BOWERS, D., FENNELL, E., ROPER, S., TROWBRIDGE, P., POIZNER, H., & HEILMAN, K. (1996) Lateralization and intrahemispheric localization studies of a familially left-handed, deaf, epileptic signer of American Sign Language. *Brain and Cognition*, 32, 335-338.
MAXWELL, M. (1998) The alphabetic principle and fingerspelling. *Sign Language Studies*, 61, 377-404.
NEVILLE, H., BAVELIER, D., CORINA, D., RAUSCHECKER, J., KARNI, A., LALWANI, A., BRAUN, A., CLARK, V., JEZZARD, P., & TURNER, R. (1998) Cerebral organization for language in deaf and hearing subjects: biological constraints and effects of experience. *Proceedings of the National Academy of Sciences USA*, 90, 922-929.
NISHIMURA, N., HASHIKAWA, K., DOI, K., IWAKI, T., WATANABE, Y., KUSUOKA, H., & KUBO, T. (1999) Sign language 'heard' in the auditory cortex. *Nature*, 397, 116.
PETITTO, L., ZATORRE, R., GAUNA, K., NIKELSKI, E., DOSTIE, D., & EVANS, A. (2000) Speech-like cerebral activity in profoundly deaf people processing signed language: implications for the neural basis of human language. *Proceedings of the National Academy of Sciences USA*, 97, 13961-13966.
POLK, T., & FARAH, M. (1998) The neural development and organization of letter recognition: evidence from functional neuroimaging computational modeling, and behavioral studies. *Proceedings of the National Academy of Sciences USA*, 95, 847-852.
PUGH, K., MENCL, W., JENNER, A., KATZ, L., FROST, S., LEE, J., SHAYWITZ, S., & SHAYWITZ, B. (2000) Functional neuroimaging studies of reading and reading disability (developmental dyslexia). *Mental Retardation and Disabilities Research Review*, 6, 207-213.
PUGH, K., SHAYWITZ, B., SHAYWITZ, S., CONSTABLE, R., SKUDLARSKI, P., FULBRIGHT, R., BRONEN, R., SHANKWEILER, D., KATZ, L., FLETCHER, J., & GORE, J. C. (1996) Cerebral organization of component processes in reading. *Brain*, 119, 1221-1238.
QUIGLEY, S., & PAUL, P. (1984) *Language and deafness*. San Diego, CA: College-Hill Press.
REED, C., DELHORNE, L., & DURLACH, N. (1990) A study of the tactual and visual reception of fingerspelling. *Journal of Speech and Hearing Research*, 33, 789-797.
SARTORI, G., & UMILTÀ, C. (2000) How to avoid the fallacies of cognitive subtraction in brain imaging. *Brain and Language*, 74, 191-212.
SAVAGE, R., EVANS, L., & SAVAGE, J. (1981) *Psychology and communication in deaf children*. Sydney: Grune & Stratton.
SUGIO, T., INUI, T., MATSUO, K., MATSUZAWA, M., GLOVER, G., & NAKAI, T. (1999) The role of the posterior parietal cortex in human object recognition: a functional magnetic resonance imaging study. *Neuroscience Letters*, 276, 45-48.
SUTCLIFFE, T. (1981) *Sign and say book 1*. London: Royal National Institute of the Deaf.
TALAIRACH, J., & TOURNOUX, P. (1988) *Co-planar stereotaxic atlas of human brain*. New York: Thieme.
WILCOX, S. (1992) *The phonetics of fingerspelling. (Studies in speech pathology and clinical linguistics: 4)* Amsterdam, Philadelphia, PA: Benjamins.

Accepted March 8, 2004.

WEEKLY TREATMENTS WITH A BURST-FIRING MAGNETIC FIELD ALTERS BEHAVIOR IN THE ELEVATED PLUS MAZE AFTER TWO SESSIONS [1]

R. E. FITZPATRICK AND M. A. PERSINGER

Laurentian University

Summary.—In a split-litter design, rats were either injected with 15 mg/kg of clomipramine or saline from postnatal Days 8 through 21. Other rats from the same litters were not injected. When the rats were 90 days of age, the rats were tested once per week for five weeks in an elevated plus maze that contained two open arms (no walls) and two walled arms. Following each test, they were exposed (total of 4 exposures) for 30 min. to a burst-firing magnetic field (1 microTesla) that has been shown to reduce depression in human beings. After two treatments, the rats exposed to the burst-firing fields spent about half the amount of time in the open arms compared to the sham-field exposed rats. The interaction between adult treatment and whether the rats had received the antidepressant before weaning was not significant statistically. These results suggest that at least two weekly sessions may be required before significant changes in behavior occur after weekly 30-min. exposures to these potentially "therapeutic" magnetic fields.

Rats exposed to a weak (1 microTesla) specifically patterned magnetic field for 30 min. after training have shown significantly diminished fear conditioning (McKay, Persinger, & Koren, 2000). This field also potentiated the deficits in contextual fear learning from concurrent administration of agmatine (McKay & Persinger, 2003). We reasoned that sensitivity to other patterned magnetic fields long after administration of a drug such as clomipramine (Prathiba, Kumar, & Karanth, 2000), that permanently altered brain chemistry, would require several exposures. We selected a burst-firing pattern presented once per week because of its utility in treating depression in human patients (Baker-Price & Persinger, 2003).

To examine the validity of our hypothesis, rats in each of five litters from albino Wistar females were injected subcutaneously with a Hamilton microliter syringe with either 15 mg/kg (15 mg/cc) of clomipramine or saline from postnatal Days 8 through weaning (Day 21). Other rats from the same litters were not injected. After weaning, they were housed in same-sex cages until about 90 days of age. Nine rats from each of the three postnatal conditions (drug, saline, not injected) were tested once per week for 5 min. on the same day of the week for five weeks in an elevated plus maze. Equal numbers of rats from each condition were tested Monday through Friday.

The elevated plus maze had four runways positioned at right angles; 50-cm high walls surrounded the arms of one axis, while the orthogonal arms were exposed to open space. The time spent in the middle of the maze, within the closed arms, and within the open arms was recorded for each rat during its 5-min. test once per week. Within 5 min. after the testing in the maze, each rat was placed for 30 min. in a plastic cube cage (1700 cc). Three pairs of solenoids in each plane delivered the burst-firing field. It was presented for 0.5 sec. to each pair of

---

[1]Send correspondence to Dr. M. A. Persinger, Behavioral Neuroscience Laboratory, Department of Psychology, Laurentian University, Sudbury, ON Canada P3E 2C6 or e-mail (mpersinger @laurentian.ca).

solenoids and then to all solenoids simultaneously (McKay, Persinger, & Koren, 2000). The burst-firing magnetic field, whose intensity within the volume of the chamber was about 1 microT, was presented once every 4 sec. Half of the rats from each postnatal condition received the field while the other half did not.

A four-way analysis of variance with one level repeated (weeks) and three between-subject levels (sex, postnatal treatment, adult magnetic field treatment) for the square root transformation of the time spent in the open arms showed a statistically significant interaction ($F_{4,60}=2.74$, $p=.04$; $\eta^2=.16$) between adult treatment and weeks of exposure. The only other statistically significant effects were differences in durations spent within the open arms per week ($F_{4,60}=14.34$, $p<.001$; $\eta^2=.49$). The predicted interaction between postnatal treatment weeks of the adult magnetic field treatment was not significant statistically ($F_{8,60}=.27$, $p>.05$).

The means for the square root of the amount of time in minutes spent in the open arms for the five weeks (first week was baseline, before magnetic field treatment) for the sham-exposed rats were 1.4, .9, .9, .9, and .3, respectively. These values for rats exposed to the burst-firing field were 1.4, 0.7, 0.4, 0.4, and 0.5, respectively. All standard errors of the mean were about 0.1.

These results did not support our hypothesis that early exposures to this antidepressant compound increased the sensitivity of the rats' maze behavior to this particular pattern of magnetic field stimulation. However, the results clearly suggest that at least *two* weekly sessions may be required before any significant behavioral effects from 30-min. exposures to these "therapeutic" treatments are evident.

REFERENCES

BAKER-PRICE, L., & PERSINGER, M. A. (2003) Intermittent burst-firing weak (1 microTesla) magnetic fields reduce psychometric depression in patients who sustained closed head injuries: a replication and electroencephalographic validation. *Perceptual and Motor Skills*, 96, 965-974.

MCKAY, B. E., & PERSINGER, M. A. (2003) Complex magnetic fields potentiate agmatine-mediated contextual fear learning in rats. *Life Sciences*, 72, 2489-2498.

MCKAY, B. E., PERSINGER, M. A., & KOREN, S. A. (2000) Exposure to a theta-burst patterned magnetic field impairs memory acquisition and consolidation for contextual but not discrete conditioned fear in rats. *Neuroscience Letters*, 292, 99-102.

PRATHIBA, J., KUMAR, K. B., & KARANTH, K. S. (2000) Effects of REM sleep deprivation on cholinergic receptor sensitivity and passive avoidance behavior in the clomipramine model of depression. *Brain Research*, 876, 243-245.

Accepted March 23, 2004.

CARRY-OVER EFFECTS OF MUSIC IN AN ISOMETRIC MUSCULAR ENDURANCE TASK [1]

LEE CRUST

Sport Science Department, Lincoln College, UK

Summary.—This study tested the effects of exposure to self-selected motivational music both prior to and during performance of a muscular endurance task. 27 male undergraduate students in sports science completed an isometric weight-holding task on two separate occasions while listening either to self-selected motivational music or white noise. Participants were assigned to one of three groups on the basis of scores on a familiarization trial. The three groups were Prior Exposure, music or white noise played immediately before task commencement; Half Exposure, conditions initiated simultaneously with task commencement but terminated approximately half-way through the trial; and Full Exposure, conditions initiated simultaneously with trial commencement and continuing until voluntary cessation. A two-way mixed-model analysis of variance yielded a significant interaction and a main effect for condition. Participants held the weight suspended significantly longer when listening to music than with white noise. For the interaction, analysis of gain scores indicated participants' performance increased more for exposure to music during the entire session, than for exposure to music prior to the session. These results suggest that exposure to music during muscular endurance trials can yield significantly longer endurance times, but that exposure to music prior to task commencement may not carry over to influence performance.

A significant amount of research supports the proposed ergogenic and psychophysical properties of music (cf. Karageorghis & Terry, 1997). In particular, more consistent findings have been noted when musical tempo is synchronised with the rhythm of continuous physical tasks such as cycling (Anshel & Marisi, 1978; Mertesdorf, 1994). The influence of asynchronous music is much less clear (Karageorghis, Terry, & Lane, 1999). Although some studies have reported longer endurance times and more physical work during progressive maximal tests (Copeland & Franks, 1991; Szabo, Small, & Leigh, 1999) and others increased volume of training (Kodzhaspirov, Zaitsev, & Kosarev, 1988) when exposed to asynchronous music, other studies have found no significant differences (Schwartz, Fernhall, & Plowman, 1990; Dorney, Goh, & Lee, 1992; Pujol & Langenfeld, 1999).

One of the limitations of previous research identified by Karageorghis and Terry (1997) is that little consideration has been given to temporal factors in the methodology. Different approaches have been evident in relation

---

[1]Address correspondence to Lee Crust, Sport Science Department, Lincoln College, Monks Road, Lincoln, LN2 5HQ, United Kingdom or e-mail (lcrust@lincolncollege.ac.uk).

to the point at which exposure to music is begun. Some researchers have exposed participants to music prior to experimental trials but switched off selections at the initiation of the task (Pearce, 1981; Dorney, et al., 1992; Becker, Brett, Chambliss, Crowers, Haring, Marsh, & Montemayor, 1994). In such cases these researchers appear to assume that the effects of musical exposure carry over to influence task performance, presumably by changes in arousal.

Support for this assumption was obtained in a tightly controlled study by Karageorghis, Drew, and Terry (1996). Participants were exposed to stimulating (arousing) music, sedative (calming) music, or white noise prior to performing a single maximal pull on a handgrip dynamometer. Analysis indicated that prior exposure to stimulating music yielded significantly higher grip-strength than either sedative music or white noise. Also, sedative music was associated with significantly lower force than white noise, which appeared to suggest the effects of music on performance were related to changes in arousal.

Becker, et al. (1994) employed music prior to a 2-min. exercise bout on a stationary cycle. Exact details of the task were not given, but it was assumed to be anaerobic in nature (Pujol & Langenfeld, 1999). Analysis showed that exposure to music was associated with performance increases. A logical explanation of these findings is that music promoted increases in arousal that led to greater effort and enhanced performance. The effects of prior exposure to music carried over to influence this task of short duration.

Some researchers have taken a different approach in exposing participants to music as the performance task is initiated (Pujol & Langenfeld, 1999; Szabo, et al., 1999) with exposure continuing until the task is completed. In one such study, Szabo, et al. (1999) manipulated musical tempo using a piece of classical music during progressive cycling to voluntary physical exhaustion. Twenty-four university students completed five experimental trials and were exposed to no music, slow music, fast music, slow to fast music, and fast to slow music. Significantly, more physical work was achieved in the slow to fast condition, when the tempo of music was doubled as participants reached 70% of their maximal heart-rate reserve. The authors suggested that the results were due to music acting as an external focus that distracted participants' attention from sensations of pain and fatigue. Doubling of the tempo was proposed to have produced changes in arousal that led to a temporary external focus sufficient to affect performance.

A key question yet to be assessed by researchers is whether the effects of prior exposure to music can carry over and influence tasks involving characteristics other than maximal strength. Given reported increases in the use of music in applied settings (Bull, Albinson, & Shambrook, 1996), it is important to know whether any beneficial effects are immediate then dissipate, or are longer lasting. Some studies have shown heart-rate increases (suggesting changes in arousal) while listening to music, but no residual effect after the music had ceased (Ellis & Brighouse, 1952; Coutts, 1964). This study manipulated the timing of exposure to music to assess whether changes in arousal or attentional focus were more salient with regards to a short-duration isometric strength-endurance task. It was hypothesised that performance changes would be greatest when music was played during rather than before the endurance-type task.

Method

Participants

Twenty-seven male undergraduate students in sport and exercise science with a mean age of 20.2 yr. ($SD = 1.7$) volunteered to participate in this investigation. Participants signed informed consent forms prior to testing.

Apparatus

A York 2.2-kg sand-filled dumbbell was used for the performance task. Music was delivered via a Sony Walkman (Model No. WM-EX 404) with shaped in-ear headphones. Volume was set and remained at a constant high level during musical exposure. A stopwatch accurate to 1/1000 sec. was used to record performance times.

Musical Selection

Participants self-selected music that conformed to the following restrictions. First, all selections were taken from popular music that had appeared within the top 40 positions of the British Music Charts over the previous two years. Secondly, only selections that possessed a fast tempo (120 beats · min.$^{-1}$) were accepted to conform to previous classifications of motivational music (Karageorghis, et al., 1999). Thirdly, duration of musical selections had to be between 180 and 270 sec. to avoid large differences in exposure times which could threaten internal validity. Fourthly, participants completed a copy of the Brunel Music Rating Inventory (Karageorghis, et al., 1999) to ensure the selected music was sufficiently motivating. This inventory has recently been shown to be a satisfactory measure of the motivational properties of asynchronous music (Karageorghis, et al., 1999; Szabo & Griffiths, 2003). Only selections scoring above the median value of 18.3 on the inventory were deemed appropriate for use in this study. Participants' selections were checked in regard to length and tempo prior to experimentation, and, where necessary, participants were asked to choose more appropriate selections.

Procedure

Prior to the experiment, participants performed the task to control for expectations and to obtain data to ensure groups were matched on level of endurance. For this purpose participants were seated at a desk in a quiet room. A visual demonstration of the task and safety instructions was given to each participant prior to the commencement of the trial. Participants were told to hold the suspended weight for as long as possible. When ready, participants lifted a York 2.2-kg dumbbell with the dominant arm using an overhand grip from the resting position on the desk to a holding position. This position required the participant to maintain a straight arm in front of the body, directly over the desk, i.e., a 90° angle established between arm and torso. Timing began once the holding position had been reached and ceased when the weight could no longer be held out and was returned to the resting position on the desktop.

Following the familiarisation trial, participants were placed into rank order based on weight-holding performance, and assigned to three groups using a matched-group technique. This process was used to ensure that each group was equivalent in regards to weight-holding performance. Two experimental trials were then completed by each group over a 2-wk. testing period with exposure to conditions randomised. The Prior Exposure group ($n=9$) were exposed to white noise (blank audio-cassette tape) or self-selected music immediately prior to initiating the same isometric weight-holding task. The trial began immediately after the Walkman was switched off. The white noise condition lasted for the same duration as the music. Those in the Half Exposure group ($n=9$) were exposed to either white noise or music simultaneously as the task commenced. With this group, exposure to conditions was halted approximately half-way through the trial, based on halving the performance time in the familiarisation trial. The participants completed the trial without white noise or music present. The Full Exposure group ($n=9$) was exposed to music or white noise as the weight reached the holding position and exposure continued throughout the entire duration of the trial.

Participants did not engage in high intensity upper body exercise within 24 hr. or eat within 2 hr. of trials. Each participant was asked to give their maximum effort in attempting to hold out the weight for as long as possible. No timing feedback was given during trials, and participants completed trials at the same time of day on the same day of the week. The time in seconds for each trial was recorded once the participant left the laboratory.

Results

Descriptive statistics showing mean performance times in seconds for groups and conditions can be viewed below in Table 1. Performance data, analysed using a two-way (3 groups × 2 conditions) mixed-model analysis of variance, indicated a significant interaction effect ($F_{2,24}=3.49$, $p<.05$) and a significant main effect for conditions ($F_{1,24}=20.97$, $p<.01$). All trials (prior, half, and full exposure) with music ($M = 102.3$ sec., $SD = 21.1$) were associated with significantly longer endurance times ($p < .01$) than trials with white noise ($M = 95.0$ sec., $SD = 20.2$).

To examine the interaction effects, mean Gain scores were calculated for each group to represent increments above white noise (see Table 1). A simple one-way analysis of variance was conducted on Gain scores which identified significant between group differences ($F_{2,24} = 3.49$, $p < .05$). A *post hoc* Tukey *HSD* test showed that Gain scores were significantly greater with full as opposed to prior exposure to music ($p < .05$). The Half Exposure group did not significantly differ in Gain scores to either Full or Prior Exposure ($p > .05$). The effect size of music was calculated for each group based upon mean differences between exposure to white noise and music. Moderate effects were evident for the Full Exposure group ($ES = 0.6$) and Half Exposure group ($ES = 0.5$) but Prior Exposure to music had little influence ($ES = 0.1$).

TABLE 1
Isometric Weight-holding Performance Times in Seconds by Group and Condition

Condition	Prior Exposure[a] M	SD	Half Exposure[b] M	SD	Full Exposure[c] M	SD
White Noise	96.6	22.7	94.0	17.4	94.4	18.8
Music	98.4	26.6	102.9	14.6	105.9	18.2
Mean Gain Score	1.6[c]	6.4	8.9	11.2	11.6[a]	6.5

Note.—Different superscripts along rows indicate significant differences between pairs of groups ($p < .05$).

Discussion

The results of this investigation support past research evidence which suggested asynchronous music could facilitate increased endurance performance (Copeland & Franks, 1991; Szabo, *et al.*, 1999). However, the fast stimulating popular musical selections used in the present study differed from the classical and soft slow music employed in the previously noted examples (Copeland & Franks, 1991; Szabo, *et al.*, 1999) and provided a more realistic accompaniment for strenuous exercise. In the present research, an attempt was made to match the stimulating music to the difficulty of the task. Also, in contrast to Copeland and Franks (1991) and Szabo, *et al.* (1999), self-selected music rated by the individual as motivational was used, based on responses to the Brunel Music Rating Inventory. This finding further supports the use of this inventory as an appropriate and useful tool in the selection of motivational music.

Furthermore, in examining the location of differences between white noise and music conditions, results seem to suggest that exposure to music during, rather than prior to, the trials had a greater effect. Although research by Karageorghis, *et al*. (1996) showed that stimulating music could be effectively employed before performance to promote increases in static strength, this finding was limited to a single maximal pull on a handgrip dynamometer. Similarly, Becker, *et al*. (1994) suggested that exposure to music before performance could enhance short-duration cycle performance, but the present research does not support this claim. The present findings suggest that the effects of prior exposure to music on subsequent performance may be relatively short-lived.

Differences between the present research and that of Becker, *et al*. (1994) might be related to the nature of experimental tasks. Whereas exposure to music before the task might have stimulated an increase in work rate (pedalling speed), the task employed in the present research involved enduring pain and sustaining effort, in conditions that were not self-paced, and would intuitively appear more suited to dissociation. The findings for exposure to music during trials seemingly offers further support to the supposition of Szabo, *et al*. (1999) that to aid performance in endurance-based activities, music must be sufficiently arousing to cause a temporary attentional shift and divert focus away from sensations of pain and fatigue.

The use of a Half Exposure group in the present study was an attempted reversal of the approach taken by previous researchers. Whereas Szabo, *et al*. (1999) switched tempo as the demands to the task increased to facilitate an attentional shift, the present study switched off the music to determine any significant detrimental effects. Finding significant performance decrements would have supported the theory of attentional shifting, as switching off the music might have expected to cause attention to be directed sharply back to sensory cues concerning pain- and fatigue-related symptoms. However, performance increments rather than decrements were observed, and these were not significantly different for the Prior and Full Exposure groups. The direction of change appears to suggest the existence of a short-term carry-over effect—although this could be due to distraction during the first half of the trial.

One of the potential limitations of the present study was the different durations of selections used in the Prior Exposure group. Although the selections were within the time scales specified in the Method section, absolute differences may have threatened internal validity. As noted by Karageorghis, *et al*. (1996) fading out of the selections might have overcome this issue but at the cost of potentially compromising the personal meaning of selections. As such, in line with Karageorghis, *et al*. (1996), a decision was made not to fade the selections.

The results of this study cast doubt on whether the effects of prior exposure to music carry over into all performance domains. Further research may be designed to assess how long the effects of prior exposure to music last using different duration tasks. In line with Karageorghis and Terry (1997), it is recommended that more consideration be given to the timing of exposure to music and that clear rationales should be forwarded and incorporate matching the type of music and timing of exposure to specific requirements of the task.

REFERENCES

ANSHEL, H. M., & MARISI, D. Q. (1978) Effect of music and rhythm on physical performance. *Research Quarterly*, 49, 109-113.

BECKER, N., BRETT, S., CHAMBLISS, C., CROWERS, K., HARING, P., MARSH, C., & MONTEMAYOR, R. (1994) Mellow and frenetic antecedent music during athletic performance of children, adults and seniors. *Perceptual and Motor Skills*, 79, 1043-1046.

BULL, S. J., ALBINSON, J. G., & SHAMBROOK, C. J. (1996) *The mental game plan: getting psyched for sport*. Eastbourne, UK: Sports Dynamics.

COPELAND, B. L., & FRANKS, B. D. (1991) Effects of types and intensities of background music on treadmill endurance. *The Journal of Sports Medicine and Physical Fitness*, 15, 100-103.

COUTTS, C. (1964) Effects of music on pulse rates and work output of short duration. *Research Quarterly*, 36(1), 17-21.

DORNEY, L., GOH, E. K. M., & LEE, C. (1992) The impact of music and imagery on physical performance and arousal: studies of co-ordination and endurance. *Journal of Sport Behavior*, 15, 21-33.

ELLIS, D. S., & BRIGHOUSE, G. (1952) Effects of music on respiration and heart rate. *American Journal of Psychology*, 65, 39-47.

KARAGEORGHIS, C. I., DREW, K. M., & TERRY, P. C. (1996) Effects of pretest stimulative and sedative music on grip strength. *Perceptual and Motor Skills*, 83, 1347-1352.

KARAGEORGHIS, C. I., & TERRY, P. C. (1997) The psychophysical effects of music in sport and exercise: a review. *Journal of Sport Behavior*, 20, 54-68.

KARAGEORGHIS, C. I., TERRY, P. C., & LANE, A. M. (1999) Development and initial validation of an instrument to assess the motivational qualities of music in exercise and sport: the Brunel Music Rating Inventory. *Journal of Sport Sciences*, 17, 713-724.

KODZHASPIROV, Y. G., ZAITSEV, Y. M., & KOSAREV, S. M. (1988) The application of functional music in the training sessions of weightlifters. *Soviet Sports Review*, 23, 39-42.

MERTESDORF, F. L. (1994) Cycle exercise in time with music. *Perceptual and Motor Skills*, 78, 1123-1141.

PEARCE, K. A. (1981) Effects of different types of music on physical strength. *Perceptual and Motor Skills*, 53, 351-352.

PUJOL, T. J., & LANGENFELD, M. E. (1999) Influence of music on Wingate Anaerobic Test performance. *Perceptual and Motor Skills*, 88, 292-296.

SCHWARTZ, S. E., FERNHALL, B., & PLOWMAN, S. A. (1990) Effects of music on exercise performance. *Journal of Cardiopulmonary Rehabilitation*, 10, 312-316.

SZABO, A., & GRIFFITHS, L. (2003) Evaluation of the motivational quality of music played during exercise in two fitness centres using the Brunel Music Rating Inventory. *Journal of Sport Sciences*, 21, 360.

SZABO, A., SMALL, A., & LEIGH, M. (1999) The effects of slow- and fast-rhythm classical music on progressive cycling to voluntary physical exhaustion. *The Journal of Sports Medicine and Physical Fitness*, 39, 220-225.

Accepted March 22, 2004.

TEST OF AN ALTERNATIVE EXPLANATION FOR EFFECTS OF AROUSAL GRADIENT ON COGNITIVE PERFORMANCE[1]

WILLIAM STANKARD

University of Connecticut

Summary.—A two-dimensional view of arousal was operationalized by controlling gradient and intensity of exercise-induced arousal in a 2 × 2 factorial design with 80 male undergraduates. Significant decrement in cognitive performance on a visual-search task occurred at a moderate arousal intensity in the steep-gradient arousal conditions. The rate at which arousal increased, not intensity of arousal, led to decrement in performance. This successful replication also eliminated the alternative explanation that increased movement and exertion caused decrement in performance. Analysis indicated no significant correlations between participants' affect and performance.

The present study replicated the third of three experiments conducted to investigate the relationship between arousal gradient and performance (Stankard, 1990) and tested an alternative explanation for previous findings. The prior experiments controlled gradient and intensity of exercise-induced arousal and resulted in significant decrement in cognitive performance on a visual-search task at moderate intensities of arousal during or shortly after steep-gradient increases in arousal. These results could not have been predicted by theories in which arousal is viewed as unidimensional. For example, the inverted-U hypothesis states that moderate arousal contributes to optimal performance and extreme arousal results in poor performance (Yerkes & Dodson, 1908; Duffy, 1957; Malmo, 1957). Cue utilization theory (Easterbrook, 1959) suggests that arousal influences the attentional processes required to perform cognitive and motor tasks. During moderate arousal, attention will be narrowed and focused on task-relevant cues, and performance will be optimal. Additional arousal causes further attentional narrowing, so that some relevant cues are not processed and performance deteriorates. Drive-theory predicts a linear function in which high arousal leads to optimal performance of well-learned tasks (Spence & Spence, 1966).

The aforementioned hypotheses operationally define and measure arousal as a scalar quantity, varying only in intensity. Arousal, however, always occurs with a potentially calculable rate of change, yet few psychologists have suggested that arousal gradient may significantly affect performance. Most of the investigations that have reported arousal gradient data are studies of the startle response (Landis & Hunt, 1939). This response is a brief,

---

[1]Send correspondence to William Stankard, Department of Psychology, Dickinson State University, 291 Campus Drive, Box 108, Dickinson, ND 58601.

involuntary, general body flexion, accompanied by an eyeblink. It occurs in response to sufficiently sudden and intense stimulation, such as a gunshot or a flash of bright light. Tomkins (1962) attributed the startle response to a critical rate of increase in the density of neural firing and asserted that the response and subsequent recovery interrupt the execution of skilled performances. Many early studies of the startle response have been successfully replicated and clearly demonstrated a relation between steep-gradient increases in arousal and the disruption of ongoing activity (Ekman, Friesen, & Simmons, 1985).

In the present study and in the experiment it replicated, variable-workload exercise protocols were employed to ensure that all participants, regardless of fitness, were at the same arousal intensity within a designated period of time prior to the presentation of a visual-search performance task. When an exercise stimulus is standardized, arousal will vary with the fitness of the participant. To standardize an arousal response to exercise, the exercise stimulus must be varied to accommodate the fitness of the participant. The reasoning behind the state-standardization approach is that all participants within conditions must be brought to the same state through manipulation of the independent variable to demonstrate that experimental control has been established and to contribute to the external validity of the laboratory experiment (Aronson & Carlsmith, 1968). The inherent pitfall of the state-standardization design is that radical differences in the arousal-stimulus parameters (exercise) can constitute an alternative explanation for significant differences in the dependent variable (performance). Depending on the condition to which they were assigned, some participants experienced much greater movement and exertion than others in the 30-sec. period prior to presentation of the performance task. An alternative explanation for the performance scores would be that participants in steep-gradient conditions performed poorly because movement and exertion demands were increased.

In the present study, one-half of the participants were required to cease all movement and exertion just prior to the presentation of the performance task. Stimuli that elicit the startle response are not usually present during response and subsequent recovery. The continuous presence of the exercise stimulus may not be necessary for an effect of arousal gradient upon performance to occur. Removal of the arousal-initiating stimulus allows evaluation of whether increased movement and exertion constitute an alternative explanation for significant differences in performance between conditions. A significant main effect of gradient upon performance was predicted.

Method

Participants

Voluntary informed consent was obtained from 80 male undergraduates enrolled in introductory psychology classes at the University of Connecticut. Participants received credit toward the course grade. Their average age was 20 yr. A medical history questionnaire was completed by each participant to identify those for whom moderate exercise was contraindicated. Guidelines of the American College of Sports Medicine (1995) were adhered to.

Apparatus

Equipment included a Tunturi bicycle ergometer, a Kodak Ektagraphic III E slide projector, a Da-Lite projection screen, a Baum blood pressure unit, a Franz electronic metronome, a Tandy microcassette recorder, a Smiths stopwatch, two Lafayette four-bank program timers, a Gerbrands tachistoscope, and a Borg scale of weight in pounds.

Performance Task

This was a visual-search task for which a target stimulus, i.e., red square, was distributed with similar objects in a matrix display. The feature-integration theory of attention (Treisman & Gelade, 1980) states that dimensions such as color and shape are processed automatically and independently of attentional capacity limits (Schiffrin & Schneider, 1977; LaBerge, 1981). However, correct target identification, i.e., blue square, requires the integration of color and shape, and the serial scanning of the other stimuli in the display. The task demands focused attention, of which we have a limited amount to allocate (Schneider & Schiffrin, 1977).

Stimulus Materials

Each of four visual-search performance task slides contained a 25-box matrix. Each box was 3- × 3-in. and contained a red or blue 2- × 2-in. triangle or square. In the center of each colored shape was a black capital letter of the alphabet. The letter Z was not used, and the box in the lower right corner of each matrix contained one letter but no colored shape. On each slide, one colored shape was a designated target. There were nine targets per slide. Targets were randomly assigned positions in the matrices with the provisions that no two could occupy vertically or horizontally adjacent boxes and that each matrix have equal numbers of colors and shapes. For example, the red triangle target slide contained 9 red triangles, 3 red squares, 3 blue triangles, and 9 blue squares. There was one demonstration slide in which colored shapes were not randomly assigned to matrix position.

Slides were presented to each participant with the explanation that the experimenter would designate a target stimulus, i.e., red triangle, a slide would be presented, and the participant must try to recall as many of the letters corresponding to the target stimulus as he could. Participants were told to respond verbally immediately after the screen went blank. The experimenter used the verbal prompt "go" immediately after the screen went blank. Each slide was presented for 2 sec., followed by a 3-sec. verbal response period.

Each of the four slides of the affect-rating scale was rated 1 to 7, using anchors of 1: positive affect and 7: negative affect. Each scale contained a different bipolar adjective combination: pleasant–unpleasant, relieved–anxious, calm–aggitated, and energized–fatigued. There was one demonstration slide which contained all four bipolar scales.

Slides were presented to each participant with the explanation that four affect-rating slides would be individually presented. Participants were to respond verbally with the number on the scale which corresponded to their feelings. Participants were told to respond verbally immediately after the screen went blank. The experimenter used the verbal prompt "go" immediately after the screen went blank. The four affect-rating slides were presented, each for 2.5 sec., followed by a 2.5-sec. verbal response period.

Procedure

This replication was a 2 × 2 factorial design in which participants were randomly assigned to one of four conditions reflecting two levels of arousal gradient (30 sec. and 120 sec. to target heart rate) and two levels of movement (pedalling and stationary). Pretest and test scores were recorded for each of five dependent variables (one performance variable and four affect-rating variables).

Each participant's age, weight, resting heart rate, and blood pressure were recorded. A target heart rate was calculated for each participant, using 60% of his functional heart-rate capacity measured from resting rate to a maximum of 220 bpm minus the participant's age. For example, a 20-yr.-old participant with a resting heart rate of 70 bpm would have a functional heart-rate range of 130 bpm. Of this range, 60% (78 bpm) would be added to the participant's resting heart rate (70 bpm) to obtain the target heart rate (148 bpm) at which the visual-search performance task and the affect-rating scales would be presented. The bicycle ergometer was adjusted for each participant so that there was a 15° bend at the knees when the feet were at the lowest point of the pedal stroke. The cardiotachometer belt was attached around the participant's chest, with the electrodes centered just below the pectoral muscles. The cardiotachometer receiver was attached around the participant's right wrist, out of his view, but within the view of the experimenter. The blood-pressure cuff was wrapped around the participant's right arm. Each participant sat six feet from the projection screen.

Training phase.—This phase consisted of the presentation of the visual-search performance task demonstration slide and the affect-rating demonstration slide. Any questions participants had regarding instructions for successful completion of the performance task and the affect ratings were answered at this time.

Pretest phase.—This phase consisted of the 30-sec. presentation of one target stimulus slide and the four affect-rating slides while each participant sat on the bicycle ergometer but did not exercise.

Test phase.—This phase consisted of the 30-sec. presentation of one target stimulus slide and the four affect-rating slides to all participants, both those who continued to exercise and those who were instructed to stop immediately after they reached their specified target heart rates. Red triangle and red square target slides were counterbalanced across pretest and test presentations.

Exercise protocols.—This design attempted to fix an average target heart rate for a 30-sec. period by varying pedalling resistance in kilopond meters (kpm) while pedalling speed in revolutions per minute (rpm) was fixed at either 50 or 72. Arousal was measured as heart rate (bpm), the primary limiting factor in the delivery of oxygen to working muscles (Noble, 1986). All participants were brought to 40% of their functional heart-rate capacity and stabilized at that level for a 2-min. period prior to the initiation of the arousal gradient protocol to which they were assigned (Fast or Slow). The following protocols were effective in producing the treatment conditions just described (Stankard, 1990):

Initial 40%: One 5-min. workload stage ranging from 300 to 750 kpm, at 50 rpm.

Slow 60%: One 2-min. workload stage ranging from 600 to 1350 kpm, at 50 rpm.

Fast 60%: One 30-sec. workload stage ranging from 900 to 1800 kpm, at 72 rpm.

Participants in the stationary conditions resumed exercise after dependent measures were recorded. Three 2-min. progressive cool-down stages followed the test period. Rpms were reduced to 40 and kpms were reduced by one-third at each stage. Blood pressure was recorded at 2-min. intervals throughout the exercise protocols and the cool-down period. Six 5-sec. heart-rate averages yielded the critical 30-sec. target heart rate during the test period. Thirty-second heart-rate averages were recorded throughout the exercise protocols and the cool-down period. Time to target heart rate and mean heart-rate increase in the 30-sec. period prior to test were calculated.

Results

Five two-way analyses of covariance (pretests as covariates) indicated a significant main effect of gradient upon performance ($F_{1,75} = 8.8$, $p = .004$). There were no significant group differences for the four affect variables. Adjusted group means for all dependent variables are shown in Table 1. There were no significant differences in mean target heart rates between Fast Gradient ($M = 148$, $SD = 6.4$) and Slow Gradient ($M = 148$, $SD = 5.5$) conditions

TABLE 1
ADJUSTED MEANS FOR ALL DEPENDENT VARIABLES

Group		Performance	Pleasant	Relieved	Calm	Energized
Fast Pedalling	M	3.3	3.4	3.7	3.9	3.4
	SD	.8	1.3	1.4	.8	1.2
Fast Stationary	M	3.5	3.1	3.1	3.3	3.1
	SD	.7	1.0	1.2	1.2	1.3
Slow Pedalling	M	3.8	3.7	3.6	3.6	3.3
	SD	.7	1.0	.8	1.0	1.4
Slow Stationary	M	4.0	3.2	3.3	3.4	3.1
	SD	.6	.7	1.1	.7	.8

($t_{78} = -0.36$, ns) at the time the performance task and affect ratings were presented. Mean times to target heart rates were 27.5 sec. ($SD = 5.9$) in the Fast Pedalling condition, 28.6 sec. ($SD = 4.1$) in the Fast Stationary condition, and 120 sec. in the Slow conditions. There were no significant differences in time to target heart rate in the Fast conditions ($t_{38} = -0.66$, ns). There were no significant differences in heart-rate increases during the 30-sec. period prior to testing in the Fast conditions ($t_{38} = -1.08$, ns). Mean heart-rate increases during the 30-sec. period prior to testing are shown in Table 2.

TABLE 2
HEART-RATE INCREASE (BPM) DURING 30-SEC. PERIOD PRIOR TO TEST

Group	M	SD
Fast Pedalling	22.7	4.8
Fast Stationary	24.5	5.4
Slow Pedalling	4.2	2.1
Slow Stationary	3.4	2.6

Using unadjusted test scores, there were no significant correlations between performance and affect for any cell.

DISCUSSION

The variable-workload exercise protocols were successful in bringing all participants to 60% of their functional heart-rate capacity within the designated period of time prior to the presentation of the visual-search performance task and the affect-rating scales. Significant differences in cognitive performance can be attributed to arousal gradient, not intensity of arousal, in this experiment. In addition, removal of the arousal-initiating stimulus just prior to performance in the Stationary conditions did not mitigate the negative effects of steep-gradient arousal on cognitive performance. Analysis indicated that movement and exertion demands did not constitute a viable alternative explanation for significant differences in cognitive performance in this experiment.

Participants appeared to have no conscious awareness of arousal gradient sensations while performing. Participants' affect was not significantly correlated with performance. These results are consistent with previous findings (Stankard, 1990) and Landis and Hunt's speculation (1939) that the human nervous systems may not be organized to discriminate between sensations of gradient and intensity.

The performance means could not have been predicted by theories that operationally define and measure physiological arousal as a scalar quantity, varying only in intensity. The rate at which arousal increased disrupted performance, not arousal intensity. Rather than abandon arousal as a psychological construct (Neiss, 1988), adoption of a two-dimensional view of arousal may lead to more accurate predictions about arousal and performance. Measurement difficulties notwithstanding, laboratory investigations of the arousal-performance relationship might profitably proceed using a controlled-gradient paradigm.

REFERENCES

AMERICAN COLLEGE OF SPORTS MEDICINE. (1995) *ACSM's Guidelines for exercise testing and prescription.* (5th ed.) Baltimore, MD: Williams & Wilkins.

ARONSON, E., & CARLSMITH, J. M. (1968) Experimentation in social psychology. In G. Lindzey & E. Aronson (Eds.), *The handbook of social psychology.* Vol. 2. (2nd ed.) Reading, MA: Addison-Wesley. Pp. 1-79.

DUFFY, E. (1957) The psychological significance of the concept of "arousal" or "activation". *Psychological Review,* 64, 265-275.

EASTERBROOK, J. A. (1959) The effects of emotion on cue utilization and the organization of behavior. *Psychological Review,* 66, 183-201.

EKMAN, P., FRIESEN, W. V., & SIMMONS, R. C. (1985) Is the startle reaction an emotion? *Journal of Personality and Social Psychology,* 49, 1416-1426.

LABERGE, D. (1981) Automatic information processing: a review. In J. Long & A. Baddeley (Eds.), *Attention and performance: IX.* Hillsdale, NJ: Erlbaum. Pp. 173-186.

LANDIS, C., & HUNT, W. A. (1939) *The startle pattern.* New York: Farrar & Rinehart.

MALMO, R. (1957) Anxiety and behavioral arousal. *Psychological Review,* 64, 367-386.

NEISS, R. (1988) Reconceptualizing arousal: psychobiological states in motor performance. *Psychological Bulletin,* 103, 345-366.

NOBLE, B. J. (1986) *Physiology of exercise and sport.* St. Louis, MO: Times Mirror/Mosby College Publ.

SCHIFFRIN, R. M., & SCHNEIDER, W. (1977) Controlled and automatic information processing: II. Perceptual learning, automatic attending, and a general theory. *Psychological Review,* 84, 127-190.

SCHNEIDER, W., & SCHIFFRIN, R. M. (1977) Controlled and automatic information processing: I. Detection, search, and attention. *Psychological Review,* 84, 1-63.

SPENCE, J. T., & SPENCE, K. W. (1966) The motivational components of manifest anxiety: drive and drive stimuli. In C. D. Spielberger (Ed.), *Anxiety and behavior.* New York: Academic Press. Pp. 291-326.

STANKARD, W. (1990) Arousal gradient and performance. *Perceptual and Motor Skills,* 71, 935-946.

TOMKINS, S. S. (1962) *Affect, imagery, consciousness.* Vol. 1. *The positive affects.* New York: Springer.

TREISMAN, A. M., & GELADE, G. (1980) A feature-integration theory of attention. *Cognitive Psychology,* 12, 97-136.

YERKES, R., & DODSON, J. P. (1908) The relation of strength of stimulus to rapidity of habit-formation. *Journal of Comparative Neurology of Psychology,* 18, 459-482.

Accepted March 22, 2004.

SEMANTIC SATIATION EFFECT IN YOUNG AND OLDER ADULTS[1]

MAURA PILOTTI

Dowling College

AYESHA KHURSHID

Mississippi State University

Summary.—Auditory and auditory+visual massed repetition served to examine semantic satiation in young and older adults and to understand the possible sources of this phenomenon. In Exp. 1, participants either heard or heard and saw prime words (ROYALTY) repeated 2, 15, or 30 times and made relatedness judgments on targets that were either semantically related (queen) or unrelated (box) to the repeated word. To distinguish satiation from general boredom, semantic satiation was operationally defined as a repetition-induced change in the difference between related and unrelated pairs (relatedness effect). Auditory massed repetition, either alone or in conjunction with prolonged visual exposure, produced semantic satiation effects in both young and older adults. In Exp. 2, participants heard the prime words of the earlier experiment, each repeated 30 times and reported perceptual changes (verbal transformations) during the repetition treatment. In this experiment, older adults were less susceptible to this type of habituation. The discussion focuses on the mechanisms that may be responsible for producing semantic satiation effects in young and older adults with different forms of massed repetition.

Excessive exposure to a stimulus produces habituation, which is generally conceptualized as a reduction in the responsiveness of the neural structures involved in processing incoming information (Sokolov, 1991; Cowan, 1995). The goal of the present study was to examine a type of habituation phenomenon referred to as semantic satiation. *Semantic satiation* is an attenuation of the meaningfulness of a word that occurs as a result of rapidly repeating a word aloud (Smith & Klein, 1990), reading it silently for a prolonged period of time (Balota & Black, 1997), or simply hearing it spoken over and over (Pilotti, Antrobus, & Duff, 1997; for satiation with other stimuli, see Lewis & Ellis, 2000). Semantic satiation reflects one of the most basic aspects of the efficient processing of linguistic information, which is the ability to minimize the allocation of processing resources to repetitive noninformative stimuli so that these resources can be tuned to information-bearing stimuli (see MacKay, 1990). Behaviorally, semantic satiation manifests itself as a slowing in participants' responses in tasks requiring conscious access to the meaning of the repeated word (see Smith, 1984; Smith & Klein, 1990; Balota & Black, 1997).

Interestingly, while there is no shortage of studies of semantic satiation

---

[1]Address correspondence to M. Pilotti, Department of Psychology, Dowling College, Oakdale, NY 11769-1999 or e-mail (pilottim@dowling.edu).

in young adults (see Esposito & Pelton, 1971; Smith, 1984; Smith & Klein, 1990), relatively little progress has been made in (1) understanding the sources of this habituation-type phenomenon in different perceptual domains and (2) examining whether aging affects one's sensitivity to semantic satiation. With respect to the first issue, the vast majority of the studies in this area of inquiry have used visual+motor vocal repetition (reading a word either aloud or silently for a prolonged period of time) to induce satiation in young adults. The findings of these studies have supported the notion that semantic satiation is a purely semantic phenomenon arising from the habituation of the meaning of a word (Balota & Black, 1997). Of course, the notion of semantic satiation as a purely semantic phenomenon is not surprising in the context of motor vocal repetition, which is known to attenuate habituation at the earlier lexical level of processing (see MacKay, Wulf, Yin, & Abrams, 1993). However, there is reason to believe that this notion would not apply to other forms of massed repetition such as listening to a word spoken over and over. This is because auditory repetition is known not only to produce semantic satiation in young adults (Pilotti, et al., 1997) but also to promote a lexical habituation effect known as verbal transformations (Warren, 1961, 1968; Warren & Warren, 1966). Therefore, it is possible that habituation arising from earlier levels of processing could account for semantic satiation induced by auditory massed repetition. With respect to the second issue, relatively little research has been devoted to the understanding of the effects of aging on semantic satiation. Indeed, only one study (Balota & Black, 1997) has examined semantic satiation in young and older adults, and its findings have provided *prima facie* evidence for the notion that older adults are less susceptible to this habituation effect. Given the different mechanisms that might produce semantic satiation with auditory and visual+motor vocal repetition, it is unclear whether the age-related decline in semantic satiation reported by Balota and Black with visual+motor vocal repetition would generalize to other perceptual domains. Therefore, the main goal of the present study was two-fold: first, to clarify the possible mechanisms underlying auditory-induced semantic satiation in young and older adults, and second, to examine the effects of aging on this phenomenon.

Conceptual Framework

Activation-based models were the conceptual framework to account for semantic satiation in young and (possibly) older adults. In general, these models postulate that word recognition and comprehension occur via the activation of units hierarchically organized into different representational levels, including those symbolizing lexical information (orthographic and phonological knowledge about words and their component units) and those representing semantic information (see Lucas, 2000). In activation models, the presentation of a spoken word produces a pattern of activation across this hierarchical structure, and how much activation of sublexical/lexical units within this structure is determined by the extent to which they match the incoming signal (Elman & McClelland, 1986; McClelland & Elman, 1986; Elman, 1989; MacKay, et al., 1993).

Word recognition is assumed to rely on the level of activation of a particular unit relative to all the other units. Accordingly, a spoken word such as ROYALTY activates its target lexical unit and, to a lesser extent, neighboring units that share with the former some phonological information, e.g., loyalty. The recognition of the word ROYALTY occurs when the amount of activation of the lexical unit which represents this word exceeds those of neighboring units. Similarly, the activation of ROYALTY leads to the activation of the unit representing its meaning and, by spreading of activation, of those units which are semantically similar (see Collins & Loftus, 1975; Anderson, 1976; Neely, 1991; McNamara, 1994). Therefore, the understanding of a word depends on the activation of the semantic representation corresponding to the lexical entry ROYALTY, and it may be facilitated by the prior presentation of semantically related words (QUEEN and DUKE).

In activation models, semantic satiation is conceptualized as a temporary decrement in the amount of activation of the semantic representation that corresponds to the repeated word (MacKay, 1990; MacKay, et al., 1993; Balota & Black, 1997). This decrement in activation of the repeated word is thought to impair not only the processing of its meaning but also its ability to spread activation to related words, and thereby facilitate their processing (Smith, 1984; Balota & Black, 1997; Pilotti, et al., 1997). Thus, the massed repetition of a prime word (ROYALTY) can slow the decision on whether ROYALTY and QUEEN are semantically related.

Within these models, semantic satiation may arise from the repeated activation (habituation) of the meaning of the repeated word, or it may reflect a repetition-induced decrement at the lexical level of processing carried onto the semantic level (see Fig. 1). Which of these two alternative sources of habituation is responsible for producing semantic satiation effects appears to be determined by the type of massed repetition used to induce satiation. Indeed, visual+motor vocal repetition has produced semantic satiation effects in young adults without concurrently inducing habituation of lexical information (Balota & Black, 1997). In contrast, auditory repetition (passively listening to a speaker saying a word repeatedly) has not only produced semantic satiation in young adults (Pilotti, et al., 1997) but also induced a habituation-type effect at the earlier lexical level of processing known as verbal transformations (Warren, 1961, 1968; Warren & Warren, 1966). Verbal transformations are illusory changes that occur as a result of listening to a word repeated over and over. For instance, upon hearing the word ROYALTY repeated over and over, listeners may report perceiving LOYALTY, intermixed with reversals to the veridical percept.

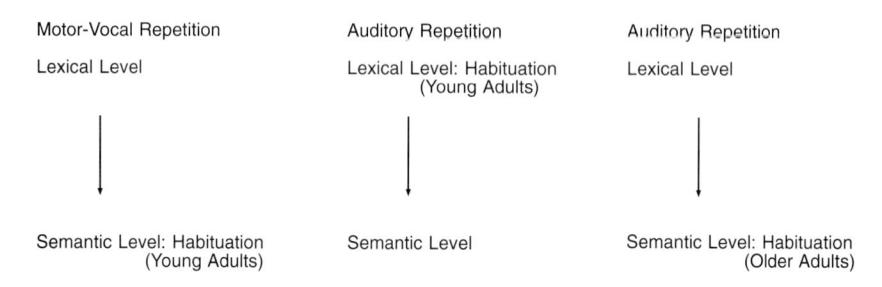

```
Motor-Vocal Repetition        Auditory Repetition           Auditory Repetition

Lexical Level                 Lexical Level: Habituation    Lexical Level
                              (Young Adults)

      |                              |                             |
      ↓                              ↓                             ↓

Semantic Level: Habituation   Semantic Level                Semantic Level: Habituation
(Young Adults)                                              (Older Adults)
```

FIG. 1. Schematic representation of the possible sources of semantic satiation effects as a function of age and modality of repetition

Within activation models, verbal transformations reflect a temporary decrement in the activation of the lexical unit that originally represented the best match for the incoming auditory signal (ROYALTY). This decrement results in other lexical units related to ROYALTY to gain relative strength. In a word-recognition system where activation levels are relative in nature, the most strongly activated unit at a given time becomes the listener's percept. Therefore, listeners who continue to be exposed to the auditory signal originally perceived as ROYALTY now experience auditory illusions, such as "loyalty," "realty," and "specialty." Listeners also experience reversal to the original percept when ROYALTY regains its original strength due either to the habituation of other lexical units or to a weakening of the habituation effect on ROYALTY when these other units become activated.

Interestingly, even though the source of semantic satiation may be different for visual+motor vocal and auditory repetition, the behavioral and neurophysiological correlates of satiation are largely the same at the semantic level. Indeed, with either form of repetition, the prime word ROYALTY can slow the decision on whether ROYALTY and QUEEN are semantically related (Balota & Black, 1997; Pilotti, et al., 1997) and influence the amplitude of an event-related potential, N400, which is a neurophysiological indicator of semantic processing (Kounios, Kotz, & Holcomb, 2000).

Age Differences in Semantic Satiation?

With respect to aging, Warren (1961, 1968), Warren and Warren (1966), and Yin and MacKay (1992) reported that older adults' lexical units are less susceptible to auditory-induced habituation, and Pilotti, Balota, Sommers, and Kurdish (2000) reported that this age-related decline does not result from hearing loss leading to less information being carried to these units from the periphery. Yet, with visual+motor vocal repetition (reading a printed word over and over), Balota and Black (1997) found no evidence of habituation of lexical units in either young or older adults, whereas they uncovered semantic satiation in young but not older adults. These findings led Balota and Black to conclude that semantic satiation effects induced by visual+motor vocal repetition arise from the habituation of semantic units, and that these units in older adults are simply less susceptible to habituation.

Of course, the lack of habituation at the lexical level of processing reported by Balota and Black is not surprising. It is well known that the activation level of lexical units is sustained rather than diminished by motor vocal repetition (see MacKay, et al., 1993). However, whether older adults' semantic units are indeed less susceptible to habituation is not entirely clear. In fact, motor vocal repetition requires the allocation of attentional resources to lexical units to maintain these units in a heightened state of activation during the satiation period. Otherwise the repeated pronunciation of a given word would be difficult, if not impossible. Given the processing capacity limitations generally attributed to aged persons (Craik, 1977), the possibility exists that the allocation of attentional resources to the lexical level of processing might have taken away resources from semantic analyses during the satiation treatment, preventing older adults' semantic units from becoming repeatedly activated and thus satiated. Of course, there is no reason to assume that the allocation of attentional resources to lexical units during the satiation treatment produced similar effects in young adults. As a result, young adults' semantic units would have become repeatedly activated and thus habituated, producing the semantic satiation effects observed in the Balota and Black study.

As noted earlier, auditory repetition as opposed to motor vocal repetition habituates lexical units (at least in young adults) so the question of interest is whether this form of habituation would attenuate or preserve the age differences in semantic satiation observed by Balota and Black with visual+motor vocal repetition. Of course, if older adults' semantic units are less likely to become habituated, the age differences in semantic satiation reported by Balota and Black should generalize to auditory massed repetition. Specifically, auditory massed repetition (listening to a word spoken over and over), as the visual+motor vocal repetition procedure in the Balota and Black study, should yield semantic satiation in young adults but not older persons. However, if satiation units preserve their ability to become habituated with aging, as evidence from a variety of techniques reporting no declines in semantic processing for aged persons would lead us to believe (see Salthouse, 1982), a different pattern of results should be expected with auditory repetition. Specifically, because auditory massed repetition is less likely to induce habituation of lexical information in older adults, the lexical unit that corresponds to the repeated word would remain activated for a longer period of time in aged persons than in young adults. As a result, the matching semantic unit would have more chances to be repeatedly activated and so habituated. In young adults, however, the lexical unit that corresponds to the repeated word would be habituated, i.e., not be available, for a longer period of time than in aged persons. Thus, the temporary inability of this unit to spread activation to its corresponding semantic representation would produce semantic satiation effects in young adults.

Of course, according to this interpretation of repetition-induced effects in the auditory domain illustrated in Fig. 1, auditory repetition, albeit in a different manner, would produce semantic satiation effects in both young and older adults. That is, young adults would be slower in deciding whether ROYALTY and QUEEN are semantically related following 30 repetitions of ROYALTY as compared to 2 repetitions because the habituation of the lexical unit that corresponds to ROYALTY impairs the activation of its semantic representation. Older adults would also be slower in making the same decision, but because the semantic representation activated by ROYALTY is habituated.

Should auditory massed repetition produce either pattern of results, an interesting question arises regarding the role of prolonged visual exposure above and beyond that of auditory repetition. As discussed earlier, Balota and Black found no evidence of habituation at the lexical level with visual+motor vocal repetition. Their null finding, however, might have arisen from motor vocal repetition, which is known to attenuate the verbal transformation effect in young adults who are listening to a word repeated over and over while concurrently saying each repetition of the word (MacKay, et al., 1993). Prolonged visual exposure, on the other hand, is known to produce perceptual distortions that are to a certain extent analogous to the fluctuations experienced in the auditory domain (Marks, 1949; Pritchard, Heron, & Hebb, 1960). Accordingly, a bimodal repetition treatment (concurrently seeing and hearing a word repeated several times) would provide the lexical unit that corresponds to the repeated word with two converging sources of bottom-up activation and thus habituation. The main question of interest is whether prolonged visual exposure would modulate auditory-induced habituation at the lexical level in young and older adults. Because the present experiment is the first attempt to examine the contribution of these two sources of bottom-up activation to the habituation of lexical units, it is unclear whether prolonged visual exposure would produce any habituation effect in young adults above and beyond that produced by auditory repetition. However, if older adults' lexical units are simply less likely to habituate, as suggested by the findings of the verbal transformation experiments, two sources of bottom-up activation (habituation) converging on the same units would not change the pattern of results obtained with auditory repetition.

In Exp. 1, we examined whether auditory massed repetition either alone or combined with prolonged visual exposure would produce semantic satiation in young and older adults. In Exp. 2, we tested the claim that older adults are less susceptible to lexical habituation with auditory massed repetition. In this experiment, we required young and older adults to report perceptual changes during the massed repetition treatment of the prime words used to induce semantic satiation in the preceding experiment.

Exp. 1: Semantic Satiation in Young and Older Adults

The main purpose of Exp. 1 was twofold: first, to examine semantic satiation effects with auditory and auditory+visual repetition in young adults, and second, to assess whether being older modulates these effects. In this experiment, participants made relatedness judgments on prime-target pairs as in the Balota and Black study (1997). In our experiment, however, participants either heard prime words (auditory-only condition) or concurrently heard and saw prime words (auditory+visual condition). The targets were always auditorily presented. Primes were repeated 2, 15, or 30 times. As in the Balota and Black study, to distinguish satiation from general boredom, semantic satiation was operationally defined as a repetition-induced change in the difference between related and unrelated trials (relatedness effect) for response latencies and accuracy, whereas boredom was defined as a generalized increment in response latencies and decline in accuracy, which would be largely the same for related and unrelated trials.

Balota and Black (1997) also manipulated the relation between primes and targets (related: yes vs unrelated: no) and its strength (high vs low) as to obtain the following sets of trials: high-strength related (ROYALTY-queen), low-strength related (ROYALTY-duke), and unrelated (ROYALTY-box or ROYALTY-pig). The latter served as controls for trials including related pairs. Trials with high strength pairs consisted of words that share several semantic features (they are clearly related) and for which a relatively shallow nonanalytic comparison is sufficient to produce a relatedness judgment. In contrast, trials with low strength pairs consisted of words that share fewer semantic features and that require a more in-depth analysis to produce a relatedness judgment. Balota and Black found that high strength pairs were as susceptible to satiation as low strength pairs in young adults, suggesting that semantic satiation depends on both the closeness of the meaning of the two words and the depth of the semantic analyses carried out on the words. In Exp. 1, we manipulated the associative strength of the prime-target relation via the same stimulus material used by Balota and Black to assess whether their findings would generalize to an auditory (or auditory+visual) satiation procedure.

Method

Participants.—Ninety-six young adults and 96 older adults from Washington University participated. Young adults' mean age was 20.7 yr. (17–33), and their mean vocabulary score was 54.5 (Wechsler, 1981). Older adults' mean age was 74.5 yr. (64–87), and their mean vocabulary score was 53.4. The two groups did not reliably differ on vocabulary scores ($t < 1.00$). All the participants reported themselves as being in a healthy condition for their age.

Participants received an abbreviated audiological evaluation to measure pure-tone air-conduction thresholds for octave frequencies between 250 and 4,000 dB HL. In this evaluation, even though young adults had lower average thresholds than older adults at all the frequencies ($F_{1,190} = 376.87$, $MSe = 230.65$), high frequency information produced the largest age group differences ($F_{4,760} = 113.47$, $MSe = 55.55$). One additional older adult was not included in the experiment because his hearing acuity was considerably lower than the hearing acuity of the other older participants at all the tested frequencies.

Stimuli and procedure.—The stimuli were the words used by Balota and Black in Exp. 1 (1997). They consisted of four sets of 96 prime-target combinations (Lorch, 1982): high-strength related pairs (ROYALTY-queen), low-strength related pairs (ROYALTY-duke), and unrelated pairs serving as controls for the previous sets (ROYALTY-box or ROYALTY-pig). The 384 prime-target pairs were organized into four lists of 96 trials. The prime words were the same in all the lists. Each list contained 24 prime-target pairs of each type of association (high-strength related, low-strength related, high-strength unrelated, and low-strength unrelated). Within a list, each subset of prime-target pairs contained eight primes repeated two times, eight primes repeated 15 times, and eight primes repeated 30 times. The counterbalancing of number of repetitions produced 12 unique lists. The stimuli, spoken by a male speaker, were recorded and digitized at a 20-kHz sampling rate, and their root-mean square amplitudes were digitally equated. Two independent raters per age group correctly identified all the stimuli prior to experimental implementation.

Each trial began with a 1000-msec. blank screen, followed by the message "PRESS ANY KEY TO BEGIN." The participant's response triggered the following events: a 400-msec. blank screen, a 600-msec./1000-Hz warning signal, a 10-msec. blank screen, and the presentation of a prime word repeated either 2, 15, or 30 times with a 100-msec. interstimulus interval between consecutive repetitions. A 100-msec. blank screen separated the last repetition of the prime and the presentation of the target. Manual responses were made on one of the two keys of an external device, appropriately labeled as YES and NO. Trials were randomized separately for each participant. There were two between-subjects conditions (each including 48 young and 48 older adults): auditory and auditory+visual. In both conditions, all the prime-target pairs were presented over headphones (at 80 dB sound-pressure level). However, in the auditory+visual condition, each prime word also appeared printed on the screen and remained on until the repetitions of that word ended. Continuous visual exposure was known to produce habituation at the lexical level (Warren, 1968), and thus it made the visual and auditory components of this repetition treatment compatible in their effects on the participants.

Each participant was given 10 practice trials and then received a list of 96 trials organized into four blocks of 24 trials each. Each block contained six trials for each prime-target relation (two per repetition level). The order in which blocks were presented was counterbalanced across participants. At the beginning of the practice session, participants were asked to pay attention to each repetition of a prime word and then decide whether a target word presented at the end of the repetition sequence was semantically related to the repeated prime. The experiment involved a 2 (age: young vs old) × 2 (modality of repetition: auditory vs auditory+visual) × 2 (relatedness: related vs unrelated) × 2 (strength: high vs low) × 3 (repetition: 2 vs 15 vs 30) mixed factorial design. Age and modality of repetition were the only between-subjects factors.

Results and Discussion

Each participant's response latencies for correct responses that were between 250 msec. and 4,000 msec. were used to calculate the participant's mean response time and standard deviation. In addition, response latencies for correct responses two standard deviations above or below the participant's mean were treated as outliers. The mean percentage outlier rates were 4% for the young adults and 6% for the older adults. A mean percentage correct was calculated for each participant in each of the within-subjects conditions. Tables 1 and 2 display the mean response latencies from stimulus onset and percentage correct as a function of the main factors included in the experimental design: age, strength, repetition, and relatedness. In these tables, the data pertaining to the two modalities of repetition were combined because, as it is to be shown, there were no reliable differences between them. The analyses reported below are significant at the point .05 level unless otherwise specified.

Response latencies.—A 2 (age) × 2 (strength) × 3 (repetition) × 2 (relatedness) × 2 (modality of repetition) mixed-factorial analysis of covariance was conducted on the z-score transform of the response latencies for correct responses. The z-score transforms were used here to control for differences

TABLE 1
Exp. 1: Young and Older Adults' Mean Response Latencies (in msec.) as a Function of Strength, Repetition, and Relatedness With Relatedness Effects (Difference Between Unrelated and Related Trials) of Interest

Age	Strength	Related Trials 2	15	30	Unrelated Trials 2	15	30	Effect 2	15	30
Young	High	1045	1050	1099	1142	1159	1180			
	Low	1092	1136	1158	1162	1170	1184			
	M	1069	1093	1129	1152	1165	1182	+83	+72	+53
Older	High	1415	1460	1494	1693	1657	1690			
	Low	1542	1581	1630	1740	1690	1729			
	M	1479	1521	1562	1717	1674	1710	+238	+153	+148
	M							+161	+113	+101

in speed between age groups and between modality of repetition conditions (see Faust, Balota, Spieler, & Ferraro, 1999) uncovered in the preliminary analyses of the raw response latencies. Hearing acuity (defined as participants' average thresholds for the better ear) served as the covariate to rule out age differences in hearing acuity as a contributor to any of the effects described below.

TABLE 2
Exp. 2: Young and Older Adults' Percentage Correct as a Function of Strength, Repetition, and Relatedness

Age	Strength	Related Trials 2	15	30	Unrelated Trials 2	15	30
Young	High	97	95	93	92	95	95
	Low	88	84	86	95	96	96
	M	92.5	89.5	89.5	93.5	95.5	95.5
Older	High	95	95	95	92	94	95
	Low	90	86	86	93	94	95
	M	92.5	90.5	90.5	92.5	94.0	95.0
	M	92.5	90.0	90.0	93.0	94.8	95.3

The analysis of the z-score transforms yielded a main effect of relatedness ($F_{1,187} = 219.09$, $MSe = 1.38$; related: 1309 msec. vs unrelated: 1433 msec.), strength ($F_{1,187} = 150.78$, $MSe = .69$; high strength: 1340 msec. vs low strength: 1401 msec.), and repetition ($F_{2,376} = 20.73$, $MSe = .87$; 2: 1354 msec. vs 30: 1396 msec.). As found by Balota and Black, there was an interaction between relatedness and strength ($F_{1,187} = 77.46$, $MSe = .67$), indicating that the difference between related and unrelated trials, i.e., relatedness effect, was larger for high strength than low strength pairs (159 msec. vs 89 msec.). Again, as found by Balota and Black, age interacted with relatedness ($F_{1,187} = 5.48$, $MSe = 1.38$), indicating that the relatedness effect was larger in older adults than in young adults (180 msec. vs 69 msec.). Most interesting for the purpose of the present investigation, repetition interacted with relatedness ($F_{2,376} = 10.10$, $MSe = .78$), indicating that the relatedness effect declined with massed repetition (161 msec. vs 113 msec. vs 101 msec.). This effect was produced by response latencies for related trials, which increased with repetition (1274 msec. vs 1307 msec. vs 1346 msec.), whereas response latencies for unrelated trials remained largely stable (1435 msec. vs 1420 msec. vs 1446 msec.). In contrast to Balota and Black who reported a repetition-induced decline in the relatedness effect that was limited to young adults, there was no evidence here that such a decline was modulated by age ($F = 1.49$; other $Fs \leq 1.91$).

Accuracy.—The analysis conducted on response latencies was replicated on the percentage correct responses. This analysis yielded a main effect of relatedness ($F_{1,187} = 60.44$, $MSe = 122.20$; related: 91% vs unrelated: 94%) and of strength ($F_{1,187} = 107.42$, $MSe = 75.58$; high strength: 94% vs low strength: 91%). Relatedness interacted with strength ($F_{1,187} = 177.60$, $MSe = 73.93$), indicating that for high strength pairs participants were more accurate on related than unrelated trials (95% vs 94%), whereas for low strength pairs the opposite was true (87% vs 95%). Age interacted with relatedness and strength ($F_{1,187} = 4.00$, $MSe = 73.93$), indicating that in unrelated trials young adults were more accurate in rejecting low strength pairs than older adults (96% vs 94%). In contrast, there were no age differences in accuracy for high strength pairs in both related and unrelated trials (for both age groups: 95% and 94%) and for low strength pairs in related trials (young: 86%; older: 87%). Relatedness also interacted with repetition ($F_{2,376} = 11.30$, $MSe = 106.35$). This effect was attributed to the tendency of the accuracy to decrease for related trials (from 92.5% with 2 repetitions to 90% with 30 repetitions) and increase in unrelated trials (from 93% with 2 repetitions to 95.3% with 30 repetitions; other $Fs \leq 2.88$).

In summary, irrespective of age, modality of repetition, and strength of the relationship between primes and targets, massed repetition affected the relatedness effect mainly by slowing and reducing the accuracy of responses to related pairs. This finding is consistent with the notion that massed repetition, by weakening the activation of the semantic representations of the repeated words, also reduces the spreading of activation to units in the semantic network that share with the repeated words some semantic features. As a result, the responses to prime-target pairs involving two related words become slower and less accurate.[2] The absence of age differences on these trials, however, should not be interpreted as suggesting that semantic satia-

---

[2]Repetition slowed and reduced the accuracy of participants' responses to related pairs, whereas it slightly increased the accuracy of responses to unrelated pairs without affecting their latencies. One could argue that this pattern of effects is also consistent with a bias account, according to which repetition leads participants to become more "reluctant" to make relatedness

tion effects in young and older adults arise from the same underlying processes. On the contrary, we propose that auditory repetition induces semantic satiation effects in young adults by habituating the lexical units of the repeated primes, making these units less able to spread activation to their matching semantic representations. In contrast, we maintain that auditory repetition in older adults does not affect the lexical units of the repeated primes as much as in young adults. As a result, older adults' lexical units have more opportunities to continue spreading activation to their matching semantic representations, thereby also giving the latter more opportunities to become habituated.

Our finding of a repetition-induced increment in young and older adults' response latencies for related trials conflicts with the results of the Balota and Black study. Why were the older adults in their study not as sensitive as ours to massed repetition in these trials? Although there is no simple answer to this question, it is reasonable to assume that motor vocal repetition, an important component of the Balota and Black satiation treatment, may have been responsible for their finding. We propose that repeating a word to oneself over and over requires that its phonological and articulatory information be preserved in an activated state for a prolonged period of time. Given the capacity limitations associated with aging (Craik, 1977), older adults' allocation of attentional resources to the lexical level of processing may have limited the flow of activation to semantic representations during the repetition treatment, preventing their repeated activation and their habituation. In contrast, young adults' allocation of attention to the lexical level is unlikely to have had the same outcome, thereby allowing semantic units to become repeatedly activated and thus habituated. Of course, if this is true, no habituation of lexical units should be observed with motor vocal repetition in both young and older adults. Indeed, Balota and Black (1997) reported that the massed repetition of words that share with their targets phonological rather than semantic information (SAME-claim) did not affect either young or older adults' rhyme-decision latencies.

The findings of Balota and Black and ours suggest that different mechanisms may be responsible for young adults' semantic satiation with motor

---

decisions (R. Klein, personal communication, March 28, 2000). This bias would slow and reduce the accuracy of responses to related pairs. It would also increase the accuracy of responses to unrelated pairs while making these responses faster. However, no evidence of faster responses to unrelated pairs was observed here. Of course, one could propose that massed repetition also reduces participants' alertness, which could offset their tendency to produce an unrelated decision quickly. Nevertheless, the issue is what in the first place could produce participants' "reluctance" to make relatedness judgments. The answer to this question brings us back to the notion of satiation as reduction in the activation level of the meaning of the repeated words and that of related words, which makes these words "less available" to participants when they are asked to make relatedness judgments.

vocal as opposed to auditory repetition. Specifically, because motor vocal repetition prevents the habituation of lexical units (as demonstrated by the Balota and Black rhyming study), semantic satiation effects induced by motor vocal repetition appear to arise from the habituation of semantic units. In contrast, because auditory repetition promotes habituation at the lexical level (as demonstrated by the verbal transformation studies), semantic satiation effects induced by this mode of repetition seem to arise from the lexical level.

Lastly, the finding that prolonged visual exposure added to auditory repetition did not change the semantic satiation effects observed with auditory repetition alone suggests that two converging sources of satiation do not produce additive effects. Of course, the encoding of visual stimuli involves the translation of visual patterns into orthographic codes before the latter can activate phonological codes (Manning, Koehler, & Hampton, 1990). Because auditory stimuli have a more direct route to phonological information, it is possible that they provided the phonological codes for the visually presented stimuli, and thus reduced the processing of the latter in our experiment. If this is true, then it is not surprising that auditory repetition played a dominant role in our experiment.

Exp. 2: Perceptual Changes During 30 Repetitions

In Exp. 1, we attributed young adults' semantic satiation effects to the habituation of lexical information and supported our claim by relying on earlier studies documenting this type of habituation with auditory massed repetition (Warren, 1961). In Exp. 2, we provided a direct test for this claim. Participants were presented with the prime words of the earlier experiment, all repeated 30 times, and were asked to indicate whether during the repetition treatment of each word they heard other words. We were interested in how many times out of 30 participants heard a word different from the repeated word. Therefore, in this experiment, perceiving a new word and later perceiving that same new word again counted as two "different words." As in Exp. 1, we adopted two repetition models: auditory and auditory+visual. In the latter condition, we asked participants to focus on the auditory presentation of the repeated word and to examine the visually presented stimulus only if there was a discrepancy between the immediately preceding word and the currently perceived word. Their task was to report a change in the auditorily presented word only if their auditory perceptions did not match the printed word. Therefore, the auditory+visual condition permitted us to control for possible age differences arising from participants forgetting the veridical stimulus during the auditory-only repetition treatment.

We predicted that if the semantic satiation effects observed in the young adults of Exp. 1 were indeed due to lexical habituation (verbal transformations), young adults should report perceiving more illusory percepts than the aged in the present experiment. Of course, we also predicted that, if age differences in participants' reports are not due to differences in forgetting, the auditory and auditory+visual study conditions should produce equivalent results.

Method

 Participants.—Thirty-six young and 36 older adults from Washington University participated. Young adults' mean age was 20.6 yr. (18–29), and their mean vocabulary score was 54.0. Older adults' mean age was 75.0 yr. (67–87), and their mean vocabulary score was 55.6. The two groups did not reliably differ on vocabulary scores ($t_{70} < 1.00$). All the participants reported themselves as being in a healthy condition for their age. As in the audiological evaluation of Exp. 1, even though young adults had lower average thresholds than older adults at all the frequencies ($F_{1,46} = 99.98$, $MSe = 389.35$), high frequency information produced the largest age group differences ($F_{4,184} = 12.97$, $MSe = 83.05$). Two additional older participants were excluded from the experiment for displaying audiometric scores reliably lower than those of the other older adults.

 Procedure and stimuli.—The 96 prime words of Exp. 1 were organized in six blocks of 16 word trials. Participants were asked to press a key to initiate a trial and were given a one-word practice trial prior to the experimental session. The participant's response triggered the following events: a 400-msec. blank screen, a 600-msec./1000-Hz warning signal, a 10-msec. blank screen, and the presentation of a prime word repeated 30 times with a 100-msec. interstimulus interval between consecutive repetitions. Therefore, the sequence of events triggered by the participant's key press at the beginning of each trial was identical to the one used in Exp. 1 with the exception that all the primes were repeated 30 times and targets were not presented. Furthermore, there were three between-subjects conditions: auditory, auditory+visual, and control. Twelve young and 12 older adults were assigned to each modality of repetition condition, and 12 young and 12 older adults were assigned to the control condition. In the auditory+visual condition, each prime word also appeared printed on the screen and remained on until the repetitions of that word ended. The control condition was similar to the auditory condition with the exception that on half of the trials there was a real change in the repeated word. A change in the repetition sequence of a word involved hearing another word (randomly selected without replacement from the remaining 95 stimuli) at some point after the first 10 repetitions of the target word. This condition was introduced to ensure that age-group differences in the reports of illusory changes could not be attributed to older adults' adopting a more conservative response criterion (response bias). In all the conditions, participants were instructed to listen carefully to each repetition and press a key of an external device every time they heard a word that was different from the word they heard at the beginning of the trial. The order of stimulus presentation was randomized separately for each participant, and a Latin square design was used to counterbalance the order in which blocks were presented.

Results and Discussion

In the auditory repetition condition, the average number of key presses per word was 2.79 ($SD=2.40$) for young adults and .15 ($SD=.21$) for older adults. In the auditory+visual condition, the average number of key presses per word was 1.89 ($SD=2.37$) for young adults and .14 ($SD=.13$) for older adults. In the control condition, both age groups reliably perceived the real changes introduced in half of the trials ($t<1.00$). With respect to the other half of the trials, which did not involve such changes, the average number of key presses (illusory reports) was 1.85 ($SD=.25$) for young adults and .18 ($SD=.12$) for older adults.

The reports of illusory changes were submitted to a two-way analysis of covariance with age and condition as factors and hearing acuity as the covariate. In this analysis, older adults produced fewer key presses than young adults ($F_{1,65}=7.94$, $MSe=1.95$; condition and interaction: $Fs<1.00$). The larger number of illusory reports by young adults suggests that the semantic satiation effects observed in the young adults of Exp. 1 were probably because they did not hear as many repetitions of the veridical form as the older adults did during the repetition period. These findings replicate the results of a recent study examining the verbal transformation effect (Pilotti, *et al.*, 2000) where older adults also reported fewer illusory changes.

GENERAL DISCUSSION

The results of the experiments presented here can be summarized in three main points. First, in both young and older adults, auditory massed repetition either alone or combined with visual repetition produced reliable semantic satiation effects. Second, young adults who listened to 30 repetitions of the prime words used in the semantic satiation experiment reported perceiving fewer instances of the repeated words than older adults. Third, prolonged visual exposure did not change the patterns of habituation effects observed with auditory repetition alone.

The present experiments provide *prima facie* evidence for a model of semantic satiation in which age differences in habituation at the lexical level of processing can nevertheless produce the same patterns of satiation effects at the semantic level. Specifically, in young adults, any repetition-induced decline in processing at the semantic level appears to be dependent on the habituation of lexical units. On the other hand, in older adults, the weak habituation of these units seems to promote habituation in their corresponding semantic representations. Our findings are consistent with earlier data (Balota & Duchek, 1988; Spieler & Balota, 2000), suggesting that age modulates lexical processing (word recognition) while having virtually no effect on the semantic level (word comprehension). Indeed, semantic priming studies have consistently reported that aging does not impair the activation of semantic units (see Cohen, 1979; Balota, Black, & Cheney, 1992). Similarly, we found that aging does not affect participants' ability to withdraw processing resources from repetitive stimuli when such stimuli are subjected to semantic analysis. Interestingly, Pilotti, et al. (2000) found that neither age-related losses in auditory acuity nor slowing in the uptake of sensory information accounted for older adults' declines in lexical habituation (as demonstrated by the verbal transformation effect). Taken together, these findings along with those of the present study suggest that the effects of aging on information-processing mechanisms are specific rather than global and centrally located rather than peripherally induced.

With respect to the issue of the sources of satiation, Kounios, et al. (2000) found that repetition-induced changes in the N400, a neurophysiological indicator of semantic processing, did not vary as a function of modality of repetition (visual vs auditory). This finding, albeit limited to young adults, is consistent with our claim that different modalities of repetition may not induce satiation in the same manner, but they nonetheless yield the same declines in processing at the semantic level. Of course, one may ask whether the lexical habituation effects observed in our young adults are simply the byproduct of habituation at earlier stages of processing (acoustic). Kounios, et al. (2000) found that physical changes in the repeated stimuli (voice or type case), intended to reduce habituation at these stages of processing, did not affect the N400. However, Pilotti, et al. (1997) reported that such changes eliminated evidence of satiation at the behavioral level. Differences in the rate of repetition between the two studies may be responsible for the discrepancy in their findings. For instance, the much slower repetition rate of the Kounios, et al. study may have allowed participants more time to override irrelevant physical changes and focus on abstract lexical information. Research should be designed to examine this possibility.

REFERENCES

ANDERSON, J. R. (1976) *Language, memory, and thought*. Hillsdale, NJ: Erlbaum.

BALOTA, D. A., & BLACK, S. (1997) Semantic satiation in healthy young and older adults. *Memory & Cognition*, 25, 190-202.

BALOTA, D. A., BLACK, S., & CHENEY, M. (1992) Automatic and attentional priming in young and older adults: re-evaluation of the two-process model. *Journal of Experimental Psychology: Human Perception and Performance*, 18, 485-502.

BALOTA, D. A., & DUCHEK, J. M. (1988) Age-related differences in lexical access, spreading activation, and simple pronunciation. *Psychology and Aging*, 3, 84-93.

COHEN, G. (1979) Language comprehension in old age. *Cognitive Psychology*, 11, 412-429.

COLLINS, A. M., & LOFTUS, E. F. (1975) A spreading activation theory of semantic processing. *Psychological Review*, 82, 407-428.

COWAN, N. (1995) *Attention and memory: an integrated approach*. New York: Oxford Univer. Press.

CRAIK, F. I. M. (1977) Age differences in human memory. In J. E. Birren & K. W. Schaie (Eds.), *Handbook of the psychology of aging*. New York: Van Nostrand Reinhold. Pp. 384-420.

ELMAN, J. L. (1989) Connectionist approaches to acoustic/phonetic processing. In W. D. Marslen-Wilson (Ed.), *Lexical representation and process*. Cambridge, MA: MIT Press. Pp. 227-260.

ELMAN, J. L., & MCCLELLAND, J. L. (1986) Exploiting lawful variability in the speech waveform. In J. S. Perkell & D. H. Klatt (Eds.), *Invariance and variability in speech processing*. Hillsdale, NJ: Erlbaum. Pp. 360-385.

ESPOSITO, N. J., & PELTON, L. H. (1971) Review of the measurement of semantic satiation. *Psychological Bulletin*, 75, 330-346.

FAUST, M. E., BALOTA, D. A., SPIELER, D. H., & FERRARO, F. R. (1999) Individual differences in information-processing rate and amount: implications for group differences in response latency. *Psychological Bulletin*, 125, 777-799.

KOUNIOS, J., KOTZ, S. A., & HOLCOMB, P. J. (2000) On the locus of the semantic satiation effect: evidence from event-related potentials. *Memory & Cognition*, 28, 1366-1377.

LEWIS, M. B., & ELLIS, H. (2000) Satiation in name and face recognition. *Memory & Cognition*, 28, 783-788.

LORCH, R. F., JR. (1982) Priming and search processes in semantic memory: a test of three models of spreading activation. *Journal of Verbal Learning and Verbal Behavior*, 21, 468-492.

LUCAS, M. (2000) Semantic priming without association: a meta-analytic review. *Psychonomic Bulletin and Review*, 7, 618-630.

MACKAY, D. G. (1990) Perception, action, and awareness: a three-body problem. In O. Neumann & W. Prinz (Eds.), *Relations between perception and action*. Berlin: Springer-Verlag. Pp. 269-303.

MACKAY, D. G., WULF, G., YIN, C., & ABRAMS, L. (1993) Relations between word perception and production: new theory and data on the verbal transformation effect. *Journal of Memory and Language*, 32, 624-646.

MANNING, S. K., KOEHLER, L., & HAMPTON, S. (1990) The effects of recoding and presentation format in recency suffix effects. *Memory & Cognition*, 18, 164-173.

MARKS, M. R. (1949) Some phenomena attendant on long fixation. *The American Journal of Psychology*, 62, 392-398.

MCCLELLAND, J. L., & ELMAN, J. L. (1986) The TRACE model of speech perception. *Cognitive Psychology*, 18, 1-86.

MCNAMARA, T. P. (1994) Theories of priming: II. Types of primes. *Journal of Experimental Psychology: Learning, Memory, and Cognition*, 20, 507-520.

NEELY, J. H. (1991) Semantic priming effects in visual word recognition: a selective review of current findings and theories. In D. Besner & G. W. Humphreys (Eds.), *Basic processes in reading: visual word recognition*. Hillsdale, NJ: Erlbaum. Pp. 264-336.

PILOTTI, M., ANTROBUS, J. S., & DUFF, M. (1997) The effect of presemantic acoustic adaptation on semantic "satiation". *Memory & Cognition*, 25, 305-312.

PILOTTI, M., BALOTA, D. A., SOMMERS, M., & KURDISH, A. (2000) Auditory habituation in young and older adults: the verbal transformation effect. *Psychology and Aging*, 15, 313-322.

PRITCHARD, R. M., HERON, W., & HEBB, D. O. (1960) Visual perception approached by the method of stabilized images. *Canadian Journal of Psychology*, 14, 67-77.

SALTHOUSE, T. A. (1982) *Adult cognition*. New York: Springer-Verlag.

SMITH, L. C. (1984) Semantic satiation affects category membership decision time but not lexical priming. *Memory & Cognition*, 12, 483-488.

SMITH, L. C., & KLEIN, R. (1990) Evidence for semantic satiation: repeating a category slows subsequent semantic processing. *Journal of Experimental Psychology: Learning, Memory, and Cognition*, 16, 852-861.

SOKOLOV, E. N. (1991) Local plasticity in neuronal learning. In L. R. Squire, N. M. Weinberger, G. Lynch, & J. L. McGaugh (Eds.), *Memory: organization and locus of change*. New York: Oxford Univer. Press. Pp. 364-391.

SPIELER, D. H., & BALOTA, D. A. (2000) Factors influencing word naming in younger and older adults. *Psychology and Aging*, 15, 225-231.

WARREN, R. M. (1961) Illusory changes in repeated words: differences between young adults and the aged. *The American Journal of Psychology*, 52, 249-258.

WARREN, R. M. (1968) Verbal transformation effect and auditory perceptual mechanisms. *Psychological Bulletin*, 70, 261-270.

WARREN, R. M., & WARREN, R. P. (1966) A comparison of speech perception in childhood, maturity, and old age by means of the verbal transformation effect. *Journal of Verbal Learning and Verbal Behavior*, 5, 142-146.

WECHSLER, D. (1981) *Manual for the Wechsler Adult Intelligence Scale–Revised*. New York: Psychological Corp.

YIN, C., & MACKAY, D. G. (1992) Auditory illusions and aging: transmission of priming in the verbal transformation paradigm. Poster presented at the Cognitive Aging Conference, Atlanta, March.

Accepted March 26, 2004.

EFFECT OF DECEPTION OF DISTANCE ON PROLONGED CYCLING PERFORMANCE[1]

S. PATERSON AND F. E. MARINO

School of Human Movement Studies
Charles Sturt University

Summary.—This study examined the effect of deception of distance end-point on prolonged cycling performance. 21 subjects were randomly allocated to three groups ($n = 7$ per group). Each group completed three self-paced time-trials separated by one day. Subjects were told that each trial was a 30-km time-trial and were required to complete the distance in the fastest time possible. Following the initial trial of 30 km, one group completed Trial 2 with a longer distance (long distance group; 36 km), another group with a shorter distance (24 km; short distance group), and the third group as control (30 km; control). Each group then completed a third time-trial of 30 km. At no time was the deception of distance in Trial 2 disclosed to the subjects, and all sources of physiological and mechanical feedback were withheld during the trials. Data from Trials 1 and 3 were analysed by repeated-measures analysis of covariance. Time to complete Trial 1 was similar among groups (~65 min.). Following the deception in Trial 2 the time to complete the 30 km in Trial 3 was increased for the short distance group, decreased for the long distance group, whilst the time for the control group remained unchanged. The times to complete the 30 km on Trials 1 and 3 were matched by changes in power output throughout the trials. It is concluded that subjects deceived of the actual distance completed will complete the subsequent performance trial based on perceived effort rather than on actual distance.

An important area of research and a key issue in sports science is the use of pacing strategies for successfully completing a sporting event. Although a strict definition for pacing is difficult to articulate, pacing during exercise performance would most likely be related to the physiological and perceptual responses of athletes and to the spatial and temporal changes occurring during the performance. Although pacing strategies are undoubtedly used in a variety of sporting events, pacing can be studied more effectively in long distance events with the best examples evident in running and cycling competition. To date, an understanding of the mechanisms related to pacing are unclear. However, Ulmer (1996) has suggested that a central "programmer" takes into consideration the requirements to complete the activity by integrating peripheral systems such as metabolic perturbations to reduce the likelihood of cellular injury or terminating the exercise bout prematurely. The ability to anticipate the impending needs for successful completion of the exercise bout has been termed teleoanticipation (Ulmer, 1996).

---

[1]Address enquiries to Frank E. Marino, Ph.D., School of Human Movement Studies, Charles Sturt University, Bathurst, NSW 2795, Australia or e-mail (fmarino@csu.edu.au).

In support of such a teleoanticipation model, the use of electromyography (EMG) during cycling exercise has shown that efferent neural command was systematically reduced over a 60-min. period whilst subjects continued to give a conscious maximal effort during cycle sprints as evidenced by the lack of change in either heart rate or perceived exertion (Kay, Marino, Cannon, St Clair Gibson, Lambert, & Noakes, 2001). However, during the final sprint, muscle activation was restored close to initial values, indicating a restoration in efferent neural command, suggesting that a "subconscious" control of efferent command must have been operating. This hypothesis is supported by the notion that in closed-loop experiments wherein the nature, length, and timing of the activity are known, subjects typically down-regulate the motor command to the skeletal muscles to prevent muscle damage (St Clair Gibson, Schabort, & Noakes, 2001). In contrast, for open-loop activity where the duration of exercise is undetermined, subjects terminate the activity voluntarily because they are exhausted or fatigued.

The teleoanticipation model also suggests that an indication of an endpoint to the exercise bout would be required *a priori* so that the organism is able to make the continuous adjustments necessary for the activity to be completed successfully. It follows that after completing a given exercise bout an "exertion template" is created so that for a subsequent and similar exercise bout the most appropriate adjustments can be made for successful completion of that activity. Others have shown that well-trained cyclists select pacing strategies based on the perceived distance of a time-trial rather than the actual distance (Nikolopoulos, Arkinstall, & Hawley, 2001). However, in this study subjects were given feedback in the form of percentage distance remaining and in one trial were permitted to view their heart-rate response throughout the ride. This provided the researchers with data to infer that pacing strategies were not modified even when physiological cues such as heart rate were available. As far as we are aware there are no studies that have evaluated the effect of deception of end-point whilst providing no external or physiological feedback to subjects during prolonged exercise.

We hypothesised that if persons were deceived or deprived of the predetermined end-point for a given bout of prolonged exercise, an adjustment to their perceived effort for the subsequent exercise bout would be made in accordance with the new and revised exertion template. Specifically, an increased distance should be perceived as more difficult compared to a shorter distance with subjects finding a subsequent shorter bout easier or harder, respectively. To test this hypothesis three separate groups of subjects were told that they were required to complete three self-paced cycling trials of a set distance (30 km). However, for two groups the distance of the middle trial was either shortened or lengthened by 6 km to deceive subjects regarding the actual end-point to the exercise bout. Thus, the time taken to complete the final trial would reflect the adjustment in the exertion template according to the difficulty of the deception trial (either short or long distance).

Method

Subjects and Experimental Design

All experimentation was approved by the Ethics in Human Research Committee of the university, and all subjects signed a letter of informed consent. Given the low risk associated with the experiment and that healthy, physically active subjects would be recruited, the Ethics Committee approved the deception of distance during experimentation provided that there was continuous monitoring of vital signs. Table 1 shows the mean subject characteristics of each group. Twenty-one (17 male and 4 female) endurance-trained cyclists participated. All subjects were apparently healthy, having completed a health history questionnaire and an incremental test to exhaustion. Prior to the first experimental session, subjects attended the Human Performance Laboratory for the purpose of familiarisation with the experimental requirements, equipment, and procedures. During this session, descriptive data such as height, body mass, and body fat by hydrostatic weighing (Siri, 1961) were recorded and an incremental test to voluntary exhaustion performed on a cycle ergometer for the determination of peak oxygen uptake (VO_2 peak) and peak power output.

TABLE 1
Subjects' Characteristics For Each Group

	Age (yr.)	Mass (kg)	Height (cm)	Body Fat (%)	VO_2 peak ($1 \cdot min.^{-1}$)	Peak Power Output (W)	HR_{peak} (beats $\cdot min.^{-1}$)
Long Distance							
M	26.9	75.9	177.4	16.1	4.3	303.4	183.4
SD	10.6	11.2	9.4	5.2	0.5	34.9	8.3
Short Distance							
M	26.0	73.8	171.6	20.0	3.8	276.6	185.3
SD	11.8	10.8	6.4	10.2	0.7	61.1	6.3
Control							
M	27.6	76.1	176.8	19.6	4.2	310.0	190.1
SD	9.0	11.0	12.5	10.2	0.4	75.3	13.1

Note.—VO_2 peak, PPO, and HR_{peak} are peak oxygen uptake, peak heart rate, and peak power output, respectively, during incremental exercise.

Before any experimental testing, all subjects were informed that the purpose of the investigation was to test physiological responses to 30-km time-trials without any external feedback. All experimental sessions were conducted at the same time of day to minimise the effects of circadian variations in core temperature. Subjects were asked to abstain from vigorous exercise throughout the period of testing and consumption of alcohol and caffeine for at least 24 hours prior to the experimental sessions. During the experimental period subjects were required to standardize eating and drinking routines in the 24 hours prior to each experimental test.

Following the familiarisation session subjects were randomly allocated to one of three experimental groups. The female subjects were randomly assigned so that each group comprised at least one female participant. Each experimental group ($n=7$) completed three self-paced time-trials each separated by one day, i.e., Monday-Wednesday-Friday. Subjects were informed that they were to complete a 30-km time-trial on each occasion. However, for Trial 2 one group was required to cycle 6 km further, i.e., 36 km; the long distance group, and another group 6 km less, i.e., 24 km; the short distance group, and the third group exactly 30 km (the control group). The manipulation of the distance in Trial 2 was not disclosed at any time during testing. Following Trial 2, subjects returned for a third and final 30-km trial. During the experimental sessions, the researcher was situated behind the participant and remained there until the trial was completed. All sources of physiological and mechanical feedback were withheld from the participants during these trials, i.e., duration, distance, heart rate, speed, and cadence, and at no time during the trial did subjects have a view of the researcher and were unaware as to the timing of measurements. At the conclusion of each trial participants were asked about the difficulty of the trial. Although none could confirm the difference in distance cycled, subjects did consider longer distance trials more difficult than the other trials. This procedure confirmed that participants were able to discriminate between trial difficulty regardless of the lack of feedback. All experimental sessions were conducted in a climate chamber, where ambient temperature and relative humidity were maintained at 22°C and 40%, respectively. Once the research was complete all subjects were debriefed as to the precise nature of the study and to the deception of the actual distance cycled.

Anthropometric Measurements and Incremental Test

Height was measured to the nearest 0.1 cm using a stadiometer (Len Blayden, Lugarno, Australia), and body mass was measured to 0.01 kg using an electronic precision balance (HW-100KAI, GEC, Avery, Ltd., Australia). Body surface area (A_D) was determined using the method described by DuBois and DuBois (1916). Hydrostatic weighing was used to determine body density for each subject, and percent body fat was estimated as descried by Siri (1961).

All subjects underwent an incremental test to exhaustion for the determination of peak power output and VO_2 peak. The subject performed this test using his own bicycle attached to an electromagnetic trainer (Tacx,

Technische Industry Tacx BV, Wassenaar, Netherlands). This was the same bicycle that was used in the subsequent experimental trials. Following a 5- to 10-min. warm-up at a self-selected intensity, the test commenced at a workload of 100W. The load was then increased by 10W each 30 sec. until the subject could no longer maintain the required power output. During these incremental tests to exhaustion, subjects were requested to remain in a seated position. During the test, subjects breathed through a two-way non-breathing valve (Series 2700, Hans Rudolph, St. Louis, MO, USA). Expired air passed via the respiratory tubing to an automated gas analyser (Quinton Instrument Company, Bothell, WA, USA). Prior to analysis, the pneumotach (Hans Rudolph, St. Louis, MO, USA) and gas analysers were calibrated using a 3 l syringe and gases of known concentration, respectively. Expired air passed through a mixing chamber of 5.5 litre volume and sampled at 15-sec. intervals. The criteria for VO_2 peak was the highest mean value obtained over a 1-min. period.

Time-trial Procedure

Prior to each time-trial, the cycle trainer was calibrated for distance by recording the number of pedal revolutions required to ride a distance of 5 km. This procedure yielded a coefficient of variation of 0.7%. During the time-trial subjects were provided a standard 250 ml of water to be consumed *ad libitum*. Before commencing the test subjects were asked to choose their starting gear and assume their natural starting position. Once relaxed, subjects were instructed to cycle the 30 km "as hard and as fast as possible." The ergometer, heart-rate monitor, and stopwatch were synchronised and started on the word "go." Throughout each time-trial, heart rate was recorded using a heart-rate monitor (Polar Vantage, Polar Electro, Kempele, Finland) at 15-sec. intervals and stored for later analysis. Instantaneous power output was sampled at the midpoint of every 6-km progression, i.e., 5.5 km, 11.5 km, 17.5 km, 23.5 km, and 29.5 km. An overall rating of perceived exertion (RPE) was recorded at the conclusion of each time-trial using Borg's scale (1982). This recording was taken at the end to avoid any external cues related to timing. As to the result of the trial, subjects were not provided any feedback until all subjects had completed all three trials.

Statistical Analysis

Since each group received a different deception in Trial 2, the results from Trials 1 and 3 were analysed by repeated-measures analysis of covariance using data from Trial 2 as the covariate as this trial differed in distance and duration between groups. This analysis was also chosen to maximize statistical power as real differences between final values may not be evident without the addition of the covariate (Huck, Cormier, & Bounds, 1974, p. 135). The time taken to cycle the given distance for Trials 1 and 3, and mean heart rate were analysed with a 3 × 2 (group × trial) repeated-measures analysis of covariance, whilst the power output was analysed with a 3 × 5 (group × distance) repeated-measures analysis of covariance. Assumptions of correlation, homogeneity of variance, and normal distribution of within cells residuals were verified for each analysis of covariance. When significant main effects or interactions were detected the resulting estimated marginal means were compared using Tukey HSD *post hoc* procedure. The level of significance was set at $p < .05$.

RESULTS

The times taken to complete the trials by each group are given in Table 2. Analysis showed a significant main effect for group ($F_{2,17} = 3.59$, $p < .01$). *Post hoc* analysis yielded no significant differences for time taken to cycle 30 km in Trial 1. The times for Trial 2 were relative to the distance cycled (Table 2). Compared with Trial 1, the long distance group cycled 30 km in Trial 3 approximately 8.9 min. faster. In contrast the short distance group increased the time taken to cycle 30 km in Trial 3 by about 8.4 min. The time taken to cycle 30 km by the control group in Trial 3 was not different compared with Trial 1. However, the time taken by the control group in Trial 3 was significantly faster by about 14.0 min. compared with the short distance group but was significantly slower by about 9.2 min. when compared with the long distance group (see Table 2).

TABLE 2
TIME (MIN.) TAKEN TO CYCLE GIVEN DISTANCES BY EACH GROUP

		Trial 1	Trial 2	Trial 3
Long Distance	M	61.5	76.1	53.3*†
	SD	3.1	2.9	2.6
Short Distance	M	66.4	53.5	74.8*†
	SD	3.4	2.4	2.1
Control	M	63.4	62.3	61.8
	SD	3.4	2.6	2.0

Note.—Trials 1 and 3 are 30 km each for long distance and short distance groups. Trial 2 is the covariate and deception trial of 36 km for the long distance group, 24 km for the short distance group, and 30 km for the control group. *$p < .05$ compared to Trial 1. †$p < .05$ amongst groups.

The power outputs during each trial are given in Table 3. There was no significant main effect for group ($F_{2,35} = 3.32$, ns). However, there was a main effect within trials ($F_{1,35} = 4.17$, $p = .01$). *Post hoc* analysis showed that on Trial 1 the power output was not significantly different among groups at any time. However, power output decreased over time in each group reaching statistical significance at the end of the trial compared with the initial power output. On Trial 1, the mean power output for the long distance group was significantly less than on Trial 3. The mean power output for the short distance group on Trial 1 was similar to that for Trial 3. However, on Trial 3 the power output for the short distance group was reduced from the initial value to that at the end of the trial. The mean power output for the control group was similar for the two trials.

TABLE 3
POWER OUTPUT (WATTS) FOR EACH GROUP DURING EACH TRIAL AT GIVEN DISTANCES

	5.5 km M	5.5 km SD	11.5 km M	11.5 km SD	17.5 km M	17.5 km SD	23.5 km M	23.5 km SD	29.5 km M	29.5 km SD
Long Distance										
Trial 1	197.7	6.7	185.4	6.6	179.3	6.5	171.0	7.9	172.0	8.2
Trial 3	195.8	6.6	192.8	5.2	198.3	5.4	192.9	7.9	200.6	8.2*
Short Distance										
Trial 1	188.4	6.8	185.4	5.1	170.7	5.4	170.1	7.9	168.0	8.2
Trial 3	193.3	6.7	190.8	5.1	179.4	5.4	170.3	7.9	165.8	8.2*†
Control										
Trial 1	195.3	6.7	190.8	5.1	189.8	5.4	184.0	7.9	176.7	8.2
Trial 3	198.2	6.7	194.3	5.1	184.0	5.4	182.1	7.9	183.6	8.2*

*$p < .05$ compared with initial power output. †$p < .05$ compared with other groups.

For RPE there was no significant main effect for group ($F_{2,15} = 3.68$, ns). RPE values for Trial 3 were comparable to those on Trial 1 for all three groups, indicating that subjects perceived their exertion to be similar in those trials. The mean heart-rate responses for each trial are shown in Table 4. There was no significant main effect for group ($F_{2,15} = 3.68$, ns) or trial ($F_{1,35} = 4.17$, ns) for mean heart-rate response.

TABLE 4
MEAN HEART-RATE RESPONSE FOR EACH TRIAL

		Trial 1	Trial 2	Trial 3
Long Distance	M	157	149	152
	SD	5	8	5
Short Distance	M	156	150	156
	SD	5	6	5
Control	M	163	165	161
	SD	6	6	4

Note.—Trials 1 and 3 are 30 km each for long distance and short distance groups. Trial 2 is covariate and deception trial of 36 km for the long distance group, 24 km for the short distance group, and 30 km for the control group.

DISCUSSION

We hypothesised that, if persons were deceived or deprived of the predetermined end-point, an adjustment to their perceived effort for the subsequent exercise bout would be made relative to the previously experienced effort. This is based on the model that subjects may regulate performance by central calculations stemming from previous experience and efferent commands that integrate metabolic and biomechanical limits of the body in relation to the immediate task (Ulmer, 1996). In the present situation this suggests that, when an initial exercise bout is followed by another more difficult bout, then a further exercise bout which is similar in perceived difficulty to the initial bout should see either a decrease in time to complete the trial or an increase in intensity of effort. Indeed, on Trial 1 when subjects were told and actually cycled 30 km, an effort template would have been set for this particular distance. However, on Trial 2 subjects were told that they would be required to reproduce the same effort as on Trial 1 but were actually deceived about the actual distance cycled. It was hypothesised that an adjustment to the effort template would be made but that adjustment would only be manifest in a subsequent trial designed to elicit similar responses as those on Trial 1. According to the present results, subjects deceived of the actual distance adjust their pacing strategy such that the time to complete the distance reflects the effort template set by the expectation. This finding alone indicates that the deception of actual distance and end-point alters the perceived effort in accordance with what is thought to be required to complete the exercise bout successfully. This point is strengthened by the fact that no deception leads to stable times for completion of the 30 km as evidenced by the control group.

The present findings are consistent with the teleoanticipation model (proposed by Ulmer, 1996) which is thought to act as a safety mechanism controlling exercise intensity by down-regulating the efferent command to muscles, attenuating the accumulation of metabolites or substrate depletion, and maintaining metabolic activity within a safe range. However, the present findings indicate that a teleoanticipation model requires insight to the impending end-point and required effort. When the end-point is not provided subjects are unable to set the appropriate effort template. This is most evident in the two groups for whom deception of distance was used, in contrast to the control group with whom no deception was used and distance remained constant for the three trials.

Although some findings of the present study are surprising, some results are in agreement with previous work. For example, in the present study power output during Trial 1 was systematically attenuated over time for each group and agrees with previous findings (Häkkinen & Komi, 1983; Crenshaw, Karlsson, Gerdle, & Friden, 1991; Gerdle, Karlsson, Crenshaw, & Friden, 1997). However, following the deception trial and compared with Trial 1, the long distance group on Trial 3 increased power output with the overall effect being a decreased time to complete the trial. In contrast, the short distance group decreased power output during Trial 3 with the cumulative effect being an increase in the total time to complete the trial compared with that for Trial 1. These data present an interesting proposition in relation to pacing strategy. That is, for the long distance group, the deception of the requirement for increased effort allowed subjects to adjust the effort template to an appropriate power output in contrast to the effort template that would have been used on Trial 1 which would not have been perceived sufficient to allow successful completion of the trial. However, for the short distance group the deception of reduced effort on Trial 2 allowed subjects to set the power output for the expectation of a shorter or easier bout, but because Trial 3 was actually more difficult than anticipated the overall effect was an increased time to complete the trial.

These data support previous findings (Kay, *et al.*, 2001) which suggest a subconscious control of efferent neural command where muscle activation was systematically reduced along with power output until the final sprint when power output was restored near initial values. In the present study a final burst or increase in power output was not evident probably because the subjects had no cue as to the remaining distance to be covered. The only available cue to the subject was past experience or an effort template set from the previous trials.

Interestingly, the heart-rate response in the present study is not completely representative of the power outputs or the intensity of each experimental condition. For all conditions the mean heart rate remained unchanged between trials. Nonetheless, these findings are consistent with previous work which shows heart rate to be similar regardless of the physiological requirements of the task, provided that the perception of effort is similar (Nikolopoulos, *et al.*, 2001). Direct evidence for this comes from a recent study where hypnotic manipulation of effort sense was used to examine cardiovascular responses (Williamson, McColl, Matthews, Mitchell, Raven, & Morgan, 2001). In that study, subjects undertook constant-load exercise under three hypnotic conditions (1) perceived level grade, (2) perceived downhill grade, and (3) perceived uphill grade. The suggestion of downhill cycling decreased RPE but not heart rate, with the suggestion of uphill cycling increasing both RPE and heart rate. The authors concluded that increases in effort sense can elevate cardiovascular responses but decreases in effort sense do not reduce cardiovascular responses below the level required to sustain metabolic needs (Williamson, *et al.*, 2001). Hence, in the present study it is possible that the effort sense may have been reduced for the short distance group and increased for the long distance group, with the heart-rate response on Trial 3 maintained at a level required for metabolic needs.

In conclusion, the present findings suggest that individuals deceived about the actual distance will select a pacing strategy based on the perceived effort. This is evidenced by the changes in power output which seem to be dependent on the expected effort and that heart rate was not altered according to the intensity but rather seemed to be adjusted to the minimal metabolic demands.

REFERENCES

BORG, G. A. V. (1982) Psychological bases of physical exertion. *Medicine and Science in Sports and Exercise*, 14, 377-381.

CRENSHAW, A. G., KARLSSON, S., GERDLE, B., & FRIDEN, J. (1991) Differential responses in intramuscular pressure and EMG fatigue indicators during low-vs-high-level isometric contractions to fatigue. *Acta Physiologica Scandinavica*, 160, 353-361.

DUBOIS, D., & DUBOIS, E. F. (1916) A formula to estimate the approximate surface area if height and weight be known. *Archives of Internal Medicine*, 17, 831-836.

GERDLE, B., KARLSSON, S., CRENSHAW, A. G., & FRIDEN, J. (1997) The relationships between EMG and muscle morphology throughout sustained static knee extension at two submaximal force levels. *Acta Physiologica Scandinavica*, 160, 341-351.

HÄKKINEN, K., & KOMI, P. V. (1983) Electromyographic and mechanical characteristics of human skeletal muscle during fatigue under voluntary and reflex conditions. *Electroencephalography and Clinical Neurophysiology*, 55, 436-444.

HUCK, S. W., CORMIER, W. H., & BOUNDS, W. C. (1974) *Reading statistics and research*. New York: Harper & Row.

KAY, D., MARINO, F. E., CANNON, J., ST CLAIR GIBSON, A., LAMBERT, M. I., & NOAKES, T. D. (2001) Evidence for neuromuscular fatigue during high-intensity cycling in warm, humid conditions. *European Journal of Applied Physiology*, 84, 115-121.

NIKOLOPOULOS, V., ARKINSTALL, M. J., & HAWLEY, J. A. (2001) Pacing strategy in simulated cycle time-trials is based on perceived rather than actual distance. *Journal of Science and Medicine in Sport*, 4, 212-219.

SIRI, W. E. (1961) Body composition from fluid spaces and density: analysis of method. In J. Brozek & A. Henschel (Eds.), *Techniques for measuring body composition*. Washington, DC: National Academy of Science. Pp. 223-224.

ST CLAIR GIBSON, A., SCHABORT, E. J., & NOAKES, T. D. (2001) Reduced neuromuscular activity and force generation during prolonged cycling. *American Journal of Physiology: Regulatory, Integrative and Comparative Physiology*, 71, R187-R196.

ULMER, H. V. (1996) Concept of an extracellular regulation of muscular metabolic rate during heavy exercise in humans by psychophysiological feedback. *Experientia*, 52, 416-420.

WILLIAMSON, J. W., MCCOLL, R., MATTHEWS, D., MITCHELL, J. H., RAVEN, P. B., & MORGAN, W. P. (2001) Hypnotic manipulation of effort sense during dynamic exercise: cardiovascular responses and brain activation. *Journal of Applied Physiology*, 90, 1392-1399.

Accepted March 22, 2004.

DECEPTION AND PERCEIVED EXERTION DURING HIGH-INTENSITY RUNNING BOUTS [1]

DAVID B. HAMPSON, ALAN ST CLAIR GIBSON, MIKE I. LAMBERT,
JONATHAN P. DUGAS, ESTELLE V. LAMBERT, AND TIMOTHY D. NOAKES

MRC/UCT Research Unit of Exercise Science and Sports Medicine
Department of Human Biology
University of Cape Town

Summary.—This investigation examined the overall and localized perceived exertion responses to repeated bouts of submaximal, high-intensity running when subjects were deceived. Well-trained male and female ($n = 40$) runners were randomly assigned to four groups who completed three 1680-m bouts of running at 80–86% peak treadmill running speed. The two experimental groups, Expected Similar and Expected Increase, were deceived of the actual run intensities while the two control groups, Control Increase and Control Similar, were informed of the actual protocol. After each run, ratings of perceived exertion (RPE) were taken for the whole body, chest, legs, head, and other areas. No significant differences were found in overall RPE between deceived and control groups. However, there was a tendency for the Expected Increase group, deceived into believing the intensity would be higher than they were subsequently made to run, to experience an attenuated increase in RPE between runs compared to the control group (Control Increase) who were honestly informed. For all groups, legs and chest were given consistently higher localized exertion scores than the head and other areas. It appears that a precise system of afferent feedback mediates the overall perceived exertion response during high-intensity running, and psychological intervention that alters pre-exercise expectations has minimal feedforward effect on exertion ratings taken postexercise.

The perception of exertion during exercise is a phenomenon that, despite being widely studied, is still not well understood. The most widely utilized scale for quantification of perceived exertion remains the Borg 15-point (ratings of perceived exertion) RPE scale introduced in 1967 (Mihevic, 1981). It has since become the standard instrument for evaluating the perception of whole body exertion during exercise and has been shown to be an accurate and reliable measure of exercise intensity (Mihevic, 1981; Robertson & Noble, 1997).

Despite widespread use of the RPE scale to prescribe and monitor exercise intensity, it is not clear how the brain interprets afferent feedback to induce the perception of exertion during exercise (Mihevic, 1981; Carton &

---

[1]Address correspondence to Alan St Clair Gibson, MRC/UCT Research Unit of Exercise Science and Sports Medicine, Department of Human Biology, University of Cape Town Faculty of Health Sciences, Sports Science Institute of South Africa, P.O. Box 115, Newlands 7725, South Africa or e-mail (agibson@sports.uct.ac.za).

Rhodes, 1985; Hampson, St Clair Gibson, Lambert, & Noakes, 2001). This feedback may be categorized, for example, as either cardiopulmonary or peripheral. Cardiopulmonary factors include such variables as respiratory rate, minute ventilation, heart rate, and oxygen consumption, while peripheral factors include lactate concentration, muscular strain, and skin temperature. It has been suggested that an integration of these sensory cues may indirectly and unconsciously influence the perception of effort during exercise (Pandolf, 1982). However, the extent to which each of these variables influences perceived exertion is not evident from the contradictory literature in this area (Mihevic, 1981).

As a conscious sensory modality, the perception of exertion and fatigue may be modifiable by psychological interventions. Several investigations have shown that exertion can be modified by hypnotic suggestion (Morgan, Raven, Drinkwater, & Horvath, 1973; Morgan, Hirta, Weitz, & Balke, 1976; Williamson, McColl, Mathews, Mitchell, Raven, & Morgan, 2001). In addition, Rejeski and Ribisil (1980) have shown an attenuated perceived exertion response when actual exercise duration is shorter than expected (Rejeski & Ribisil, 1980). However, the above investigations utilized low to moderate exercise intensities. It has been suggested that psychological factors become less important at high exercise intensities, and afferent sensations become the predominant mediator of effort perception (Noble & Robertson, 1996).

To our knowledge, no study has examined how perceived exertion is altered during high-intensity exercise when actual exercise intensity is different from expected intensity. So, the purpose of this study was to examine physiological and psychological responses both when subjects were made aware of changes in running speed and when subjects expected an increase in running speed, when in fact, running velocity was held constant. If a feedforward system controlled the perception of fatigue and this system was centrally modifiable, an athlete's perception of fatigue would be affected by psychological manipulations. However, if a precise system of afferent feedback regulation is in place to prevent reaching the body's physiological limits, the strong afferent signals derived from high-intensity exercise should override any psychological influence on perception. Accordingly, this study examined whether subjects' RPE would be modulated by deception of exercise intensity, or whether the subjects would exhibit a similar RPE response irrespective of whether they were consciously aware of the exercise intensity or were deceived.

Method

Pilot Testing

Prior to recruitment of our subjects, a series of pilot tests were conducted on volunteer runners ($n = 4$) to specify the appropriate range of intensities for the experimental trial. Based on this pilot testing, three speeds (80%, 83%, and 86% peak treadmill running speed) were selected for the experimental trials. This was a range large enough to produce differences in perceived exertion and heart rate, but narrow enough to deceive the subjects that they were running at any of the three intensities within that range.

Subjects

Trained runners ($n=40$) who currently ran three or more times per week were recruited for this study. Their training status was confirmed by a training questionnaire subjects were asked to complete. This study was approved by the Ethics and Research Committee of the Faculty of Health Sciences, University of Cape Town, and all subjects completed a written informed consent prior to any testing procedures. The total subject pool was randomly divided into two experimental ($n=10$) and two control ($n=10$) groups. Upon recruitment, subjects were informed that they would participate in a repeatability study involving a VO_2 max test and a trial of three 1680-m running bouts at submaximal speeds with 10 min. standing recovery between each. Subjects randomized into Experimental Group 1 (Expected Similar) were told that all 1680-m running bouts would be run at 83% of peak treadmill running speed, when in fact they were made to run at intensities of 80%, 83%, and 86% of peak treadmill running speed. In contrast, subjects randomized into Control Group 1 (Control Increase) were informed of the true protocol, which included 1680-m runs at 80%, 83%, and 86% peak treadmill running speed. Exercise intensities were presented in random order for subjects in Expected Similar and Control Increase groups. This was done to examine the perception of exercise intensity separately from the perception of fatigue. Subjects in Experimental Group 2 (Expected Increase) were told that they would run at 80%, 83%, and 86% of peak treadmill running speed, while they were actually made to run at 83% peak treadmill running speed for all three run bouts. Control Group 2 (Control Similar) included subjects who were correctly informed that all runs would be completed at 83% peak treadmill running speed. Thus, subjects in Expected Similar and Control Increase ran at the same intensities (80%, 83%, and 86% peak treadmill running speed) as did subjects in Expected Increase and Control Similar (83% peak treadmill running speed for each run) groups. To our knowledge, all subjects were unaware of the true nature of the trial for the duration of the trial.

To ensure that all subjects would be able to complete the session, they were instructed not to conduct any long or intense training the day preceding each running trial.

Exertion Scales

Experienced subjective exertion was quantified on two different scales, the Borg 15-point RPE scale and the Borg category-ratio scale. Printed instructions were provided to familiarize subjects with each scale prior to the VO_2 max test. Instructions were given for the RPE scale as suggested by Pandolf (1982). Subjects were asked to provide a single appropriate score on the 15 point scale that was the best representation of an overall level of exertion. No assistance was given by the researcher in translating their feelings into numerical ratings on the RPE scale. The Borg category-ratio exertion scale was used to quantify exertion localized to the head, chest, legs, and other areas. The category-ratio scale was selected to measure localized exertion because the growth of this scale more closely parallels the exponential increase in many of the parameters associated with peripheral exertion, i.e., ventilation, respiratory rate, lactate, and perceived muscular strain (Noble, 1982; Noble, Borg, Jacobs, Ceci, & Kaiser, 1983; Hassmén, 1990). As suggested by Borg (1973), subjects were instructed to use decimals where appropriate, as well as produce ratings below and above the limits of the scale (0.5 to 10) if necessary (Noble, et al., 1983).

Subjects were familiarized with these exertion scales twice prior to the experimental trial, once during the maximal treadmill run, and once during the track familiarization run.

VO_2 peak Measurements and Peak Treadmill Running Speed

Determination of each subject's peak oxygen consumption (VO_2 peak) and peak treadmill running speed were completed during their first visit to the laboratory following a standard protocol (Noakes, Myburgh, & Schall, 1990). The testing procedure involved an easy 10- to 15-min. warm-up period on the treadmill at the subject's chosen pace, followed by a 5-min. rest. The maximal test then began on a horizontal treadmill grade with a starting speed of 12 km · hr.$^{-1}$. The starting speed was maintained for 60 sec., followed by an increase in speed of the treadmill belt of 0.5 km · hr.$^{-1}$ each 30 sec. until volitional fatigue occurred. Subjects were given verbal encouragement throughout the test to ensure maximal effort. The peak speed maintained 30 sec. prior to test termination was taken as the peak treadmill running speed. Throughout the test, the volume and composition of gases expired were measured by indirect calorimetry using an automated gas analysis system (Oxycon Alpha®, Enrich JAEGER, Wuerzburg, Germany). The system was calibrated against known standards prior to each test. The gas meters were calibrated with a 3-litre syringe (Hans Rudolf), and the gas analyzers were calibrated with a gas mixture containing 4.5% CO_2, with the remainder made up of a N_2/O_2 mixture. The VO_2 peak was defined as the highest rage of oxygen consumption recorded during a 30-sec. average. Maximum heart rate was recorded on a telemetric heart-rate monitor (Polar® Heart Rate Monitors, Finland). After termination of the test, subjects were asked to rate their overall sensation of exertion for the level which coincided with fatigue utilizing Borg's 15-point RPE scale. Exertion was quantified on the Borg category-ratio scale for the head, legs, and chest. Subjects were also asked to report on any other relevant area in which they felt localized exertion.

Familiarization Trial

Subsequent to the VO_2 peak test, but on the same day, subjects completed a familiarization trial of running on the indoor track with the pacing lights utilized during the experimental trial. The pacing lights were placed on the inner circumference of the track at an interval of 5 m and were linked to a digital control panel which could be set such that the lights would blink sequentially at a given running velocity. The runner followed the blinking series of lights to run at the required velocity. However, since this was a novel experience for many runners, it was important they familiarized themselves with this technique before the experimental trial. The pacing lights were set to blink coinciding with a velocity of 70% peak treadmill running speed, and subjects completed 10 min. of continuous running. Subsequent to the run, subjects rated their exertion on the overall and localized RPE scales. This was done to give subjects further practice utilizing these scales.

Submaximal Running Trials

Subjects were asked to report back to the laboratory within 7 to 10 days of the VO_2 max test for the submaximal running trial. These running trials were conducted on a 140-m indoor track, and velocity was set with the pacing light system as described above. Just prior to each trial, subjects completed a standardized 1400-m warm-up at 60% peak treadmill running speed, followed by a 5-min. rest. The three 1680-m running bouts were run at speeds of 80%, 83%, and 86% peak treadmill running speed presented in random order for Expected Similar and Control Increase groups. Expected Increase and Control Similar groups completed all runs at 83% peak treadmill running speed. During the trials, heart rate was measured with a portable heart-rate monitor (Polar® Heart Rate Monitors, Finland) that could be downloaded to a computer software program for analysis. Prior to initiating the trial and during the 3-min. rest between runs subjects rated their exertion on the RPE and localized scales.

Statistical Analysis

All data were analyzed using a statistical software package (Statistica©, StatSoft, Inc., Tulsa, OK, USA). A one-way analysis of variance was conducted to compare group means for descriptive characteristics. Given the nature of the protocol (exercise intensity was presented in random order for

Expected Similar and Control Increase but not for Expected Increase and Control Similar groups), comparisons in outcome measures could not be made among all four groups. Differences between Expected Similar and Control Increase and Expected Increase and Control Similar were analyzed with a two-way analysis of variance for repeated measures. *Post hoc* analysis was conducted with Scheffé's test. An alpha level of .05 was taken as statistically significant.

RESULTS

Descriptive characteristics of subjects are shown in Table 1. Twenty-eight men and 12 women participated in the trial. The mean age of all the subjects was 28 ± 10 yr. There were no significant differences between groups for age, weight, height, percentage body fat, peak treadmill running speed, maximum heart rate, or VO_2 peak.

TABLE 1
SUBJECTS' CHARACTERISTICS BY GROUP

	Expected Similar M	Expected Similar SD	Control Increase M	Control Increase SD	Expected Increase M	Expected Increase SD	Control Similar M	Control Similar SD
Age, yr.	31.2	11.5	28.4	11.3	28.8	10.1	25.1	8.0
Weight, kg	66.4	12.6	66.7	13.6	67.4	10.4	67.8	6.9
Body fat, %	15.8	6.3	18.2	5.5	16.1	5.3	16.9	6.4
Peak treadmill running speed, km/hr.	18.7	1.8	17.9	1.8	19.6	3.1	18.3	2.5
Max heart rate, bpm	186	12	183	10	185	10	185	17
VO_2 peak, ml · kg · min.$^{-1}$	62.6	4.5	59.5	5.7	64.5	11.0	60.2	10.8

Heart rate and RPE responses for all groups and all runs are displayed in Table 2. There were no significant differences between Expected Similar and Control Increase or Expected Increase and Control Similar groups for variables of heart rate, RPE overall, RPE chest, RPE legs, RPE head, and RPE other. For Expected Similar and Control Increase groups there were differences between intensities for heart rate, RPE overall, RPE chest, RPE legs, and RPE head. No significant differences were found between runs for RPE other. For Expected Increase and Control Similar groups there were differences between runs for heart rate and RPE overall. Only Expected Increase showed no differences between runs for RPE chest and RPE legs. No significant differences were found between runs for either group for RPE head and RPE other. No significant correlation was found between heart rate and RPE ($r = .19$) when the data from all runs for the four groups were combined.

TABLE 2
HEART RATE AND RPE VALUES FOR THREE DIFFERENT RUNS

		Run 1 M	Run 1 SD	Run 2 M	Run 2 SD	Run 3 M	Run 3 SD	Significant Comparisons*
Heart Rate	Expected Similar	164	14	167	12	169	12	1 v 2, 1 v 3, 2 v 3
	Control Increase	173	12	176	11	178	11	1 v 2, 1 v 3, 2 v 3
	Expected Increase	173	10	177	9	178	10	1 v 2, 1 v 3
	Control Similar	179	17	183	17	184	17	1 v 2, 1 v 3
RPE Overall	Expected Similar	12.9	1.7	14.0	1.8	15.3	1.3	2 v 3, 1 v 3
	Control Increase	14.2	2.0	15.3	1.8	16.6	1.8	1 v 3, 2 v 3
	Expected Increase	13.6	1.5	14.0	1.8	14.0	2.8	1 v 3
	Control Similar	12.5	2.1	14.1	2.7	15.3	2.4	1 v 3
RPE Chest	Expected Similar	4.0	1.5	4.9	1.9	5.9	2.2	1 v 2, 1 v 3
	Control Increase	4.7	1.9	5.6	2.0	6.7	1.7	1 v 2, 1 v 3
	Expected Increase	4.1	2.1	4.4	2.0	4.4	2.0	
	Control Similar	3.9	1.7	4.4	2.1	5.1	1.9	1 v 3
RPE Legs	Expected Similar	4.1	1.3	5.1	1.5	5.8	1.4	1 v 2, 1 v 3
	Control Increase	4.8	1.8	5.8	1.7	6.4	1.5	1 v 2, 1 v 3
	Expected Increase	4.6	2.8	4.3	2.2	4.5	2.7	
	Control Similar	3.4	2.0	4.3	2.0	5.1	2.0	
RPE Head	Expected Similar	2.4	1.7	2.9	1.0	3.8	2.4	1 v 2
	Control Increase	2.8	2.8	3.5	3.1	4.2	3.4	1 v 2
	Expected Increase	2.1	2.1	2.2	2.1	2.5	2.2	
	Control Similar	2.3	2.5	2.3	2.1	2.7	2.7	
RPE Other	Expected Similar	1.0	2.0	1.9	2.8	2.1	3.1	1 v 2
	Control Increase	1.2	2.0	1.8	2.6	2.7	2.7	1 v 2
	Expected Increase	1.5	3.2	1.0	2.3	0.6	1.9	
	Control Similar	0.3	0.5	1.0	1.6	1.6	2.5	

*$p < .05$.

DISCUSSION

Humans are able to perceive accurately the intensity at which they are exercising under normal circumstances, although the biological mechanisms underlying this ability are poorly understood. The aim of this study was to determine whether the accuracy of perception during high-intensity exercise would be perturbed by deception. The hypothesis was that, if a feedforward system originating in cognitive brain structures controlled the overall perception of fatigue, this perception would be modifiable by psychological manipulations. The alternate hypothesis was that, if a precise system of afferent feedback regulation was responsible for controlling the perception of fatigue, the afferent signals derived from high-intensity exercise should override any psychological influence of perception.

The most significant finding was that all subjects had a similar overall RPE and heart-rate response irrespective of whether they were honestly informed or deceived of the actual run intensity. This suggests a precise system of afferent feedback interpretation to monitor high-intensity exercise at a subconscious level, and this interpretation mediates the conscious perception of effort.

These results contrast the finding that perceived exertion can be modified in a feedforward manner with psychological interventions. Morgan, *et al.* (1973, 1976) and Williamson, *et al.* (2001) conducted several studies in which subjects cycled at a constant workload under hypnosis while being told that they were cycling up a steep grade, cycling on level terrain, or coasting downhill. The subjects' perceived exertion changed in accord with each hypnotic suggestion. Furthermore, Pelah and Barlow (1996) showed that immediately after running on a treadmill, a sensation of accelerated self-motion occurred during postexercise walking. Differences between the results of these investigations and the present study may be a consequence of differences in perception or afferent sensory interpretation in the hypnotic vs waking state. Deception may thus be more likely to influence perception when the subject is under hypnosis. Further, in our study, it is impossible to speculate what contribution feedforward commands made to the perceptual and physiological responses, as RPE measures were only taken immediately after each run. At this point, any initial feedforward effect on effort perception may have been overridden by afferent feedback. Nevertheless, a mild feedforward effect is suggested by the nonsignificant attenuation of chest and legs RPE response between running bouts for the Expected Increase group. In contrast, there was a significant increase in RPE between running bouts for the Control Similar group. Because subjects in the Expected Increase group expected the intensity to be more difficult with each subsequent run, they may have interpreted the afferent input differently when it was less intense than expected. Similarly, Rejeski and Ribisil (1980) have shown an attenuated RPE response when exercise duration is shorter than expected. In their investigation, when subjects who were told they would be running for 30 min. were stopped at 20 min., they produced a lower exertion rating during that period than subjects who were honestly informed of the 20-min. trial duration. Taken together, these results suggest that, when a stimulus is presented at a lower grade (workload, duration, etc.) than was originally expected, it may be consciously perceived as less intense than it would be perceived if the stimulus matches the expected gradation.

It has been suggested that afferent input from different areas of the body induces a perception of exertion that causes the individual to stop exercise or reduce work output before ever reaching a maximal physiological capacity (Hampson, et al., 2001). Termination of exercise with a physiological reserve is suggested by the finding that individuals terminate exercise at altitude with a reduction in cardiac output, muscle recruitment, and lactate accumulation compared with sea level values (Sutton, Reeves, Wagner, Groves, Cymerman, Malconian, Rock, Young, Walter, & Houston, 1988; Kayser, Narici, Binzoni, Grassi, & Cerretelli, 1994), that the decrements in force output during maximal sprints are coupled with reduced muscle recruitment (Kay, Marino, Cannon, St Clair, Lambert, & Noakes, 2001; St Clair Gibson, Schabort, & Noakes, 2001), that ATP levels never fall below 60–70% of resting values during exercise (Spriet, Soderlund, Bergstrom, & Hultman, 1987; Fitts, 1994), and consequently rigor does not develop during maximal exercise under any circumstances (Noakes, 2000). Were such a protective mechanism in place, afferent sensory feedback would become the primary determinant of effort perception at high exercise intensities at which the individual encroaches upon a maximal capacity. This may also explain why, in the present study where exercise intensities of 80–86% peak treadmill running speed were utilized, psychological intervention (deception) had little or no effect on postexercise overall perceived exertion measures.

A secondary finding of this study is that there were distinct differences in the localized areas in which exertion was perceived. The afferent signals which may have the most influence on effort perception during high-intensity exercise appear to be derived from the chest and the legs. This is not a surprising finding, as previous investigations have related perception of effort to both cardiopulmonary and peripheral factors (Hampson, et al., 2001). Other research has yielded a relationship between RPE and minute ventilation (Noble, Metz, Pandolf, & Cafarelli, 1973; Robertson, 1982), respiratory rate (Noble, Metz, Pandolf, & Cafarelli, 1973), heart rate (Borg & Linderholm, 1967; Bar-Or, Skinner, Buskirk, & Borg, 1972; Borg, 1973; Skinner, Hutsler, Bergsteinova, & Buskirk, 1973; Stamford & Noble, 1976), oxygen consumption (Skinner, et al., 1973; Robertson, Gilcher, & Metz, 1979), blood lactate (Edwards, Melcher, Hesser, Wigertz, & Ekelund, 1972; Gamberale, 1972; Hetzler, Seip, Boutcher, Pierce, Snead, & Weltman, 1991), and muscular strain (Noble, Metz, Pandolf, Bell, Cafarelli, & Sime, 1973; Skinner, et al., 1973; Stamford & Noble, 1974; Takai, 1998). However, studies of perceived exertion have not isolated a single variable associated with RPE in all circumstances. Accordingly, it may be concluded that conscious perception of exertion is a consequence of the integration of multiple afferent signals and that the primary determinants of RPE arise from the chest and active muscle mass.

An additional important finding was the low correlation between heart rate and RPE. The Borg scale was developed as a category scale to reflect the linear relationship between RPE and heart rate during incremental exercise. Borg suggested that the heart rate should be about 10 times the RPE for healthy middle-aged men at moderate to hard intensities (Borg, 1973). Other studies have yielded a significant correlation between heart rate and RPE across sexes (Skinner, et al., 1973; Stamford & Noble, 1976), exercise modality, and intermittent or continuous exercise protocols. (Edwards, et al., 1972). The lack of a correlation in the present study may be explained by the limited range of intensities utilized, steady-state nature of the exercise, and duration of the run bouts. The above studies utilized a wider range of intensities and short bouts of exercise. In addition, other studies have shown that heart rate can be dissociated from RPE (Ekblom & Goldbarg, 1971; Pandolf, Cafarelli, Noble, & Metz, 1972; Kamon, Pandolf, & Cafarelli, 1974; Pandolf, Kamon, & Noble, 1978; Davies & Sargeant, 1979). Thus, heart rate is likely indirectly related to RPE or only one of multiple mediators of perceived exertion.

It must be noted that a relatively small sample was used for this study. Further, as with all psychophysiological testing, a problem is that the body is only approximated by measured physiological indices, and perceptual state is only approximated by these physiological indices. Thus the results of any psychophysiological study using correlations between physiological changes and perceptual states should be interpreted with caution.

In summary, these results demonstrate that, at high exercise intensities, the overall perception of exertion is primarily a consequence of afferent sensory feedback. Psychological deception that influences pre-exercise expectations has a limited role in postexercise effort perception and appears to have a mild influence on RPE only when the workload (intensity) is lower than expected. A limit of the present design was that exertion measures were only taken at the completion of each run. Any feedforward effect deception may have had on the initial perception of exertion would only have been apparent if perceived exertion measures were taken early in the exercise session. Subsequent designs in this area of effort perception should include measures of exertion during the initial seconds of the exercise bout to isolate a feedforward effect. A greater understanding of the role of psychological and physiological variables in the perception of exertion is an important step towards elucidating how human exercise performance is regulated by effort perception such as to avoid premature fatigue or overexertion.

REFERENCES

BAR-OR, O., SKINNER, J. S., BUSKIRK, E. R., & BORG, G. (1972) Physiological and perceptual indicators of physical stress in 41- to 60-year-old men who vary in conditioning level and body fatness. *Medicine and Science in Sports*, 4, 96-100.

BORG, G. A. (1973) Perceived exertion: a note on "history" and methods. *Medicine and Science in Sports*, 5, 90-93.

BORG, G. A., & LINDERHOLM, H. (1967) Perceived exertion and pulse rate during graded exercise in various age groups. *Acta Medica Scandinavica*, (Suppl. 472), 194-206.

CARTON, R. L., & RHODES, E. C. (1985) A critical review of the literature on ratings scales for perceived exertion. *Sports Medicine*, 2, 198-222.

DAVIES, C. T., & SARGEANT, A. J. (1979) The effects of atropine and protolol on the perception of exertion during treadmill exercise. *Ergonomics*, 22, 1141-1146.

EDWARDS, R. H., MELCHER, A., HESSER, C. M., WIGERTZ, O., & EKELUND, L. G. (1972) Physiological correlates of perceived exertion in continuous and intermittent exercise with the same average power output. *European Journal of Clinical Investigation*, 2, 108-114.

EKBLOM, B., & GOLDBARG, A. N. (1971) The influence of physical training and other factors on the subjective rating of perceived exertion. *Acta Physiologica Scandinavica*, 83, 399-406.

FITTS, R. H. (1994) Cellular mechanisms of muscle fatigue. *Physiological Review*, 74, 49-94.

GAMBERALE, F. (1972) Perceived exertion, heart rate, oxygen uptake and blood lactate in different work operations. *Ergonomics*, 15, 545-554.

HAMPSON, D. B., ST CLAIR GIBSON, A. C., LAMBERT, M. I., & NOAKES, T. D. (2001) The influence of sensory cues on the perception of exertion during exercise and central regulation of exercise performance. *Sports Medicine*, 31, 935-952.

HASSMÉN, P. (1990) Perceptual and physiological responses to cycling and running in groups of trained and untrained subjects. *European Journal of Applied Physiology*, 60, 445-451.

HETZLER, R. K., SEIP, R. L., BOUTCHER, S. H., PIERCE, E., SNEAD, D., & WELTMAN, A. (1991) Effect of exercise modality on ratings of perceived exertion at various lactate concentrations. *Medicine and Science in Sports*, 23, 88-92.

KAMON, E., PANDOLF, K., & CAFARELLI, E. (1974) [The relationship between perceptual information and physiological responses to exercise in the heat]. *[Journal of Human Ergology (Tokyo)]*, 3, 45-54.

KAY, D., MARINO, F. E., CANNON, J., ST CLAIR GIBSON A., LAMBERT, M. I., & NOAKES, T. D. (2001) Evidence for neuromuscular fatigue during high-intensity cycling in warm humid conditions. *European Journal of Applied Physiology*, 84, 115-121.

KAYSER, B., NARICI, M., BINZONI, T., GRASSI, B., & CERRETELLI, P. (1994) Fatigue and exhaustion in chronic hypobaric hypoxia: influence of exercising muscle mass. *Journal of Applied Physiology*, 76, 634-640.

MIHEVIC, P. M. (1981) Sensory cues for perceived exertion: a review. *Medicine and Science in Sports*, 13, 150-163.

MORGAN, W. P., HIRTA, K., WEITZ, G. A., & BALKE, B. (1976) Hypnotic perturbation of perceived exertion: ventilatory consequences. *American Journal of Clinical Hypnosis*, 18, 182-190.

MORGAN, W. P., RAVEN, P. B., DRINKWATER, B. L., & HORVATH, S. M. (1973) Perceptual and metabolic responsivity to standard bicycle ergometry following various hypnotic suggestions. *International Journal of Clinical and Experimental Hypnosis*, 21, 86-101.

NOAKES, T. D. (2000) Physiological models to understand exercise fatigue and the adaptations that predict or enhance athletic performance. *Scandinavian Journal of Medicine and Science in Sports*, 10, 123-145.

NOAKES, T. D., MYBURGH, K. H., & SCHALL, R. (1990) Peak treadmill running velocity during the VO_2 max test predicts running performance. *Journal of Sports Science*, 8, 35-45.

NOBLE, B. J., BORG, G. A., JACOBS, I., CECI, R., & KAISER, P. (1983) A category-ratio perceived exertion scale: relationship to blood and muscle lactates and heart rate. *Medicine and Science in Sports*, 15, 523-528.

NOBLE, B. J., METZ, K. F., PANDOLF, K. B., BELL, C. W., CAFARELLI, E., & SIME, W. E. (1973) Perceived exertion during walking and running: II. *Medicine and Science in Sports*, 5, 116-120.

NOBLE, B J., METZ, K. F., PANDOLF, K. B., & CAFARELLI, E. (1973) Perceptual responses to exercise: a multiple regression study. *Medicine and Science in Sports*, 5, 104-109.

NOBLE, B. J., & ROBERTSON, R. J. (1996) *Perceived exertion*. Champaign, IL: Human Kinetics.

PANDOLF, K. B. (1982) Differentiated ratings of perceived exertion during physical exercise. *Medicine and Science in Sports*, 14, 397-405.

PANDOLF, K. B., CAFARELLI, E., NOBLE, B. J., & METZ, K. F. (1972) Perceptual responses during prolonged work. *Perceptual and Motor Skills*, 35, 975-985.

PANDOLF, K. B., KAMON, E., & NOBLE, B. J. (1978) Perceived exertion and physiological responses during negative and positive work in climbing a laddermill. *Journal of Sports Medicine and Physical Fitness*, 18, 227-236.

PELAH, A., & BARLOW, H. B. (1996) Visual illusion from running. *Nature*, 381, 283.

REJESKI, W. J., & RIBISIL, P. M. (1980) Expected task duration and perceived effort: an attributional analysis. *Journal of Sport Psychology*, 2, 227-236.

ROBERTSON, R. J. (1982) Central signals of perceived exertion during dynamic exercise. *Medicine and Science in Sports*, 14, 390-396.

ROBERTSON, R. J., GILCHER, R., & METZ, K. (1979) Central circulation and work capacity after red blood cell reinfusion under normaloxia and hypoxia in women. *Medicine and Science in Sports*, 98. [Abstract]

ROBERTSON, R. J., & NOBLE, B. J. (1997) Perception of physical exertion: methods, mediators, and applications. *Exercise and Sport Science Review*, 25, 407-452.

SKINNER, J. S., HUTSLER, R., BERGSTEINOVA, V., & BUSKIRK, E. R. (1973) Perception of effort during different types of exercise and under different environmental conditions. *Medicine and Science in Sports*, 5, 110-115.

SPRIET, L. L., SODERLUND, K., BERGSTROM, M., & HULTMAN, E. (1987) Anaerobic energy release in skeletal muscle during electrical stimulation in men. *Journal of Applied Physiology*, 62, 611-615.

STAMFORD, B. A., & NOBLE, B. J. (1974) Metabolic cost and perception of effort during bicycle ergometer work performance. *Medicine and Science in Sports*, 6, 226-231.

STAMFORD, B. A., & NOBLE, B. J. (1976) Validity and reliability of subjective ratings of perceived exertion during work. *Ergonomics*, 19, 53-60.

ST CLAIR GIBSON, A., SCHABORT, E. J., & NOAKES, T. D. (2001) Reduced neuromuscular activity and force generation during prolonged cycling. *American Journal of Physiology: Regular and Integrative Comparative Physiology*, 281, R187-R196.

SUTTON, J. R., REEVES, J. T., WAGNER, P. D., GROVES, B. M., CYMERMAN, A., MALCONIAN, M. K., ROCK, P. B., YOUNG, P. M., WALTER, S. D., & HOUSTON, C. S. (1988) Operation Everest: II. Oxygen transport during exercise at extreme simulated altitude. *Journal of Applied Physiology*, 64, 1309-1321.

TAKAI, K. (1998) Cognitive strategies and recall of pace by long-distance runners. *Perceptual and Motor Skills*, 86, 763-770.

WILLIAMSON, J. W., MCCOLL, R., MATHEWS, D., MITCHELL, J. H., RAVEN, P. B., & MORGAN, W. P. (2001) Hypnotic manipulation of effort sense during dynamic exercise: cardiovascular responses and brain activation. *Journal of Applied Physiology*, 90, 1392-1399.

Accepted March 26, 2004.

IMPROVING ACCURACY OF VERACITY JUDGMENT THROUGH CUE TRAINING[1]

MARIA SANTARCANGELO, ROBERT A. CRIBBIE

York University

AMY S. EBESU HUBBARD

University of Hawaii at Manoa

Summary.—The ability to make judgments of veracity was investigated to see if training individuals on visual, vocal, or verbal content cues of deception would increase their ability to judge whether a message was truthful. The overall rate of accuracy of judging veracity was significantly greater for subjects trained on verbal content cues. More specifically, for detecting truthful messages, subjects trained on verbal content cues had significantly greater accuracy than subjects who received no cue training, whereas for detecting deceptive messages, there were no significant differences in accuracy among conditions.

Within daily interactions people often come across instances in which they must make judgments of veracity, i.e., evaluate whether someone is lying or telling the truth. Previous studies examining the rate of accuracy of human lie detection have shown the average accuracy barely exceeds chance expectations (Hocking & Leathers, 1980; DeTurck & Miller, 1985; Kohnken, 1987; DePaulo, Tornqvist, & Cooper, 2002). Even when the individuals who were detecting the deception were friends of the person communicating the message, the rates of accuracy were not significantly greater than chance (Anderson, DePaulo, & Ansfield, 2002). Stiff and Miller (1986) found that, when making judgments about the veracity of a message, individuals relied on a number of visual, vocal, and verbal cues unrelated to the actual veracity of the message. Research examining the cues used by individuals to make judgments of veracity has indicated little correspondence between the cues individuals perceive to be related to deception and the actual cues related to deception (DePaulo, Rosenthal, Rosenkrantz, & Green, 1982; DeTurck & Miller, 1985; Fiedler & Walka, 1993; Anderson, DePaulo, Ansfield, Tickle, & Green, 1999; DePaulo, Tornqvist, & Cooper, 2002). Zuckerman, Koestner, and Driver (1981) and Zuckerman, Koestner, and Colella (1985) investigated the beliefs about cues associated with deception and found that there are common stereotypes people hold about cues for deception and that these stereotyped cues were minimally correlated with actual cues for deception.

Beliefs about deception cues are often attributed to arousal theories of deception. Detecting deception is based on the assumption that a person

---

[1]Address correspondence to Robert A. Cribbie, Department of Psychology, York University, Toronto, ON Canada M3J 1P3 or e-mail (cribbie@yorku.ca).

who is being deceptive will experience increased physiological arousal compared to a person who is telling the truth. This arousal is an indicator of the guilty feelings, anxiety, embarrassment, or nervousness associated with lying. It is also assumed that arousal is an indicator of stress associated with cognitive attempts to construct believable messages or efforts to avoid mistakes (Hocking & Leathers, 1980; DeTurck & Miller, 1985; Fiedler & Walka, 1993). Detecting deception is made possible through the display of physiological arousal. Deception-induced arousal can be detected in physical, vocal, and verbal displays. However, a person who is being deceptive will deliberately try to control their behavioral displays to avoid suspicion (Hocking & Leathers, 1980; Zuckerman, *et al.*, 1981). According to Kraut (1978), "one should believe most in those aspects of a person's performance that the person is least able to deliberately and consciously control" (p. 381). Research has supported this statement and has found that there are behavioral displays unique to deception-induced arousal. DeTurck and Miller (1985) investigated the behavioral differences between people being deceptive and aroused truth-tellers and found that adaptors (such as scratching, stroking), hand gestures, speech errors, pauses, response latency, and message duration reliably distinguished people being deceptive from unaroused truth-tellers and also from aroused truth-tellers.

Training individuals on the behavioral cues related to deception-induced arousal has increased the rate of accuracy of detecting deception (DeTurck & Miller, 1990; Fiedler & Walka, 1993). Training improved the ability to detect deception in those who were high self-monitors and who had rehearsed their lies. These are two groups whose deception is difficult to detect (DeTurck & Miller, 1990). DePaulo, Lassiter, and Stone (1982) found that subjects merely instructed to pay attention to tone of voice or words were more accurate at detecting deception than those who were told to pay attention to visual cues. On the other hand, Kohnken (1987) trained police officers to detect deception and found subjects who were trained were no more accurate than subjects in the control group who received no training. Kohnken concluded that cue training may have led to information-processing overload. Subjects in this study had to learn an extensive set of behavioral cues which hindered their detection of deception. By using fewer cues, observers may more fully utilize the cue information and make more accurate judgments.

Research on deception has often focused on examining the behaviors associated with deception communication. Results of these studies indicate that there are consistent verbal and nonverbal cues related to actual deception. For the purpose of this study, these cues have been categorized into verbal content cues, vocal cues, and visual cues.

Verbal Content Cues

Little research has focused on the verbal content cues related to deception. This is due to the belief that verbal content can be monitored and controlled by the speaker (Kraut, 1978; DePaulo, Rosenthal, Rosenkrantz, & Green, 1982). However, research on verbal content cues has indicated that cues within the speech content of people being deceptive (and those telling the truth) can actually be more reliable in detection of deception than nonverbal cues. DePaulo, Rosenthal, Rosenkrantz, and Green (1982) reported that speech can reliably indicate whether deception is occurring and that perceivers are often strongly influenced by speech in their judgments about deceit. In a study comparing verbal cues, vocal cues, and visual cues, only one verbal cue (verbal content) was related to actual deception (Stiff & Miller, 1986). Kraut's study (1978) on verbal content cues and nonverbal cues identified six of nine behavioral cues as actually related to deception, of which four were verbal content cues. The four verbal content cues related to veracity of a message are plausibility, concreteness, consistency, and clarity. Research has found that people being deceptive give less plausible, less concrete, less consistent, and less clear responses.

Vocal Cues

Vocal cues are defined as the cues within speech, excluding meaning. Research has found that twice as many vocal behaviors as opposed to nonverbal behaviors distinguished people being deceptive from those telling the truth and has consistently shown vocal behaviors to be more reliable indices of deception than nonverbal behaviors (DeTurck & Miller, 1985). These include response duration, pauses, speech errors, and response latency. These four cues have been consistently related to actual deception. People being deceptive produced shorter responses, more pauses during speech, more speech errors, and longer response latency (DeTurck & Miller, 1985; Stiff & Miller, 1986; Kohnken, 1987).

Visual Cues

Visual cues have received the most attention in research and yet have yielded the most inconsistent findings. Several studies yielded increases in the number of visual cues during deception, and in other studies decreases in the number of visual cues in deception have been noted. The increases in visual cues have been linked to the hypothesis that deception elicits arousal, for example, increased nervousness results in more hand gestures and foot movements (Vrij, 1995). The decreases in visual cues can be explained by people being more deceptive believing that movements give their lies away so they tend to avoid movements not strictly essential. This control results in an unusual rigidity and inhibition (Hocking & Leathers, 1980; Vrij, 1995). Research has also found that observers largely rely on visual cues when making judgments of deception, and possibly these visual cues may serve as distractors in the process of detecting deception (Stiff & Miller, 1986; Stiff, Miller, Sleight, Mongeau, Rogan, & Garlick, 1989). The visual cues consistently related to actual deception are self-adaptors (scratching, grooming, stroking the face, etc.), hand gestures, foot and leg movements, and postural shifts. A person who is being deceptive engages in more of these behaviors.

The purpose of this study is to investigate whether providing short-term training to individuals on behavioral cues related to deception will increase their correct judgment of veracity compared to individuals who received no training. This study investigated the behavioral cues related to judgments of veracity to assess which set of cues is most effective in improving judgment of veracity. It was hypothesized that participants who received cue training would have a higher proportion of correct judgments of veracity than those participants who received no cue training. For participants who received cue training, it was hypothesized that participants trained on verbal content cues would have the highest accuracy of judgments of veracity.

METHOD

Participants

Ninety-seven first-year undergraduate psychology students volunteered to participate in the study and received course credit for their participation. There were 16 men and 81 women, ranging in age from 18 to 43 years ($M = 20.8$).

Materials

A stimulus videotape of interviews with 60 subjects, 45 minutes long, was adapted from videotapes utilized by Ebesu and Miller (1994) who had individuals produce one of four different messages within different scenarios: (1) lie, (2) misdirection, (3) implying the truth, and (4) telling the truth. Subjects were videotaped so that their entire bodies were seen easily. The truth and lie message conditions were extracted from these videotapes with permission for use in this study. Specifically, 30 subjects giving truth messages and 30 different subjects giving lie messages were randomly selected and ordered, producing a 45-min. videotape of 60 subjects, each one telling either the truth or a lie.

Handouts were created for the three experimental conditions and the control condition. For the experimental conditions, the handout consisted of a training sheet and a response sheet. The training sheets for the verbal content, visual, and vocal cues consisted of four cues, each defined and explained with examples. Subjects in the verbal content cue condition were trained to be sensitive to the plausibility, concreteness, consistency, and clarity of the statements. Subjects in the visual cue condition were trained to be sensitive to the presence of self-adaptors (such as rubbing your face), hand gestures, foot/leg movements, and postural shifts. Lastly, subjects in the vocal cues condition were trained to be sensitive to response duration, the presence of pauses, speech errors, and response latency, i.e., hesitation before speaking.

Procedure

Participants were randomly assigned to one of the four conditions. Participants were seated before a television screen on which the stimulus videotape was presented. Participants in the cue training conditions were given the corresponding training sheets to study and, in addition, the experimenter read each behavioral cue with associated definitions and examples. Participants were provided an opportunity to ask for clarification on any of the behavioral cues. Participants in the control condition received no written or oral information on behavioral cues related to deception. Participants in both experimental and control conditions were instructed that they would be shown a 45-min. videotape of 60 individuals, each of whom was either telling the truth or a lie. After viewing each individual, the participants were instructed to indicate on their response sheet whether they judged the individual to be telling the truth or a lie.

RESULTS

Means and standard deviations for each training condition across each type of message are displayed in Table 1. An alpha level of .05 was adopted for all tests of significance. Distribution shapes were approximately normal in form for each message type within each condition. All tests of mean differences were performed with Welch's heteroscedastic two-sample and omnibus statistics, respectively (1938, 1951; cf. Keselman, Huberty, Lix, Olejnik, Cribbie, Donahue, Kowalchuk, Lowman, Petoskey, Keselman, & Levin, 1998). Where necessary, the Games-Howell heteroscedastic pairwise multiple comparison procedure (Games & Howell, 1976) was utilized (in essence,

TABLE 1
MEAN ACCURACY AND STANDARD DEVIATIONS FOR TRAINING CONDITIONS BY CORRECT JUDGMENT OF ALL, TRUTHFUL, AND DECEPTIVE MESSAGES

Condition	n	\multicolumn{6}{c}{Correct Judgment of Message}
		All 60		30 True		30 Lie	
		M	SD	M	SD	M	SD
No Cue Training	30	38.8	5.5	21.0	4.9	17.6	2.7
All Cue Training	67	41.3	4.8	23.6	4.1	17.7	3.6
Visual Cues	21	40.4	4.6	23.7	4.4	16.7	3.6
Vocal Cues	20	40.4	5.9	22.8	4.9	17.6	4.2
Verbal Content Cues	26	42.9	3.7	24.3	3.1	18.6	2.8

Tukey's honestly significant difference familywise error control with the Welch heteroscedastic statistic). In addition, recent research has reported that model-testing procedures, which eliminate intransitivity and provide a more logical method for evaluating pairwise mean differences, can also be much more likely to detect the true underlying population mean configuration than traditional pairwise multiple comparison procedures (e.g., Dayton, 1998, 2003; Cribbie, 2003; Cribbie & Keselman, 2003). Thus, the model-testing procedure proposed by Dayton (1998) was also utilized in evaluating differences in the means of the conditions. With this procedure the model with the lowest Akaike Information Criteria value (see Dayton, 1998, 2003) was retained as the most probable population mean configuration (assuming the omnibus test of mean difference was statistically significant, see Cribbie & Keselman, 2003). In essence, the Dayton model-testing procedure conducts pairwise comparisons of the means but does so in a way that is transitive, i.e., a condition/group cannot be drawn from two distinct populations, and wholistic, i.e., the results are interpretable within the framework of a population model rather than within isolated two-group comparisons.

To assess whether training individuals on behavioral cues related to deception would improve their correct judgment of the truthfulness of a message, a two-sample Welch test was conducted to compare the overall detection by participants who received cue training with that of participants who received no cue training. There was a significant mean difference in accuracy between participants who received cue training and those who did not ($t_{49.87} = 2.13$, $p = .04$, $\eta^2 = .09$), with the former having a higher proportion of correct judgments of veracity than the latter. The significant mean difference between the experimental and control groups indicates that, as predicted, training individuals on behavioral cues related to deception improved their overall detection. More specifically, there was a significant mean difference in accuracy between participants who received cue training and those who did not receive cue training for detecting when subjects were telling the truth ($t_{48.31} = 2.63$, $p = .01$, $\eta^2 = .13$), showing those who received cue training had a higher proportion of correct judgments. However, there was no significant difference between participants who received cue training and those who did not receive cue training for detecting when subjects were not telling the truth ($t_{71.36} = 0.18$, ns, $\eta^2 < .01$).

To examine the relative importance of each set of behavioral cues in judging the message's veracity, an omnibus Welch test was conducted to compare the overall detection of participants trained on verbal content cues, visual cues, and vocal cues with that of individuals who received no cue training. There was a significant mean difference in accuracy between these two groups of participants ($F_{3, 48.01} = 3.77$, $p = .016$, $\eta^2 = .09$). Pairwise comparisons indicated that the participants trained on verbal content cues had a significantly higher proportion of correct judgments of veracity than the participants who received no cue training. Dayton's model-testing procedure (1998) indicated that subjects who were trained to be sensitive to verbal content cues were drawn from a population distinct from those who had no training or who were trained to be sensitive to vocal or visual cues (see Table 2).

TABLE 2
Dayton's Model Testing Procedure (1998): Results For Eight Potential Transitive Population Mean Configurations

Mean Population Configuration*	Akaike Information Criteria†	
	Overall	Truth
[Control, Vocal, Visual, Verbal Content]	595.29	570.57
[Control] [Vocal, Visual, Verbal Content]	592.01	564.43†
[Control, Vocal] [Visual, Verbal Content]	592.00	565.34
[Control, Vocal] [Visual] [Verbal Content]	590.96	567.14
[Control, Vocal, Visual] [Verbal Content]	589.49*	568.54
[Control] [Vocal] [Visual, Verbal Content]	592.83	565.17
[Control] [Vocal, Visual] [Verbal Content]	589.79	565.49
[Control] [Vocal] [Visual] [Verbal Content]	591.79	566.97

*Conditions enclosed within brackets represent distinct populations. †The model with the lowest Akaike Information Criteria value is retained as the most likely mean population configuration.

The effect of cue training on detection was further investigated by examining the detection of message type. To assess whether training individuals on cues related to deception would improve their detection of truthful messages, an omnibus Welch test was conducted, comparing the proportion of correctly judged truthful messages of individuals in each training condition. There was a significant mean difference in accuracy ($F_{3,47.58} = 3.21$, $p = .031$, $\eta^2 = .09$), and pairwise comparisons showed participants who received training on verbal content cues had a significantly higher proportion of correct truth judgments than those who received no cue training. Dayton's model-testing procedure (1998) indicated subjects who were trained to be sensitive to any of the cues related to deception were drawn from a population distinct from those who had no training in the cues related to deception (see Table 2).

Whether training individuals on cues related to deception would improve their detection of deceptive messages was tested with an omnibus Welch test comparing the proportion of correctly judged deceptive messages in each condition. There was no significant mean difference in accuracy in detection of deceptive messages between participants in the four training conditions ($F_{3,46.60} = 1.42$, ns, $\eta^2 = .04$).

Discussion

The present study investigated judgments of the truth or falsehood of a message. The primary purpose was to investigate the effect of short-term cue training on individuals' judgments of this veracity. It was hypothesized that cue training would increase detection accuracy. Participants who received cue training were more accurate at judging veracity than the participants in the control condition, who received no cue training. Participants who received information on cues associated with actual deception (and how to use these cues effectively in making judgments) were significantly better than the control group on the overall detection of truthful and deceptive messages. It was also hypothesized that participants trained on verbal content cues would be more accurate in judging veracity of a message than would the other cue sets and control condition. The results, both in terms of traditional pairwise comparison analyses and the preferable model-testing procedure of Dayton (1998), confirmed that verbal content cues were the most effective training cues. Short-term training in the detection of plausibility, concreteness, consistency, and clarity cues significantly improved correct judgments of veracity relative to judgments of subjects in the control condition. This finding is consistent with results of Stiff and Miller (1986), Kraut (1978), and others, as well as with the results of a large meta-analysis by DePaulo, Lindsay, Malone, Muhlenbruck, Charlton, and Cooper (2003), wherein verbal content cues (such as the plausibility, logical structure, discrepancy/ambivalency, or amount of detail), unlike most other cues investigated in the literature on deception, significantly increased accuracy of judgments of veracity. These findings support the use of verbal content training for individuals, e.g., police officers, who are routinely required to differentiate between truthful and untruthful messages, although it is important to acknowledge that accuracy rates are still below 70%, and more research should be done into factors that help improve overall accuracy; see DePaulo, *et al.* 2003 for an extensive discussion on this topic.

In detection of truthful statements, participants trained on verbal content cues had a significantly higher accuracy rate than the control condition, and Dayton's model-testing procedure indicated all training conditions produced better performance than that of the control condition. In detecting untruthful statements, no significant differences in accuracy were found among the conditions as rates of accuracy were only minimally above chance performance. The poor accuracy rate for detecting deceptive messages is consistent with previous research showing deception detection is no greater than chance expectation (Hocking & Leathers, 1980; DeTurck & Miller, 1985; Kohnken, 1987). This could be a result of the truthfulness bias, that incorrectly judging a deceptive statement as truthful is more likely than judging a truth statement as deceptive (Kohnken, 1987; Anderson, *et al.*, 2002).

The participants who did not receive cue training illustrate that humans' judgments of veracity do not exceed chance expectations. These individuals were significantly less accurate at detecting truthful statements and at making overall judgments of veracity.

One weakness of this study was that subjects were judging the truthfulness of individuals who were sanctioned to lie or tell the truth. The individuals who were presented in the videotape may not have been displaying the physiological arousal associated with deception because they were enacting imaginary scenarios that led to no serious consequences of their deception. These individuals may not have been experiencing the guilt and anxiety typically associated with deception that would have otherwise possibly been evident. This could also explain why the deceptive messages were so difficult to detect by the training conditions, as there may not have been significant displays of cues for subjects to make accurate judgments. However, another way to interpret this is that, even though the cues for detecting deception were not highly evident, the subjects trained even briefly on detecting verbal content cues were still more likely to make accurate judgments of veracity. In this manner, it may be possible that subjects who are more extensively trained to detect verbal content cues may be even more accurate in detecting the truthfulness of a message, relative to subjects with no cue training or with training in identifying other types of behavioral cues, when the individual whom they judged to be lying or telling the truth is, in reality, actually telling the truth or lying and not a confederate of the experiment.

REFERENCES

ANDERSON, D. E., DEPAULO, B. M., & ANSFIELD, M. E. (2002) The development of deception detection skill: a longitudinal study of same-sex friends. *Personality and Social Psychology Bulletin*, 28, 536-545.

ANDERSON, D. E., DEPAULO, B. M., ANSFIELD, M. E., TICKLE, J. J., & GREEN, E. (1999) Beliefs about cues to deception: mindless stereotypes or untapped wisdom? *Journal of Nonverbal Behavior*, 23, 67-89.

CRIBBIE, R. A. (2003) Pairwise multiple comparisons: new yardsticks, new results. *Journal of Experimental Education*, 71, 251-265.

CRIBBIE, R. A., & KESELMAN, H. J. (2003) Pairwise multiple comparisons: a model comparison approach versus stepwise procedures. *British Journal of Mathematical and Statistical Psychology*, 56, 167-182.

DAYTON, C. M. (1998) Information criteria for the paired-comparisons problem. *The American Statistician*, 52, 144-151.

DAYTON, C. M. (2003) Information criteria for the pairwise comparisons. *Psychological Methods*, 8, 61-71.

DEPAULO, B. M., LASSITER, G. D., & STONE, J. I. (1982) Attentional determinants of success at detecting deception and truth. *Personality and Social Psychology Bulletin*, 8, 273-279.

DEPAULO, B. M., LINDSAY, J. J., MALONE, B. E., MUHLENBRUCK, L., CHARLTON, K., & COOPER, H. (2003) Cues to deception. *Psychological Bulletin*, 129, 74-118.

DEPAULO, B. M., ROSENTHAL, R., ROSENKRANTZ, J., & GREEN, C. R. (1982) Actual and perceived cues to deception: a closer look at speech. *Basic and Applied Social Psychology*, 3, 291-312.

DEPAULO, B. M., TORNQVIST, J. S., & COOPER, H. (2002) Accuracy at detecting deception: a meta-analysis of modality effects. (Unpublished manuscript, Univer. of Virginia)

DeTurck, M. A., & Miller, G. R. (1985) Deception and arousal: isolating the behavioral correlates of deception. *Human Communication Research*, 12, 181-201.

DeTurck, M. A., & Miller, G. R. (1990) Training observers to detect deception: effects of self-monitoring and rehearsal. *Human Communication Research*, 16, 603-620.

Ebesu, A. S., & Miller, M. D. (1994) Verbal and nonverbal behaviors as a function of deception type. *Journal of Language and Social Psychology*, 13, 418-442.

Fiedler, K., & Walka, I. (1993) Training lie detectors to use nonverbal cues instead of global heuristics. *Human Communication Research*, 20, 199-223.

Games, P. A., & Howell, J. F. (1976) Pairwise multiple comparison procedures with unequal n's and/or variances. *Journal of Educational Statistics*, 1, 113-125.

Hocking, J. E., & Leathers, D. G. (1980) Nonverbal indicators of deception: a new theoretical perspective. *Communication Monographs*, 47, 119-131.

Keselman, H. J., Huberty, C. J., Lix, L. M., Olejnik, S., Cribbie, R., Donahue, B., Kowalchuk, R. K., Lowman, L. L., Petoskey, M. D., Keselman, J. C., & Levin, J. R. (1998) Statistical practices of educational researchers: an analysis of their ANOVA, MANOVA, and ANCOVA analyses. *Review of Educational Research*, 68, 350-386.

Kohnken, G. (1987) Training police officers to detect deceptive eyewitness statements: does it work? *Social Behavior*, 2, 1-17.

Kraut, R. E. (1978) Verbal and nonverbal cues in the perception of lying. *Journal of Personality and Social Psychology*, 36, 380-391.

Stiff, J. B., & Miller, G. R. (1986) "Come to think of it": interrogative probes, deceptive communication, and deception detection. *Human Communication Research*, 12, 339-357.

Stiff, J. B., Miller, G. R., Sleight, C., Mongeau, P., Rogan, R., & Garlick, R. (1989) Explanations for visual cue primacy in judgments of honesty and deceit. *Journal of Personality and Social Psychology*, 56, 555-564.

Vrij, A. (1995) Behavioral correlates of deception in a simulated police interview. *The Journal of Psychology*, 129, 15-28.

Welch, B. L. (1938) The significance of the difference between two means when population variances are unequal. *Biometrika*, 29, 350-362.

Welch, B. L. (1951) On the comparison of several mean values: an alternative approach. *Biometrika*, 38, 330-336.

Zuckerman, M., Koestner, R., & Colella, M. J. (1985) Learning to detect deception from three communication channels. *Journal of Nonverbal Behavior*, 9, 188-194.

Zuckerman, M., Koestner, R., & Driver, R. (1981) Beliefs about cues associated with deception. *Journal of Nonverbal Behavior*, 6, 105-114.

Accepted March 31, 2004.

MODELING JUDGMENTS OF LINEAR EXTENT [1]

ERNEST GREENE AND WILLIAM FRAWLEY

Department of Psychology
University of Southern California
Neuropsychology Foundation, Los Angeles

Biostatistics Group, University of Texas
Southwestern Medical Center at Dallas

Summary.—Subjects were asked to make judgments of linear extent, specifically, to assess and reproduce the span between dots, with distances that ranged from 0.5 to 8° of visual angle. The errors of judgment were modeled by regressing against linear and Fourier components, yielding a model for each of the 25 subjects who participated in the five experiments and for each session in which the subjects were tested. Most of the models manifested a complex profile of underestimates and overestimates of span as a function of the span being judged. Successive cycles of under- and overestimation of spans appeared as quasiperiodic oscillations in some of the models. We hypothesize that spatial position is encoded by neuron receptive fields that are organized as a mosaic, and these judgment errors may reflect defects in or competitive interaction among these receptive fields.

In previous work, we found strange anomalies in judgment of spatial position that suggested defects in the position encoding process at various levels of scale (Greene, Frawley, & Swimm, 2000; Greene & Frawley, 2001a, 2001b).[2] In those studies, we were examining collinearity judgments, wherein one stimulus dot varied its angular position around a second stimulus dot, and the subject was asked to mark a location in open space that was collinear to the two dots. We observed deviations of error judgment, i.e., clockwise and counterclockwise error bias, that was a function of the angular position of the eccentric dot. These errors were modeled with Fourier analysis, that is, regression against harmonic components, and the resulting models showed very complex profiles of error tendency as a function of the angular position of the eccentric dot.

These models manifested significant deviations from accurate judgment, designated as "excursions," that could plunge from positive (counterclockwise) to negative (clockwise) when angular position had changed by only 10–15°. Alternatively, an excursion might show the same direction of error bias across a much larger range of angles. The shape of the error profile varied from one subject to the next, but tests administered across successive sessions showed substantial similarity for a given subject.

---

[1]This research was supported, in part, by the Neuropsychology Foundation. Address reprint requests to Ernest Greene, Department of Psychology, University of Southern California, Los Angeles, CA 90089-1061 or e-mail (egreene@usc.edu).
[2]Acrobat pdf copies of these and related articles can be found at http://www-rcf.usc.edu/~egreene.

These results implied localized defects in the encoding of stimulus position and seemed consistent with a concept that the nervous system was specifying spatial location through selective activation of receptive fields. The fact that the excursions might cover a large range of angular positions or be restricted to a narrow range could reflect the contribution of receptive fields of various sizes. We thought it possible and offered the hypothesis that spatial position was being registered by a nested mosaic of receptive field sizes.

It is conceivable that such anomalies are specific for judgment of collinearity or angular position. To determine whether effects are more general, here we examined judgments of linear extent, i.e., length, span. We used stimulus and task protocols similar to those of Greene and Frawley (2001a, 2001b). Subjects were required to judge the span between the two dots, and then (using one of the dots as an anchor), mark a location in open space that provided a comparable span (designated as a *response span*[3]). Errors in the response span as a function of true span were modeled using an adaptation of harmonic analysis. The results indicate a common trend for progressive underestimation as the span to be judged increased in length, but the models also manifested numerous local excursions.

We briefly discuss these results in relation to potential neural substrates, and suggest that the errors reflect a mosaic of position-encoding fields that tile the visual field and provide coordinates for control of action.

Experiment 1

Method

Subjects.—Six University of Southern California undergraduates served in the first experiment, hereafter designated as S1 through S6. All were naive to the phenomenon under investigation. Each was tested for acuity using a Snellen Eye Chart and was found to have 20/20 visual acuity without correction. By self-report all were right-handed, and all held a pencil in the right hand when executing the task demands.

Stimulus materials.—An example of the stimulus configuration used for the experiment is shown in Fig. 1. The configuration consisted of a pair of dots (positions specified in detail below), that were presented on 8.5- × 11-in. sheets. A round, white *display field* was provided at the center of each test sheet. This field was created by printing a circular rim on the sheet, the inner portion of the rim having a radius of 12° of visual angle. [Hereafter, degrees of visual angle is abbreviated as *arc°*.] It was black outside the rim, extending to the edges of the sheet. Thus the central zone of the sheet appeared as a large white disk, upon which the stimulus material to be judged,

---

[3]Operational definitions and terms of art are shown in italics at the point where they are most clearly specified.

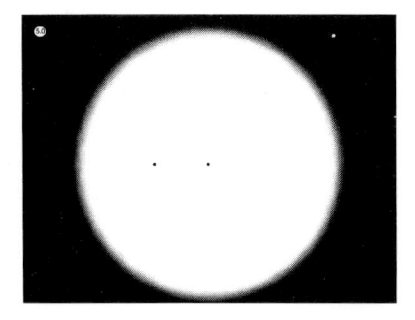

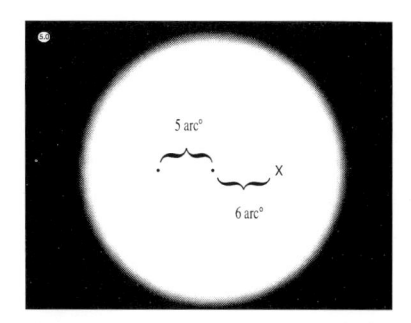

FIG. 1. An example of the stimulus configuration is provided in the left panel. Dot 1 was always presented at the center of the display field, and dot 2 was presented at various distances to the left of center. Here dot 2 lies at 5 arc°, this distance being designated as the "stimulus span." Subjects were told to mark a response dot to the right of center at a distance that was equivalent to the stimulus span, and an X has been placed at a location which might be selected. It lies at 6 arc° from the center, i.e., providing an error of +1 arc°. [Dot size has been increased for purposes of illustration.]

i.e., the dot pair, was printed. The rim of the display field consisted of a gradient of gray levels, being lightest at the 12 arc° radius and transitioning to black at 12.1 arc°. The gray gradient provided an indefinite boundary at the rim of the display field, reducing the ability to use the rim itself as an anchor in judging stimulus span.

The members of the dot pair were designated as dot 1 and dot 2, each having a diameter of 12 arc′. *Dot 1* was always positioned at the center of the display field, and *dot 2* was placed to the left of center, on the horizontal axis of the display field, at specified distances from the center. We used left displacements only so that the right-handed subjects would not be required to reach across the sheet, potentially obstructing their view of the position of the stimulus dots. The goal was to require a response that was very similar across all stimulus conditions.

The span between the two dots was designated as *rho* (ρ). *Rho* was varied in 0.5 arc° increments, with the minimum stimulus span being 0.5 arc° and the maximum being 8.0 arc°. Thus there were 16 levels of this treatment condition. To facilitate sorting and tabulation of the results, these levels were specified in a small white oval printed outside the display field at one corner of the test sheet.

There were six replications for each of the 16 treatment levels, so the complete *stimulus set* consisted of 96 sheets.

The order of stimulus presentation was determined as follows. First, a computer-based algorithm was used to order the sheets of the stimulus set. This order was random except for the restriction that one could not follow a given treatment level (a specific stimulus span) with the same level and not with one that was immediately adjacent. This restriction was designed to reduce redundancy of successive judgments.

The stimulus set was then divided into six subsets, with each subset being comprised of successive blocks of 16 sheets that followed the semirandom order discussed above. Copies of these subsets provided the *test set* for each of the subjects, using a random order for inclusion of the subsets. By this two-stage randomization procedure, each subject was presented with a different ordering of stimulus sheets.

Test protocols.—Subjects judged the stimulus displays with both eyes, with the aid of a stand that maintained a constant viewing distance (as detailed by Greene, *et al.*, 2000). Each subject was told that this was a test of accuracy and reliability for judging the span between the two stimulus dots. Each was further instructed to mark each test sheet with a *response dot* at a location to the right of the center dot, selecting a distance that was equivalent to the span between the stimulus dots. Note that we use the term "span" as a simple method for describing the encoding of stimulus positions and responding to those positions. It is possible to make a distinction between a mechanism that is based on the spatial position of each stimulus dot (perhaps as coordinate addresses), and a mechanism that extracts the relative distance between the two dots. Here we make no effort to separate these alternatives.

The instructions emphasized that if an initial response did not appear to provide an equivalent span, it could be erased and marked again. It appears that subjects used this option on very few of the judgments. Once the task demands had been explained, each subject proceeded through the test set at a self-selected pace. Subjects completed the experimental session in about 40 minutes.

Results

Measuring and conditioning the data.—The distance between dot 1 and the response dot was measured in units of visual angle with a resolution of 3 arc′. Judgment error, i.e., the difference between this measure and the stimulus span being judged, was designated as *eta* (η).

The variability of the span errors increased markedly as a function of the span being judged. When performing linear regression analysis, it is important to determine whether the variance of the observations is homogeneous. If it is not, then the observations should be weighted inversely proportional to their variance. Since the true variances are unknown in any practical situation, typically a simple, e.g., linear or quadratic, weighting function is estimated from sample observations.

For the present experiments the variances of the error observations are so different across the range of span that weighting in this fashion would amount to effectively disregarding all but the smallest observations—hardly a satisfying approach. However, by using proportional error as a temporary data transform, we were able to derive an acceptable level of homogeneity across the range being tested.

For this transform, we simply divided the error observation by the true length, which converts absolute error into relative error. We found that the sample standard deviations of the relative error decreased in an approximately linear fashion from the smallest to the largest span. The standard deviation associated with the smallest span was roughly two times that associated with the largest span, a range much more satisfactory than with the absolute error observations. This held across subjects.

By performing the simple weighting and subsequent linear regression with relative error observations, the predictions and confidence bounds emanating from the resulting model could be inverse-transformed back to absolute error. In other words, the final models shown here reflected a Euclidean metric.

Modeling protocols.—Our goal was to determine whether eta error varied as a function of the stimulus span, and to model these errors. The scale of the span variable is open ended and nonperiodic. Further, the error deviations did not begin and end at zero. Nonetheless, it was possible to use a Fourier series to model the data in conjunction with a linear component.

To be specific, the proportion-transformed data were regressed against a subset of sine and cosine components for each harmonic up to the Nyquist limit (Nyquist, 1928/2002), a constant, and a linear component. This precludes problems arising from the fact that the full design matrix is singular. We then computed estimates of each component coefficient, and the probability that the component should be judged to be zero. The data from 16 treatment levels allowed for extraction of components up to the eighth harmonic.

Components were included in the selected subset if they served to minimize the Mallows Cp statistics (Hocking, 1976). This statistic is a cost function that seeks to balance between over- and under-selection of independent variables. It adds a penalty if the most important components are not being included in the model and also if one is including unimportant components. This statistic commonly includes components that have an associated probability of less than .15 of being, in fact, zero, and on this basis we could describe each component as being "significant." It should be clear that the model combines at least several of these components such that the overall probability is much smaller than this, almost all being at $p < .0001$.

Components that minimized the Cp statistic constituted the model for the proportional error. From this model one could derive a prediction of the 95% confidence intervals for the mean proportional error at each span. An inverse proportion transform returned the model to Euclidean space.

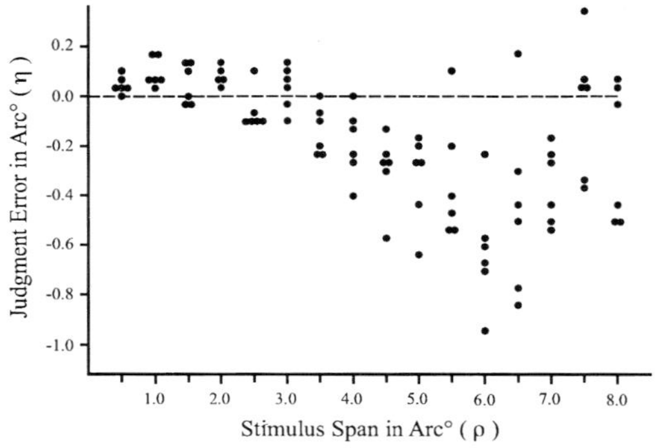

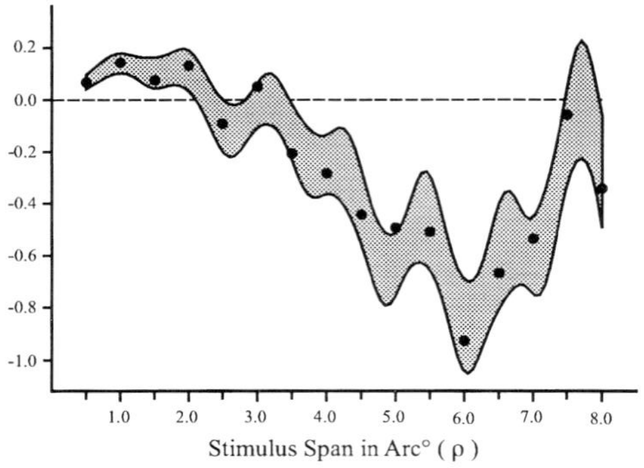

Coefficient	Value	Probability
constant	−.03	.0001
linear	−.03	.0001
1st cosine	.07	.0001
1st sine	.02	.14
2nd cosine	.02	.02
4th sine	−.02	.09
7th sine	−.02	.007

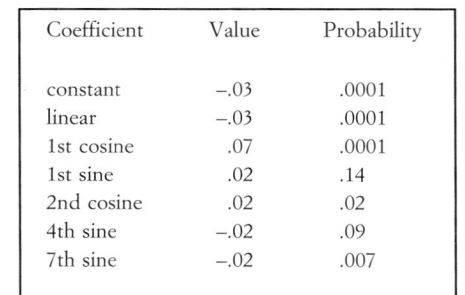

FIG. 2. The results from S1 are used to demonstrate the modeling procedure. The upper left panel shows the raw data for this subject. The tendency to over-estimate short spans and to underestimate long ones is clear from the position of the data points. The lower left panel shows the table of coefficients that met the Mallows Cp criterion. These coefficients were then used in an inverse construction to derive the model of effect. The 95% confidence interval for this model is shown in the upper right panel, along with mean error at each stimulus span.

Fig. 2 illustrates key elements of the modeling, using the first subject as an example. The raw data is plotted in the upper left panel, consisting of six judgments at each of the 16 stimulus spans. Accurate judgment of the span would place the data point on the dashed horizontal line, i.e., at zero error. At a number of stimulus spans one can see that many or all of the data points fall far from this zero line. At small spans the errors tend to be positive, meaning that the distance has been overestimated, but at large spans the judgments tend to be underestimates.

The right panel of Fig. 2 shows the model that was derived from these data. Actually, we have provided the 95% confidence interval for the model, and the model itself would lie at the center of this interval. Because the model is derived from functions having continuous distributions, i.e., the sine, cosine, and linear components, the model predicts not only the value at spans that were sampled, but also the intermediate positions throughout the range.

Also, in the right panel of Fig. 2 we have plotted the mean that was observed at each of the 16 stimulus spans. Although the confidence interval properly specifies only the values of the model prediction itself, one would expect that most of the means would be contained within this interval. With rare exception, this was the case for all the models in each of the five experiments.

In Fig. 2, lower left panel, we report the key values that were derived from the regression for S1, including the amplitude and significance levels of model coefficients. The data for this subject showed a number of coefficients of low probability, most notably the constant, the linear component, the first harmonic cosine, and the seventh harmonic sine. Except for the few trends noted above, there was little consistency across subjects as to which component was significant, or with the associated probabilities. Thus there seems to be little benefit in reporting these details.

Regression Fs and R^2 *values.*—For each model, a regression F statistic can be calculated, along with a probability that specifies the extent to which the model should be attributed to chance. For the six models of Exp. 1 the probabilities were all less than .0001.

For each model, we can also calculate an R^2 value that indicates how much of the overall variance in the data is accounted for by the model. Table 1 provides the R^2 value for each of the models of Exp. 1 (and those of the experiments that follow). One can see from the table that the models accounted for a substantial portion of the variance.

Idiosyncratic error profiles.—The models for the six subjects of Exp. 1 are shown in Fig 3, S1 being plotted again to facilitate comparison. Each subject shows a consistent trend wherein the variance (reflected in the width of the confidence interval) tends to increase as the span being judged be-

TABLE 1
THE R^2 VALUE FOR EACH MODEL*

Exp. 1		Exp. 2			Exp. 3					Exp. 4		Exp. 5	
S1	.51	S7	.24	.25	S13	.40	.31	.26	.37	S17	.70	S23H	.69
S2	.70	S8	.43	.30	S14	.34	.29	.28	.25	S18	.15	S23D	.67
S3	.33	S9	.50	.32	S15	.59	.35	.53	.52	S19	.54	S24H	.40
S4	.36	S10	.48	.40	S16	.59	.43	.42	.57	S20	.70	S24D	.57
S5	.20	S11	.37	.57						S21	.47	S25H	.79
S6	.64	S12	.80	.65						S22	.32	S25D	.85

*Where a given subject was tested for more than one session, the successive sessions are shown in a row to the right of the subject number.

comes larger. While the overall tendency is for greater width with larger spans, one should not assume that the function is consistently monotonic.

The second conspicuous feature of the models is that each shows large excursions from accurate judgment, i.e., from the zero line. Most of the excursions are significant—nonrandom—departures, as reflected in the fact that the 95% confidence interval does not include the zero line.

Several of the subjects tended to overestimate small stimulus spans, and most subjects underestimated large spans through a major portion of the range. This tendency was manifested primarily in the amplitude of the linear component, one end of the line being positive and the other end being negative.

There was also some consistency with respect to the first harmonic cosine that was significant for four of the six subjects. Mostly, however, the set of coefficients which were significant varied substantially from one subject to the next. This resulted in models that varied in the amplitude, position, and number of error excursions, and the overall profile of each model appeared to be idiosyncratic.

Evaluation

For most of the subjects of the first experiment, the dominant trend was for judgments to underestimate the stimulus span. A similar tendency is found for saccadic eye movements (Hallett, 1978), for which the metrics of stimulus position are specified relative to the fovea. This is consistent with our view of the judgment process, wherein the position of the central dot is specified relative to the fovea, and then the position of the eccentric dot is encoded as a vector. [See Discussion for details.]

In addition to the linear trend, each of the models displayed conspicuous large and small excursions, with each subject manifesting a unique and idiosyncratic profile for these excursions across the 8 arc° range. The excursion amplitudes in the present work were modulated by the span being judged, but otherwise these effects are similar to what we have reported with collinearity judgments (Greene, *et al.*, 2000; Greene & Frawley, 2001a, 2001b).

As indicated in the Introduction, we thought it possible that perceived span might show localized defects, consistent with the hypothesis that a receptive field mosaic provides the mechanism for encoding spatial position. Nonetheless, we were prepared to model the data using tools that seemed most appropriate. In early analysis we examined the data using a polynomial (Taylor) series but found a better fit when harmonic components were included. In the end, the best models were provided using only a linear component in addition to the harmonics.

We have no hypothesis as to the basis for the linear component—the progressive underestimation of the span as it is increased. What we are emphasizing, therefore, is the presence of localized excursions in the error models. They suggest that the mechanism for registering spatial position may be comprised of encoding elements that vary in size and may be configured as a mosaic across the visual field.

Experiment 2

It would be useful to determine whether the profile of the model for a given subject is stable across repeated testing. If the excursions are due to fixed anomalies in the position encoding system, it is possible that the same profile would be manifested across two separate test sessions. If the excursions were more labile, one might argue for changes in attention, preferred fixation site, or other kinds of dynamic influence. The goal of the second experiment, therefore, was simply to test and model the judgment errors across two separate test sessions.

Method

Six new subjects, designated as S7 through S12, served as subjects for the second experiment. Each was tested and showed 20/20 vision without correction, and all were right-handed.

Stimulus material and task protocols were identical to those of Exp. 1, except that the subjects judged stimulus sets in two test sessions—one in the morning and one in the afternoon of the same day. Each stimulus set consisted of six replications across 16 spans, i.e., 96 sheets, presented to each subject in a different semirandom order as described in Exp. 1.

Results

Measurement of the errors and modeling of the resulting data was done the same as described in Exp. 1. All the models were significant at $p < .0001$ and carried R^2 values in the same range as those of Exp. 1 (see Table 1). Models are presented in Fig. 4, with the two sessions for a given subject being plotted together to facilitate comparison.

As was true for the subjects of Exp. 1, the dominant tendency across most of the range was for the stimulus span to be underestimated. However,

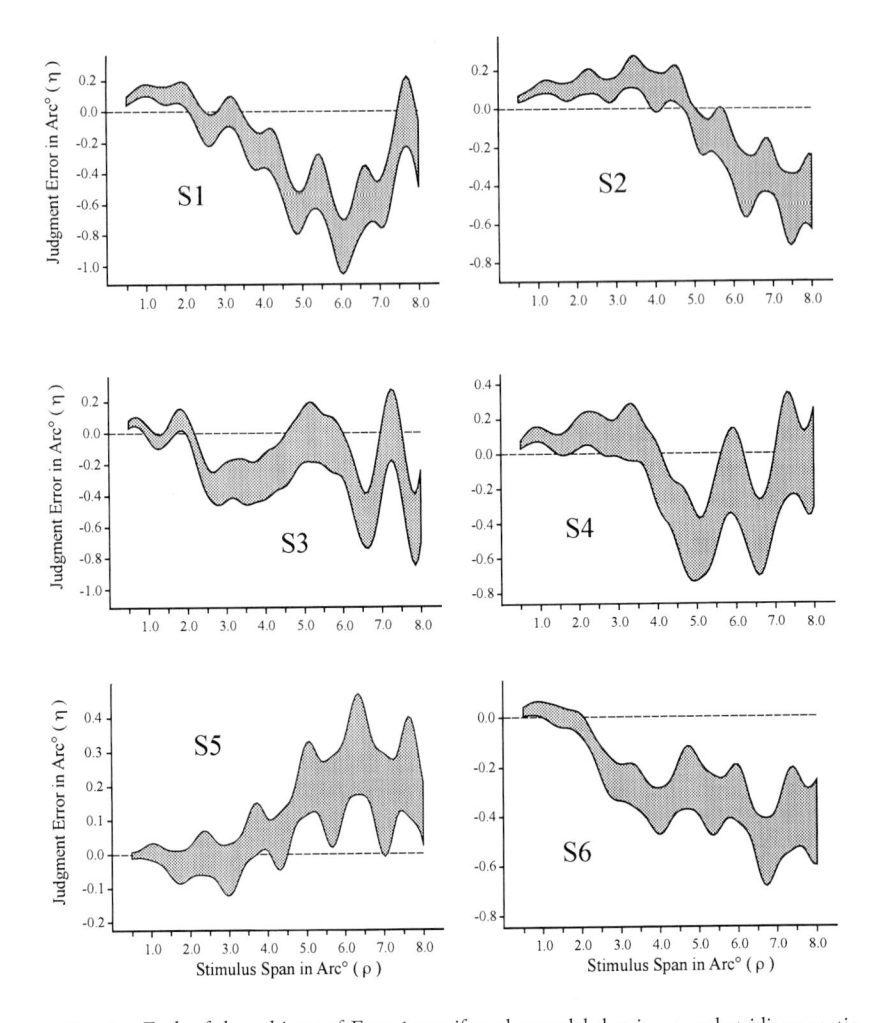

FIG. 3. Each of the subjects of Exp. 1 manifested a model that is somewhat idiosyncratic. Each model includes a general sweep, most often reflecting an underestimation of the true span as that span is increased. But, additionally, each model contains a number of short excursions that may reflect localized sources of error.

for several of the subjects there were large excursions that reflected either overestimation at some stimulus spans, or at least a substantial reduction in the magnitude of underestimation. As before, each subject manifested excursions across the full range of spans being judged.

The models for a given subject showed some consistency across the two test sessions, but there were also major differences. The curves for S10 look quite similar, except for some shift in the length at which the major excur-

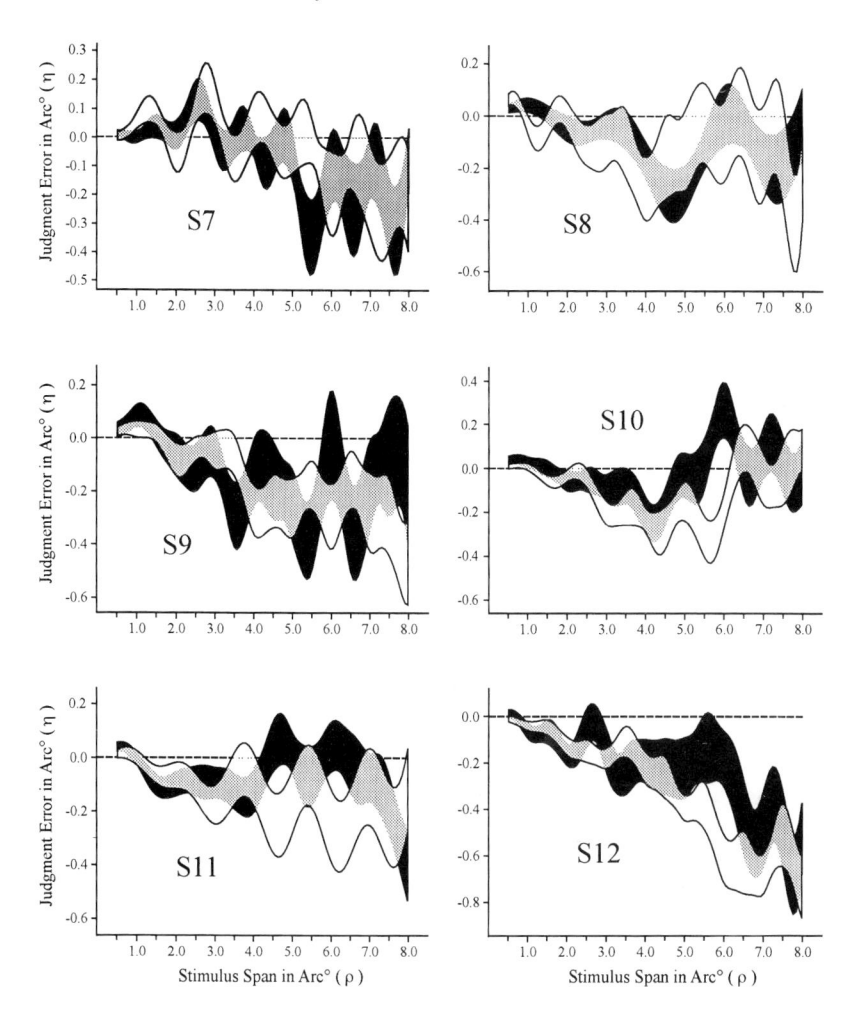

FIG. 4. For each subject of Exp. 2 the model for the first session is shown in white, and the model for the second session is shown in black. For each subject, there were major trends and excursions that were the same across the two sessions. There were, however, some conspicuous differences.

sions peak. For S8, both sessions show similarities in the large components. For S12, a large negative-going linear trend with very small excursions is conspicuous for both models; for S7, each shows similar amplitudes of excursion across the full range. On the other hand, for none of the six subjects could the models of the two sessions be considered a very close match.

To provide a more quantitative index of comparability, we calculated Pearson correlations for each session pair, using the means at each of the 16 sampled positions as the raw data. The analysis yielded one *isocombic correlation* for each subject, wherein the means from the first session were compared against the means from the second session. Additionally, it provided 10 *metacombic correlations* for each subject, these being the comparison of each session for that subject against the corresponding session of the other five subjects.

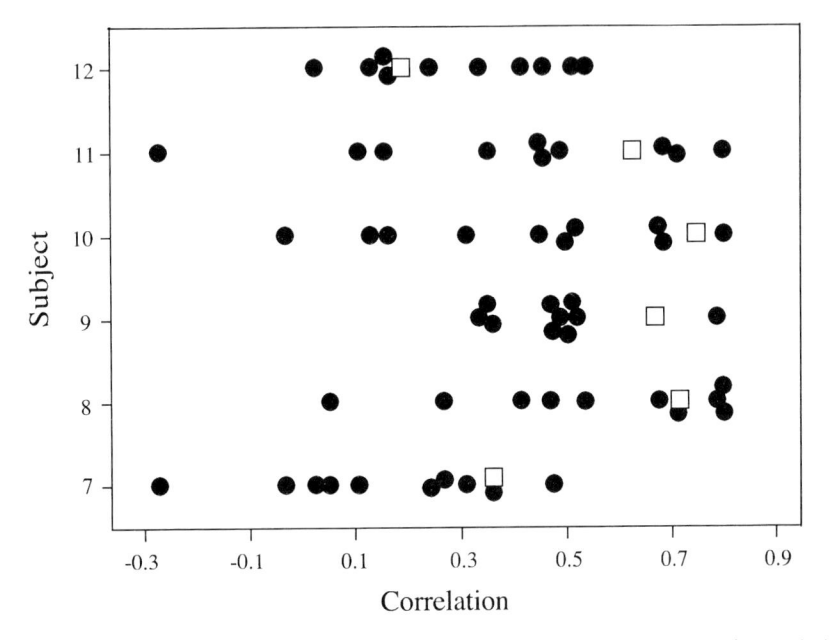

FIG. 5. Isocombic (self-self) correlations (□) and metacombic (self-other) correlations (●). Most of the isocombic correlations were high, and near the top of the range. Only S12 provided an isocombic correlation which was very low and near the bottom of the range of values. The fact that most isocombic correlations were near the top of the range supports the view that the error profile is fairly idiosyncratic.

These correlation values are plotted in Fig. 5. For S7 the isocombic correlation was just above .30, but this was well above the level for most of the metacombic correlations. For S8–S11 the isocombic correlations were high (approximately .70) and also near the top of the distribution of values. Only for S12 was there a disparity, with the isocombic correlation being very low and below most of the metacombic correlations. This result seems at odds with the impression provided by Fig. 4, in that the strong negative-going trend line of S12 is similar for the two sessions and seems considerably different from the profiles of most other subjects.

Evaluation

The results of Exp. 2 indicate some similarity of error profiles across two test sessions. Some portion of the error profile, therefore, should be considered to be a stable, idiosyncratic attribute of a given subject. However, there were conspicuous differences for each pair of models that reflect labile sources of effect.

This result differs somewhat from what was found with collinearity judgments (Greene, et al., 2000; Greene & Frawley, 2001a, 2001b). The Greene and Frawley (2001a) article is especially pertinent. For that work we used a circular display field and asked for judgment of two dots, one of which was positioned at the center of the field. The major difference was in the positioning of the eccentric dot and in the judgment that was required. The angular position of the eccentric dot was varied through 360°, and subjects were asked to place a response dot to be collinear (aligned) with the two stimulus dots. When tested across three or more sessions, the isocombic correlations were uniformly high, and all were well above the values found for metacombic correlations.

At first blush, therefore, collinearity judgments (Greene, et al., 2000; Greene & Frawley, 2001a, 2001b) appear to be more stable and consistent than are judgments of span, although this might be an artifact of the span that was probed. Varying the angular position of an eccentric dot provides a linear displacement that is more than six times greater than the maximum span used here. To be specific, here the maximum span was 8 arc°, which happens to match the distance between the center and eccentric dot for the Greene and Frawley (2001a) experiments. The linear displacement for the range of angular positions consists of the circumference of a circle having a radius of 8 arc°, i.e., $2\pi r = 50$ arc°.

The differential in length may be critical if position is encoded by an array of fields that have a lower limit of resolution. One would expect the smallest encoding elements to show the least stability in their output, or perhaps, to be sampled with lower reliability due to variation of fixation. Certainly in the studies of collinearity, the smaller excursions were manifested less reliably than were the large ones (Greene & Frawley, 2001a). By sampling the 8 arc° across 16 levels, we are essentially probing small-scale sources. Finding that the resulting models have only modest correspondence is not inconsistent with the results of collinearity judgment.

Experiment 3

The results from Exp. 2 suggested a modest level of consistency across test sessions. It would be good to test across additional sessions to confirm whether a stable profile will develop.

Method

Four new subjects, designated as S13–S16 were tested and showed normal, uncorrected visual acuity. All were right-handed.

Stimulus and test conditions were identical to those of Exp. 1, except that the subjects were tested for four sessions—once in the morning and once in the afternoon on successive days. As before, in each test session the subject received a test set consisting of the six replications of 16 spans, provided in a semirandom order according to the protocol explained previously. The test apparatus was the same as that in the first two experiments. Test instructions were given prior to the first session and were not required thereafter.

Results

Analysis of data, including regression Fs, correlations, and modeling were identical to the methods used in prior experiments. The probabilities of the regression Fs were less than .0001 for each session for each subject, and R^2 values were all in an acceptably high range (see Table 1 above).

Models were extracted for each of the sessions, and for the average of the four sessions. These are designated as *session models* and the *average model*, respectively. Fig. 6 displays the session models as an array on the left and plots the average model on the right for each of the subjects. First, one might note certain similarities in the profiles of the average models for the four subjects. All showed a strong linear trend for the first 4 arc°. At the longer spans, S14 and S15 have large excursions that are fairly similar, and the overall trends are not unlike those of S13. These commonalities tend to undermine the tentative conclusion that the error profiles are idiosyncratic. Rather, it is possible that earlier differences among the models could reflect the lability that is evident for a given session.

With respect to the session models, the differences seem more conspicuous than do the similarities. To emphasize the latter, one could note that Sessions 2 and 4 for S13 look comparable, which is true also for Sessions 1 and 4 for S15. Additionally, the major trend line, i.e., the linear component, is consistent for most of the subjects. On balance, however, the session models for each subject differ in terms of the positioning, amplitude, and number of excursions.

Given the apparent instability of the models with repeated testing, we should address the question of whether we could be modeling noise. In reporting the results from Exp.1, we outlined the modeling criteria and noted that many of the model components were found to have respectable significance levels. [See, for example, the table in Fig. 2 above.] We have not provided comprehensive tables of the coefficients (and their significance levels), feeling that this might imply some functional reality for the individual components.[4] Given the variability across sessions, however, it would be

---

[4]The point being that the errors are modeled by the combination of all the components, and we have no reason to believe that the sources of error correspond to the individual components.

MODELING JUDGMENTS OF LINEAR EXTENT 1063

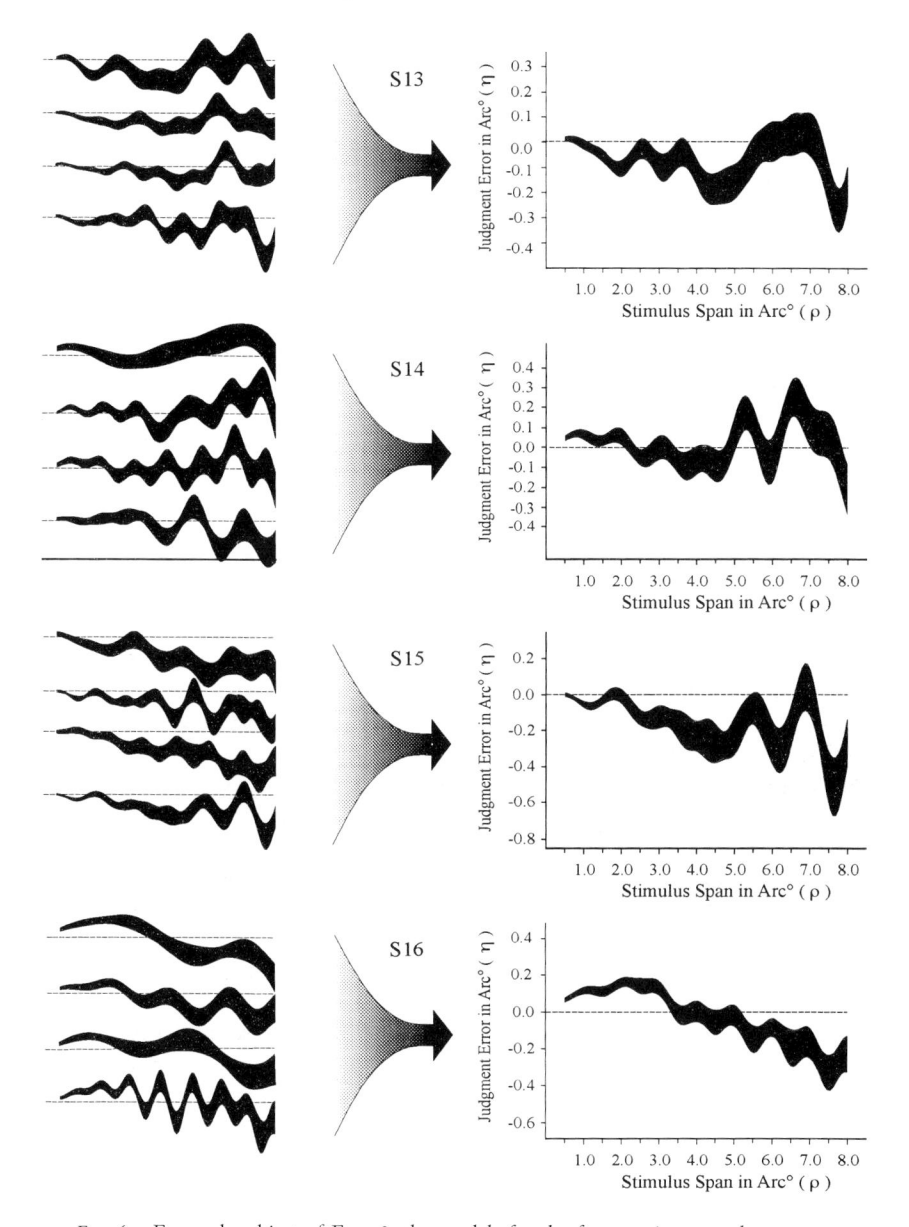

FIG. 6. For each subject of Exp. 3, the models for the four sessions are shown as an array, with the models for each subject being displayed at the same scale. For each array, Session 1 is shown at the top and Session 4 at the bottom. The model for the average of the four sessions is shown on the right. There was substantial variation of the model profile across sessions, but most of the models display small-scale oscillations. Among other possibilities (see text), these oscillations might be due to mispositioning of neural elements within a mosaic that encodes the spatial position of stimuli.

good to provide additional evidence that the model for a given session is not spurious.

Eighty-nine coefficients were used to construct the 16 session models represented in Fig. 6. The p values associated with these coefficients were all less than .15. We tabulated the observed significance levels for these coefficients, and found the following number of coefficients to be significant as follows: 21 at .0001; 12 at .001; 10 at .01; 26 at .05.[5] Thus 69 of the 89 coefficients are significant at .05 or smaller, with most carrying very small probabilities.

A more concrete example might be useful. An extreme case is Session 4 for S16. As shown in Fig. 6, the model for the fourth session is dominated by large sawtooth excursions. Such tendencies were not shown to a substantial extent in the first three sessions. Sessions 1 and 3 show only a few, gently sweeping excursions. Session 2 has additional excursions but nothing like the sharp deflections being manifested in Session 4. Given these results, there may be some doubt as to whether the model for Session 4 really represents the error profile of the data.

To further evaluate this issue, in Fig. 7 we present the model again and have superimposed the observed means. The mean at 1.0 arc° lies just outside the confidence limits for the model, but the other 15 means lie within the confidence interval. The values of these means vary in amplitude in a sawtooth manner, beginning at a span of 1.5 arc° and continuing to the final value at 8.0 arc°. The only values showing a monotonic trend are the first four—the means that lie between 0.5 and 2.0 arc°. Further, starting at 3.0 arc° the errors swing from overestimation of span to underestimation of span for nine successive means. Most of these transitions are large. At the extreme, the judgments at 4.0 and 4.5 arc° show a total error difference of 0.5 arc°. In other words, at 4.0 the span is overestimated by approximately a quarter of a degree of visual angle, and at 4.5 it is underestimated by that amount. Given the level of consistency indicated by the confidence interval, this is not likely a chance outcome.

There was additional concern about the low probability provided by the model shown in Fig. 7. Any significance might be due to the overall sweep of the judgments—overestimation at short spans and underestimation at long spans. To evaluate this possibility, we conducted a *post hoc* test of the null hypothesis that the coefficients of the components above the first harmonic are equal to zero (Graybill, 1961). The resulting F value was significant at $p < .0001$. This indicates that the combined contributions of com-

---

[5]Decimal digits to the right of the categories shown were rounded to the nearest whole number and then assigned to the category that lies at or above this value. Thus, .00012 would be tallied as .0001, and .017 would be tallied as .05.

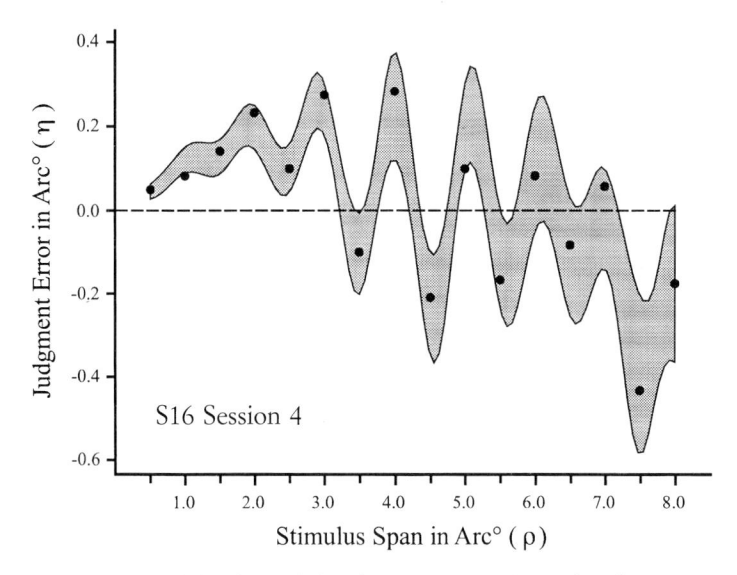

FIG. 7. The means of the observed data for S16 (Session 4) are plotted, superimposed on the model. A *post hoc* test suggests that the localized excursions reflected in the model and the means are not likely due to chance (see text).

ponents from the second harmonic and above are modeling highly localized sources of position error.

Evaluation

The small probability that is associated with the regression F for each session, as well as the number of significant harmonic components for each model, indicate that we are not modeling noise. This begs the question of what might be the source of variability across session.

We think it likely that there are small changes in preferred fixation site for making the judgments of span, and this alters the position of the stimulus dots on small-scale position encoding fields. This could have the effect of producing a mismatch between the spacing of stimulus dots and the spacing of the encoding mosaic, i.e., aliasing. At some fixation positions the mismatch might augment errors, and at other it might serve to cancel error tendency. If fixation changed from one session to the next, one would see inconsistency in the model profiles.

EXPERIMENT 4

One can reduce the effects of aliasing by sampling at smaller increments of span. But there is a practical limit to the number of data points one can collect without the risk of fatigue or boredom on the part of the subject. As a means for getting smaller increments within a single session, we chose to sample over a shorter range of spans.

Method

Six new subjects, designated as S17 through S22 showed normal, uncorrected visual acuity. All were right-handed.

Stimulus and task conditions were identical to those of Exp. 1, except that the spans ranged only from 4 arc° to 8 arc° in 0.1-arc° increments, each increment being represented three times within the test set. For this experiment, the spans from 0.5–4.0 arc° were not evaluated. Each of the six subjects judged just one test set in a single session.

Results and Evaluation

The data were regressed against a constant, a linear component, and the first 18 Fourier harmonics. However, to provide additional protection against Type I error, i.e., to reduce the chance for erroneous inclusion of noise, we required a $p < .10$ for entry/exit of a component into a stepwise linear regression model. The resulting models are presented in the six panels of Fig. 8. The model probability values were all less than .0001, except for S18 ($p = .0007$), and the R^2 values, shown in Table 1, are all in a relatively high range.

A very large number of extremely regular excursions is a conspicuous feature of each model. Indeed, over major portions of the tested range, i.e., between 4.0 arc° and 8.0 arc°, each model displays many excursions that appear very similar in amplitude and spacing.

The major purpose of reducing the spacing of the sampled positions was to determine whether the excursions seen in earlier experiments were due to aliasing. From the results of this experiment it would appear that they are not. We continue to see large excursions, with the influence of the closer spacing being, if anything, to make the excursions more regular. Given this result, we think it unlikely that simple aliasing is the source of these excursions.

To assess whether there are treatment effects that should be attributed to higher harmonic components, i.e., those other than the constant, the linear term, and the first harmonics, we again conducted *post hoc* tests. This was done by computing an F statistic composed of the adjusted mean sum of squares due to the second harmonics and above, divided by the mean square error under the full model. The probabilities provided by these *post hoc* tests, for S17–S22, were .002, .03, .001, .0001, .001, and .001, respectively. This affirms that the higher harmonics, i.e., the second harmonic and above, are registering patterns in the data that reflect real sources of error and that those sources have a fairly regular spacing across the range of stimulus spans. While these results do not demand a mosaic substrate, the results provide encouragement to our hypothesis that stimulus position is encoded by receptive fields that tile the visual field in such a manner.

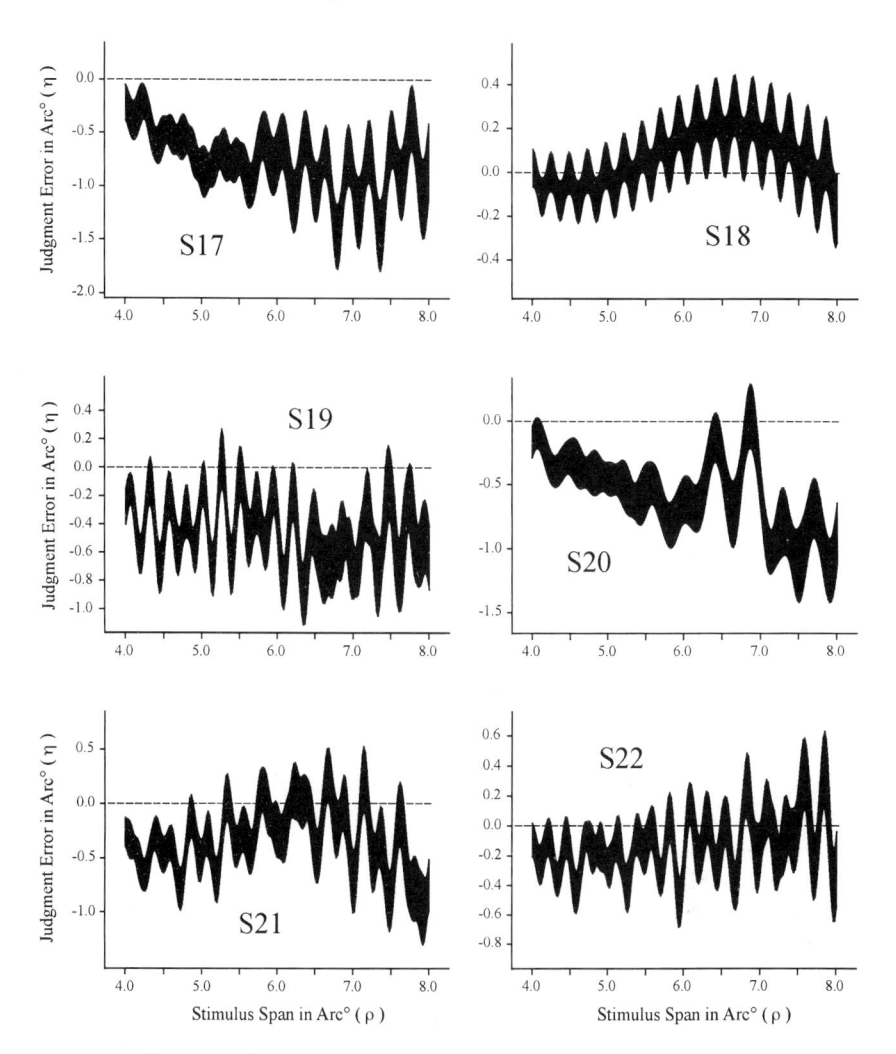

FIG. 8. The range of spans from 4.0 arc° to 8.0 arc° was sampled in 0.1-arc° increments. The models of error show very sharp excursions, with amplitudes and spacing being very regular across some portions of the range. It is possible that these excursions are reflecting the hypothesized position encoding mosaic of the visual system (see Discussion).

Experiment 5

Consistent with a well known phenomenon commonly described as the "oblique effect," in each of our previous studies of collinearity judgment we found that error models had larger excursions and were more variable for oblique than for cardinal (horizontal and vertical) angles (Greene, et al., 2000; Greene & Frawley, 2001a, 2001b). Perhaps the fields that register stimulus position have a tighter spacing along the cardinal axes than is true for the diagonal.

Method

To test this issue we tested three new subjects, designated as S23, S24, and S25. Each showed normal, uncorrected visual acuity and was right-handed.

The stimulus and task conditions were identical to those of Exp. 4, except for the addition of an orientation condition with two levels, designated as horizontal and diagonal. For each condition we sampled with three replications every 0.1 arc° from 4.0 to 8.0 arc° of span between the two dots. For the Horizontal condition the dots were aligned with a horizontal axis that crossed through the center of the display field. For the Diagonal condition the axis which passed through the dots was at 45° from the horizontal, and the eccentric dot was down and to the left of center. For each condition, the subjects were asked to judge the span and provide a response dot that was at the same span from center, and approximately in line with the other two.

The sheets from each condition were presented in a different random order for each subject, using the method specified in Exp. 1. For each subject the resulting test set was divided in two and was administered over two sessions, one in the morning and the other in the afternoon of the same day. The data from the two sessions were recombined for purposes of analysis and modeling.

Results and Evaluation

Models were extracted as in Exp. 4, and are shown in Fig. 9. The regression probabilities were all less than .0001, and the R^2 values are reported in Table 1 above. There was nothing in the models that would suggest a differential of effect, so the application of a two-way analysis of variance to determine whether Horizontal and Diagonal conditions produced a differential effect seemed unwarranted.

We thought it possible that the diagonal condition would yield models that had greater spacing among the excursions, and possibly the excursions would be larger than for the horizontal condition. This was based on an extrapolation from the angular position results (Greene, *et al.*, 2000; Greene & Frawley, 2001a, 2001b), where judgments were more accurate and less variable when the stimulus material was aligned with a cardinal axis. Bouma and Andriessen (1970), among others, have suggested that precision could be based on the relative density of overlapping receptive fields—the more fields available, the better the average that they can deliver. And, if there are fewer receptive fields along an oblique axis, e.g., at the 45° diagonal used here, then one might expect judgments to be less precise and show large excursions. The present results do not support this line of speculation, as the

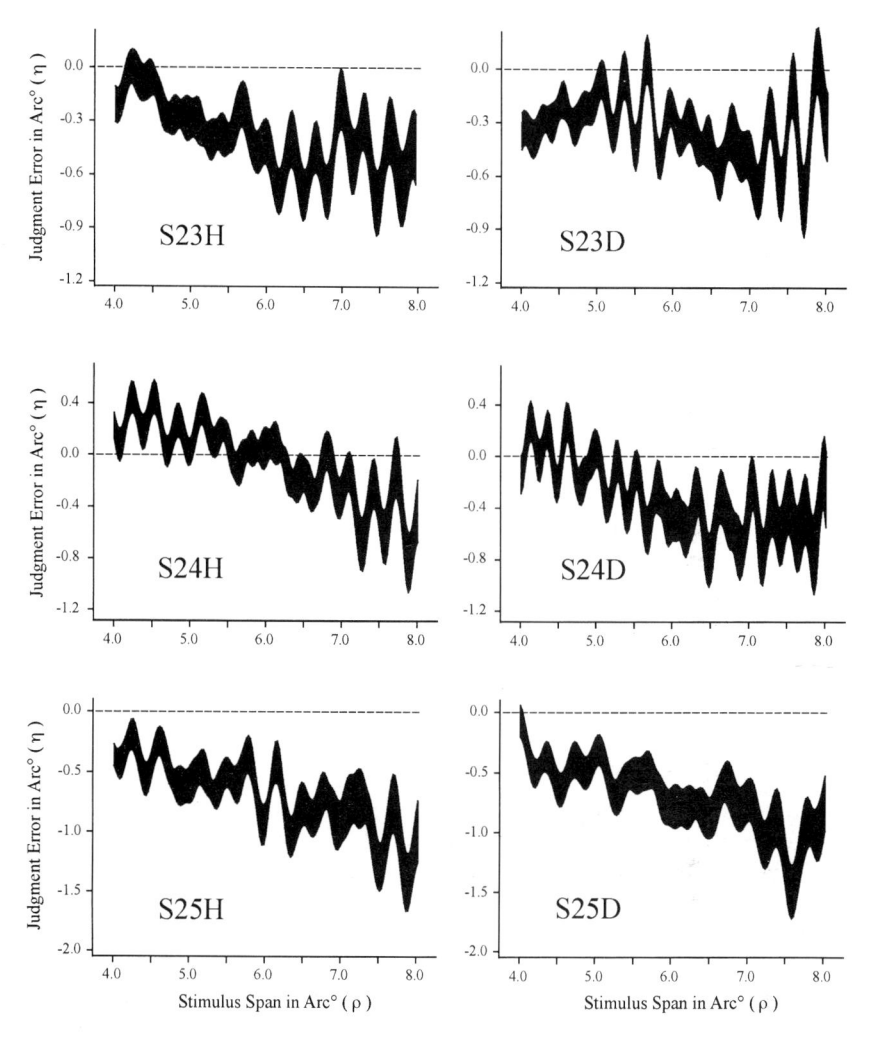

FIG. 9. The three subjects of Exp. 3 judged spans wherein the dots were aligned either on the horizontal axis (H) or on the 45° diagonal axis (D). The models of judgment error all show small scale excursions, i.e., changes of the amplitude of error over very short distances. However, there was no indication that the models were different for horizontal versus diagonal judgments. It does not appear, therefore, that these judgments are subject to the "oblique effect."

models for the Horizontal and Diagonal conditions appear to be very comparable.

Although there was no Horizontal vs Diagonal treatment effect, we note that for each condition and for each subject the models show unambiguous variation in judgment error. Further, there appears to be considerable regularity to the excursions, to the point where one might describe them as oscillations. Such oscillations suggest a regular spacing in the mechanism that registers spatial position, that mechanism being a mosaic of position encoding fields.

Discussion

It seems reasonable that the judgments of span would be derived from a common retinocentric mapping of stimulus position(s). In selecting a spot that is judged to be an equivalent span, the subject first looks to a potential target location in open space and then reaches to mark that location. The visual selection of the target site is essentially an antisaccade (Everling & Fischer, 1998), wherein the values for control of the action are drawn from the vector(s) of the visible stimulus material.[6]

It is not clear, however, how the spatial position of a stimulus element is specified by the nervous system. The process is most often viewed as involving a simple mapping, wherein the locations on the retina are transferred by the bundle of optic nerve fibers to the other brain structures, preserving adjacency among the image points. Such a mapping might seem sufficient, given the fact that each optic nerve contains over a million fibers. One can see each fiber as specifying a discrete spatial position, such that selective activation of a specific fiber or a set of adjacent fibers would provide the basis for knowing the spatial position of the stimulus.

One problem with this view is that our perception of spatial position, as reflected in various perceptual judgments, is partly a function of the stimulus configuration itself. For example, we misperceive the length of the span between two dots when fins are added at one end of the span being judged (Greene & Nelson, 1997; Nelson & Greene, 1998). The perceptual error is a function of the length of the fins and the angle between them. This begs the question of whether the activation of specific fibers can be the basis for one's awareness of position. If the fins can bias perceived position of one or both dots, how can "location" be determined solely by the activity of the fibers that were directly stimulated by the dots?

But focusing on the demands of the present judgment task, one finds that simple mapping concepts can carry one's thinking only so far. Such mapping can be used to link sensory location with motor response where the action is triggered directly by the stimulus. In the superior colliculus, for example, there is a mapping of motor neurons in juxtaposition to the sensory map. These neurons command actions appropriate for responding to

---

[6]The simplest case is one in which a subject fixates on the center dot and then must select a point that is opposite to the eccentric dot. But if one allows for the calculation of difference vectors, the required action can be specified with fixation at an arbitrary location.

that location, and a stimulus can trigger a saccade that results in the stimulus being fixated. [For a review of saccadic control in the superior colliculus, see Guitton (1991), Sparks and Hartwich-Young (1989), or Wurtz (1996).]

In practice, however, even with the best example of such a system—saccade control in superior colliculus—one finds that the output of the motor neurons do not specify the muscle contractions that will effect the response. Rather, one is forced to hypothesize a subsequent stage of processing in which the motor command is respecified as horizontal and vertical responses, which can be seen as coordinate values.

Further, a mapping concept does not provide a plausible basis for a number of voluntary eye movements. Subjects can be asked to perform an antisaccade, wherein they look to a location which is at the same distance as the trigger stimulus but in the opposite direction (see Everling & Fischer, 1998). Or they can execute a sequence of two saccades which calls for a "difference vector" that is not directly provided by the trigger stimuli (Hallett & Lightstone, 1976). Without elaborating, the basic concept is that the simple juxtaposition of sensory and motor maps will not explain these responses. Instead, it would seem that the location of a stimulus is specified on the basis of calculated values, i.e., coordinates.

It is not clear, however, how such coordinates could be derived from an array of neurons. We suggest a multiscale encoding concept, wherein the visual field is tiled with "position encoding fields" that vary in size—a separate tiling across the entire field at each level of scale.[7] These fields are contrast insensitive, and they deliver values that specify large or small spans according to the dimensions of a given field. The large-scale excursions could be generated by anomalies in large fields, and small-scale excursions by anomalies in small fields. The values provided by adjacent fields would be subject to bias through mutual interaction, which might be manifested under illusion-inducing conditions. Further, if the fields overlap, cross-computation could be required to resolve encoding conflicts. Small changes in fixation would alter the exact positioning of a stimulus within overlapping fields, which might alter this balance and produce some variation in perceived position.

Whether our multiscale encoding hypothesis is correct, the small, localized excursions that can be seen in the models suggest the presence of perceptual modules and, possibly, the neural substrates for the perceptual judgments.

We find no precedent for a finding of small, regularly spaced variations

---

[7]One can derive the formal equivalent of a tile by combining the output from a pool of lower elements. Thus, the specification of "fields" and a "mosaic" of such fields should be taken as functional concepts.

in error tendency for judgments of linear extent. The closest parallel comes from the reports that angular position judgments show such variation (see Greene, et al., 2000). It seems possible that the model reflects localized sources of judgment control and that the local sources are juxtaposed in a mosaic. If so, then the specificity of match between stimulus dimensions and the spacing of that mosaic will determine what kind of aliasing is produced. In other words, the variation in spacing for a given individual may interact with the spacing of the stimulus to produce larger excursions, or the canceling of error tendency.

If the present results are not based on a mosaic of localized sources, we are at a loss to explain what kind of perceptual mechanism would produce the lumpy models we have observed. We think the most parsimonious explanation is that position judgments are provided by neural modules which tile the visual field, and the summary from these position encoding fields is subject to discretizing errors.

There is solid evidence for the existence of a mosaic at the beginning stages of image encoding, i.e., in the spacing of ganglion cells in the retina. This is reviewed by Wassle and Boycott (1991), but for more recent findings see DeVries and Baylor (1997) and Rockhill, Euler, and Masland (2000). Whether the regular tiling by ganglion cells provides the basis for deriving an index of spatial position, i.e., a coordinate address, remains to be seen.

The major source of insight about the mechanism for position encoding may come from direct study of the tissue, but we are intrigued by the possibility that the activity of neural modules can be inferred from the judgments of human subjects.

REFERENCES

Bouma, H., & Andriessen, J. J. Induced changes in the perceived orientation of line segments. *Vision Research*, 1970, 10, 333-349.

DeVries, S. H., & Baylor, D. A. Mosaic arrangement of ganglion cell receptive fields in rabbit retina. *Journal of Neurophysiology*, 1997, 78, 2048-2060.

Everling, S., & Fischer, B. The antisaccade: a review of basic research and clinical studies. *Neuropsychologia*, 1998, 36, 885-899.

Graybill, F. A. *An introduction to linear statistical models*. Vol. 1. New York: McGraw-Hill, 1961.

Greene, E., & Frawley, W. Evaluating models of collinearity judgment for reliability and scale. *Perception*, 2001a, 30, 543-558.

Greene, E., & Frawley, W. Idiosyncratic profiles of collinearity error using segments and dot pairs. *Psychological Research*, 2001b, 65, 260-278.

Greene, E., Frawley, W., & Swimm, R. Individual differences in collinearity judgment as a function of angular position. *Perception & Psychophysics*, 2000, 62, 1440-1458.

Greene, E., & Nelson, B. Evaluating Müller-Lyer effects using single fin-set configurations. *Perception & Psychophysics*, 1997, 59, 293-312.

Guitton, D. Control of saccadic eye and gaze movements by the superior colliculus and basal ganglia. In R. H. S. Carpenter (Ed.), *Vision and visual dysfunction, eye movements*. London: Macmillan, 1991. Pp. 244-276.

Hallett, P. E. Primary and secondary saccades to goals defined by instructions. *Vision Research*, 1978, 18, 1279-1296.

HALLETT, P. E., & LIGHTSTONE, A. D. Saccadic eye movements to flashed targets. *Vision Research*, 1976, 16, 107-114.

HOCKING, R. R. The analysis and selection of variables in linear regression. *Biometrics*, 1976, 32, 1-50.

NELSON, B., & GREENE, E. Similar Müller-Lyer effects from operant and comparison modes. *Perceptual and Motor Skills*, 1998, 86, 499-511.

NYQUIST, H. Certain topics in telegraph transmission theory. *Proceedings of the IEEE*, 2002, 90, 280-305. [Reprinted from Transactions of the A.I.E.E., 1928(Feb.), 617-644]

ROCKHILL, R. L., EULER, T., & MASLAND, R. H. Spatial order within but not between types of retinal neurons. *Proceedings of the National Academy of Sciences*, 2000, 97, 2303-2307.

SPARKS, D. L., & HARTWICH-YOUNG, R. The deep layers of the superior colliculus. In R. H. Wurtz & M. E. Goldberg (Eds.), *The neurobiology of saccadic eye movements, reviews of oculometer research*. Vol. 3. Amsterdam: Elsevier, 1989. Pp. 213-256.

WASSLE, H., & BOYCOTT, B. B. Functional architecture of the mammalian retina. *Physiological Reviews*, 1991, 71, 447-480.

WURTZ, R. H. Vision for the control of movement. *Investigative Ophthalmology and Visual Science*, 1996, 37, 2131-2145.

Accepted March 23, 2004.

EFFECTS OF FOOT-PEDAL POSITIONS BY INEXPERIENCED CYCLISTS AT THE HIGHEST AEROBIC LEVEL [1]

DUANE MILLSLAGLE, SARA RUBBELKE, TOM MULLIN,
JOHN KEENER, AND RYAN SWETKOVICH

University of Minnesota at Duluth

Summary.—The purpose of this study was to assess whether the platform foot-pedal position affected maximal oxygen intake (VO_2 max) at the highest aerobic demand in cycling. 21 inexperienced cyclists completed two exercise tests, one in the "normal" platform foot-pedal position and the other in the Biopedal™ forefoot varus foot-pedal position, cycling on an exercise ergometer. The time between tests ranged from 1 to 3 days depending on the subject's reported fatigue and muscle soreness. The highest aerobic demand was the subject's VO_2 max at the point just below the subject's anaerobic threshold. A one-way analysis of variance indicated that the subject's VO_2 max performance was similar between the foot-pedal positions. These results did not support the assumption that the Biopedal™ forefoot varus foot-pedal position would enable the cyclist to be more efficient at the highest aerobic demand when compared to a standard platform foot-pedal position.

According to Garbalosa, McClure, Catlina, and Wooden (1994), 87% of the cycling population has a misalignment in the foot structure known as "forefoot varus" wherein the foot tilts up to the inside position. In the same study, an additional 9% of the cycling population have another misalignment known as "forefoot valgus" in which the foot tilts to the outside when the ankle joint is in its neutral position.

Conventional or standard platform foot-pedal systems are designed for the cyclist to be positioned on the pedal flat-footed. This is ideal for those 4% of the cycling population who do not have forefoot varus or valgus misalignment in the foot structure. Varus or valgus misalignment causes a side-to-side motion of the knee during the pedal cycle instead of the ideal straight up and down motion. The side-to-side motion of the knee during the pedal cycle has been assumed to contribute to patella femoral knee pain and loss of power in cycling (Burke, 1995).

Given the potential connection between foot-pedal position on the pedal and the effects of varus or valgus misalignment on cycling, a number of pedals have been developed to correct the misalignment. One such orthopedic pedal is called the Biopedal™ (Biosport, Inc., 1988) which allowed adjustment of the cyclist's foot-pedal position in three planes of movement: forefoot varus/valgus, toe-in/toe-out, and leg length.

---

[1]Send correspondence to Dr. Duane Millslagle, Health, Physical Education, and Recreation Department, SpHc 115, 1216 Ordean Court, 10 University Avenue, University of Minnesota at Duluth, Duluth, MN 55812 or e-mail (dmillsla@d.umn.edu).

Researchers have studied foot-pedal position as a mechanical factor in cycling (Hannaford, Moran, & Hlavac, 1985; Moran, 1988; Moran, Robertson, & Einhorn-Dicks, 1992) using the specially designed orthopedic Biopedal™. These researchers have assessed whether different foot positions balance the structure and dynamic function of the limb throughout the cycling stroke. Findings have indicated that muscle recruitment patterns changed with variation in forefoot varus/valgus foot-pedal alignment. Furthermore, knee pain in cyclists was minimized when foot-pedal position allowed the tibial tubercle to track in a linear path during the cycling stroke. These studies support the assumption that for the cyclists there is an optimal foot-pedal position which produced less skeletomuscular and ligament stress on the knees during the cycling stroke.

Moran and McGlinn (1995) examined foot-pedal position effects on cyclists' production of maximum anaerobic power and aerobic cycling efficiency. The aerobic and anaerobic performances of 10 cyclists were measured when the Biopedal™ was positioned in the forefoot varus foot-pedal position versus a standard platform foot-pedal position. Aerobic cycling efficiency was measured by assessing maximum aerobic power (VO_2 max) during steady-state cycling that simulated intensity similar to that of a 20–40 mile ride. Production of maximum anaerobic power was measured by a 30-sec. Wingate cycling test. The results indicated that aerobic performance between the two different pedal positions did not differ significantly, but production of maximum anaerobic power differed significantly. Nine of the 10 subjects showed an increase in anaerobic power with the pedals in a forefoot varus-adjusted foot-pedal position. A limitation of this study is the sample size of the competitive subjects which resulted in a low effect size (.10) and power (.05).

Moran and McGlinn suggested that the lack of difference in aerobic performance between the foot-pedal positions was because differences may only be manifested at the subjects' aerobic VO_2 max at the point just below the subjects' anaerobic threshold. Also, this point represents the highest demand on aerobic ability while performing. The purpose of this study was to examine whether forefoot varus foot-pedal position would produce different maximal aerobic power compared to standard foot-pedal position at the highest aerobic demand.

Foot-pedal research using experienced and inexperienced cyclists indicated that foot-pedal cadence and force application in cycling did not differ with training (Sanderson, Hennig, & Black, 2000). Regardless of the riding experience, cyclists used similar foot-pedal strategies at increasing intensities of power output. In a review of cycling research Atkinson, Davison, Jeukendrup, and Passfield (2003) reported that there is a poor understanding of what happens to VO_2 max for both the nontrained and trained cyclists at high intensities.

Given prior research which indicated similarity between nontrained and trained cyclists' foot-pedal strategies, the poor understanding of what happens to VO_2 max at a high intensity for the nontrained cyclist, and the difficulty in recruiting a representative sample of suitable size from competitive cyclists who had a forefoot-varus alignment in both feet, this study recruited inexperienced cyclists as subjects. The hypothesis tested in this study was that a higher VO_2 max would be produced by inexperienced cyclists who assume the adjusted forefoot-varus position not the standard foot-pedal position at the point of the highest aerobic power.

METHOD

Subjects

Forty-six subjects volunteered to participate. Twenty-one inexperienced cyclists (10 men and 11 women) who required a self-adjusted Biopedal™ varus position in both feet were subjects. Their mean age was 22 ± 2 yr., and mean body weight was 71 ± 7 kg. The subject group was comprised of undergraduate students at the University of Minnesota at Duluth who were active, cycled less than twice a week, and had no competitive cycling experience. All were volunteers, and subjects' assent to participte in the study was gained prior to testing. Human subject approval to conduct the study was approved by the Institution Review Board of the University of Minnesota.

Platform and Biopedal™ Positions

A Biopedal™ was mounted to each pedal spindle of a Monark 818-cycle ergometer. The Biopedal™ enabled the researchers to set each foot of the subject into either the platform foot-pedal position or the self-adjusted Biopedal™ position. In the platform pedal position, the forefoot varus/valgus and toe-in/toe-out planes were set at 0°, and leg length plane was set at 0 in. Front and back increments marked on each Biopedal™ provided the researchers the ability to set the left and right pedals in the forefoot-valgus/varus position (0 to 12°), toe-in/toe-out planes (0 to 5°) and leg-length plane from 0- to 1-in. range. The self-adjusted method of setting the Biopedal™ involved each subject riding for 10 or more minutes at a typical training pace where the pedal is in a free floating mode until the cyclist assumes a position in which the tibular insertion of patella is directly over the top of the position on the ball of the foot. This position provided a direct up and down line of force during cycling (Biosports, Inc., 1988). Once the neutral foot-pedal position of power and efficiency was achieved, an assistant would tighten the platform bolts that locked the subject's foot in this pedal position. Each subject's Biopedal™ forefoot-varus setting was recorded and assumed for the exercise test.

Procedure

Each subject completed two graded cycling ergometer tests, one for each foot-pedal position (platform or forefoot varus). A one- to three-day recovery period was given depending upon the subject's reported muscular soreness and fatigue. Prior to each test, a Parvo Medics True One 2400 metabolic system was calibrated to assure proper measurement of metabolic performance. The Parvo Medics True One 2400 system (Parvo Medics, Sandy, UT) is a complete, integrated metabolic measurement system used to assess oxygen uptake, carbon dioxide output, minute ventilation, respiratory rate, and heart rate. These data were used to calculate ventilatory equivalent for O_2 and CO_2, and VO_2 max. Data were used to set these values at each 30-sec. period during both work tests.

Birkholz and Jones's guidelines (1991) were used to establish each subject's seat height, fore-aft, and ball of foot positions prior to testing using the Monark-880 cycle ergometer. Optimal seat position was established between 25 to 30° of knee flexion. This allows for adequate decompression of the knee during the pedal stroke and an optimum position of the leg in which it is most capable of applying force to the pedals (Burke, 1995). The subject's fore-aft position of each leg was based on a plumb line that fell from tibular insertion of each patella and intersected the spindle of each pedal. Each subject's foot was positioned so the axle of the pedal was directly under the ball of the foot that allowed maximal leverage without straining the toes. The subject's seat height, fore-aft, and ball of the foot positions were recorded to assure the seat height and ball of foot positions were standardized across both tests.

The order of the pedal positions was randomly assigned for each subject. A 10-min. warm-up and cool-down pedaling period at a cadence of 60 rotations per minute (RPM) with no resistance was given before and after each test.

After the warm-up period, the subject was fitted with a head support, nose clip, and mouthpiece. The respiratory tubing attached to the mouthpiece and head support was then fitted to the Parvo Medics TrueMax 2400 metabolic system. The American College of Sport Medicine (2000) bike protocol for unfit or sedentary adults was used in each graded cycle ergometer test. The initial workload was 1 kg and was increased by .5 kg for each subsequent 2-min. interval. The subjects were instructed to maintain a cadence of 60 RPM throughout the test and continue to cycle until they were unable to maintain the 60-RPM cadence for three consecutive seconds.

The technique for identifying anaerobic threshold involved monitoring both the ventilatory equivalent for oxygen (VE/VO_2) and the ventilatory equivalent for carbon dioxide (VE/VCO_2), which is the ratio of the amount of air breathed to the amount of carbon dioxide produced (Wilmore & Costill, 1999). The anaerobic threshold was automatically assessed using Parvo Medics TrueMax 2400 metabolic system software which objectively identifies the point at which VE/VO_2 shows a sudden increase while VE/VCO_2 stays relatively stable. Of interest in this study was the subjects' VO_2 max just below the identified anaerobic threshold, which represented the subject's highest aerobic output.

RESULTS

The two tests differed by the type of foot-pedal position, platform or varus. The dependent variable measured in both tests was the subjects' VO_2 max just below the anaerobic threshold. VO_2 max was recorded in milliliters of oxygen consumed per kilogram of body weight ($ml/O_2/kg$). A one-way analysis of variance ($\alpha = .05$) was calculated to judge whether foot-pedal position affected the subjects' cycling aerobic performance. The one-way analysis of variance indicated a nonsignificant foot-pedal position effect ($F_{1,40} = 2.98, p > .05$). The statistical effect size was moderate (.32) with a low power rating (.38) as determined by Cohen's formulas (1988). The means and standard deviations for the two foot-pedal positions involving the subjects' VO_2 max are reported in Table 1. Also reported in Table 1 are the mean workloads, which were similar for both foot-pedal types at the groups' mean VO_2 max.

TABLE 1
DESCRIPTIVE STATISTICS FOR FOOT-PEDAL POSITION INVOLVING
VO_2 MAX ($ml/O_2/kg$) AND WORKLOAD (KG)

Foot-pedal Type	M VO_2 max	Workload M	Workload SD
Varus	29.1	2.5	4.5
Platform	27.2	2.5	6.1

DISCUSSION

This study examined how varying foot-pedal position (varus and platform) affected high aerobic cycling performance with inexperienced cyclists. Moran and McGlinn (1995) suggested that differences between the foot-pedal positions in the cyclists' aerobic ability might occur at a point near the cyclists' anaerobic threshold or highest aerobic output. In this study, no statistically significant effect was found between the self-adjusted Biopedal™ forefoot-varus and platform-pedal positions at the highest aerobic ability.

A particular limitation of this study and of the Morgan and McGlinn study is the reliance on small samples, producing low statistical power and nonsignificant aerobic power findings. According to Cohen (1992), studies with a moderate effect size with low power can lead to misleading inferential statistics and can cause major problems in the control of Type I errors in statistical tests. The only solutions available to researchers are to increase the sample size which increases the statistical power or to use sample size and power as a descriptive statistic to enable interpretation of the importance of the findings (Mullineaux, Bartlett, & Bennett, 2001).

A moderate effect size and low power were found in this study, which means this study cannot rule out other plausible alternatives of accepting a null hypothesis. According to Garbalosa, *et al.* (1994), 87% of the cycling population has a forefoot-varus misalignment in one or both feet. In this study, this percentage was much lower (46%) because only subjects with *both* feet needing a forefoot-varus correction were included. The difficulty in obtaining a sample size which meets the recommended power involving inexperienced or experienced cyclists using a corrected varus foot-pedal position in both feet and having them perform a difficult and demanding test is a limitation in foot-pedal position research and will be a challenge for those planning to conduct research on foot-pedal position.

The cycling performance of the subjects performing at their highest aerobic output was not altered when using the self-adjusted Biopedal™ varus position. Each subject required a varus correction such that the tibial tubercle tracked a linear path during the cycling stroke. This correction during the cycling stroke causes less skeletomuscular and ligamentous stress on the knees during the cycling stroke (Hannaford, *et al.*, 1985; Moran, 1988). One important implication of this study is that cyclists who require a corrected forefoot-varus position can still cycle at their highest aerobic output with a lower skeletomuscular and ligamentous stress on the knees when in the forefoot varus-pedal position.

This study used inexperienced cyclists, who required a forefoot-varus correction, performing a VO_2 max test for sedentary adults pedaling at an optimal cadence of 60 RPM. Burke (1995) indicated that a competitive cyclist's optimal cadence is between 80 to 90 RPM. Further foot-pedal research could be conducted to assess whether different foot-pedal variations (varus, valgus, toe-out, or toe-in) involving inexperienced or experienced cyclists pedaling at their optimal cadence would produce similar or different findings from those of this study.

REFERENCES

AMERICAN COLLEGE OF SPORTS MEDICINE. (2000) *Guidelines for exercise testing and prescription.* (6th ed.) Philadelphia, PA: Lippincott, Williams, & Wilkins.
ATKINSON, G. A., DAVISON, R., JEUKENDRUP, A., & PASSFIELD, L. (2003) Science and cycling: current knowledge and future directions of research. *Journal of Sport Sciences*, 21, 767-787.
BIRKHOLZ, D., & JONES, C. C. (1991) *Coaches cycling specific manual.* Colorado Springs, CO: United States Cycling Federation.
BURKE, E. (1995) *High tech cycling.* Champaign, IL: Human Kinetics.

COHEN, J. (1988) *Statistical power analysis for the behavioral sciences.* (2nd ed.) Hillsdale, NJ: Erlbaum.

COHEN, J. (1992) A power primer. *Psychological Bulletin*, 112, 155-159.

GARBALOSA, J. C., MCCLURE, M. H., CATLINA, P. A., & WOODEN, M. J. (1994) The frontal plane relationship of the forefoot to the rearfoot in a symptomatic population. *Journal of Orthopedic and Sports Physical Therapy*, 20, 200-206.

HANNAFORD, D. R., MORAN, G. T., & HLAVAC, H. F. (1985) Video analysis and treatment of overuse knee injury in cycling: a limited cyclist study. In J. Terauds & J. Barham (Eds.), *Biomechanics in sport*. Delmar, CA: Academic Press. Pp. 134-139.

MORAN, G. T. (1988) Biomechanics of cycling: the role of the foot pedal interface and cycling pathomechanics. In E. Kreighbaum & A. McNeill (Eds.), *Biomechanics in sport: VI*. Bozeman, MT: International Society of Biomechanics in Sports. Pp. 43-49.

MORAN, G. T., & MCGLINN, G. H. (1995) The effect of variations in the foot pedal interface on the efficiency of cycling as measured by aerobic power and anaerobic power. In A. Barabas & G. Fabian (Eds.), *Biomechanics in sport: XII*. Budapest, Hungary: International Society of Biomechanics in Sports. Pp. 105-109.

MORAN, G. T., ROBERTSON, R. N., & EINHORN-DICKS, S. (1992) The use of biomechanical adjustable cycling pedals in the development of rehabilitation protocols for ankle and knee injuries. In R. Redano, G. Ferrigno, & G. Santambrogio (Eds.), *Proceedings of International Society of Biomechanics in Sport*. Milan, Italy: International Society of Biomechanics in Sport. Pp. 288-292.

MULLINEAUX, D. R., BARTLETT, R. M., & BENNETT, S. (2001) Research design and statistics in biomechanics and motor control. *Journal of Sport Science*, 19, 739-760.

SANDERSON, D. J., HENNIG, E. M., & BLACK, A. H. (2000) The influence of cadence and power output on force application and in-shoe pressure distribution during cycling by competitive and recreational cyclists. *Journal of Sports Science*, 18, 173-181.

WILMORE, J. H., & COSTILL, D. L. (1999) *Physiology of sport and exercise.* (2nd ed.) Champaign, IL: Human Kinetics.

Accepted March 25, 2004.

SENSITIVITY TO DIFFERENCES IN THE EXTENT OF NECK-RETRACTION AND -ROTATION MOVEMENTS MADE WITH AND WITHOUT VISION[1]

HAEJUNG LEE, LESLIE L. NICHOLSON, AND ROGER D. ADAMS

University of Sydney

Summary.—19 subjects (10 men, 9 women) ages 19 to 30 years ($M = 23.2$, $SD = 3.3$) volunteered to participate in a study to investigate the just-noticeable-difference in movement extent for neck retraction and neck rotation. Testing was carried out with stopped movements, conducted according to the method of constant stimuli, and repeated both with and without vision in a comfortable seated position. Sensitivity was greatest for neck-retraction movements, which had lower just-noticeable-difference than either left or right rotation movements. Having full vision available gave no significant advantage in any direction when discriminating between different extents of midrange head movements.

To maintain task validity in laboratory research on the control of limb movements, proprioception has been studied by the method of selectively rather than completely obscuring vision, so that general vision is available for maintaining balance, but no visual information is available about the point of contact between the limb and its target (Smyth & Marriott, 1982; Waddington & Adams, 1999; Cameron, Adams, & Maher, 2003). Currently, there is still a lack of a widely agreed upon definition of proprioception (Beard & Refshauge, 2000). The definition employed here is that proposed by Dickinson (1974, p. 10), of proprioception as "... the appreciation of movement and position of the body and parts of the body based on information from other than visual, auditory or superficial cutaneous sources." For active movement, this definition incorporates the concept of corollary discharge, as well as many afferent sources, all providing information when judgments are made of active movement extent. The study of the use of proprioception in neck movements has a unique difficulty, in that the source of vision (the eyes) are located in the body part being moved (the head). Indeed, visual, vestibular, and cervical proprioceptive information all normally contribute to neck-movement control (Gimse, Tjell, Bjorgen, & Saunte, 1996), and it has been suggested that there is a hard-wired association between the visual and cervical proprioceptive systems (Rosenhall, Tjell, & Carlsson, 1996; Heikkila & Wenngren, 1998). However, there are presently

---

[1]Address correspondence to Haejung Lee, School of Physiotherapy, Faculty of Health Sciences, University of Sydney, P.O. Box 170, Lidcombe NSW 1825, Australia or e-mail (hlee3652@mail.usyd.edu.au).

no data available regarding the consequences of judging neck movements with vision, compared to not having vision during the movement.

From an ecological standpoint, Gibson (1986) has proposed that to assess any discrimination ability, the test should be functional and conducted under normal sensory conditions. An implication of assessing movements of specific body parts in an ecologically valid fashion is that other limbs or segments are not restrained with straps or clamps. Russell (1976) noted that a continuously updated representation of the body in space was needed for all movements, so that, for example, directed arm movements would have to take any trunk movement into account. Even though a movement being assessed is primarily made at one joint from one limb, it could still be regarded as part of a movement grouping or synergy (Kelso, 1995). For these reasons, a functional test of neck movements should not involve restraint or fixing of any body part. Accordingly, an apparatus was developed to assess neck-movement discrimination which would enable the subject to move the neck actively without any equipment attached to the head or other body part.

Midrange movements made from physical contact to physical contact were employed. Rotation and retraction movements were chosen, as rotation is the movement most commonly used when exploring the external environment, and retraction is the neck movement most affecting posture (Taylor & McCloskey, 1988; Rubin, Woolley, Dailey, & Goebel, 1995; Hanten, Olson, Russell, Lucio, & Campbell, 2000).

The measure of sensitivity to the extent of neck movements employed here was the just-noticeable-difference. This is defined as that distance either side of the standard distance which can be discriminated from this standard on at least 50% of the trials (Magill & Parks, 1983; Choi, Meeuwsen, & Arnhold, 1995). The aim of this study was to investigate: (1) any difference in sensitivity between various directions of neck movement: neck retraction, and left and right rotations and (2) whether the just-noticeable-difference for extent is affected when neck movements are made with vision or without vision.

Method

Nineteen volunteers (10 men, 9 women) took part, all of whom were students at the University of Sydney and ages 18 to 30 years ($M=23.2$, $SD=3.3$). The advertisements placed on noticeboards sought subjects over 18 years of age, with no experience of neck, upper back, or spinal problems that had resulted in a restriction of normal activity or any time off from work, and having no current neck symptoms. Subjects who had sought medical attention for neck pain or related problems within the last 6 months were excluded from participation in the study, as was anyone with any medical condition likely to affect mobility of the cervical spine, e.g., ankylosing spondylitis. Approval for the study was obtained from the Human Ethics Committee of the University of Sydney, and each subject gave informed consent prior to testing.

As in Magill and Parks' (1983) study of arm movements, the method of constant stimuli was used to determine the difference threshold for neck movements, as a measure of neck-movement sensitivity. With this method, the subject judges pairs of movement stimuli, one the standard and the other the variable stimulus (Woodworth & Schlosberg, 1954). Comparisons between each of the six variable movements and the standard movement were presented in random order. After carrying out both movements, the subject told the experimenter which of the two movements appeared to be the greater in extent. All movement sets were performed once with and once without vision. Retraction and rotation directions of movement were tested on separate occasions, with order of testing randomly arranged.

The apparatus used to measure discrimination of neck rotation movements is shown in Fig. 1. A stepper motor (RS Components Pty. Ltd., 129-137 Beaconsfield St., Silverwater, NSW 2141, Australia) was clamped to a height-adjustable bar attached across two fixed poles and connected to a laptop computer. The program allowed the stepper motor shaft to move in and out to any one of seven preset positions. Before moving to the test position,

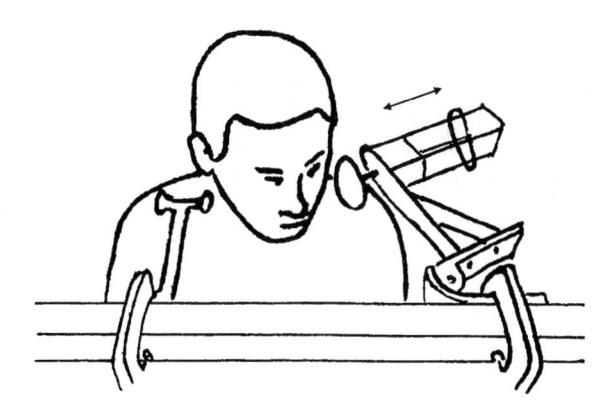

FIG. 1. Testing positions for rotation movements. *Note.*—The subject sat on a chair in a comfortable sitting position with the stepper motor shaft moving the mushroom-shaped contact backward and forward as indicated by the arrowheads.

the stepper motor was programmed to make additional movements of randomly ordered duration, to remove any auditory cues which could aid in judgments of distance moved to the test location. There was a fixed plate on the opposite side to the motor and shaft, for the subjects to contact as the test starting position.

The subject sat comfortably on a height-adjustable chair, with the feet placed flat on the floor at 90° of knee flexion and the hands resting in the lap. For starting the left rotation test, the subject's right cheek was to contact the fixed plate, which was adjusted for each subject's neutral sitting position. The movable end plate, which was fixed on the stepper-motor shaft was located in the target range, i.e., between 25° and 41° of rotation. From the starting position, the subject was asked to rotate the head to the left till the left cheek touched the movable plate. Then, the subject returned the head back to the starting position while the stepper motor progressed the movable mushroom-shaped contact either closer to or further from the original position. The subject then repeated the task, touching the variable plate in the new position and touching the standard, before making a judgment. The task was always to compare two movements to decide which of the two was further from the starting position, i.e., the response given was that the 'first one' or 'second one' was 'further away' from the starting position. For the right rotation test, the movable plate was located to the subject's right side. The test procedure was then the same as for left rotation.

For testing retraction movements, the subject was positioned parallel to the crossbar, such that their forehead (glabella) contacted the fixed plate when they were in their neutral sitting position. The hinged stepper motor was swung around so that the direction of travel of the shaft was also parallel to the crossbar, and the movable plate which was attached to the shaft was located in the target movement range, i.e., between 1.0 and 1.9 cm. Starting with the forehead against the fixed contact, the subject was asked to pull the head backward from the neutral position while tucking in the chin until the back of the head touched the movable plate. After each pair of retraction movements, the subject was asked which movement was 'further from' the starting position.

Random allocation determined whether vision or no vision was used in the initial session. During testing, all six pairs of movements were presented 12 times in random order. Therefore, the subject moved the head a total of 144 times for both the vision and no-vision tests. There was a 5-min. break so that subjects were able to rest before commencing the next session. Each session took 20 min. to complete.

For retraction, the six variable positions were 1.00, 1.15, 1.30, 1.60, 1.75, and 1.90 cm, with the standard position at 1.45 cm. The set of lengths from the stepper-motor shaft used in testing was the same in both retraction and rotation movements. The six variable positions used for rotation were therefore the same linear translations, corresponding to 25.0°, 28.0°, 31.0°, 37.0°, 40.0°, and 43.0° of rotation, with the standard position always at 34°. Each test set in the rotation and retraction directions was in midrange, so as not to cause any stress on the neck. For this subject population, the average total ranges for left and right rotations have been reported as 73.1° and 71.7°, respectively, and for retraction, average total range was 2.9 cm (Lee, Nicholson, & Adams, 2004).

RESULTS

Raw scores for the 'further from' judgment category were collated, and data were analysed using Probit, a SPSS-Windows subroutine (SPSS for Windows, Release 10.05, 233 Wacker Drive, 11th floor, Chicago, IL 60606). The just-noticeable-difference was defined as that movement extent difference which could be discriminated 75% of the time (Coren, Ward, & Enns, 1994). Each subject's just-noticeable-difference was obtained for both retraction and rotation movements, under the vision and no-vision conditions.

TABLE 1
JUST-NOTICEABLE-DIFFERENCE (MM) FOR THREE NECK-MOVEMENT DIRECTIONS OBTAINED FROM SESSIONS WITH AND WITHOUT VISION

Condition	Retraction M	SD	Left Rotation M	SD	Right Rotation M	SD	All Movements M	SD
Vision	1.9	0.5	2.7	0.8	2.7	1.0	2.4	0.5
No vision	2.2	0.6	3.2	0.3	2.7	0.8	2.7	0.7
All conditions	2.1	0.3	3.0	0.9	2.7	0.8		

A 2 (vision: yes, no) × 3 (movement direction: retraction, left rotation, right rotation) repeated-measures analysis of variance using orthogonal planned contrasts (Winer, Brown, & Michels, 1991) was performed on the just-noticeable-differences. Means and SDs of just-noticeable-difference with and without vision for each of the neck movements are shown in Table 1. There was a significant difference between the mean just-noticeable-difference for retraction and combined left and right rotation movements ($F_{1,17} = 16.40$, $p < .001$), but not between left and right rotations ($F_{1,17} = 1.48$, ns). The mean just-noticeable-differences for retraction and combined rotations were 2.1 and 2.8 mm, respectively. As a lower value represents better discrimination, retraction movements were better discriminated than rotation movements. For each subject, the difference between their rotation and retraction just-noticeable-difference values was calculated and plotted in Fig. 2.

From the vision/no-vision comparison, vision showed no significant advantage in the discrimination of movements ($F_{1,17} = 2.47$, ns). The individual subject differences between movement sensitivity with vision and without vision can also be seen in Fig. 2. Subject ranks refer to each plot separately, so the subject with the largest difference between scores for vision conditions is not the same subject with the largest difference on direction conditions. Retraction is more sensitive than rotation, as most subjects' differences in just-noticeable-difference are positive, whereas there is no signifi-

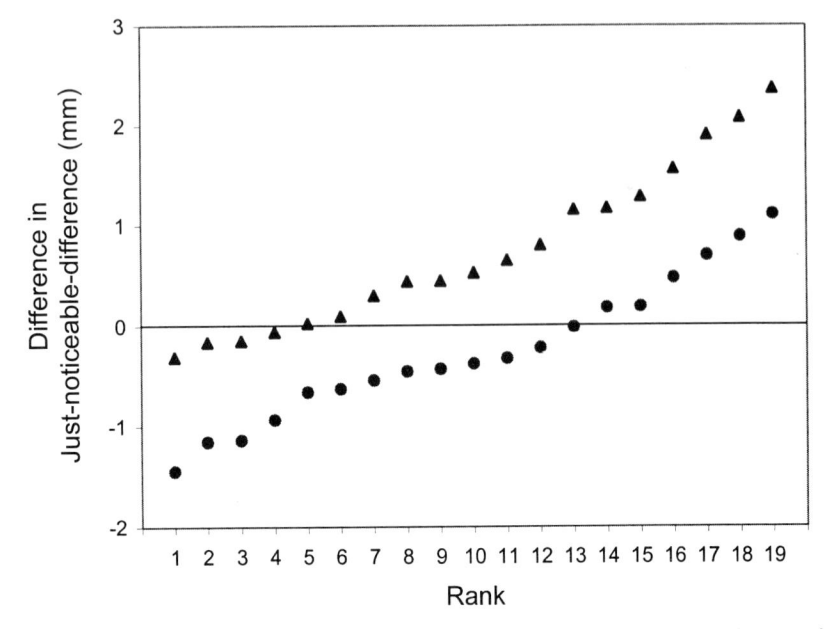

FIG. 2. Individual subjects' data for differences between the just-noticeable-differences for rotation and retraction movements (▲), and between vision and no-vision conditions (●), ranked across subjects. Retraction is more sensitive than rotation (most subjects' differences in just-noticeable-difference are positive), whereas there is no significant sensitivity advantage from having vision available during testing (differences between the conditions are more distributed over negative and positive). Subject ranks refer to each difference plot separately.

nificant sensitivity advantage from having vision available during testing, as differences between the conditions are more evenly distributed over negative and positive. Negative differences show a vision advantage.

DISCUSSION

Although the neck may be regarded as the movable platform for vision, having vision available when judging the extent of neck-rotation or -retraction movements did not significantly improve discrimination accuracy. As Delgado-Garcia (2000) has noted, the eyes are not pasted onto the head like postage stamps but move separately. Head-rotation movements are immediately accompanied by compensatory eye movements in the opposite direction (Gibson, 1986). If the rotation movement continues, the eyes then swing to a fixation in the new forward direction. In the absence of novel objects coming into view after turning to different extents, this automatic opposite-direction eye movement may be what makes 'visual proprioception' (Lishman & Lee, 1973) an insignificant source of additional information for extent of head-turning movements.

Compensatory eye movements do not occur during head retraction, but without novel objects coming into view for deeper retractions, the expansion of the visual field accompanying neck retraction over the range employed here does not give significant useful additional information, over the 'feel' of the retraction movement. For some subjects, having vision during judgment of neck movements may have distracted attention from cervicocephalic proprioception, through the operation of visual dominance (Lee & Aronson, 1974; Klein, 1976).

Kinesthetic sensitivity, or proprioception, in the neck has been dependent on input from proprioceptors in joint tissues (capsule and ligaments) and from muscle receptors (Golgi organs and spindles) (McCloskey, 1978; Gandevia, McCloskey, & Burke, 1992). In the midrange, as used in the current study, muscle receptors are considered to be the major sensory sources for the discrimination of movement, since several studies have shown that muscle spindles are sensitive to stretch over a wide range of muscle lengths including the midrange (Boyd & Roberts, 1953; McCall, Farias, Williams, & BeMent, 1974; Clark & Burgess, 1975; McCloskey, 1978). Therefore, it is likely that subjects rely primarily on cervicocephalic kinesthesia to make their judgments about the extent of head movements, whether or not vision is available.

In terms of absolute sensitivity, retraction movements showed smaller just-noticeable-difference values than right or left neck-rotation movements. An explanation of this effect can be put forward which considers the need to balance the head on the neck. The weight of the head is more destabilizing when it is retracted or protracted, as it moves the center of mass of the head closer to the balance periphery than when the head is rotated. For this reason, maintaining upright balance may require greater sensitivity of judgment of movement extent for retraction and protraction movements than for head-rotation movements. It has been found previously that there is a very high density of muscle spindles in the neck retractor muscles compared to the neck rotator muscle group (Peck, Buxton, & Nitz, 1984). This factor may allow backward movements of the head to be better controlled and better detected than other directions of neck movement.

The apparatus employed here permits a psychophysical method (constant stimuli) previously used to determine the accuracy of forearm and whole arm movements (Magill & Parks, 1983; Carlton & Newell, 1985; Choi, et al., 1995; Naughton, Adams, & Maher, 2002) to be employed in the measurement of sensitivity to movement extent at the neck. Previous testing of sensitivity to neck-movement differences has involved blindfolding subjects in order to assess cervicocephalic kinesthetic sensitivity (Revel, Andre-Deshays, & Minguet, 1991; Kristjansson, Dall'Alba, & Jull, 2001). Neither a main effect nor interaction effect involving vision was detected in the current analysis, suggesting that there was no movement direction where having vision available made a significant difference to sensitivity scores and, therefore, that testing of proprioception at the neck can be carried out without blindfolding. Further studies can now evaluate this method of measurement of neck-movement discrimination sensitivity with different populations, e.g., neck-injured subjects.

REFERENCES

BEARD, D., & REFSHAUGE, K. (2000) Effects of ACL reconstruction on proprioception and neuromuscular performance. In S. M. Lephart & F. H. Fu (Eds.), *Proprioception and neuromuscular control in joint stability*. Champaign, IL: Human Kinetics. Pp. 213-224.

BOYD, I. A., & ROBERTS, T. D. M. (1953) Proprioceptive discharges from stretch-receptors in the knee-joint of the cat. *Journal of Physiology*, 122, 38-58.

CAMERON, M., ADAMS, R., & MAHER, C. (2003) Motor control and strength as predictors of hamstring injury in elite players of Australian football. *Physical Therapy in Sport*, 4, 159-166.

CARLTON, L. G., & NEWELL, K. M. (1985) A psychophysical examination of the perception of movement extent under passive movement conditions. *Journal of Human Movement Studies*, 11, 35-47.

CHOI, S. O., MEEUWSEN, H. J., & ARNHOLD, R. W. (1995) On the psychophysics of arm-positioning movements. *Perceptual and Motor Skills*, 80, 1163-1169.

CLARK, F. J., & BURGESS, P. R. (1975) Slowly adapting receptors in cat knee joint: can they signal joint angle? *Journal of Neurophysiology*, 38, 1448-1463.

COREN, S., WARD, L. M., & ENNS, J. T. (1994) *Sensation and perception*. (4th ed.) New York: Harcourt Brace College Publ.

DELGADO-GARCIA, J. M. (2000) Why move the eyes if we can move the head? *Brain Research Bulletin*, 52, 475-482.

DICKINSON, J. (1974) *Proprioceptive control of human movement*. Princeton, NJ: Princeton Book Co.

GANDEVIA, S., MCCLOSKEY, D., & BURKE, D. (1992) Kinaesthetic signals and muscle contraction. *Trends in Neurosciences*, 15, 62-65.

GIBSON, J. J. (1986) *The ecological approach to visual perception*. Hillsdale, NJ: Erlbaum.

GIMSE, R., TJELL, C., BJORGEN, I. A., & SAUNTE, C. (1996) Disturbed eye movements after whiplash due to injuries to the posture control system. *Journal of Clinical and Experimental Neuropsychology*, 18, 178-186.

HANTEN, W. P., OLSON, S. L., RUSSELL, J. L., LUCIO, R. M., & CAMPBELL, A. H. (2000) Total head excursion and resting head posture: normal and patient comparisons. *Archives of Physical Medicine and Rehabilitation*, 81, 62-66.

HEIKKILA, H. V., & WENNGREN, B. I. (1998) Cervicocephalic kinesthetic sensibility, active range of cervical motion, and oculomotor function in patients with whiplash injury. *Archives of Physical Medicine and Rehabilitation*, 79, 1089-1094.

KELSO, J. A. (1995) *Dynamic patterns: the self-organization of brain and behavior*. Cambridge, MA: MIT Press.

KLEIN, R. M. (1976) Attention and movement. In G. E. Stelmach (Ed.), *Motor control*. New York: Academic Press. Pp. 143-173.

KRISTJANSSON, E., DALL'ALBA, P., & JULL, G. (2001) Cervicocephalic kinaesthesia: reliability of a new test approach. *Physiotherapy Research International*, 6, 224-235.

LEE, D. N., & ARONSON, E. (1974) Visual proprioceptive control of standing in human infants. *Perception & Psychophysics*, 15, 529-532.

LEE, H., NICHOLSON, L., & ADAMS, R. (2004) Cervical range of motion association with low-level neck pain. *Spine*, 29, 33-40.

LISHMAN, J. R., & LEE, D. N. (1973) The autonomy of visual kinaesthesis. *Perception & Psychophysics*, 2, 287-294.

MAGILL, R. A., & PARKS, P. F. (1983) The psychophysics of kinesthesis for positioning responses: the physical stimulus-psychological response relationship. *Research Quarterly for Exercise and Sport*, 54, 346-351.

McCall, W. D., Jr., Farias, M. C., Williams, W. J., & BeMent, S. L. (1974) Static and dynamic responses of slowly adapting joint receptors. *Brain Research*, 70, 221-243.

McCloskey, D. I. (1978) Kinesthetic sensibility. *Physiological Reviews*, 58, 763-820.

Naughton, J., Adams, R., & Maher, C. (2002) Discriminating overhead points of contact after arm raising. *Perceptual and Motor Skills*, 95, 1187-1195.

Peck, D., Buxton, D. F., & Nitz, A. (1984) A comparison of spindle concentrations in large and small muscles acting in parallel combinations. *Journal of Morphology*, 180, 243-252.

Revel, M., Andre-Deshays, C., & Minguet, M. (1991) Cervicocephalic kinesthetic sensibility in patients with cervical pain. *Archives of Physical Medicine and Rehabilitation*, 72, 288-291.

Rosenhall, U., Tjell, C., & Carlsson, J. (1996) The effect of neck torsion on smooth pursuit eye movements in tension-type headache patients. *Journal of Audiological Medicine*, 5, 130-140.

Rubin, A. M., Woolley, S. M., Dailey, V. M., & Goebel, J. A. (1995) Postural stability following mild head or whiplash injuries. *American Journal of Otology*, 16, 216-221. [Comment]

Russell, D. G. (1976) Spatial location cues and movement production. In G. E. Stelmach (Ed.), *Motor control: issues and trends*. New York: Academic Press. Pp. 67-85.

Smyth, M. M., & Marriott, A. M. (1982) Vision and proprioception in simple catching. *Journal of Motor Behavior*, 14, 143-152.

Taylor, J. L., & McCloskey, D. I. (1988) Proprioception in the neck. *Experimental Brain Research*, 70, 351-360.

Waddington, G., & Adams, R. (1999) Discrimination of active plantarflexion and inversion movements after ankle injury. *Australian Journal of Physiotherapy*, 45, 7-13.

Winer, B. J., Brown, D. R., & Michels, K. M. (1991) *Statistical principles in experimental design*. (3rd ed.) New York: McGraw-Hill.

Woodworth, R. S., & Schlosberg, H. (1954) *Experimental psychology*. (3rd ed.) London: Methuen.

Accepted March 23, 2004.

USE OF THE SAME AND A LONGER TIME SERIES TO REPLICATE DAVID LESTER'S STUDY OF SUICIDE AND BIRTH RATES IN CANADA[1]

F. STEPHEN BRIDGES AND L. CAROLYN PEARSON

The University of West Florida

Summary.—This is a replication of Lester's work (2000) using the time series 1970–1990 to study associations between age-standardized rates of suicide and crude birth rates in the 10 Canadian provinces were also examined between 1961 and 1999.

Durkheim (1951) postulated that the rates of suicide varied inversely with social integration. Stack (1980a, 1980b) among others provided analysis generally supporting Durkheim's proposition, i.e., high rates of birth are seen as increasing social integration in a society. According to Lester (2000), in sociological studies of suicide some researchers have reported correlations over different geographic regions (Stack, 1981), or over a series of years (Lester & Yang, 1998), or over a mix of regions and years (Trovato & Jarvis, 1986). Lester's correlations (2000) between the rates of suicide and birth in the 10 Canadian provinces (see Table 1 for list) from 1970 to 1990, estimated using three different methods (over time, over space, and mixed), were small and negative. The source of Lester's data (2000) was not reported nor was each province listed or any of Canada's three territories mentioned.

The present study examined correlations obtained with these methods using age-standardized suicides (P. Tully, custom tabulation from Deaths database, August 2002, Health Statistics Division, Statistics Canada, Ottawa) and crude birth rates (per 100,000 population) for the 10 provinces in Canada from 1961 to 1999. Rates of birth by province were calculated for data obtained from the Federal Government of Canada (Statistics Canada, 2002; K. Hung, personal communication, March 2002, Research and Statistics Division, Department of Justice, Ottawa).

Pearson correlations over 39 years for each province ranged from –.84 to .29 and averaged –.43. These correlations and their 95% confidence intervals are provided in Table 1. Similarly, over 21 years, i.e., 1970–1990, for each province Lester (2000) reported very similar correlations ranging from –.82 to .28, with an average of –.29. Interestingly, further analysis of a subset of our data for the years 1970 to 1990 produced correlations ranging from

---

[1]Please send enquiries to Dr. F. Stephen Bridges, Division of Health, Leisure, and Exercise Science, The University of West Florida, 11000 University Parkway, Pensacola, FL 32514-5750 or e-mail (fbridges@uwf.edu).

TABLE 1
CORRELATIONS AND 95% CI FOR SUICIDE† AND BIRTH RATES OVER 10 PROVINCES FOR EACH OF 39 YEARS AND OVER 39 AND 21 YEARS‡ BY CANADIAN PROVINCE

Suicide and Birth Rates For Each of 39 Years

Year	Pearson r	95% CI	Year	Pearson r	95% CI
1961	−.58	−.89, .08	1981	.04	−.61, .65
1962	−.60	−.89, .05	1982	.22	−.47, .75
1963	−.69*	−.92, −.10	1983	.17	−.52, .72
1964	−.64*	−.90, −.01	1984	.46	−.23, .85
1965	−.61	−.90, −.03	1985	−.06	−.67, .59
1966	−.73*	−.93, −.18	1986	.30	−.41, .78
1967	−.78**	−.95, −.30	1987	.23	−.47, .75
1968	−.69*	−.92, −.11	1988	.37	−.34, .81
1969	−.76*	−.94, −.26	1989	.39	−.32, .82
1970	−.44	−.84, .26	1990	.54	−.14, .87
1971	−.61	−.89, .04	1991	.55	−.12, .88
1972	−.65*	−.91, −.04	1992	.62	−.02, .89
1973	−.76*	−.94, −.25	1993	.26	−.44, .76
1974	−.68*	−.92, −.10	1994	.31	−.40, .79
1975	−.62	−.90, .02	1995	.17	−.52, .72
1976	−.39	−.82, .32	1996	.28	−.43, .77
1977	−.46	−.84, .24	1997	.37	−.34, .81
1978	−.43	−.83, .27	1998	.18	−.50, .73
1979	−.36	−.80, .35	1999	.10	−.57, .68
1980	−.10	−.69, .56			

Suicide and Birth Rates Over 39 and 21 Years by Province

Province	39 Years Pearson r	95% CI	21 Years Pearson r	95% CI
Newfoundland	−.58**	−.76, −.32	−.45*	−.74, −.02
Prince Edward Island	−.27	−.54, .06	.25	−.20, .62
Nova Scotia	−.72**	−.85, −.53	−.14	−.54, .31
New Brunswick	−.77**	−.88, −.61	−.68**	−.86, −.34
Quebec	−.84**	−.92, −.72	−.55*	−.70, −.16
Ontario	−.01	−.33, .31	.44*	.01, .73
Manitoba	−.33*	−.59, −.02	.17	−.29, .56
Saskatchewan	−.41*	−.64, −.10	.20	−.26, .58
Alberta	−.61**	−.77, −.36	−.04	−.46, .40
British Columbia	.29	−.03, .55	.44*	.01, .73

†Age-specific suicide rates underlying the age-standardized suicide rates were calculated with June 1 population estimates for 1950 to 1970 and with July 1 population estimates for 1971 to 1999. 1950 to 1970 population estimates were not adjusted for net census undercoverage and do not include nonpermanent residents; 1971 to 1999 estimates do. ‡For 1970–1999 as reported by Lester (2000). *p<.05. **p<.01.

−.68 to .44, with an average of −.04. This difference might possibly be attributed to a different data source(s) used by Lester (2000) than used in the present study or rounding error. Also, the correlations over provinces for each of our 39 years ranged from −.78 to .62 and averaged −.16. For the years 1970–1990, Lester (2000) reported correlations that ranged from −.73 to .46 and averaged −.16. Our analysis of a subset of our data from 1970–1990 produced correlations very similar to those of Lester (2000), ranging from −.76 to .46, with an average of .14.

Over all 210 data points (10 provinces by 20 years) the correlation was −.21 (cf. Lester's average correlation of −.25). Further, for the subset from 1970–1990 mean r was −.10. Thus each procedure led to the conclusion that the association was small and negative as Lester (2000) previously reported. Further interpretation of these data would require other data as well as those for suicide.

REFERENCES

DURKHEIM, E. (1951) *Suicide: a study of sociology.* (J. A. Spaulding & G. E. Simpson, Eds.) Glencoe, IL: Free Press.

LESTER, D. (2000) Comparing correlations over time and space. *Perceptual and Motor Skills*, 91, 758.

LESTER, D., & YANG, B. (1998) *Suicide and homicide in the 20th Century.* Commack, NY: Nova Science.

STACK, S. (1980a) Domestic integration and the rate of suicide: a comparative study. *Journal of Comparative Family Studies*, 11, 249-260.

STACK, S. (1980b) Family integration and suicide: a comparative analysis. Presented at the North Central Sociological Association. [Abstract]

STACK, S. (1981) Suicide and religion. *Sociological Focus*, 14, 207-220.

STATISTICS CANADA. (2002) *Table 053-001: vital statistics, births, deaths, and marriages, quarterly (number).* CANSIM II. Ottawa, Canada: Demography and Health Statistics Divisions.

TROVATO, F., & JARVIS, G. K. (1986) Immigrant suicide in Canada. *Social Forces*, 65, 433-457.

Accepted March 31, 2004.

BODY SATISFACTION IN COLLEGE WOMEN AFTER BRIEF EXPOSURE TO MAGAZINE IMAGES[1]

ELIZABETH M. CAMERON AND F. RICHARD FERRARO

University of North Dakota

Summary.—Female undergraduates were divided into groups based on their rated body dissatisfaction ($n = 45$ operationally defined as Satisfied, $n = 45$ as Dissatisfied). These groups were then randomly assigned to one of three magazine categories: fashion, fitness-and-health, and news. Measures of Body Satisfaction, Depression, Anxiety, Self-esteem, Fear of Fat, Eating Attitudes, and Control of Weight were taken. Significant group main effects were found on Depression, Trait Anxiety, Eating Attitudes, Fear of Fat, and Self-esteem. A significant main effect for media was found for scores on Body Satisfaction, with the fitness-and-health Dissatisfied group reporting decreased body satisfaction following magazine exposure. No interactions were found. It appears women who are dissatisfied with their bodies may be at risk for a further decrease in body satisfaction after even a 15-min. exposure to fitness and health magazines but further follow-up measures were not made.

    The incidence of eating disorders in the general population has increased steadily over the past 30 years (Harrison & Cantor, 1997), with female cases outnumbering male cases 10 to 1 (Andersen & DiDomenico, 1992). The most widely accepted and developed theory of eating disorders is the sociocultural model (Thompson & Heinberg, 1999), which model emphasizes the role of multiple sociocultural factors contributing to the formation of eating disorders in a social environment in which thinness is valued. Through many channels society can promote an ideal standard of beauty, the most popular being mass media (Silverstein, Perdue, Peterson, & Kelly, 1986; Vandenberg, Thompson, Obremski-Brandon, & Coovert, 2002; Palladino-Green & Pritchard, 2003).

    One major avenue by which the media can portray the ideal physical form is through magazine images and content. Garner, Garfinkel, Schwartz, and Thompson (1980) evaluated Playboy centerfolds over a 20-yr. period from 1959–1978 and found that the bust and hip ratios of the models decreased significantly while their height increased. Weight analyses indicated that the centerfolds exhibited a weight that is significantly below that of the average woman during the same period.

    Subsequently, Garner, *et al.* (1980) evaluated the number of articles about dieting and weight loss in six women's magazines (Good Housekeeping, Harper's Bazaar, Ladies Home Journal, McCall's, Vogue, Woman's

---

[1]Address correspondence to F. Richard Ferraro, Ph.D., Department of Psychology, University of North Dakota, Grand Forks, ND 58202 or e-mail (f_ferraro@und.nodak.edu).

Day) for the same period. They found an increase in the number of magazine articles relating to dieting and weight loss over the period, with a significant increase over the last 10 years. This study provides evidence for a systematic portrayal in printed media of an increasingly thin ideal; women may attempt to emulate the ideal image which becomes increasingly difficult to obtain as the divergence between the ideal woman and the average woman increases, creating potential for the development of an eating disorder.

Wiseman, Gray, Mosimann, and Ahrens (1992) replicated and extended the work of Garner, *et al.* in an analysis of measurements of Playboy centerfolds over the 10-yr. period 1979–1988. The measurements remained at the low body weight found in previous research. More importantly, however, was that 60% of the centerfolds reported a weight 15% or more below their expected weight according to actuarial tables. This raised concern about the media's portrayal of women, especially since a weight 15% or more below an expected weight is one of the major criteria for anorexia nervosa (American Psychiatric Association, 1994).

Wiseman, *et al.* (1992) also examined the same magazines as did Garner, *et al.* (1980). They recorded the number of articles related to dieting for weight loss, exercise articles and diet-and-exercise articles for the years 1959–1988. They found an increase in the number of diet, exercise, and diet-and-exercise articles; however, the number of exercise articles from 1980–1988 was larger than the number on a diet. Because there was still an emphasis on thinness, Wiseman, *et al.* speculated that these exercise articles were merely weight-loss articles "in disguise."

Previous research has focused mainly on the effects of fashion magazines (e.g., Turner, Hamilton, Jacobs, Angood, & Dwyer, 1997), with analyses showing adverse effects on body satisfaction following exposure to fashion magazines. However, if the assertion made by Wiseman, *et al.* (1992) is correct, that exercise articles are actually only diet articles "in disguise," then it becomes increasingly important to study fitness and health magazines as well because a disturbance of body image is one of the four criteria for a diagnosis of either anorexia or bulimia (American Psychiatric Association, 1994).

The current study assessed the effects of fashion and fitness-and-health magazines on body satisfaction and related variables in college-age women. Two groups of women were studied, those satisfied (or not) with their bodies. It was hypothesized that the women who were initially dissatisfied with their bodies would report a decrease in body satisfaction after exposure to the fashion and fitness-and-health magazines. An additional group for each category of women read news magazines; this group served as the control group. No difference was expected for the group response to news magazines.

Method

Participants

Subjects were 90 undergraduate women from a large midwestern university. Based on the results of screening, 45 participants were assigned to one of two categories based on body satisfaction, i.e., Satisfied, Dissatisfied. Each group of 45 women was further divided randomly into three 15-subject magazine subgroups: fashion, fitness-and-health, news. Participation was voluntary, and subjects were given research credit for their time. Power calculations indicated that a relatively small effect size could be observed.

Materials

Magazines.—The 15 magazines used in the present study were chosen based on results of a pilot study, in which 50 participants, none of whom participated in the present experiment, indicated their preferred fashion, fitness-and-health, and news magazines. The selected magazines were taken from the September-November 2000 issues, as follows: Fashion, Cosmopolitan, Glamour, In Style, Mademoiselle, Vogue; Fitness-and-Health, Fitness, Health, Self, Shape, Sports Illustrated for Women; News, The Atlantic Monthly, Business Week, Newsweek, Time, U.S. News and World Report.

Questionnaires.—To measure Body Satisfaction/Dissatisfaction, the 99-item Body Image Questionnaire (Berscheld, Walster, & Bohanstedt, 1972) was used. The questionnaire consists of items used to measure individuals' satisfaction with their bodies. Only Questions 1–25 were scored for this study. The other questions served as distractor or filler questions. These 25 questions ask subjects to indicate how satisfied they are with different parts of their bodies. Subjects rate each question, using a 6-point scale using anchors of 1 = Extremely Satisfied and 6 = Extremely Dissatisfied. The possible range of scores across the 25 questions was 0–150. Scores of 1–75 were defined as body Satisfaction, and scores of 76–150 were defined as body Dissatisfactions.

The Geriatric Depression Scale–Short Form (Ferraro & Chelminski, 1996) is a 15-item questionnaire to assess depressive symptoms. In samples of young adults, the scale scores correlate strongly with the Beck Depression Inventory ratings ($r = .86$) and are easier to implement. Cronbach alpha (Brink, Yesavage, Lum, Heersema, Adey, & Rose, 1982) was reported to be .94.

The State-Trait Anxiety Inventory (Spielberger, 1983) measured both stable aspects of anxiety, e.g., how subjects generally feel, and fluctuating aspects of anxiety, e.g., how subjects feel right now. This inventory has test-retest correlations for college students between .27 and .86. Also, scores correlate with other anxiety measures at $rs = .52$ and .86.

Rosenberg's Self-esteem inventory (Rosenberg, 1965) is a 10-item measure with which subjects' self-esteem was assessed. Subjects respond to the 10 attitude statements by marking the anchors of 1 = Strongly Agree and 4 = Strongly Disagree. Five statements are reverse-scored and then summed with responses to the other statements. The possible range of scores is 10–40, with 10 indicating higher self-esteem. This measure has a test-retest reliability of .85 (Demo, 1985).

The Eating Attitudes Test (Garner, Olmsted, Bohr, & Garfinkel, 1982) is a 26-item measure designed to evaluate behaviors and attitudes characteristic of anorexia nervosa, e.g., "Become anxious prior to eating." Subjects are asked to respond to the questions using anchors of 1 = Always and 6 = Never. The 26 items are summed, with lower scores being indicative of eating disordered behavior. Cronbach alpha has ranged from .83 to .90.

The Attention to Body Shape Scale (Beebe, 1995) is a 7-item test measuring subjects' preoccupation with the shape of their bodies, e.g., "I place a great deal of importance on my body shape." Subjects respond with a 5-point scale, with anchors of 1 = Definitely Disagree and 5 = Definitely Agree. One item is reverse-scored. Higher scores indicate more attention to body shape. Adequate reliability and validity coefficients have been reported, and internal consistency estimates have ranged between .70 and .82 (Beebe, 1995).

The Goldfarb Fear of Fat Scale (Goldfarb, Dykens, & Gerrard, 1985) has 10 items to assess subjects' concern with weight gain, e.g., "I am afraid to gain even a little weight." Subjects respond on a 4-point scale with anchors of 1 = Very Untrue and 4 = Very True. The responses are summed, with higher scores indicating greater concern with body weight. This scale has been reported (Goldfarb, et al., 1985, p. 329) to have a Cronbach alpha of .85.

Procedure

Women were tested in groups of five and were instructed that the study involved a discussion about magazine content. When the women arrived at the testing center, they were asked to sit around a large table. Five magazines were placed on the table according to the group to which they were assigned, and each subject freely selected one magazine. The women were told that there would be a discussion following to ensure that they would look through and/or read the magazine thoroughly. No further information was presented regarding the content of the discussion, so as not to influence subjects' approach to reading or looking through the magazine. When the allotted time of 15 min. expired, subjects were told to place their magazines in the middle of the table, open their folders, and complete the questionnaires. Following completion of questionnaires, subjects were given a copy of the consent form they initially signed along with the contact numbers of the researchers in case of further questions or concerns.

Results

Demographic Information

Groups did not differ on age, height, desired weight, or desired height ($Fs < 3.21$, $ps > .07$). Significant demographic differences appear in Table 1.

TABLE 1
MEANS AND STANDARD DEVIATIONS FOR DEMOGRAPHIC INFORMATION BY GROUP

Demographic Variable	Satisfied M	Satisfied SD	Dissatisfied M	Dissatisfied SD	$F_{1,90}$
Current Weight	137.7	20.9	144.1	29.1	10.88†
Geriatric Depression Scale–Short Form	1.5	2.3	2.8	1.8	5.35*
State Anxiety	37.1	2.8	44.1	2.0	11.63†
Trait Anxiety	39.4	2.0	46.2	1.9	14.87†

*$p < .05$. †$p < .01$.

Group × Media Analyses of Variance

Following magazine exposure, several 2 (Group: Satisfied, Dissatisfied) × 3 (Media: Fashion, Fitness-and-Health, News) analyses of variance were performed on rating scores from the Depression, State Anxiety, Trait Anxiety, Attention to Body Shape, Self-esteem, Eating Attitudes, Fear of Fat, and Body Satisfaction. Means and standard deviations appear in Table 2. There were no significant interactions. Analyses of covariance using the demographic measures listed above as covariates did not change the overall pattern of results.

TABLE 2
MEANS AND STANDARD DEVIATIONS WITH MAIN EFFECTS OR INTERACTIONS
BY GROUP AND MEDIA AFTER MAGAZINE EXPOSURE

Measure	Satisfied M	Satisfied SD	Dissatisfied M	Dissatisfied SD	F
Main Effects of Group ($df = 1,90$)					
Geriatric Depression Scale–Short Form	1.5	2.8	2.6	2.6	5.87*
Trait Anxiety	37.0	1.9	42.4	2.7	8.01†
Eating-disordered Behavior	112.2	3.9	120.2	5.7	4.81*
Fear of Fat	19.4	2.9	23.4	3.2	12.68†
Self-esteem	20.9	1.8	17.4	2.0	13.30†
Main Effect of Media					
Body Satisfaction (Change)	2.06		–3.02		3.41*

*$p < .05$. †$p < .01$.

Discussion

The significant main effect for media was based on the decline in Body Satisfaction after exposure to fitness-and-health magazines. Group differences detected on Depression, Trait Anxiety, Eating Attitudes, Fear of Fat, and Self-esteem indicated a higher propensity for the Dissatisfied group to report adverse characteristics, as expected. In the Fashion-magazine condition, neither the Satisfied nor the Dissatisfied group showed any significant change in Body Satisfaction scores. In the Fitness-and-Health magazine condition, body-image scores remained similar, yet the Dissatisfied group showed a decrease in Body Satisfaction after the 15-min. exposure. Consistent with Cusumano and Thompson (1997), exposure to the thin ideal was not related to decreased Body Satisfaction for women who were exposed to and presumably read fashion magazines.

While the 15-min. exposure appeared to be too brief to detect many group differences or interactions, it is of some interest that those women classified as dissatisfied with their bodies appear to be at risk for further decreases in body dissatisfactions scores even after only a 15-min. exposure. We did not follow these women over time so the question of whether the dissatisfaction was temporary awaits further study.

An important limitation of the study was the subject pool: college-age women were selected for the study because of availability and convenience. However, the internalization of the thin ideal seems to happen often during adolescence when self-concepts are still being formed (Brenner & Cunningham, 1992). Although some have reported an effect of media exposure on body satisfaction (Turner, *et al.*, 1997; King, Touyz, & Charles, 2000), others have not (Cusumano & Thompson, 1997).

The present study did indicate that women dissatisfied with their bodies reported a further decrease in rated body satisfaction following a 15-min. exposure to fitness-and-health magazines. While those magazines attempt to encourage healthy lifestyles, they may instead stimulate greater distress for readers already dissatisfied with their bodies. How long such a decrease might last remains to be studied.

REFERENCES

AMERICAN PSYCHIATRIC ASSOCIATION. (1994) *Diagnostic and statistical manual of mental disorders*. (4th ed.) Washington, DC: Author.

ANDERSEN, A. E., & DIDOMENICO, L. (1992) Diet vs. shape content of popular male and female magazines: a dose-response relationship to the incidence of eating disorders? *International Journal of Eating Disorders*, 11, 283-287.

BEEBE, D. W. (1995) The Attention to Body Shape Scale: a new measure of body focus. *Journal of Personality Assessment*, 65, 486-501.

BERSCHELD, E., WALSTER, E., & BOHANSTEDT, G. (1972) Body image. *Psychology Today*, 21(6), 57-63.

BRENNER, J. B., & CUNNINGHAM, J. G. (1992) Gender differences in eating attitudes, body concept, and self-esteem among models. *Sex Roles*, 27, 413-437.

BRINK, T. L., YESAVAGE, J., LUM, O., HEERSEMA, P. H., ADEY, M., & ROSE, T. S. (1982) Screening tests for geriatric depression. *Clinical Gerontologist*, 1, 37-43.

CUSUMANO, D. L., & THOMPSON, J. K. (1997) Body image and body shape ideals in magazines: exposure, awareness, and internalization. *Sex Roles*, 37, 701-727.

DEMO, D. H. (1985) The measurement of self-esteem: refining our methods. *Journal of Personality and Social Psychology*, 48, 63-74.

FERRARO, F. R., & CHELMINSKI, I. (1996) Preliminary normative data on the Geriatric Depression Scale–Short Form (GDS–SF) in a young adult sample. *Journal of Clinical Psychology*, 52, 443-447.

GARNER, D. M., GARFINKEL, P. E., SCHWARTZ, D., & THOMPSON, M. (1980) Cultural expectations of thinness in women. *Psychological Reports*, 47, 483-491.

GARNER, D. M., OLMSTED, M. P., BOHR, Y., & GARFINKEL, P. E. (1982) The Eating Attitudes Test: psychometric features and clinical correlates. *Psychological Medicine*, 12, 871-878.

GOLDFARB, L. A., DYKENS, E. M., & GERRARD, M. (1985) The Goldfarb Fear of Fat Scale. *Journal of Personality Assessment*, 49, 329-332.

HARRISON, K., & CANTOR, J. (1997) The relationship between media consumption and eating disorders. *Journal of Communication*, 47, 40-67.

KING, N., TOUYZ, S., & CHARLES, M. (2000) The effect of body dissatisfaction on women's perceptions of female celebrities. *International Journal of Eating Disorders*, 27, 341-347.

PALLADINO-GREEN, S., & PRITCHARD, M. E. (2003) Predictors of body image dissatisfactions in adult men and women. *Social Behavior and Personality*, 31, 215-222.

ROSENBERG, M. (1965) *Society and the adolescent self-image*. Princeton, NJ: Princeton Univer. Press.

SILVERSTEIN, B., PERDUE, L., PETERSON, B., & KELLY, E. (1986) The role of the mass media in promoting a thin standard of bodily attractiveness for women. *Sex Roles*, 14, 519-532.

SPIELBERGER, C. D. (1983) *Manual for the State-Trait Anxiety Inventory*. Palo Alto, CA: Consulting Psychologists Press.

THOMPSON, J. K., & HEINBERG, L. J. (1999) The media's influence on body image disturbance and eating disorders: we've relived them, now can we rehabilitate them? In P. A. Katz (Ed.), *Journal of Social Issues*, 27, 339-353.

TURNER, S. L., HAMILTON, H., JACOBS, M., ANGOOD, L. M., & DWYER, D. H. (1997) The influence of fashion magazines on the body image satisfaction of college women: an exploratory analysis. *Adolescence*, 32, 603-614.

VANDENBERG, P., THOMPSON, J. K., OBREMSKI-BRANDON, K., & COOVERT, M. (2002) The tripartate influence model of body image and eating disturbance: a covariance structure investigation testing the mediational role of appearance comparison. *Journal of Psychosomatic Research*, 53, 1007-1020.

WISEMAN, C. V., GRAY, J. J., MOSIMANN, J. E., & AHRENS, A. H. (1992) Cultural expectations of thinness in women: an update. *International Journal of Eating Disorders*, 11, 85-89.

Accepted March 23, 2004.

DETERMINANTS OF PGA TOUR SUCCESS: AN EXAMINATION OF RELATIONSHIPS AMONG PERFORMANCE, SCORING, AND EARNINGS[1]

PETER S. FINLEY AND J. JASON HALSEY

University of Northern Colorado

Summary.—Professional Golf Association (PGA) statistics for the 2002 season were analyzed to estimate the relationships between performance variables, scoring, and earnings. Two newly considered variables, Scrambling and Bounce Back percentages, showed meaningful correlation to Simple Scoring Average ($rs = -.69$ and $-.40$, respectively), and each made a significant contribution to a regression model. While the full model of performance variables explained most of the variance in Simple Scoring Average ($R^2 = .94$), an adjusted scoring figure, accounting for the performance of the full field of players in each round, better correlated with Earnings over a PGA Tour season ($r = .77$).

A number of studies have been conducted to identify which one skill or combination of skills best explains the variance in scoring averages and money earned among professional golfers (Davidson & Templin, 1986; Hale & Hale, 1990; Jones, 1990; Belkin, Gansneder, Pickens, Rotella, & Striegel, 1994; Wiseman, Chatterjee, Wiseman, & Chatterjee, 1994; Engelhardt, 1995, 1997; Moy & Liaw, 1998; Dorsel & Rotunda, 2001). The skills generally included were measures of putting, driving accuracy, driving distance, total driving, sand saves, and greens hit in regulation.

Davidson and Templin (1986) first attempted to explain variance in money earned and scoring averages using measures of Driving Proficiency, combining distance and accuracy, Greens in Regulation, Sand Saves, Putts Per Round, and Number of Events Entered. Greens in Regulation correlated highest with success ($rs = -.63$ for scoring and .43 for earnings), with Driving Proficiency next ($rs = -.34$ for scoring and .40 for earnings). The other variables correlated less strongly. Season statistics were used from 119 of the top 125 money winners on the PGA tour.

Jones (1990) supported the saying that players "drive for show and putt for dough." He used PGA statistics from 99 of the top 100 players in 1988 to identify that Putts Per Round best predicted success ($rs = .36$ for earnings and $-.27$ for scoring). Conversely, Engelhardt (1995) reported that Total Driving, combining Driving Distance and Driving Accuracy, better correlated with Earnings than did Greens in Regulation. Hale and Hale (1990)

---

[1]Address correspondence to Peter S. Finley, 2590 Gunter Hall, Box 39, University of Northern Colorado, Greeley, CO 80639 or e-mail (peter_finley@hotmail.com).

examined the various skills using statistics from the European Tour from 1984 to 1988. After computing the correlations and finding that the skill most highly correlated with earnings changed over the years, they concluded, "Whatever the attributes of gifted golfers, they are not revealed by these kinds of analyses" (Hale & Hale, 1990, p. 164). It is noteworthy, however, that this study only examined the top players each year, ranging from 14 to 20 subjects, so it can be expected, as Belkin, et al. (1994) discussed, that variances from this sample are small.

Engelhardt (1997) stated that the only areas of significant difference between top-10 and bottom-10 money earners on the PGA Tour were Driving Distance and Total Driving. In a replication of this study using data from the European Tour, Jiménez and Fierro-Hernández (1999) found significant differences in Driving Distance, Total Driving, Greens in Regulation, and Sand Saves. Engelhardt (1999) responded that this finding may indicate there is "more intense, closer parity in competition" (p. 1028) on the American PGA Tour.

While the aforementioned studies used earnings as a dependent variable, this practice may be inappropriate, "given the skewness of that distribution... that is, the assumption of a normally distributed array is violated" (Belkin, et al., 1994, p. 1276).

Wiseman, et al. (1994) were able to explain 93% of the variance in Senior Tour average scores for 43 players using only Greens in Regulation and Putting Performance. These same independent variables explained 88% of the variance of average scores among 50 Ladies Professional Golf Tour members. However, using a four variable model, including Greens in Regulation, Putting, Driving Accuracy, and Driving Distance, could only explain 67% of the scoring variance in a sample of 113 PGA tour players. The researchers believed that they might have failed to include one or more key skills in the four-variable model.

As the nature of golf evolved, with new technology allowing for longer drives than ever before, research regarding the stability of the contribution of variables was needed. Davidson and Templin (1986) posed the question of whether skills might shift in importance over time. Engelhardt (1995) claimed that a PGA resolution to increase the difficulty of pin placements may have led to an increased importance in driving skill. This supported similar findings by Belkin, et al. (1994), who found an increasing importance in driving skill over a 3-yr. period. In addition, Dorsel and Rotunda (2001) found that driving accuracy was more important than driving distance, challenging the widely held belief that longer is necessarily better. Over three PGA seasons, hitting greens in regulation and putting skills continued to be important for achieving desired results (low scores), suggesting that the variables were stable.

While research in this area has done much to describe the correlation between performance skills and success, there is room for further exploration. The PGA is currently keeping statistics that reflect the percentage of times a player saves par after missing a green in regulation, referred to as Scrambling. Further, the percentage of times players follow a bogey or worse (taking strokes beyond par) immediately with a birdie or better (taking less strokes than par) is recorded as Bounce Back.

The present study is guided by three distinct research goals: (1) estimate the contribution that abilities to Scramble and Bounce Back made in predicting score when considered alongside historically used variables; (2) use the performance variables to account for the variance of average scores (two calculations of scores were considered, Simple Scoring Average and Adjusted Scoring Average) and (3) evaluate whether Simple Scoring Average or Adjusted Scoring Average correlates better with Earnings.

Method

Sample

The data came from performances of professional golfers on the PGA Tour in 2002, collected from aggregated tournament results. All players who finished on the money list played a minimum of 15 tournaments and had complete season statistics available via PGATour.com were included ($N = 196$).

Materials

PGA Tour statistics were collected from the official PGA Tour web site. Seven of the statistical categories were considered performance variables. Driving Distance is the average length of tee shots recorded on two holes per round. Driving Accuracy is the percentage of tee shots on par four and five holes that land in the fairway. Greens in Regulation is the percentage of greens reached in two shots less than par for the hole. Putts Per Round is the average number of putts per round played. Sand Saves are recorded as the percentage of pars saved after landing in a greenside sand trap (bunker). Scrambling is the percentage of pars saved after failing to land on the green in regulation. Bounce Back is the percentage of birdies or better made immediately following a bogie or worse.

Scoring average, computed by two distinct formulas, were considered as outcomes of the performance variables and as predictors of Earnings. Simple Scoring Average is the sum of all scores divided by the total holes played. The PGA refers to this as Stroke Average (Actual). Adjusted Scoring Average is a weighted average that takes the stroke average of the field into account. The PGA refers to this as Stroke Average, and it helps compensate for weather conditions and course difficulty in comparing scores across tournaments. Earnings is the total sum of money earned in PGA events during the season.

While the PGA Tour also records putting average, this variable was not used because it does not account for putts taken on greens not hit in regulation. Further, while other researchers have examined Total Driving, this variable was not used for several reasons. First, using Driving Distance and Driving Accuracy allow examination of the unique contribution made by each. Second, Total Driving is the combination of players' rank in Driving Distance and Driving Accuracy. There is concern the rankings obscure the magnitude of differences between players' performances. Third, Driving Distance is measured only twice per round, while Driving Accuracy is generally measured 14 times per round. This disparity in measurement frequency is not addressed when rankings are combined to create the Total Driving variable.

Procedure

Pearson product-moment correlation coefficients were generated for all 10 variables in the study. It was then judged whether the seven performance variables better explained the variance in Simple Scoring Average or Adjusted Scoring Average. The R^2 Selection Method was employed to examine the predictive power of all possible performance variable models in relation to Simple Scoring Average.

RESULTS AND DISCUSSION

The correlation matrix (Table 1) showed that Greens in Regulation was the performance variable most highly correlated with scoring. Scrambling correlated nearly as highly. Driving Accuracy and Bounce Back showed similar correlations, followed by Putts Per Round, Sand Saves and Driving Distance.

While both of the newly considered variables made a significant unique

TABLE 1
PEARSON CORRELATIONS AMONG PERFORMANCE VARIABLES,
SCORING AVERAGES, AND EARNINGS ($N = 196$)

Variable	1	2	3	4	5	6	7	8	9	10
1. Driving Distance		−.45*	−.25*	−.25*	.18	−.24*	.25*	−.18	−.15	.16
2. Driving Accuracy			.45*	−.03	−.01	.41*	.03	−.43*	−.36*	.18
3. Greens in Regulation				−.13	.35*	.28*	.18	−.73*	−.63*	.46*
4. Sand Saves					−.53*	.51*	.13	−.23*	−.30*	.32*
5. Putts Per Round						−.55*	−.27*	.34*	.36*	−.26*
6. Scrambling							.13	−.68*	−.67*	.50*
7. Bounce Back								−.40*	−.41*	.27*
8. Simple Scoring Average									.94*	−.68*
9. Adjusted Scoring Average										−.77*
10. Earnings										

†$p < .005$.

contribution to the regression model (Table 2), it is clear that Scrambling is a more important variable to consider. This is not surprising, given that players on the PGA Tour miss an average of approximately six greens per round. Players consistently losing strokes on these holes would not last long on the PGA Tour, so it is crucial they be able to chip the ball close to the hole and convert most of their par-saving putts.

TABLE 2
R^2 For Predicting Simple Scoring Averages With Unique Contributions of Performance Variables

Variable	R^2	F
Greens in Regulation	.53	622.73†
Putts Per Round	.92*	277.15†
Scrambling	.93*	32.39†
Driving Distance	.94*	18.17†
Bounce Back	.94*	7.64*
Driving Accuracy	.94*	1.81
Sand Saves	.94*	.42

Note.—All R^2 account for variance in Simple Scoring Average using a regression model including the variable and all variables listed above it. For example, the best three-variable model includes the independent variables Greens in Regulation, Putts Per Round, and Scrambling ($R^2 = .93$). *$p < .01$. †$p < .0001$.

The seven performance variables accounted for the variance in Simple Scoring Average ($R^2 = .94$) better than the variances in Adjusted Scoring Average ($R^2 = .81$). Adjusted Scoring Average correlated better with Earnings ($r = -.77$) than did Simple Scoring Average ($r = -.68$).

The models generated with the R^2 Selection Method (Table 2) indicated that a simple two-variable model, including Greens in Regulation and Putts Per Round, could explain nearly as much of the variance in Simple Scoring Average ($R^2 = .92$) as could the full seven-variable model ($R^2 = .94$). Table 2 reflects the contributions of each variable to the full model, and variables are listed in order of importance. Five variables, including the newly considered Scrambling and Bounce Back measures, made significant unique contributions to the full model ($p < .05$).

Examining the difference between Simple Scoring Average and Adjusted Scoring Average enhances the understanding of how performance variables, scores, and earnings relate. The performance variables and Simple Scoring Average are both measures of actual play, so it is not surprising that nearly all of the variance in scoring could be explained. Adjusted Scoring Average, on the other hand, is a manipulated figure by definition, weighing individual scores against the average score of the field. Given the intentionally skewed distribution of Earnings (Belkin, et al., 1994), it has proven difficult to predict Earnings using performance variables; however, Adjusted Scoring Average offers a substantial correlation ($r = -.77$).

The relationship between Earnings and scoring warrants a closer look. Although consistent play is required to earn and retain a Tour Card, the PGA Tour greatly rewards brilliant play over mere consistency. A particular scoring average, achieved by two or more players, can have markedly different values depending on how the average is achieved. For example, consider this hypothetical scenario using real dollar figures from 2003 events: Player A and Player B both average 70 strokes per round during consecutive tournaments. Player A scores a 275 total at the U.S. Open, followed by a 285 total at the Buick Classic. Player B cards 282 and 278 totals in the same events, respectively. Given the same stroke averages over eight tournament rounds, Player A has earned $662,340, compared to Player B's $160,859. Amazingly, over $500,000 separates the players because Player A would have a second place in the U.S. Open to his credit. By using the scoring average of the field as a covariate, Adjusted Scoring Average increases or diminishes real scores to yield a figure that better defines the value of a particular performance. Therefore, it is not surprising this figure correlates substantially with Earnings.

Although other research has used Total Driving, the examination of Driving Distance and Driving Accuracy variables separately yielded interesting findings. Driving Accuracy and Greens in Regulation have a moderate correlation ($r = .45$), whereas Driving Distance and Greens in Regulation have a negative correlation ($r = -.25$). Further, there is a negative correlation between Driving Distance and Driving Accuracy ($r = -.45$). Given that the eventual goal of driving the ball is to reach the green in regulation on subsequent shots, the findings indicated that a sacrifice of yardage for the sake of accuracy may be rewarded.

Scrambling and Bounce Back were meaningful performance variables in the analysis of golf scores among PGA Tour players and should be utilized in subsequent research. Performance variables can explain most of the variance in Simple Scoring Average; however, Adjusted Scoring Average correlated better with Earnings than did Simple Scoring Average because of the adjustments made for the overall performance of the fields. Although recent research has used one measure of driving performance, Total Driving, examining Driving Distance and Driving Accuracy as unique variables provides an interesting and potentially more accurate alternative.

REFERENCES

Belkin, D. S., Gansneder, B., Pickens, M., Rotella, R. J., & Striegel, D. (1994) Predictability and stability of Professional Golf Association Tour statistics. *Perceptual and Motor Skills*, 78, 1275-1280.

Davidson, J. D., & Templin, T. J. (1986) Determinants of success among professional golfers. *Research Quarterly for Exercise and Sport*, 57, 60-67.

Dorsel, T. N., & Rotunda, R. J. (2001) Low scores, top 10 finishes, and big money: an analysis of Professional Golf Association Tour statistics and how these relate to overall performance. *Perceptual and Motor Skills*, 92, 575-585.

ENGELHARDT, G. M. (1995) "It's not how you drive, it's how you arrive": the myth. *Perceptual and Motor Skills*, 80, 1135-1138.

ENGELHARDT, G. M. (1997) Differences in shot-making skills among high and low money winners on the PGA Tour. *Perceptual and Motor Skills*, 84, 1314.

ENGELHARDT, G. M. (1999) Is American PGA Tour more competitive than European tour? Reply to Jiménez and Fierro-Hernández. *Perceptual and Motor Skills*, 89, 1028.

HALE, T., & HALE, G. (1990) Lies, damned lies and statistics in golf. In A. Cochran (Ed.), *Science and golf: Proceedings of the first World Scientific Congress of Golf*. London: E & FN Spon. Pp. 159-164.

JIMÉNEZ, J. A., & FIERRO-HERNÁNDEZ, C. (1999) Are European and American golf players different? Reply to Engelhardt (1997). *Perceptual and Motor Skills*, 89, 417-418.

JONES, R. (1990) A correlation analysis of the Professional Golf Association (USA) statistical rankings for 1988. In A. Cochran (Ed.), *Science and golf: Proceedings of the first World Scientific Congress of Golf*. London: E & FN Spon. Pp. 165-167.

MOY, R., & LIAW, T. (1998) Determinants of professional golf tournament earnings. *American Economist*, 42, 65-70.

WISEMAN, F., CHATTERJEE, S., WISEMAN, D., & CHATTERJEE, N. (1994) An analysis of 1992 performance statistics for players on the U.S. PGA, Senior PGA, and LPGA tours. In A. J. Cochran & M. R. Farrally (Eds.), *Science and golf: II. Proceedings of the World Scientific Congress of Golf*. London: E & FN Spon. Pp. 199-204.

Accepted April 8, 2004.

Finno-Ugrians, Blood Types, and Suicide: Comment on Voracek, Fisher, and Marusic: David Lester and Sergei V. Kondrichin 814

Handedness and Writing Performance: F. Vlachos and F. Bonoti 815

Elevated Nociceptive Thresholds in Rats With Multifocal Brain Damage Induced With Single Subcutaneous Injections of Lithium and Pilocarpine: M. A. Galic 825

Diagnosing Estimate Distortion Due to Significance Testing in Literature on Detection of Deception: M. T. Bradley and G. Stoica 827

Corsi's Block-tapping Task: Standardization and Location in Factor Space With the WAIS–R For Two Normal Samples of Older Adults: Aristide Saggino, Michela Balsamo, Anna Grieco, Maria Rosaria Cerbone, and Nicla Nicolina Raviele 840

Effectiveness of Video of Conspecifics as a Reward For Socially Housed Bonnet Macaques (Macaca radiata): Elizabeth M. Brannon, Michael W. Andrews, and Leonard A. Rosenblum 849

"The Sound Must Seem an Echo to the Sense": Pope's Use of Sound to Convey Meaning in His Translation of Homer's Iliad: Cynthia Whissell 859

Spatial Visualization of Undergraduate Education Majors Classified by Thinking Styles: Haitham M. Alkhateeb 865

Handedness and Hobby Preference: Orestis Giotakos 869

Influence of Alcohol Intake on the Parameters Evaluating the Body Center of Foot Pressure in a Static Upright Posture: Masahiro Noda, Shinichi Demura, Shunsuke Yamaji, and Tamotsu Kitabayashi 873

Influence of Music and Distraction on Visual Search Performance of Participants With High and Low Affect Intensity: Lee Crust, Peter J. Clough, and Colin Robertson 888

Retention of Practice Effects on Simple Reaction Time For Peripheral and Central Visual Fields: Soichi Ando, Noriyuki Kida, and Shingo Oda 897

Differential Effects of Laughter on Allergen-specific Immunoglobulin and Neurotrophin Levels in Tears: Hajime Kimata 901

Exact Goodness-of-fit Tests For Unordered Equiprobable Categories: Kenneth J. Berry, Janis E. Johnston, and Paul W. Mielke, Jr. 909

Optimal Handle Angle of the Fencing Foil For Improved Performance: Fang-Tsan Lin 920

Prevalence of University Students' Sufficient Physical Activity: a Systematic Review: Jennifer D. Irwin 927

Influence of Color on Number Perseveration in a Serial Addition Task: Hariklia Proios and Peter Brugger 944

Resistance Training is Associated With Improved Mood in Healthy Older Adults: Charles L. McLafferty, Jr., Carla J. Wetzstein, and Gary R. Hunter 947

Geophysical Variables and Behavior: XCIX. Reductions in Numbers of Neurons Within the Parasolitary Nucleus in Rats Exposed Perinatally to a Magnetic Pattern Designed to Imitate Geomagnetic Continuous Pulsations: Implications For Sudden Infant Death: M. J. Dupont, B. E. McKay, G. Parker, and M. A. Persinger 958

On a General Class of Chi-squared Goodness-of-fit Statistics: Tarald O. Kvålseth 967

Perceptual Encoding of Fingerspelled and Printed Alphabet by Deaf Signers: an fMRI Study: André Dufour, Renaud Brochard, Olivier Després, Christian Scheiber, and Christel Robert 971

Weekly Treatments With a Burst-firing Magnetic Field Alters Behavior in the Elevated Plus Maze After Two Sessions: R. E. Fitzpatrick and M. A. Persinger 983

Carry-over Effects of Music in an Isometric Muscular Endurance Task: Lee Crust 985

Test of an Alternative Explanation For Effects of Arousal Gradient on Cognitive Performance: William Stankard 992

Semantic Satiation Effect in Young and Older Adults: Maura Pilotti and Ayesha Khurshid 999

Effect of Deception of Distance on Prolonged Cycling Performance: S. Paterson and F. E. Marino 1017

Deception and Perceived Exertion During High-intensity Running Bouts: David B. Hampson, Alan St Clair Gibson, Mike I. Lambert, Jonathan P. Dugas, Estelle V. Lambert, and Timothy D. Noakes 1027

Improving Accuracy of Veracity Judgment Through Cue Training: Maria Santarcangelo, Robert A. Cribbie, and Amy S. Ebesu Hubbard 1039

Modeling Judgments of Linear Extent: Ernest Greene and William Frawley 1049

Effects of Foot-pedal Positions by Inexperienced Cyclists at the Highest Aerobic Level: Duane Millslagle, Sara Rubbelke, Tom Mullin, John Keener, and Ryan Swetkovich 1074

Sensitivity to Differences in the Extent of Neck-retraction and -rotation Movements Made With and Without Vision: Haejung Lee, Leslie L. Nicholson, and Roger D. Adams 1081

Use of the Same and a Longer Time Series to Replicate David Lester's Study of Suicide and Birth Rates in Canada: F. Stephen Bridges and L. Carolyn Pearson 1090

Body Satisfaction in College Women After Brief Exposure to Magazine Images: Elizabeth M. Cameron and F. Richard Ferraro 1093

Determinants of PGA Tour Success: an Examination of Relationships Among Performance, Scoring, and Earnings: Peter S. Finley and J. Jason Halsey 1100

NOTICE

June issues of PERCEPTUAL AND MOTOR SKILLS and PSYCHOLOGICAL REPORTS for 2004 are in two parts. The special issue appears as Part 2 for June. Pages are consecutive with those in Part 1 and articles appear in the indexes for the first volumes of 2004.

THE EDITORS

PERCEPTUAL AND MOTOR SKILLS

ISSN 0031-5125　　　　　　　　　　　　　　　　　　　　　　　June 2004, Part 2

SPECIAL ISSUE

Mental Rotation and Simulation of a Reaching and Grasping Manual Movement: GERARD OLIVIER, JEAN LUC VELAY, GUY LABIALE, CAROLE CELSE, AND SYLVANE FAURE 1107
Using Computer-scored Measures of Emotion and Style to Discriminate Among Disputed and Undisputed Pauline and Non-Pauline Epistles: CYNTHIA WHISSELL 1117
Geomagnetic Activity During the Previous Day is Correlated With Increased Consumption of Sucrose During Subsequent Days: Is Increased Geomagnetic Activity Aversive?: M. A. GALIC AND M. A. PERSINGER 1126
Assessing Potentially Gifted Students From Lower Socioeconomic Status With Nonverbal Measures of Intelligence: ELIZABETH SHAUNESSY, FRANCES A. KARNES, AND YOLANDA COBB 1129
Elite Athletes' Differentiated Action in Trampolining: a Qualitative and Situated Analysis of Different Levels of Performance Using Retrospective Interviews: DENIS HAUW AND MARC DURAND 1139
Random Number Generation in Native and Foreign Languages: HANS STRENGE AND JESSICA BÖHM 1153
Understanding Air Force Members' Intentions to Participate in Pro-environmental Behaviors: an Application of the Theory of Planned Behavior: MARK S. LAUDENSLAGER, DANIEL T. HOLT, AND STEVEN T. LOFGREN 1162
... n High Level Athletes: CHRISTINA D. DAVLIN 1171
...sponsibility and Semantic Task in the Language of Adults With Dementia: ROBERT GOLDFARB ... GOLDBERG 1177
...ion and Inhibition of Negative Emotions on Health, Mood States, and Salivary Secretory ...ulin A in Japanese Mildly Depressed Undergraduates: SHIZUKA TAKAGI AND HIDEKI OHIRA 1187

continued inside back cover

PERCEPTUAL AND MOTOR SKILLS

Perceptual and Motor Skills is published bimonthly, two volumes a year, the first with issues in February, April, and June, and the second with issues in August, October, and December, from Box 9229, Missoula, Montana, 59807-9229. Subscriptions are accepted only for full calendar years. A minimum of 2600 pages is planned for 2004. Subscription rate is $370.00 per year plus postage and handling ($25.00, outside USA $30.00). Single issues are $45.00 plus postage ($5.00, outside USA $25.00).

The purpose of this journal is to encourage scientific originality and creativity. Material of the following kinds is carried: experimental or theoretical articles dealing with perception or motor skills, especially as affected by experience; articles on general methodology; new material listings and reviews. All material of scientific merit will be taken in some form. An attempt is made to balance critical editing with specific suggestions from multiple referees of each paper as to changes. The approach is interdisciplinary, including such fields as perception, anthropology, physical education, physical therapy, orthopedics, time and motion study, and sports psychology. Four copies of an article should be submitted to one of the editors at Box 9229, Missoula, Montana 59807-9229. Each article must have a carefully prepared summary of appropriate length to aid readers and abstractors.

Publication is in order of receipt of proof from the authors. Authors pay for preprints, plus costs of figures and special composition, e.g., tables, mathematics. There are three publication arrangements.

(1) *Regular articles.* These are articles which require from 3 through 20 printed pages. Authors receive 200 preprints. Preprint charge is $27.50 per page in multiples of four pages. Additional preprints can be ordered.

(2) *Brief articles.* This arrangement is useful where the author does not intend to do further work in the area but feels that preliminary findings should be put on record, where it is expected that it will be several years before the final study is completed and reported, where the author submits a summary of a study accompanied by the full report for filing with the Archive for Psychological Data, or where a particular finding can be reported completely in one page. Authors receive 50 preprints. Preprint charge is $27.50. Additional preprints can be ordered.

(3) *Monograph supplements.* Certain papers printing to more than 20 pages are published as monograph supplements. These are distributed to subscribers of *Perceptual and Motor Skills* as parts of regular issues. Authors receive 200 preprints of the monographs with covers. Preprint charge is $27.50 per page in multiples of four pages. Additional preprints can be ordered.

Articles should be prepared carefully, following the form suggested for publications of the American Psychological Association (see 1983, 1994 revision, or earlier versions). During 2003 and 2004 either the old or the new APA form will be acceptable. Proof is mailed to the author within approximately three weeks of acceptance of the article, and preprints are mailed within approximately five weeks of receipt of proof from the author.

It is the policy of this journal to file raw data with the Archive for Psychological Data whenever possible. Authors should submit appropriate tables with their articles. In this way, a permanent file of data available to all researchers could be accumulated.

Responsibility for address changes rests with the subscriber. Claims for missing issues must be made within two months of publication.

PERCEPTUAL AND MOTOR SKILLS
ISSN 0031-5125

Vol. 98, No. 3, Part 2   June 2004

SENIOR EDITORS   R. B. Ammons and C. H. Ammons   *Ammons Scientific, Ltd.*

EDITORS   Bruce Ammons, Douglas Ammons, S. A. Isbell

ASSOCIATE EDITORS

Marian Annett
University of Leicester

Clark D. Ashworth
NE Washington Family Counseling

Richard W. Bohannon
University of Connecticut

Willard L. Brigner
Appalachian State University

Josef Brožek
St. Paul, MN

Peter Brugger
University Hospital Zurich

Ross H. Day
La Trobe University, Bundoora

Robert Didden
Katholieke Universiteit Nijmegen

G. William Domhoff
University of California, Santa Cruz

Christopher C. Dunbar
Brooklyn College of CUNY

John Eliot
University of Maryland, College Park

H. J. Eysenck
University of London

Ann M. Filinger
Hagerstown, MD

Bernard Fine
Weston, MA

Robert Fudin
Long Island University

David M. Furst
San Jose State University

Richard Gajdosik
The University of Montana

K. O. Götz
Kunstakademie Düsseldorf

E. Rae Harcum
The College of William & Mary

Julian Hochberg
Columbia University

Alan S. Kaufman
Yale University School of Medicine

Johannes Kingma
University Hospital Groningen

Marcel Kinsbourne
Boston University

Muriel Lezak
Oregon Health Sciences University

Paul Naitoh
San Diego, California

Kent B. Pandolf
U.S. Army Research Institute

J. Timothy Petersik
Ripon College

Paul Roodin
SUNY College at Oswego

Leon E. Smith
St. Thomas University, Miami

Arthur E. Stamps III
Institute of Environmental Quality

D. L. Streiner
Baycrest Center for Geriatric Care

Stephan Swinnen
Katholieke Universiteit Leuven

Üner Tan
Cukurova University

James M. Vanderplas
Washington University

Min Q. Wang
University of Maryland

Paul R. Yarnold
Northwestern Univer. Medical School

Published bimonthly by Perceptual and Motor Skills, Box 9229, Missoula, Montana; printed by Ammons Scientific, Ltd., 1911-17 South Higgins Avenue, Missoula, Montana 59801-1911. Please address correspondence and changes of address to Box 9229, Missoula, Montana 59807-9229. POSTMASTER: Send address changes to *Perceptual and Motor Skills*, P.O. Box 9229, Missoula, Montana 59807-9229.

Copyright 2004   Perceptual and Motor Skills

Permission to Copy Material in this Journal

It is the policy of this journal to obtain and hold the copyrights for all articles published, with the exception of a very few articles or parts of articles in the public domain. Authors are allowed and encouraged to make copies of their articles for any scholarly purpose of their own. Other scholars are hereby given permission to make single or multiple copies of single articles for personal scholarly use without explicit written permission, providing that no such copies are sold or used for commercial purposes. We consider it the obligation of any user to acknowledge sources explicitly and to obtain permission of the authors if extensive use is to be made of materials or information contained in an article. Extensive use of copy privileges in such a way as to substitute for a subscription to this journal is not intended or permitted. Such use would be unethical and, in the long run, self-defeating, since it would destroy the very basis for publication.

These policies are proposed on a trial basis and will be followed until further notice.

C. H. Ammons, Editor

R. B. Ammons, Editor

January 1, 1978

Perceptual and Motor Skills has been printed on acid-free paper since 1962, Vol. 14, No. 1 (February). See the following references.

Ammons, R. B., & Ammons, C. H. Permanent or temporary journals: are PR and PMS stable? *Perceptual and Motor Skills*, 1962, 14, 281.

Ammons, C. H., & Ammons, R. B. Permanent or temporary journals: PR and PMS become stable. *Psychological Reports*, 1962, 10, 537.

Disclaimer

This Journal is not responsible for the statements of any contributor. Statements or opinions expressed in the journal reflect the views of the authors and not the Editors, Associate Editors, or special reviewers. Publication should not be construed as endorsement. Contributing authors are expected to follow ethical procedures and sound scientific principles.

MENTAL ROTATION AND SIMULATION OF A REACHING AND GRASPING MANUAL MOVEMENT[1]

GERARD OLIVIER

Experimental and Quantitative Psychology Laboratory
University of Nice Sophia–Antipolis

JEAN LUC VELAY

Institute of Physiological and Cognitive Neurosciences
CNRS, Marseille

GUY LABIALE

Memory and Cognition Experimental Psychology Laboratory
University of Montpellier

CAROLE CELSE AND SYLVANE FAURE

Experimental and Quantitative Psychology Laboratory
University of Nice Sophia–Antipolis

Summary.—This paper deals with the kind of manual movement subjects mentally simulate when solving a left-right judgment task that requires rotating images of hands. 50 female students were asked to judge the laterality of drawings of rotated hands presented successively to the right and left visual hemifields by clicking on a mouse using either the right or left hand. Reaction times and accuracy of judgment were recorded. Analysis showed performances varied with the rotation angle at which the stimulus was presented, indicating that the subjects mentally simulated a rotation process. An interaction occurred between the visually presented hand and the responding hand, which suggests that the mental rotation process involved the simulation of a hand movement. Performance improved when the drawing of a hand was presented in the 'palm-up' position, and to the visual hemifield opposite with respect to the hand the subject moved mentally. The latter two findings suggest that the subjects performed a simulated reaching and grasping movement rather than a simulated positioning movement.

Since Shepard and Metzler's original work on mental imagery (1971), studies of mental rotation have been placing increasing importance on motor factors. Performances in visual-recognition tasks involving rotated stimuli were thought initially to depend on a purely perceptual factor, the rotation angle at which the stimulus was presented (Shepard & Cooper, 1982). Kosslyn (1994) subsequently proposed that mental rotation may involve anticipating the consequences of executing a movement. Recent studies have now suggested that this anticipatory process is sometimes based on the mental simulation of a movement (Wexler, Kosslyn, & Berthoz, 1998; Olivier &

---

[1]Address correspondence to Gerard Olivier, Experimental and Quantitative Psychology Laboratory, Pôle Universitaire Saint Jean d'Angely, 24 Avenue des Diables Bleus, Nice 06357, France or e-mail (olivierg@unice.fr).

Juan de Mendoza, 2000). Besides, when the stimuli are drawings of hands, subjects are supposed to rotate their corresponding hands mentally to match the stimulus position (Sekiyama, 1982; Parsons, 1987, 1994). It is generally held that the subjects imagine themselves "in the computer's shoes," as if the hand presented was their own hand, and they simulate the positioning movement which would enable them to rotate the corresponding hand to fit the configuration presented to them (Parsons, 1987). However, when the hand stimulus mimics a shaking hand, it is also possible that the subjects may imagine that the hand presented belongs to someone else and that they may simulate a grasping movement directed towards this hand, as if they wanted to shake it (see Fig. 1). Indeed, a grasping movement simulation sometimes occurs during the visual recognition of graspable objects (i.e., Tucker & Ellis, 1998; Craighero, Fadiga, Umilta, & Rizzolatti, 1999).

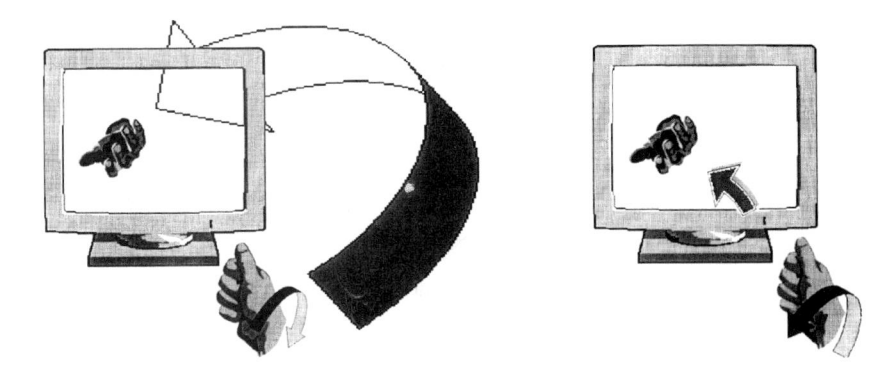

FIG. 1. Opposite wrist rotations triggered by a given hand stimulus. In this example, the stimulus was a right hand rotated at an angle of −135°. A real 'palm-up' hand like this could be reached and grasped by the subject by performing a wrist pronation with the right hand (right drawing), whereas if the subject imagined herself "in the computer's shoes," the spatial position of the hand could be imitated performing a wrist supination with the same hand (left drawing).

To check whether subjects mentally simulate a grasping manual movement rather than a positioning one when the presented hand stimulus mimics a shaken hand, we controlled the two following experimental factors.

Firstly, we exposed the hand stimulus onto either the right or left visual hemifield with respect to a central fixation point. The idea was that if the subjects imagined they were shaking the hand stimulus as if it belonged to someone else, then their performance would depend on the familiarity with the direction of the shaking movement. More precisely, in everyday life, shaking someone's hand generally requires being located in front of that person, and in this position, the hand movement is directed toward the middle saggital plane. Consequently, the hand stimuli presented to the visual hemifield contralateral to the corresponding subject's hand (right hand stimulus in left visual hemifield and left hand stimulus in right visual hemifield) are probably associated with more familiar hand-shaking movements than the hand stimuli presented to the ipsilateral hemifield.

Hypothesis 1

We therefore predicted an interaction would occur between the hand stimulus (right or left) and the visual hemifield. More precisely, the subject's performances would improve when the hand stimulus is presented to the visual hemifield contralateral to the subject's corresponding hand.

Secondly, some pictures of hands were presented palm up and others palm down. As can be seen in Fig. 2, these orientations of the hand stimulus can be adopted by making the opposite wrist rotations (pronation or supination), depending on the type of movement simulated (positioning vs grasping). The important point here is that supinated wrist rotations are characterized by more biomechanical constraints than pronated wrist rotations: one

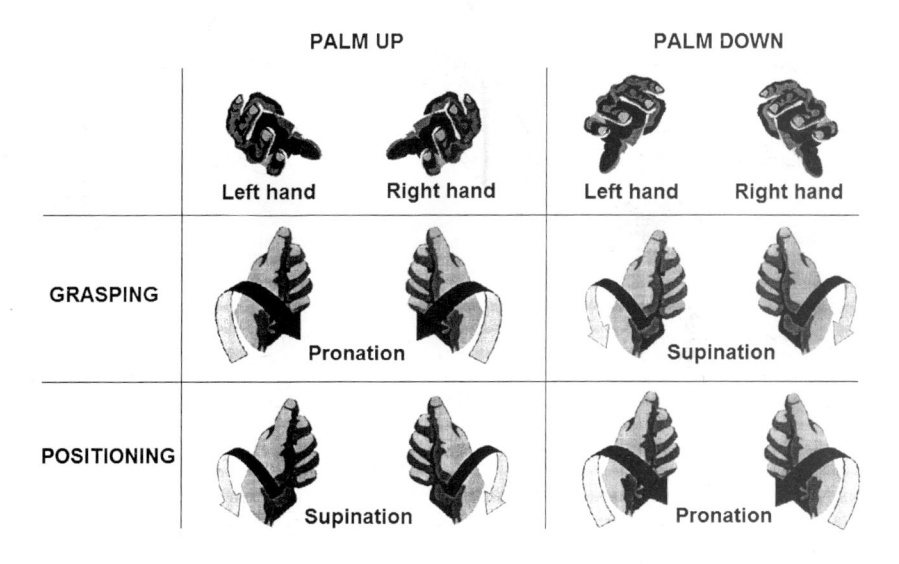

FIG. 2. Wrist rotation imposed by the hand stimulus as a function of the stimulus orientation ('palm up' vs 'palm down') and the kind of movement mentally simulated by the subject's corresponding hand ('grasping' vs 'positioning'). It can be seen here that to place the corresponding hand in the stimulus position ('positioning' row), it is necessary to perform two opposite wrist rotations: a supination movement to imitate the 'palm-up' stimulus position, and a pronation movement to imitate the 'palm-down' stimulus position. Note that an additional awkward shoulder abduction is necessary to imitate the palm-up stimulus position, but not to imitate the palm-down stimulus position. By contrast, grasping 'palm-up' stimuli requires a pronation of the corresponding hand, whereas grasping 'palm-down' stimuli requires a supination. Note that an additional awkward shoulder abduction is necessary to grasp 'palm-down' stimuli, as compared with 'palm-up' stimuli.

can adopt these orientations of the hand stimulus by making a pronated wrist rotation without reaching the limits of comfortable pronation (Johnson, 2000). Conversely, an additional awkward shoulder abduction is necessary to perform the complete supination (see Fig. 2). Moreover, it is by now generally recognized that imagined movements obey the same rules and have the same temporal characteristics as actual movements (i.e., Jeannerod, 1997; Papaxanthis, Pozzo, Skoura, & Schieppati, 2002). In particular, actual and imagined movements are sensitive to biomechanical constraints: awkward postures are not only difficult to physically adopt but also to mentally simulate (Parsons, 1994; Johnson, 2000). We therefore assumed that the time required to decide whether the hand presented was a right or left hand would be shorter when it involved mentally simulating a pronation rather than a supination. The association of the fastest performances either with 'palm-up' or 'palm-down' hand stimuli could provide some information about the nature of the manual movement being mentally simulated (grasping vs positioning).

Hypothesis 2

Since we supposed that a grasping movement would be simulated, we predicted that the fastest performances would be associated with the 'palm-up' hand stimuli (versus 'palm-down' hand stimuli).

Method

Participants

Fifty women (M age = 21.7 yr.), studying psychology at Nice University volunteered to participate. Women were chosen simply for the sake of convenience (most psychology students are women). All the participants were right-handed for writing, throwing darts, and brushing their teeth. They all reported normal or corrected-to-normal visual acuity.

Materials

The experiments were run by a microcomputer. The presentation was controlled using the 'Director 7' software program (Macromedia). The stimuli were 60-mm high, 35-mm wide drawings of a right or left hand (see Fig. 3). Left and right hands were identical mirror images of each other. In these drawings the hands were either vertical or rotated 45°, 135°, –135°, or –45°.

Procedure and Design

All subjects were tested individually. Each was seated in front of a screen placed 1 m before the subject, and the gaze was at the level of the center of the screen. The task was to decide whether the hand displayed on the computer screen was a right or left hand. They were instructed to click on the left mouse button in response to a left hand stimulus and on the

-135°   -45°   0°   45°   135°

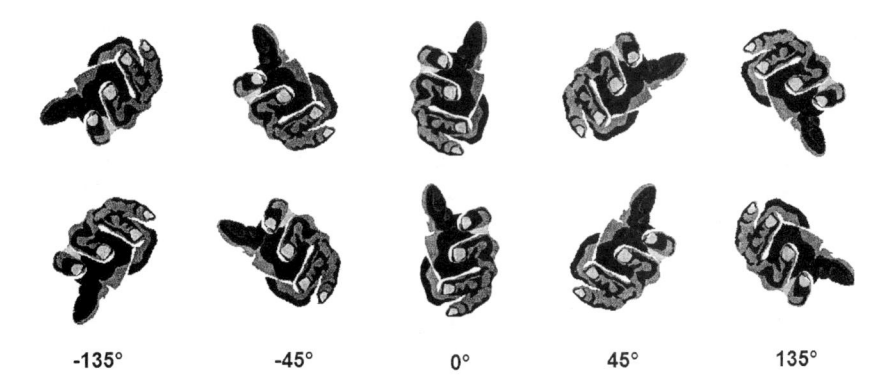

FIG. 3. The five rotation angles at which the right hand stimuli (upper row) and left hand stimuli (lower row) were presented.

right mouse button in response to a right hand. They were asked not to make any head movements and to keep their hands still while deciding. A set of hands was randomly presented to either the right or left visual hemifield. The center of the hand drawings was positioned at the level of the horizontal middle of the screen, 7 cm laterally from the fixation point (corresponding to an eccentricity of 4°). Prior to each trial, the subjects were instructed to hold the mouse with either the right or left hand and to put the other hand closed on the table with the thumb "at eleven o'clock (right hand) or "at one o'clock" (left hand). A central fixation point appeared on the screen for 1 sec. A hand stimulus was then briefly displayed (125 msec.) to prevent any visual saccades from occurring. The participants were asked to respond as quickly and accurately as they could. No references to using imagery in solving the task were made. Reaction times (RT) and accuracy were recorded. The hand used by a subject to click on the mouse, the visual hemifield to which the stimulus was presented, the laterality of the hand stimulus, and the rotation angle at which the stimulus was presented were the four independent variables. The experimental condition was started by a practice block of 20 trials. After this familiarization phase, a randomized series of hand stimuli composed of the 40 possible combinations of the four independent variables was run in a single experimental block.

Results

A 2 × 2 × 2 × 5 analysis of variance was conducted on the RTs and on the correct responses with the following factors: responding hand (right, left) × visual hemifield (right, left) × stimulus (right hand, left hand) × rotation angle (−135°, −45°, 0°, 45°, 135°). The only significant main effect indicated by the analysis of variance was an effect of the stimulus rotation angle on both the response time ($F_{4,196} = 14.79$, $p < .00001$, $MSE = 1.54$, partial

$\eta^2 = .23$, power = 1) and the number of correct responses ($F_{4,196} = 7.27$, $p < .00005$, $MSE = 0.24$, partial $\eta^2 = .13$, power = .99). As expected from classic results on mental rotation, RT increased with the stimulus rotation angle (see Table 1). Thus, the mean RTs differed significantly between −135° and −45° angles ($F_{1,49} = 11.65$, $p < .001$, $MSE = 0.33$, partial $\eta^2 = .19$, power = .92), between −45° and 0° angles ($F_{1,49} = 13.03$, $p < .001$, $MSE = 0.31$, partial $\eta^2 = .21$, power = .94), between 0° and 45° angles ($F_{1,49} = 8.35$, $p < .006$, $MSE = 0.30$, partial $\eta^2 = .15$, power = .81), and between 45° and 135° angles ($F_{1,49} = 12.57$, $p < .001$, $MSE = 0.44$, partial $\eta^2 = .20$, power = .94). As shown in Table 1, correct response rates decreased only when the hand stimulus was rotated ± 135°. Thus, correct response rates differed significantly between −135° and −45° angles ($F_{1,49} = 12.38$, $p < .001$, $MSE = 0.05$, partial $\eta^2 = .20$, power = .93) and between 45° and 135° angles ($F_{1,49} = 13.25$, $p < .001$, $MSE = 0.06$, partial $\eta^2 = .21$, power = .94).

TABLE 1
MEAN REACTION TIMES AND MEAN CORRECT RESPONSE RATES OBTAINED WITH THE RIGHT- AND LEFT-HAND STIMULI AS A FUNCTION OF STIMULUS ROTATION ANGLE

Measure and Stimulus	−135° M	−135° SD	−45° M	−45° SD	0° M	0° SD	45° M	45° SD	135° M	135° SD
Reaction Times, sec.										
Right hand	2.36[a]	1.45	2.19	1.55	1.75	.87	2.19	1.29	2.55[b]	1.60
Left hand	2.64[b]	1.65	2.28	1.37	2.00	1.41	2.12	1.46	2.43[a]	1.58
Both hands	2.50	1.55	2.22	1.51	1.93	1.23	2.16	1.37	2.49	1.58
Correct Responses, %										
Right hand	63	48	69	47	72	45	71	46	66	48
Left hand	60	49	78	41	73	44	76	43	55	50
Both hands	61	49	73	44	73	45	73	44	62	49

[a]Values corresponding to 'palm-up' stimuli (−135° rotated right hand and 135° rotated left hand). [b]Values corresponding to 'palm-down' stimuli (−135° rotated left hand and 135° rotated right hand).

In the frame of Hypothesis 1, the predicted interaction between the hand stimulus and the visual hemifield significantly affected the correct responses ($F_{1,49} = 7.19$, $p < .01$, $MSE = 0.19$, partial $\eta^2 = .13$, power = .75) but not the RTs ($F_{1,49} = .31$, $p = .58$, $MSE = 0.58$, partial $\eta^2 = .006$, power = .08). As shown in Table 2, the subjects gave more correct responses when the left-hand stimulus was presented to the right versus the left visual hemifield [$F_{1,49} = 4.56$, p (one-tailed) < .02, $MSE = .59$, partial $\eta^2 = .08$, power = .55] and when the right-hand stimulus was presented to the left versus the right visual hemifield, but this last result was not statistically significant [$F_{1,49} = 2.53$, p (one-tailed) < .06, $MSE = 0.22$, partial $\eta^2 = .05$, power = .34].

As predicted by Hypothesis 2, an interaction between the hand stimu-

TABLE 2
MEAN CORRECT RESPONSE RATES (%) OBTAINED WITH LEFT- AND RIGHT-HAND STIMULI IN LEFT AND RIGHT VISUAL HEMIFIELDS AND FOR LEFT AND RIGHT MANUAL RESPONSES

Stimulus	Visual Hemifield		Manual Response	
	Left	Right	Left	Right
Left Hand				
M	64	73	66	71
SD	48	45	47	47
Right Hand				
M	69	67	71	65
SD	46	47	46	48

lus factor and ±135° angles occurred for RTs ($F_{1,49}=9.37$, $p<.004$, $MSE=0.87$, partial $\eta^2=.16$, power=.85) but not for correct responses ($F_{1,49}=1.06$, ns, $MSE=0.34$, partial $\eta^2=.02$, power=.17). As shown in Table 1, after a right-hand stimulus display, the RTs were longer when the stimulus was rotated 135° (palm down) than when it was rotated −135° (palm up) [$F_{1,49}=5.85$, p (one-tailed) $<.01$, $MSE=1.50$, partial $\eta^2=.11$, power=.66]. Conversely, after a left-hand stimulus display, the RTs were longer when the stimulus was rotated −135° (palm down) than when it was rotated 135° (palm up) [$F_{1,49}=4.33$, p (one-tailed) $<.03$, $MSE=1.50$, partial $\eta^2=.08$, power=.53]. The interaction between the hand stimulus factor and ±45° angles was not significant in the RTs ($F_{1,49}=.39$, ns, $MSE=2.22$, partial $\eta^2=.01$, power=.09).

Finally, a significant interaction between hand stimulus and responding hand was found for correct responses ($F_{1,49}=8.09$, $p<.007$, $MSE=0.18$, partial $\eta^2=.18$, power=.80). As shown in Table 2, after a right-hand stimulus display, the participants gave fewer correct responses when they clicked on the mouse with the right hand than when they clicked with the left hand ($F_{1,49}=5.05$, $p<.03$, $MSE=0.43$, partial $\eta^2=.09$, power=.59). Conversely, after a left-hand stimulus display, the participants gave fewer correct responses when they clicked on the mouse with the left hand than when they clicked with the right hand, but this last result was not statistically significant ($F_{1,49}=3.03$, ns, $MSE=0.16$, partial $\eta^2=.06$, power=.40).

DISCUSSION

The present experiment was designed to assess if, when solving a left-right judgment task that required rotating images of hands, subjects might be mentally simulating a manual grasping movement. The first two steps were to check (1) whether subjects might simulate a rotation process when attempting to recognize the rotated hand, and (2) whether this rotation process relied on the mental simulation of a manual movement. The first assumption was supposed by the classical increase in the RTs with the stimulus rotation angle (Shepard & Cooper, 1982, see Table 1), accompanied by a decrease in the correct response rate, when the stimuli were presented at an angle of ±135°. The second assumption was supported by the interaction between hand stimulus and responding hand (see Table 2). In particular, when the subject was preparing to click on the mouse with her right hand, the visual presentation of a right-hand stimulus generated fewer correct responses than when a left-hand stimulus was presented. This finding could be easily explained if the task elicited the mental simulation of a movement of the subject's corresponding hand (i.e., Craighero, Bello, Fadiga, & Rizzolatti, 2002). As in Tucker and Ellis's second experiment (1998), it looks as if the performance dropped when the subject was simultaneously preparing and mentally simulating two different movements with the same hand.

These initial results suggest that subjects rely on a rotation process based on an internally simulated hand movement. However, it is not yet possible at this stage to specify what type of movement was simulated. The following result provides some information about the nature of the mentally simulated manual movement. The significant visual hemifield by hand stimulus interaction observed here indicated that, for a hand stimulus presented to a given visual hemifield, performance was better when this hand corresponded to the opposite body side (a right hand presented to the left visual hemifield, and *vice versa*). This finding could be easily explained if the simulated movement was a handshaking movement: this interaction might result from the familiarity of the movement direction. In fact, in handshaking, the hand to be grasped is generally located on the opposite side from the subject's hand, and the shaking movement is directed toward the middle sagittal plane. In this familiar direction, the grasping movement would be easier to simulate, and this might explain why the responses were more accurate when the hand presented was on the opposite side from the "shaking hand" of the subject. This result is compatible with the "grasping hypothesis," but for all that it does not exclude the "positioning hypothesis." Indeed, one could argue that the spatial position of the hand presented with respect to the subject could as well influence her performance if she simulated a positioning movement. For instance, to simulate a positioning movement with the right hand, the subject must rotate her hand in space to match the stimulus hand and therefore the simulated position of her hand will correspond to a hand stimulus presented in her left visual hemifield. However, we feel that the next result provides a more convincing argument in favor of the "grasping hypothesis."

'Palm-up' hands were recognized more quickly than 'palm-down' hands. In other words, the subjects simulated hand movements more quickly when the hands were presented palm up than when they were presented palm down. As mentioned above, for biomechanical reasons, palm-up stimuli were easier to "grasp" than to "imitate" through a positioning movement, whereas palm-down stimuli were easier to imitate than to grasp. Since mentally simulated movements seem to obey the same biomechanical rules and have the same temporal characteristics as actual ones (Decety & Jeannerod, 1996; Sirigu, Duhamel, Cohen, Pillon, Dubois, & Agid, 1996) and since this is known to be true of wrist movements (Johnson, 2000), we reasoned that if the subjects simulated grasping movements, fastest performance should be associated with palm-up stimuli. Therefore, since response times were shorter with palm-up stimuli than with palm-down ones, it can be concluded that the subjects simulated a grasping movement as if they wanted to shake the hand presented to them and did not make a positioning movement. Additional work is needed to determine under what conditions the subjects consider the hand presented on the computer screen is their own or, on the contrary, belongs to someone else. One could also compare the present results with the performance of schizophrenic patients who, in similar experimental conditions, tend to attribute the stimulus hand to themselves (i.e., Daprati, Franck, Georgieff, Proust, Pacherie, Dalery, & Jeannerod, 1997).

In conclusion, the mental simulation of manual movements set off a "motor-recognition" process that facilitated the identification task (Jeannerod, 1997). The particular nature of the hand stimulus presented (mimicking a hand held out to be shaken) may have elicited the mental simulation of a reaching and grasping movement, rather than a positioning movement as in Parsons' experiment (1994). More generally, the present results support the idea that motor processes are involved in the mental rotation of body parts.

REFERENCES

CRAIGHERO, L., BELLO, A., FADIGA, L., & RIZZOLATTI, G. (2002) Hand action preparation influences the responses to hand pictures. *Neuropsychologia*, 40, 492-502.

CRAIGHERO, L., FADIGA, L., UMILTA, C., & RIZZOLATTI, G. (1999) Action for perception: a motor-visual attentional effect. *Journal of Experimental Psychology: Human Perception and Performance*, 25, 1673-1692.

DAPRATI, E., FRANCK, N., GEORGIEFF, N., PROUST, J., PACHERIE, E., DALERY, J., & JEANNEROD, M. (1997) Looking for the agent: an investigation into consciousness of action and self-consciousness in schizophrenic patients. *Cognition*, 65, 71-86.

DECETY, J., & JEANNEROD, M. (1996) Fitts' law in mentally simulated movements. *Behavioral Brain Research*, 72, 127-134.

JEANNEROD, M. (1997) *The cognitive neuroscience of action*. Oxford, UK: Blackwell.

JOHNSON, S. H. (2000) Thinking ahead: the case for motor imagery in prospective judgements of prehension. *Cognition*, 74, 33-70.

KOSSLYN, S. M. (1994) *Image and brain*. Cambridge, MA: MIT Press.

OLIVIER, G., & JUAN DE MENDOZA, J. L. (2000) Motor dimension of visual mental image transformation processes. *Perceptual and Motor Skills*, 90, 1008-1026.

PAPAXANTHIS, C., POZZO, T., SKOURA, X., & SCHIEPPATI, M. (2002) Does order and timing in performance of imagined and actual movements affect the motor imagery process? The duration of walking and writing task. *Behavioral Brain Research*, 134, 209-215.

PARSONS, L. M. (1987) Image spatial transformations of one's body. *Journal of Experimental Psychology: General*, 116, 172-191.

PARSONS, L. M. (1994) Temporal and kinematic properties of motor behavior reflected in mentally simulated action. *Journal of Experimental Psychology: Human Perception and Performance*, 20, 709-730.

SEKIYAMA, K. (1982) Kinesthetic aspects of mental representations in the identification of left and right hands. *Perception & Psychophysics*, 32, 89-95.

SHEPARD, R. N., & COOPER, L. A. (1982) *Mental images and their transformations.* Cambridge, MA: MIT Press.

SHEPARD, R. N., & METZLER, J. (1971) Mental rotation of three dimensional objects. *Science*, 171, 701-703.

SIRIGU, A., DUHAMEL, J. R., COHEN, L., PILLON, B., DUBOIS, B., & AGID, Y. (1996) The mental representation of hand movements after parietal cortex damage. *Science*, 273, 1564-1568.

TUCKER, M., & ELLIS, R. (1998) On the relations between seen objects and components of actions. *Journal of Experimental Psychology: Human Perception and Performance*, 24, 830-846.

WEXLER, M., KOSSLYN, S. M., & BERTHOZ, A. (1998) Motor processes in mental rotation. *Cognition*, 68, 78-94.

Accepted March 30, 2004.

USING COMPUTER-SCORED MEASURES OF EMOTION AND STYLE TO DISCRIMINATE AMONG DISPUTED AND UNDISPUTED PAULINE AND NON-PAULINE EPISTLES [1]

CYNTHIA WHISSELL

Laurentian University

Summary.—The Dictionary of Affect in Language that allows measurement of Pleasantness, Activation, and Imagery in texts and a computer program that provides several additional stylistic measures were used to score samples from Disputed ($n = 22$ samples) and Undisputed ($n = 40$) Pauline epistles and from Other New Testament epistles ($n = 16$). All samples came from an English translation. Several significant mean differences were noted between samples from Disputed and Undisputed epistles. A discriminant function predicting Disputed or Undisputed authorship limited to five predictors was 85% successful in assigning samples to either category. The majority of samples from Other epistles were classified as Disputed, i.e., less likely to have been written by Paul. Undisputed Pauline samples were predicted to be those with lower Imagery, shorter words, less frequent words, greater repetitiveness, and greater Pleasantness. There were significant differences in patterns of word use (vocabulary) between Disputed and Undisputed samples.

There are a number of epistles or letters in the New Testament of the Christian Bible whose authorship has at one time or another been attributed to the Apostle Paul. Although this attribution has been questioned in almost every case (Selby, 1962), current analysts place the epistles into three main categories (Ehrman, 2000, p. 262). The first category includes the undisputedly Pauline epistles, where the consensus for authorship is strongest (Romans, 1 and 2, Corinthians, Galatians, Philippians, 1 Thessalonians, and Philemon). The second category includes the disputed Pauline epistles (Ephesians, Colossians, 2 Thessalonians) which were written in the manner of Paul, but possibly not by him. The third category includes the pastoral epistles (those written to pastors: 1 and 2 Timothy and Titus). It has been suggested that these epistles are pseudonymous. Analysts base this conclusion on their contents and style.

This paper describes research that employed techniques associated with the Dictionary of Affect in Language (Whissell, 1999) and with stylistic analysis (Whissell, 1996) to discriminate among the Undisputed (first category) and Disputed (second and third categories) Pauline epistles. Non-Pauline New Testament epistles, namely, those of Jude, Peter, James, and John, and the book of Hebrews were used in the research for comparative purposes.

---

[1]Address correspondence to Cynthia Whissell, Ph.D., Psychology Department, Laurentian University, Ramsey Lake Road, Sudbury, ON, Canada P3E 2C6.

Stylistic analysis can be used descriptively or, in more detailed treatments, as a way of establishing authorship. This paper takes a descriptive approach. Although such clues as there might be to authorship are examined, definitive assignments cannot be made because original Greek documents are not treated. The question underlying this research is therefore most accurately rendered as: "What are the differences in emotion and style between the different categories of Pauline epistles and the remaining epistles of the New Testament?" A close stylistic analysis of a variety of epistles including those of Paul has been reported by Neumann (1990, p. 130) who used the original Greek texts. The analysis in this report benefitted in comparison to Neumann's from the employment of emotional and imaging variables along with stylistic variables, and from the utilization of computerized scoring that did not depend on ongoing human judgments, but it fell short of Neumann's because it was based on a current English translation rather than the original Greek. The translation used was that of Clontz (Common Edition New Testament, Copyright ©Timothy E. Clontz, 1999. All rights reserved.). Clontz affirmed that one of his guiding principles in translation was accuracy in comparison to the Greek originals: the whole text of this translation is available at present on the Internet through the Gutenberg project (www.promo.net/pg/). The use of translated materials was mandated by the fact that the emotional measures and computer programs employed had been developed for English materials. Problems associated with the translation of Biblical documents from one language to another are compounded by those associated with the subtle editing enacted by those who have guarded the canon for the last two millennia. Epistles, for example, were often preserved as copies of copies, and each act of copying allowed for both intentional and unintentional redactions.

Method

The Dictionary of Affect in Language includes people's mean ratings for the Pleasantness, Activation, and Imagery of close to 9,000 words. The first two ratings represent the two main dimensions of emotional space (Whissell, 1996), while the third represents people's assessment of "how easily it is to form a mental picture" of a word. Concrete words such as "Bible" score higher on imagery than abstract ones such as "faith." Research has shown that Dictionary scores are a valid indicator of people's reactions to texts (Whissell, 2003). The stylistic measures employed in this research were Word Length (number of letters), Sentence Length (number of words), Word Frequency (per third of a million words), Repetitiveness (proportion of words or tokens that occurred more than once in the sample), the proportional use of Very Common Words (those with frequencies greater than 100 in a third of a million), and the use of particular classes of words (the verb "To Be," Negatives such as "no" and words ending in "n't," forms of the word "Love," and words describing Nature such as "sea" and "sky").

All the emotional and stylistic measures have been used in previous research, for example, to differentiate among the styles and emotions of the Romantic poets (Whissell, 1999, 2003) or between the styles and emotions of the Beatles lyricists McCartney and Lennon (Whissell, 1996). They are arguably "blind" measures, as none of them were specifically developed for the comparisons conducted in this study, and none of them had been developed on the basis of known peculiarities of Pauline style. A computer program was used to score text samples from the Undisputed, Disputed, and Non-Pauline epistles in terms of the above variables. Emotional and imagery scores were calculated on the basis of the mean ratings of matched words, i.e., words found in the Dictionary of Affect, in each sample. Most of the remaining variables were calculated using some counting procedure (of letters, words, or particular classes of words). Word Frequency and the identification of Very Common Words were scored with the help of information from a broadly sampled corpus of a third of a million English words (Whissell, 1998). This corpus included words from essays, newspaper stories, televised news broadcasts, televised situation comedies, magazines, and similar widely dispersed sources.

Each epistle included in the research was divided into samples of close to 800 words (exact mean = 784) by the process of blindly advancing a fixed number of lines down the computer text and finding the closest beginning of a paragraph (above or below). At no point was a reading of the text used in making judgments as to sample separation, which was dependent on length of sample not content. The shortest epistles, e.g., Philemon, 2 John, each constituted a single sample. Some epistles of limited length were divided into several slightly smaller samples in preference to fewer over-large samples. This process produced a total of 78 samples, 40 Undisputed Pauline, 22 Disputed (including Hebrews), and 16 from Other epistles. Hebrews was classified with the disputed epistles *a priori* because of its long history as a supposed Pauline epistle. This history suggests the presence of at least some similarities between Hebrews and the Pauline corpus. All the books of the New Testament mentioned above were included in their entirety.

Results and Discussion

The normative matching rate for the Dictionary of Affect is 90%: for the samples in this research the mean was 92% with a standard deviation of 2%, indicating that by far the majority of words in each sample could be scored in terms of their emotions and imagery. Means and standard deviations for each group on all variables are reported in Table 1. There were several significant mean differences between samples from the Undisputed

TABLE 1
MEANS AND STANDARD DEVIATIONS FOR SAMPLES FROM UNDISPUTED ($n = 40$)
AND DISPUTED PAULINE ($n = 22$) AND NON-PAULINE ($n = 16$) EPISTLES

Variable	Pauline Samples Undisputed* M	SD	Disputed M	SD	Other or Non-Pauline Samples M	SD
Pleasantness (Dictionary of Affect)	1.86	.029	1.86	.030	1.87	.039
Activation (Dictionary of Affect)	1.65	.018	1.66	.022	1.67	.032
Imagery (Dictionary of Affect)	1.44	.036	1.47	.036	1.47	.034
Use of word Love (Proportion)	.002	.004	.004	.005	.009	.011
Use of negatives (Proportion)	.021	.008	.015	.008	.019	.008
Use of nature words (Proportion)	.0005	.002	.000	.000	.0019	.004
Repetitiousness (Proportion)	.66	.04	.61	.05	.61	.09
Sentence length (No. of words)	21.87	5.18	28.66	6.86	23.30	7.14
Use of verb To Be (Proportion)	.054	.012	.045	.009	.045	.010
Word length (No. of letters)	3.97	.11	4.13	.11	4.06	.22
Word frequency (per 1/3 of a million words)	2865	227	2971	296	2931	238
Use of very common words (Proportion)	.71	.022	.70	.025	.70	.055

*Samples for Undisputed epistles were taken from the New Testament books of Romans, 1 and 2 Corinthians, Galatians, Philippians, 1 Thessalonians, and Philemon. Samples for Disputed epistles were taken from Hebrews, Colossians, Ephesians, 2 Thessalonians, 1 and 2 Timothy, and Titus. Samples for Other or Non-Pauline epistles were taken from all the epistles of Peter, James, John, and Jude.

Pauline and Disputed epistles. According to univariate F tests ($df = 1, 60, p < .05$), the Undisputed Pauline samples had lower Imagery scores (1.44 vs 1.47) and were more Repetitious (66% vs 61%). They contained more Very Common Words (71% vs 70%), and used Shorter Words (3.97 letters vs 4.13 letters). Negatives (2.1% vs 1.5%) and the verb To Be (5.5% vs 4.5%) were more common in the Undisputed Pauline samples. Sentences in samples from the Undisputed epistles were shorter than in those from the Disputed epistles (21.87 vs 28.66 words). The largest differences were those for Word Length, Sentence Length, and Repetitiousness: means for the two groups of samples were at least one standard deviation apart for these variables. On the basis of these results, it is possible to infer that St. Paul's (undisputed) writing style was admonitory (more Negatives), crisp, clear, pointed (shorter and more common words), and repetitive, though somewhat abstract (lower Imagery, greater use of the verb To Be). The simultaneous complexity and simplicity of St. Paul's style is acknowledged by analysts (Guthrie, 1970, p. 389) who regard it as closer to vernacular than to literary language, but not quite "common" in its Greek form (*koine* or common Greek would be that spoken by the man-in-the-street of Paul's day).

A discriminant function analysis (Wilks stepwise method, limited to five significant predictors) was used in an attempt to discriminate Undisputed

Pauline from Disputed samples. Discrimination was successfully accomplished with a canonical correlation of .77 (Wilks lambda = .41), and 85% of the samples were correctly classified as Undisputed Pauline or Disputed. The standardized canonical discriminant function coefficients (D weights) indicated that membership in the Undisputed Pauline group was a function of shorter Word Length (–.77), lower Imagery (–.78), and lower Word Frequency (–.57) in combination with greater Repetitiousness (.43) and greater Pleasantness (.36). Correct placement was equivalent for Disputed and Undisputed groups—86% and 85%, respectively.

When the non-Pauline or Other (Peter, etc.) epistles, which had not been included in the samples that defined the function, were classified by the same formula, 11 were classified as Disputed and five as Undisputed Pauline. There was therefore a 69% correct identification of these epistles as not belonging to the group clearly written by Paul, which provides some independent confirmation for the function and suggests that Paul's style was distinct not only from that of those possibly writing in his name but also from those of the other writers.

Samples from Undisputed Pauline sources that were misclassified as belonging to Disputed sources in this analysis came from the books of Romans (four samples: the first, third, and last two samples) and Philippians (the last two samples). Ehrman (2000, p. 319) noted that the book of Romans is "unlike all of Paul's other letters: it is written to a congregation Paul did not establish, in a city that he had never visited". A goodly portion of the misclassified samples from Romans dealt with salutations, exhortations, and parting instructions to this congregation. With respect to Philippians, some analysts consider it likely that the ending portions of the epistle, which included the misclassified samples, were portions of a different letter (Ehrman, 2000, p. 313).

Disputed samples that were misclassified as Undisputed Pauline came from 2 Thessalonians (second of two samples) and Hebrews (two nonadjacent samples from the middle of the book). According to Ehrman (2000, pp. 344-345), 2 Thessalonians is the Disputed epistle whose style most closely matches that of Paul. The book of Hebrews was included in the Christian New Testament canon only because early Christians became convinced that Paul had written it, although modern critics use the contents of this book to help reach the firm conclusion that he did not.

Acknowledged Non-Pauline samples incorrectly classified as Undisputed Pauline were all three samples from 1 John, one sample from 2 Peter, and one from James. Paul's emotion and style most closely matched those of the author of the first epistle attributed to John. 1 John lacks the literary conventions of an epistle (which are present in 2 John and 3 John) and resembles rather a persuasive essay (Ehrman, 2000, p. 164). It may be the persuasiveness which characterizes Paul's writing that forms the bridge between the two authors' epistles. Guthrie (1970, p. 864) characterized 1 John as having the same combination of profundity of thought and simplicity of style that have been used to describe the work of Paul.

D scores are the composites whose weights were described above: they are used to classify samples in the discriminant analysis. Some of the lowest of all D score means were obtained for the books of Ephesians and Colossians, indicating that these epistles were extremely unlike the Undisputed Pauline corpus in terms of their emotion and style. The highest D mean did not in fact belong to a Pauline epistle at all but to 1 John, whose similarity to the Pauline corpus has been noted. When ranked in terms of mean D scores, the books in descending order (from most Undisputed Pauline in style and emotion to least Pauline) were 1 John (D = 2.02), 1 Corinthians (1.28), 1 Thessalonians (1.26), 2 Corinthians (1.16), Galatians (.79), Romans (.66), Philemon (.04), 2 Thessalonians (–.13), 3 John (–.16), Philippians (–.19), 2 John (–.44), 1 Timothy (–.52), Titus (–.87), 2 Timothy (–1.02), James (–1.29), 1 Peter (–1.34), Hebrews (–1.69), Ephesians (–1.88), Colossians (–2.73), 2 Peter (–2.74), and Jude (–4.61). Like Ephesians and Colossians, Hebrews holds a very low rank in this list. The work least similar in style and emotion to Paul's writings was the epistle of Jude.

When the steps of the discriminant function were not limited, it carried on to include nine significant predictors, with a canonical correlation of .82 and 92% correct prediction. In this scheme, 13 of the 16 non-Pauline samples (81%) were classified in the Disputed category. Accurate classification of samples within the function and without the function therefore both improved somewhat with the addition of predictors. This likely occurred because the means for Other samples in Table 1 are generally closer to the means for Disputed samples (eight variables) than to those for Undisputed samples (three variables).

A study of the total vocabulary of any author is especially vulnerable to biases that characterize the process of translation. For example, there are several words for "but" in Greek, and certain Greek rhetorical forms cannot be translated word for word into English equivalents. Results of vocabulary comparisons for the translated epistles must, therefore, be regarded as merely exploratory: they are best used to point out areas for further research with the Greek originals. A computer program was used to examine the entire vocabulary of the translated Disputed and Undisputed Pauline epistles and to perform significance tests (z test for proportions, $p < .001$, two-tailed) comparing them word by word against each other. Punctuation marks were included in the comparison. Table 2 lists all words and punctuation marks that were used at significantly different rates in Disputed and Undisputed epistles. Words that occurred significantly more often in the Undisputed

TABLE 2
Words and Punctuation Marks Used at Significantly Different Rates in Undisputed and Disputed Pauline Epistles (z test, $p < .001$, two-tailed)

Word†	Frequency* in Epistles Disputed	Frequency* in Epistles Undisputed	Word	Frequency* in Epistles Disputed	Frequency* in Epistles Undisputed
I	685.59	1822.44	reap	33.80	.00
?	120.70	646.50	stumbling	33.80	.00
you	1506.37	2341.24	zeal	33.80	.00
law	86.91	343.20	above	57.94	7.98
not	965.62	1553.73	created	43.45	2.66
but	709.73	1226.49	of	3316.92	2769.57
we	574.55	1003.01	teach	67.59	10.64
if	275.20	587.97	appeal	38.62	.00
!	9.66	130.36	asleep	38.62	.00
written	14.48	127.70	Cephas	38.62	.00
am	106.22	284.67	cup	38.62	.00
what	207.61	415.04	natural	38.62	.00
;	511.78	803.47	seed	38.62	.00
do	400.73	641.18	sorrow	38.62	.00
are	632.48	917.87	unbelievers	38.62	.00
is	1255.31	1633.54	wait	38.62	.00
spirit	159.33	316.60	wrote	38.62	.00
my	265.55	449.62	heavenly	62.77	7.98
rejoice	4.83	66.51	mystery	62.77	7.98
man	125.53	258.07	angels	82.08	15.96
brethren	101.39	223.48	ever	82.08	15.96
			house	72.42	10.64
discipline	38.62	2.66	must	178.64	66.51
husbands	38.62	2.66	these	178.64	66.51
inheritance	38.62	2.66	deeds	67.59	7.98
pleasure	38.62	2.66	faithful	86.91	15.96
his	646.97	438.98	eats	43.45	.00
days	53.11	7.98	idols	43.45	.00
once	96.56	29.27	really	43.45	.00
everything	101.39	31.93	trespass	43.45	.00
made	202.78	95.78	Savior	53.11	2.66
offer	48.28	5.32	covenant	91.73	15.96
sound	48.28	5.32	–	125.53	31.93
abundance	33.80	.00	crucified	48.28	.00
Achaia	33.80	.00	danger	48.28	.00
believes	33.80	.00	tongue	48.28	.00
foolishness	33.80	.00	wish	48.28	.00
freedom	33.80	.00	enter	57.94	2.66
jealousy	33.80	.00	sacrifices	57.94	2.66
letters	33.80	.00	place	82.08	10.64
pass	33.80	.00	having	159.33	47.89

(continued on next page)

*The frequencies are reported as occurrences per 100,000 words. †Cases are arranged in descending order of how well they match the Undisputed Pauline sample, with the first 21 exemplars being more common in this sample and the remainder being more common in the Disputed sample.

TABLE 2 (CONT'D)
Words and Punctuation Marks Used at Significantly Different Rates in Undisputed and Disputed Pauline Epistles (z test, $p < .001$, two-tailed)

Word†	Frequency* in Epistles Disputed	Frequency* in Epistles Undisputed	Word	Frequency* in Epistles Disputed	Frequency* in Epistles Undisputed
baptized	53.11	.00	tongues	72.42	.00
boasting	53.11	.00	vain	72.42	.00
reckoned	53.11	.00	Jews	77.25	.00
sins	125.53	26.60	man's	77.25	.00
he	1120.12	747.60	which	564.89	247.43
belong	62.77	.00	myself	111.05	.00
certainly	67.59	.00	and	3500.39	2421.05
blood	130.36	21.28			

*The frequencies are reported as occurrences per 100,000 words. †Cases are arranged in descending order of how well they match the Undisputed Pauline sample, with the first 21 exemplars being more common in this sample and the remainder being more common in the Disputed sample.

epistles include "I," "you," "we," "not," and "but," as well as "Spirit" and "rejoice." The question mark (?), exclamation mark (!), and semicolon (;) were more frequently used in these epistles. The Disputed epistles made significantly more frequent use of words such as "and," "vain," "Savior," and "crucified." They also included more dashes (–). In general, the tone of words which predominate in the Disputed epistles is more negative, e.g., sins, stumbling, unbelievers, sorrow, foolishness, jealousy, than that of those which predominate in the Undisputed epistles. If the Disputed epistles were written by more than one person, which is what several analysts propose, then it is no surprise that there is a wider vocabulary which significantly characterizes them (74 words and one punctuation mark), and a smaller, tighter one which characterizes Paul (18 words and three punctuation marks). Some of the results reported above (the use of shorter words, more Very Common Words) are exemplified by the Undisputed Pauline vocabulary in Table 2.

The results of this study allow the strong conclusion that there are stylistic, vocabulary, and emotional differences between the Disputed and Undisputed Pauline epistles in Clontz' translation. These same differences are frequently noted in comparisons of the Undisputed and Other (non-Pauline) epistles. Measures of emotion and imagery (specifically emotional Pleasantness and overall Imagery) played a significant role in the classification of samples as Undisputed Pauline. Successful discrimination among samples from Disputed and Undisputed epistles was achieved entirely on the basis of measures taken by computer programs which operated very much at arm's length from the epistles.

Certain inferences cannot be drawn from the results described in this study. A difference in style does not always indicate a difference in authorship, and similarity of style does not confirm unitary authorship. Letters written by the same author to different recipients may well differ in style from one another, as was the case for portions of Romans. As well, measures of emotional tone are not necessarily the best evidence of authorship since various situations invite different emotional reactions. The highly Pauline style of 1 John is not proof that Paul authored this epistle, although it does encourage a closer comparison of the work with his. An overlap of some findings between Neumann's research (1990) and the present research (e.g., for word length, p. 213) suggests that the translated versions of the epistles studied conveyed many of the same important facts noted in the Greek originals.

This study adds to the considerable mass of information available about the epistles attributed to Paul (e.g., in Selby, 1962; Guthrie, 1970; Neumann, 1990; Ehrman, 2000). In evaluating the implications of this research, it is important to note that Christians do not study the books of the New Testament primarily in terms of literary style (Guthrie, 1970, p. 387) and that it is the books "themselves and not their sources or origins which have moulded Christian history" (Guthrie, 1970, p. 13).

REFERENCES

EHRMAN, B. D. (2000) *The New Testament: a historical introduction to the early Christian writings.* New York: Oxford Univer. Press.

GUTHRIE, D. (1970) *New Testament introduction.* Downers Grove, IL: Inter-Varsity Press.

NEUMANN, K. J. (1990) *The authenticity of the Pauline epistles in the light of stylostatistical analysis.* Atlanta, GA: Scholar's Press.

SELBY, J. D. (1962) *Toward the understanding of St. Paul.* Englewood Cliffs, NJ: Prentice-Hall.

WHISSELL, C. (1996) Traditional emotional and stylometric analysis of the songs of Beatles Paul McCartney and John Lennon. *Computers and the Humanities,* 30, 257-265.

WHISSELL, C. (1998) A parsimonious technique for the analysis of word use patterns in English texts and transcripts. *Perceptual and Motor Skills,* 86, 595-613.

WHISSELL, C. (1999) Dimensions of linguistic and emotional style: computerized analysis of the prototypical romantic poets. (Conference paper, NASSR)

WHISSELL, C. (2003) Readers' opinions of Romantic poetry are consistent with emotional measures based on the Dictionary of Affect in Language. *Perceptual and Motor Skills,* 96, 990-992.

Accepted March 30, 2004.

GEOMAGNETIC ACTIVITY DURING THE PREVIOUS DAY IS CORRELATED WITH INCREASED CONSUMPTION OF SUCROSE DURING SUBSEQUENT DAYS: IS INCREASED GEOMAGNETIC ACTIVITY AVERSIVE?[1]

M. A. GALIC AND M. A. PERSINGER

Laurentian University

Summary.—In five separate blocks over a period of several months for 33 female rats the amount of geomagnetic activity during the day before *ad libitum* access to 10% sucrose or water was positively correlated with the volume of sucrose consumed per 24-hr. period. The strength of the correlation (.62 to .77) declined over the subsequent 10 days from between .12 to –.18 and resembled an extinction curve. In a subsequent experiment four rats exposed to 5 nT to 8 nT, 0.5-Hz magnetic fields that ceased for 30 min. once every 4 hr. for 4 days consumed 11% more sucrose than the four rats exposed to no field. We suggest that the initial consumption of 10% sucrose may have been reinforced because it diminished the aversive physiological effects associated with the increased geomagnetic activity. However, over the subsequent days, as geomagnetic activity decreased or habituation occurred, negative reinforcement did not maintain this behavior.

Galic and Persinger (2002) found that female rats, when allowed free access to either water or 10% sucrose, consumed 150 to 200 cc of sugar water per day for weeks even though their typical daily intake of fluids (water) was between 25 and 30 cc. Many of the behaviours of the female rats resembled those exhibited by addicted humans. Persinger (2004) suggested that increases in geomagnetic activity result in "negative" physiological states that contribute to affectively related behaviors such as aggression, disruptions in attention (hence increased traffic, industrial, and aviation accidents), and sleep disturbances.

If increased geomagnetic activity induces a negative hedonistic state within some animals and the consumption of sucrose reduces this state, then there should be strong positive correlations between increased geomagnetic activity and the amounts of sucrose consumed. The relationship between sucrose consumption and geomagnetic activity should reflect the principle of negative reinforcement, with the geophysical stimulus being the aversive stimulus and the consumption of sucrose being the response that attenuates the magnitude of the consequences of this stimulus.

In five replicates or blocks starting on different days over a 5-mo.

---

[1]Send correspondence to Dr. M. A. Persinger, Behavioral Neuroscience Laboratory, Departments of Biology and Psychology, Laurentian University, Sudbury, ON Canada P3E 2C6.

period 33 4-mo.-old Wistar albino female rats (3 to 8 per block) were given continuous access to two 250-cc bottles containing water or 10% sucrose. The rats were housed singly in plastic shoebox cages containing 1/4-in. corn-cob bedding. Purina rat chow was available *ad libitum*. The amounts of water and sucrose-water consumed were measured daily and refreshed. Direct measurements of geomagnetic activity by a MEDA FM 300 magnetometer within the cages were correlated more than .90 with various indices of global daily geomagnetic activity, obtained from Geomagnetic Indices Bulletin (Boulder).[2]

The averages of the maximum and minimum A values for each of the three days before, the day of, and for each of the three days after the beginning of each block were correlated (using Spearman *rho* because the sample was small) with the mean values of the sucrose consumed during the first 10 days of the block. The strongest correlation ($r = .72$) occurred between the geomagnetic activity the day before the block began and the amount of sucrose consumed on the first and second days of the block. Regression analysis indicated about 100 cc of the consumption was associated with the range of average daily global activity between 12 nT and 62 nT.

The strengths of the Spearman *rho* correlations between the geomagnetic activities during the day before the blocks began and the amounts of sucrose consumed during subsequent days declined conspicuously. These values for Days 1 through 12 were .62, .77, .52, .52, .51, .43, .40, .25, .35, .12, .30, and –.08, respectively. The means and standard deviations for the average planetary A indices of the day before the beginning of the block were 18.4 and 6.2. These values for the first four days of the blocks were 19.2 ($SD = 11.7$), 18.0 ($SD = 8.9$), 15.6 ($SD = 6.2$), and 19.0 ($SD = 7.1$), respectively.

To discern whether results could be simulated experimentally four female rats were exposed during a quiet (geomagnetic) period to a 0.5-Hz, 5- to 8-nT magnetic field that was disrupted for 30 min. every 4 hr. for four days while four other female rats were exposed to a control coil (see Dupont, McKay, Parker, & Persinger, 2004). Our prediction that sucrose consumption would increase in the group exposed to the geomagnetic-simulated field compared to change for the control animals was supported ($F_{1,6} = 4.28$, $p < .05$; one-tailed, $\eta = .65$). They drank about 14 cc more sucrose per day than the control group. Group differences for the subsequent four days of sucrose consumption were not statistically significant ($F_{1,6} = 2.35$, $p > .05$).

We interpret both sets of results as supportive of the hypothesis that increased geomagnetic activity induces a negative hedonistic state. Any re-

---

[2]www.dxlc.com/solar/indices.html.

sponse that reduces this negative condition will be maintained (negative reinforcement). Because the strength of the association between daily sucrose consumptions after the first day of consumption (novelty) and the geomagnetic activity the day before the first consumption declined during subsequent days, either this hypothesized physiological state was no longer aversive or the effectiveness of sucrose consumption for attenuating this aversive state may have declined ("tolerance").

REFERENCES

DUPONT, M. J., MCKAY, B. E., PARKER, G., & PERSINGER, M. A. (2004) Geophysical variables and behavior: XCIX. Reductions in numbers of neurons within the parasolitary nucleus in rats exposed perinatally to a magnetic pattern designed to imitate geomagnetic continuous pulsations: implications for Sudden Infant Death. *Perceptual and Motor Skills*, 98, 958-966.

GALIC, M. A., & PERSINGER, M. A. (2002) Voluminous sucrose consumption in female rats: increased "nippiness" during periods of sucrose removal and possible oestrus periodicity. *Psychological Reports*, 90, 58-60.

PERSINGER, M. A. (2004) Weak-to-moderate correlations between daily geomagnetic activity and reports of diminished pleasantness: a nonspecific source for multiple behavioral correlates? *Perceptual and Motor Skills*, 98, 78-80.

Accepted April 6, 2004.

ASSESSING POTENTIALLY GIFTED STUDENTS FROM LOWER SOCIOECONOMIC STATUS WITH NONVERBAL MEASURES OF INTELLIGENCE [1]

ELIZABETH SHAUNESSY

University of South Florida

FRANCES A. KARNES AND YOLANDA COBB

The University of Southern Mississippi

Summary.—The screening and identification of gifted students has historically been conducted using verbal measures of intelligence. However, the underrepresentation in gifted programs of culturally diverse children, who may have limited English proficiency or cultural values different from those measured in traditional intelligence tests, has prompted researchers to consider other measures. Nonverbal measures of intelligence have been utilized to increase the number of gifted children from diverse backgrounds. Researchers in the current study sought to increase the number of culturally diverse gifted students at a rural public school enrolling predominantly African-American students from low socioeconomic homes. 169 students in Grades 2 through 6 were assessed using three nonverbal measures of intelligence: the Culture-Fair Intelligence Test, the Naglieri Nonverbal Abilities Test, and the Raven Standard Progressive Matrices. The scores on these nonverbal measures indicated that the Culture-Fair Intelligence Test and the Raven Standard Progressive Matrices identified more students than the Naglieri Nonverbal Abilities Test. A discussion of the results and implications for research are presented.

The challenge of identifying and serving culturally diverse and disadvantaged students has persisted for at least three decades (Marland, 1972), with recent research indicating a continued need to identify and include gifted students from underrepresented populations, especially gifted students who are culturally diverse and from disadvantaged backgrounds (Frasier, 1987; Davis & Rimm, 1989; Ford, 1994). Efforts have focused on the education of culturally diverse students with learning difficulties rather than on directing attention and services to culturally diverse and underrepresented students "with outstanding ability from these backgrounds" (Gallagher & Gallagher, 1994, p. 409).

Verbal measures of intelligence have been the traditional means of identifying students for gifted programs. However, given cultural challenges in some of these assessments, as well as the tests' emphases on linguistic intelligence, students who possess strengths in visuospatial intelligence and do not

---

[1]Address enquiries to E. Shaunessy, Ph.D., Coordinator, Gifted Education Program, University of South Florida, 4202 East Fowler Avenue, Tampa, FL 33620-5650.

manifest giftedness through verbal skills may be overlooked. To increase the representation of culturally diverse students in gifted programs, nonverbal tests of intelligence have been recommended for screening potentially gifted children from these groups (Baska, 1986; Matthews, 1988; Mills, Ablard, & Brody, 1993) since these assessments offer measures with reduced cultural bias or tests less dependent on knowledge of language symbols (Johnsen & Corn, 2001). Research has indicated that various groups, such as the culturally diverse, approach problem solving very differently than other groups. Furthermore, their performance may be lower on verbally loaded assessments since the measures are constructed to evaluate the cultural values of the dominant culture, such as response speed rather than other skills valued by culturally diverse communities, such as associative thinking (Gallagher & Gallagher, 1994).

Nonverbal assessments have been claimed to present unbiased measures for identifying potentially gifted students (Gagné, 1985; Gardner, 1993). Such tests allow screening and identification practices that may increase the representation of culturally diverse groups through incorporation of preliminary practice items, untimed testing conditions, use of abstract content rather than reading passages, use of test items that require problem-solving or reasoning rather than factual knowledge, and use of novel problems to avoid recall of previously mastered information (Johnsen & Corn, 2001).

Several studies have examined the use of nonverbal measures in identifying gifted children. However, the construct of giftedness and the definitions of intellectual giftedness vary, as each state may develop its own criteria for identifying gifted children. Many states requires an intelligence score of at or above the 98th percentile on individual measures of intelligence, which is typically 130 or above on a specific verbal measure. Other states require a score of 120 or above as one criteria for identification. This variability in identification criteria and intelligence scores renders comparison of studies challenging. However, the results of these studies indicate that the use of nonverbal measures of intelligence shows promise in addressing the underrepresentation of culturally diverse students in gifted programs.

With the goals of locating cost-and-time-effective screening procedures, Fitz-Gibbon (1974) investigated the use of the Raven Standard Progressive Matrices (Raven, 1960) and Advanced Progressive Matrices (Raven, 1962) in identifying gifted disadvantaged African-American students. In a study of students from a predominantly African-American urban community in California, 800 eighth-grade students were selected for the gifted program. Teachers' nominations of students considered to be gifted were solicited, then the Standard Progressive Matrices, the California Test of Mental Maturity, and the California Achievement Test were given to intact classes of eighth-grade students. The Advanced Progressive Matrices was then administered to students who met any of the following criteria: students scoring above 48 on the Standard Progressive Matrices, students scoring in the top 2% on the California Test of Mental Maturity or California Achievement Test, students nominated by teachers, or a random sample of students. The selection of students for individual assessment using the Wechsler Intelligence Scale for Children was based on a rank-order of scores on the Standard Progressive Matrices, California Test of Mental Maturity, California Achievement Test, or teachers' nominations. The top 2% ($n=18$ students) were then administered the Wechsler Intelligence Scale for Children. Nine students scored at 114 or above on the WISC Performance subscale.

Analysis indicated that five of the eight identified gifted students had scored at or above the top 2% on the Standard Progressive Matrices, and five had been nominated by teachers. When dividing the students into two groups of high or low scoring Wechsler Intelligence Scale for Children groups and performing a step-wise discriminant analysis, all means (except those on the mathematics concepts test) for the students identified as gifted were higher, but only three were significant at the .05 level, with the largest difference in mean scores found on the Advanced Progressive Matrices. This finding led Fitz-Gibbon to conclude that "the SPM could be used alone [to screen potentially gifted students], but the addition of the [APM] permits an increase in the efficiency and fairness of the selection procedure" (1974, p. 65).

Robinson, Bradley, and Stanley (1990) investigated ethnic differences in performance between 78 elementary students (22 African American, 56 Caucasian), who were participants in a mathematically talented after-school program (experimental group), and 183 alternate participants (40 African American, 140 Caucasian, 3 other) (comparison group). Both African-American and Caucasian students were from middle and lower middle income families. Students were identified in several steps. First, student nominations from teachers and parents based on mathematics achievement and gifted characteristics were solicited. Then a local committee screened students nominated based on demonstrated mathematics achievement and need. Students recommended by this committee were then asked to complete three assessments: the Math Applied to Novel Situations test (Hebert, 1984), the Sequential Tests of Educational Progress, and the Raven Standard Progressive Matrices (Raven, 1960). Scores on these assessments, prior mathematics achievement, and minority status were considered by the committee in selecting participants.

Robinson, *et al.* (1990) considered the ethnic differences among participants through multiple regression analyses. The independent variables were the Sequential Tests of Educational Progress, the Raven Standard Progressive Matrices (Raven, 1960), and status (participants or control group). The

Math Applied to Novel Situations, a standardized mathematics problem-solving measure, was the dependent variable. Analysis of the Standard Progressive Matrices scores indicated a statistically significant difference between African-American ($M = .21$) and Caucasian ($M = .85$) groups. Using a multiple regression analysis, Robinson, Bradley, and Stanley found the identification procedures using the Standard Progressive Matrices "contribute[d] less to the prediction of mathematics performance for [African Americans] than for [Caucasians]" (Robinson, et al., 1990, p. 10). The regression analysis of scores for only African-American students indicated that they benefitted from participation in an enriched mathematics program. The researchers found that using mathematics achievement and nonverbal reasoning were effective in identifying mathematically talented African-American students for a special program.

To identify a pool of students who may be gifted, Stephens, Kiger, Karnes, and Whorton (1999) administered the Culture-Fair Intelligence Test (Cattell & Cattell, 1965), Standard Progressive Matrices (Raven, Court, & Raven, 1996), and the Naglieri Nonverbal Abilities Test (Naglieri, 1996) to intact classes of 189 rural, economically disadvantaged, African-American (91%) and Caucasian (9%) elementary school students in Grades 3 through 8 to identify culturally diverse, potentially gifted students. All students participated in the free or reduced-cost lunch program. Scores on each of the three assessments were categorized into 5-point ranges, beginning with the 80th percentile to identify a group of high-scoring students. When compared to the number of students scoring at or above the 80th percentile on each measure, analysis indicated that the Standard Progressive Matrices identified the most students scoring at the 80th percentile or higher ($n = 15$); 10 students on the Naglieri Nonverbal Abilities Test (grade), 6 students on the Naglieri Nonverbal Abilities Test (age), and 8 students on the Culture-Fair Intelligence Test scored at or above the 80th percentile. A few students scored at or above the 80th percentile on more than one assessment; a total of 39 scores on the three tests were at the 80th percentile or higher; these scores were for 26 students.

Lewis (2001) reported a replication of the Stephens, et al. (1999) study. The Standard Progressive Matrices, Culture-Fair Intelligence Test, and Naglieri Nonverbal Abilities Test were administered to 270 Grade 3–8 students representing Hispanic (99 students), Caucasian (160 students), and Other (11 students) (Lewis & Michaelson Grippin, 2000), none of whom had been identified previously for a gifted program. As in the Stephens, et al. study, scores were ranked in increments of five, beginning with 80th% for the purpose of identifying a group of high-scoring potentially gifted students for additional study. Of the 89 students scoring at or above the 80th percentile, 25.8% were Hispanic (23 students) and 68.5% were Caucasian (61 students).

The majority of students were identified on either the Standard Progressive Matrices or the Culture-Fair Intelligence Test (57.6% of scores). Lewis and Michaelson Grippin (2000) found that the Culture-Fair Intelligence Test identified more Hispanic students (17) than the Standard Progressive Matrices (12 students) or Naglieri Nonverbal Abilities Test (4 students). However, overall, the Culture-Fair Intelligence Test and Standard Progressive Matrices identified almost the same number of students, 58 and 59, respectively.

Naglieri and Ronning (2000) examined differences among three matched samples of African American ($n=2,306$) and Caucasian ($n=2,306$), Hispanic ($n=1,176$) and Caucasian ($n=1,176$), and Asian American ($n=466$) and Caucasian ($n=466$) children from 22,620 within the Naglieri Nonverbal Abilities Test standardization sample. Participants were matched on type of school setting (private or public), socioeconomic status, ethnicity, and geographic region. Minimal differences were found between Caucasian and Asian (difference ratio = .02) and Caucasian and Hispanic groups (difference ratio = .17). Similarly, a significant but small difference was found between scores for Caucasian and African-American samples (difference ratio = .25). Scores on the Naglieri Nonverbal Abilities Test were correlated with reading (.52) and mathematics (.63) across the samples.

The Naglieri Nonverbal Abilities Test was used in a study of culturally diverse minority students in Pennsylvania to increase the representation in the gifted and talented program, which had historically identified less than 1% of its school's population (Lidz & Macrine, 2001). In Grades 1 through 5 473 students, 63% of whom were African-American, Hispanic-American, Asian-American, and East European immigrant students, were assessed. Those students scoring in the upper 10th percentile range on at least two of the screening measures, which included a teachers' checklist (Gifted and Talented Evaluation Scales) (Gilliam, Carpenter, & Christensen, 1996), achievement test scores in mathematics and reading (Iowa Test of Basic Skills) (Hoover, Hieronymus, Frisbie, & Dunbar, 1993), researcher-constructed peer and parent questionnaires, and class observations (Group Dynamic Assessment Procedure) (Lidz & Greenberg, 1997; Lidz, Jespen, & Miller, 1997).

Following the screening, researchers selected a pool of students who scored in the 90th percentile on a minimum of two screening measures, which yielded 85 students or 18% of students in Grades 1 through 5. These students were then individually assessed on either the Kaufman Assessment Battery for Children (K–ABC) (Kaufman & Kaufman, 1983) or the Naglieri Nonverbal Abilities Test, modified for individual and dynamic administration. Analysis indicated that 23 of the 25 identified students scored at the 97th percentile or better on the Naglieri Nonverbal Abilities Test posttest. The assessors used a dynamic assessment model, which included "a test—

intervene—posttest format" (Lidz & Macrine, 2001, p. 82) for the administration of the Naglieri Nonverbal Abilities Test. Examination indicated that this posttest significantly predicted gifted status (scoring at or above the 97th percentile on two measures, including the Kaufman Assessment Battery for Children, Naglieri Nonverbal Abilities Test, or Iowa Test of Basic Skills when controlling for immigrant group as well as pretest on the Kaufman Assessment Battery for Children and Naglieri Nonverbal Abilities Test pretest. Ultimately 60% of the 25 identified students were from either ethnic minority or immigrant backgrounds.

The purpose of this study was to assess culturally diverse, economically disadvantaged students from a rural elementary school using three nonverbal measures of intelligence to identify potentially gifted students.

Method

Previous studies had considered nonverbal measures of intelligence as tools in the identification of culturally diverse gifted students. The purpose of the current study was to specify which screening measure, the Standard Progressive Matrices, Naglieri Nonverbal Abilities Test, or Culture-Fair Intelligence Test, yielded the greatest number of culturally diverse students in this setting for additional investigation at the school district level. Thus, the researchers assessed 169 students enrolled in Grades 2 through 6 of a rural elementary school in a southern state, in which the average daily attendance was 359. Of the enrolled students, 93% were African American, and 96% were classified as students of low socioeconomic status since they qualified to receive free or reduced-cost lunches. Of the 169 students assessed, only two participated in their district's gifted program.

Researchers administered the Standard Progressive Matrices (Raven, *et al.*, 1996), Culture-Fair Intelligence Test (Cattell & Cattell, 1965), and Naglieri Nonverbal Abilities Test (Naglieri, 1996). The first is an untimed nonverbal assessment that measures higher-level thinking skills. It is designed for students Ages 6 through adult and has 60 questions divided into five Sets (A, B, C, D, and E), each containing 12 items that become progressively more difficult. Administration takes approximately 20 to 45 min. A question format excludes "a portion of a diagram, and the task is to determine which of several options best fits in the location" (Naglieri & Prewett, 1990, p. 358). Internal consistency investigations report split-half reliability estimates or KR–20 estimates ranging from .60 to .98, with a minimum estimate of .90 (Raven & Summers, 1986; Robinson, *et al.*, 1990).

The Naglieri Nonverbal Abilities Test (Naglieri, 1996) is a group or individually administered scale for use with kindergarten through Grade 12 students. It requires "students to rely on reasoning and problem-solving skills rather than verbal skills" (Stephens, *et al.*, 1999). The test has been designed for seven levels, including Level A for kindergarten, Level B for Grade 1, Level C for Grade 2, Level D for Grades 3 and 4, Level E for Grades 5 and 6, Level F for Grades 7, 8, and 9, and Level G for Grades 10, 11, and 12. Each level has 39 questions. The test has been normed on a national sample of 100,000 children by grade and adults. It has been studied for use with special populations, including the gifted, learning disabled, and hearing-impaired students. Cross-cultural studies also validated its use with Hispanic, Asian, and other ethnic groups. Internal reliability coefficients range from .83 to .93, and the median internal reliability has been reported at .87 (Naglieri, 1997). Administration time is estimated at 30 to 45 min. One proctor is recommended for each group of 25 students.

The Culture-Fair Intelligence Test (Cattell & Cattell, 1965) was developed to measure fluid intelligence, purportedly influenced by biological factors in distinction to crystallized intelligence, which is developed through cultural factors (Nenty, 1986). Studies of the test (Kidd, 1962) indicate "a high saturation on general ability factor and a relative independence from cultural experiences" (Nenty, 1986, p. 11). Two levels are available, Scale 1 for Ages 4 through 8, which measures general mental capacity for g, and Scale 2 for Ages 8 through 13, which measures general intelligence. The test may be administered to groups or individuals, using Scale 1 of eight subtests and Scale 2 of four subtests of perceptual tasks. Administration times vary from 22 min. for Scale 1 to 12.5 min. for Scale 2. The test has been standardized on over 4,000 boys and girls from various U.S. regions. Both scales have estimates of construct, concurrent, and predictive validity. Cattell and Cattell (1965) reported consistency reliability, based on split-half and internal consistency formulae as .91 for Scale 1 and .87 for Scale 2.

All assessments were administered to intact groups of students by grade in a regular classroom. Statistical analyses were performed using SPSS for Windows Version 11.0 (2002), subprograms for descriptive statistics, analysis of variance, and frequencies.

RESULTS AND DISCUSSION

The descriptive statistics for the Culture-Fair Intelligence Test, the Standard Progressive Matrices, and Naglieri Nonverbal Abilities Test are reported in Table 1. The standard scores (z scores) for the Standard Progressive Matrices were obtained by subtracting the mean from each raw score and dividing by the standard deviation. Although the total number of students tested was 169, given absences the total number of students was fewer than 169. To identify a pool of high-scoring students, the scores were categorized into 5-point ranges beginning at the 80th percentile. These data are reported in Table 2. It should be noted that the total number of scores at the 80th percentile or higher was 62; however, the scores were actually ob-

TABLE 1
Descriptive Statistics For Three Scores

Score	n	Range	M	SD
Culture-Fair Intelligence Test Standard Score IQ	165	18–165.00	99.65	23.74
Naglieri Nonverbal Abilities Test Ability Index	167	50–135	81.86	15.92
Ravens z Score	166	−1.99–1.98	.00	1.00

tained from only 45 different students. Compared with the Raven Standard Progressive Matrices and the Naglieri Nonverbal Abilities Test, the scores on the Culture-Fair Intelligence Test identified the largest number (36) of students scoring at the 80th percentile or higher.

TABLE 2
Percentiles by Range

Measure	80–84 n	80–84 %	85–89 n	85–89 %	90–94 n	90–94 %	95–99 n	95–99 %	Total
Culture-Fair Intelligence Test	4	2.4	9	5.5	7	4.3	16	9.7	36
Naglieri Nonverbal Abilities Test									
Age	1	.6	0		0		2	1.2	3
Grade	3	1.8	0		0		2	1.2	5
Standard Progressive Matrices	4	2.4	2	1.2	6	3.6	6	3.6	18
Total	12		11		13		26		62

As documented in the work of Stephens, *et al.* (1999) with predominantly low socioeconomic status, African-American students from a rural school, more students scored at or above the 80th percentile on the Standard Progressive Matrices than on the Culture-Fair Intelligence Test or Naglieri Nonverbal Abilities Test. However, these results are somewhat different from findings of Lewis (2001), whose study of Hispanic and Caucasian students showed more Hispanic students scoring in this range on the Culture-Fair Intelligence Test, but more Caucasian children scoring at or above the 80th percentile on the Standard Progressive Matrices.

Multiple measures for assessing potentially gifted youth are advised. Forty-nine students scored at or above the 80th percentile. As previously mentioned, the Culture-Fair Intelligence Test identified 36; of these students, nine had high scores on one of the other measures as well. Analysis of the results of nonverbal assessments of students from lower socioeconomic backgrounds can yield helpful information for researchers, psychometrists, school psychologists, teachers of the gifted, and potentially gifted students. Additional studies of this model of testing all students in a class with nonverbal measures are recommended. While this investigation indicated that this population of students might be best identified for gifted programs through the use of the Standard Progressive Matrices, these findings may not be generalizable to other groups of students of different ethnic backgrounds, socioeconomic status, or locales.

Further investigations of screening culturally diverse students using nonverbal measures in intact classes followed by individual nonverbal assessments, such as the Leiter–R or the Universal Nonverbal Intelligence Test (Bracken & McCallum, 2001) are also recommended. This sequence of group to nonverbal assessments must also be considered within the contexts of school district guidelines to identify students for gifted programs; however, some district policies, such as required grade point averages, achievement test scores, and teachers' checklists of gifted behavior, may limit the inclusion of students identified on both group and individual nonverbal assessments. While each of the previously mentioned identification criteria may identify students not typically found on measures of intelligence, very frequently these criteria can serve as gatekeepers for students who do not perform well in school settings. Nonverbal measures of intelligence provide these underrepresented and underidentified students the opportunity to be recognized for such programs.

REFERENCES

Baska, L. (1986) Alternatives to traditional testing. *Roeper Review*, 8, 181-184.

Bracken, B. A., & McCallum, R. S. (1997) *The Universal Nonverbal Intelligence Test.* Chicago, IL: Riverside.

Cattell, R. B., & Cattell, K. S. (1965) *Manual for the Culture-Fair Intelligence Test, Scale 2.* Champaign, IL: Institute for Personality and Ability Testing.

Davis, G. A., & Rimm, S. B. (1989) *Education of the gifted and talented.* (2nd ed.) Englewood Cliffs, NJ: Prentice-Hall.

Fitz-Gibbon, C. T. (1974) The identification of mentally gifted, "disadvantaged" students at the eighth grade level. *Journal of Negro Education*, 43, 53-66.

Ford, D. Y. (1994) *The recruitment and retention of African-American students in gifted education programs: implications and recommendations.* Stoors, CT: The National Research Center on the Gifted and Talented, Univer. of Connecticut.

Frasier, M. M. (1987) The identification of gifted black students: developing new perspectives. *Journal for the Education of the Gifted*, 10, 155-180.

Gagné, F. (1985) Giftedness and talent: reexamining a reexamination of the definitions. *Gifted Child Quarterly*, 29, 103-112.

Gallagher, J. J., & Gallagher, S. A. (1994) *Teaching the gifted child.* Needham Heights, MA: Allyn & Bacon.

Gardner, H. (1993) *Creating minds.* New York: Basic Books.

Gilliam, J. E., Carpenter, B. O., & Christensen, J. R. (1996) *Gifted and Talented Evaluation Scales: examiner's manual.* Austin, TX: Pro-Ed.

Hebert, M. (1984) *Comprehensive School Mathematics Program: final evaluation report.* St. Louis, MO: Mid-Continent Research Education Lab, Inc. (ERIC Document Reproduction Service No. ED243654)

Hoover, H. D., Hieronymus, A. N., Frisbie, D. A., & Dunbar, S. B. (1993) *Iowa Test of Basic Skills.* Chicago, IL: Riverside.

JOHNSEN, S. K. & CORN, A. L. (2001) *Screening assessment for gifted elementary and middle school students.* (2nd ed.) Austin, TX: Pro-Ed.

KAUFMAN, A. S., & KAUFMAN, N. L. (1983) *K–ABC: Kaufman Assessment Battery for Children.* Circle Pines, MN: American Guidance Service.

KIDD, A. H. (1962) The culture-fair aspects of Cattell's Test of *g*: culture-free. *Journal of Genetic Psychology*, 101, 343-362.

LEWIS, J. (2001) Language isn't needed: nonverbal assessments and gifted learners. (ERIC Document Reproduction Service No. ED453026)

LEWIS, J., & MICHAELSON GRIPPIN, R. (2000) Screening for gifted: identifying diverse students. (Univer. of Nebraska at Kearney, unpublished data)

LIDZ, C. S., & GREENBERG, K. H. (1997) Criterion validity of a group dynamic assessment procedure with rural first grade regular education students. *Journal of Cognitive Education*, 6, 88-89.

LIDZ, C. S., JESPEN, R. H., & MILLER, M. A. (1997) Relationships between cognitive processes and academic achievement: application of a group dynamic assessment procedure with multiply handicapped adolescents. *Education and Child Psychology*, 14, 56-67.

LIDZ, C. S., & MACRINE, S. L. (2001) An alternative approach to the identification of gifted culturally diverse learners: the contribution of dynamic assessment. *School Psychology International*, 22, 74-96.

MARLAND, S. P., JR. (1972) *Education of the gifted and talented.* Vol. 1. Report to the Congress of the United States by the U.S. Commissioner of Education. Washington, DC: U.S. Government Printing Office.

MATTHEWS, D. (1988) Raven's Progressive Matrices in the identification of giftedness. *Roeper Review*, 10, 159-162.

MCCALLUM, S., BRACKEN, B., & WASSERMAN, J. D. (2001) *Essentials of nonverbal assessment.* New York: Wiley.

MILLS, C. J., ABLARD, K. E., & BRODY, E. (1993) The Raven's Progressive Matrices: its usefulness for identifying gifted/talented students. *Roeper Review*, 15, 183-187.

NAGLIERI, J. A. (1996) *Naglieri Nonverbal Abilities Test—directions for administering.* San Antonio, TX: Harcourt Brace.

NAGLIERI, J. A. (1997) *NNAT multilevel technical manual.* San Antonio, TX: Psychological Corp.

NAGLIERI, J. A., & PREWETT, P. N. (1990) Nonverbal intelligence measures: a selected review of instruments and their use. In C. R. Reynolds & R. W. Kamphaus (Eds.), *Handbook of psychological and educational assessment of children.* New York: Guilford. Pp. 348-370.

NAGLIERI, J. A., & RONNING, M. E. (2000) Comparison of White, African American, Hispanic, and Asian children on the Naglieri Nonverbal Abilities Test. *Psychological Assessment*, 12, 328-334.

NENTY, H. J. (1986) Cross-cultural bias analysis of Cattell Culture Fair Intelligence Test. (ERIC Document Reproduction Service No. ED274668)

RAVEN, J. C. (1960) *Guide to the Standard Progressive Matrices.* New York: Psychological Corp.

RAVEN, J. C. (1962) *Guide to the Advanced Progressive Matrices.* New York: Psychological Corp.

RAVEN, J. C., COURT, J. H., & RAVEN, J. (1996) *Manual for Raven's Progressive Matrices and Vocabulary Scales.* Oxford, UK: Oxford Psychologists' Press.

RAVEN, J. C., & SUMMERS, B. (1986) *Manual for Raven's Progressive Matrices and Vocabulary Scales Research Supplement No. 3: a compendium of North American normative and validity studies.* San Antonio, TX: Psychological Corp.

ROBINSON, A., BRADLEY, R. H., & STANLEY, T. D. (1990) Opportunity to achieve: identifying mathematically gifted black students. *Contemporary Educational Psychology*, 15, 1-12.

SPSS. (2002) *SPSS for Windows 11.0.* [Computer software] Chicago, IL: SPSS.

STEPHENS, K., KIGER, L., KARNES, F. A., & WHORTON, J. E. (1999) Use of nonverbal measures of intelligence in identification of culturally diverse gifted students in rural areas. *Perceptual and Motor Skills*, 88, 793-796.

Accepted April 7, 2004.

ELITE ATHLETES' DIFFERENTIATED ACTION IN TRAMPOLINING: A QUALITATIVE AND SITUATED ANALYSIS OF DIFFERENT LEVELS OF PERFORMANCE USING RETROSPECTIVE INTERVIEWS [1]

DENIS HAUW AND MARC DURAND

LIRDEF
University Institute for Teacher Education of Montpellier

Summary.—Using a situated cognition approach, this study analyzed elite athletes' actions, i.e., behaviors link to cognitions, during competitive trampoline performances, which are evaluated from a succession of 10 acrobatic movements characterized by flight time and fall risk. 27 exercises performed by 10 elite athletes were ranked poor, average, or good and analyzed. Self-confrontation interviews were conducted and transcribed in relation with behavioral descriptions derived from video recordings. Qualitative analysis was performed to identify units of meaningful action and their components. The succession of units describing the stream of actions was used to identify differentiated organization of trampolinists' performances. Three patterns, corresponding to performance levels, were distinguished by (a) an increasing number of meaningful actions occurring at the same time, (b) a reduction in actions of waiting, and (c) the emergence of new actions aimed at interaction with the situation. These results suggest that differentiation in performance level is linked with meaningful actions modified through interaction with the context.

Research on elite performance in sport psychology has principally focused on how different dimensions of athletes' psychological processes influence the results in competitive settings (Weinberg & Gould, 1999). The emphasis of this research is on the subjective experience athletes report after competitions. The methodologies employed, interviews, questionnaires, phone interviews, and so on, however, limit analysis of the behaviors actually performed during competition. Thus, athletes' psychological processes or cognitions have been investigated with only a general view of the situation in which they occurred and with indirect connection to specific actions. Also, the cognitions of elite athletes that have been consecutively investigated are those that overdetermine performance. For example, using these methodologies, concentration and confidence have emerged as major psychological processes in athletes. However, the studies neglect the direct effect of specific sport constraints or the resources implicit in the setting and conceal the relationships with the cognitions during competition.

---

[1]This research was supported by a grant from the French Ministry of Sport and the French National Federation of Gymnastics. Address correspondence to Denis Hauw, Université Montpellier 1, Faculté des Sciences du Sport et de l'EP, 700 avenue du Pic Saint Loup 34090 Montpellier, France or e-mail (d.hauw@univ.montp1.fr).

Several studies have already analyzed the situated actions, i.e., the relations among cognitions, behavior, and specific situations, of elite table tennis players (Sève, Saury, Theureau, & Durand, 2002; Sève, Saury, Ria, & Durand, 2003), sailing coaches (Saury & Durand, 1998), archery athletes and coaches (D'Arripe-Longueville, Saury, Fournier, & Durand, 2001), and trampolinists (Hauw & Durand, 2001; Hauw, Berthelot, & Durand, 2003). All of these researchers analyzed the stream of actions by the athletes (or coaches) and showed that their concerns, perceptions, and knowledge were transformed as situations unfolded, which in turn became resources for action. In this line of research, the study of elite trampolinists was particularly informative because, although it is a major form of acrobatic sport, trampolining is highly dynamic and has received little research in sport psychology (Hauw & Durand, 2001; Hauw, *et al.*, 2003). Trampolining is a sport of high accuracy because it requires the athletes to control their movements to stay on the center of the trampoline bed despite jumping up to eight meters into the air. Accuracy is crucial because a small error may have immediate and catastrophic consequences. Trampolinists perform exercises made up of 10 consecutive acrobatic movements. Scoring takes into account the difficulty and quality of execution of the movements. Difficulty is mainly based on the number of lengthwise and sideways turns performed during a jump. There are two major types of execution errors, (a) travel away from the cross or the square imprinted, respectively, in the middle or at the edges of the trampoline bed and (b) deviation of the trampolinists's body and limb positions with respect to a coded standard, e.g., lower limbs aligned with chest and head for a layout position. The studies of elite trampolinists have indicated that their typical actions consisted of regularly alternating between actions of transforming the body position and actions of assessing these transformations in relation to the trampoline bed. Trampolinists' actions during an exercise also consisted of preparing for the next movement while still in the midst of the current movement, orienting themselves in the general unfolding of the exercise to decide whether to modify movements that have already been planned and assessing generally how certain parts of the exercise have been performed. These results were counterintuitive because they indicated that elite trampolinists' actions comprised a wide range of adaptations to the unfolding situation. Generally, trampolining has been considered to require closed skills as in diving, gymnastics, or other acrobatic sports, where little adaptation to the situation is expected (Higgins & Spaeth, 1972). These results, however, confirmed the great knowledge possessed by practitioners, coaches, and judges about the field of possible accurate adjustments that trampolining situations allow. These studies, moreover, helped to define the typical nature of elite trampolinists' actions, but they were limited in their ability to explain how different levels of performance could be linked to differentiated situated actions. If we conceive of the trampolinist's real time adjustments as a process that relies on the possibilities offered by the unfolding situation, it should be possible to find a highly differentiated organization of those actions that characterize the most successful performances.

These studies analyzed the situatedness of actions by using the course of action theory (Theureau, 1992). A course of action is defined as "the activity of a given actor engaged in a given physical and social environment belonging to a given culture, where the activity is meaningful for the actor, that is, he can show it, tell it, and comment upon it to an observer-listener at any instant during its unfolding" (Theureau & Jeffroy, 1994, p. 19). The principal assumption of this theory is that human activity is semiotic, that it is a process of construction meaning in action (Kirshner & Whitson, 1997). Course of action theory relies on three types of data in the form of statements that express this fundamental semiotic process and correspond to the triadic sign from Peirce's thought-sign model (1931–1935). A triadic sign links an Object to a Representamen through an Interpretant (Peirce, 1931–1935). The Object is the intentional state of actors which corresponds to the field of possible actions they can undertake. For example, during flight in trampolining, the Object might be a focus on the unfolding of the rotation, i.e., an executive concern, a search to locate oneself in relation to the trampoline bed as quickly as possible, i.e., perceptual concern, or a question as to which movement one will perform next, i.e., a decisional concern. In the beginning, the Object is undetermined, but it is then specified by one or more Representamens, which are situation-related judgments of a perceptual or recall-based nature. The Representamen is the contextual element to which actors give meaning—what stands out, what they are focusing on. In the previous example, these would be the body sensations when taking off from the trampoline, the recall of movements already performed, or the realization that one is arriving at the end of an exercise, and one is performing the last movements which close the Object and orient it toward executive, perceptual, or decisional action. The Object is related to a Representamen by one or more Interpretants. The Interpretant is an element of knowledge drawn from past cognition that actors being to bear in the here and now. For example, trampolinists know how to interpret the sensations experienced during the take-off. They are thus able to make estimations concerning the rest of the unfolding exercise and to turn from perceptual actions to engage in decisional actions. Trampolinists also mobilize knowledge about how to change the order of movements during an exercise or to simplify a movement during its execution. When these elementary components are linked, an Elementary Unit of Meaning emerges (Theureau, 1992). This represents the smallest unit of action that is meaningful for actors at a given moment. For example, during the rising phase of the third movement, i.e., a given moment, while concentrating on the way they are performing the movement, i.e., object, trampolinists may decide to modify the exercise, i.e., elementary unit of meaning, because they feel that the take-off was unsatisfactory, i.e., representamen, and they know that they must be in the best possible condition to finish the exercise, i.e., interpretant. The course of action is the flow of these elementary units representing their activity in relation to the unfolding situation.

Even though each action is unique, there are basic units that can be identified in all actions, such that no action is ever totally new. An action is also a construction or a reconstruction within each occurrence of a more general structure or situation, corresponding to an elementary unit of meaning-type (Rosch, 1999).

The reconstruction of courses of action is generally performed with self-confrontation interviews (Von Cranach, Kalbermatten, Indermühle, & Gugler, 1982; Theureau, 1992). Based on Ericsson and Simon's conceptualization of thoughts and feelings (1993) as sequential states of heeded information, this form of retrospective report uses visual aids to enhance and situate the recall. During the interview, athletes thus confront the physical traces of their action (in most cases, videotapes) and show, tell, and comment on the episode they have experienced. With the aid of these self-confrontation interviews, researchers can identify the meaningful behaviors and cognitions experienced by the athletes. The interviews are recorded with a video camera to ensure transcription of the verbal reports in relation to the behaviors and characteristics. In trampolining, for example, this methodology is used to define and situate athletes' meaningful actions in relation to their exhibited behaviors, e.g., raising the two arms over the head, moving sideways, and the temporal and spatial characteristics, e.g., on the trampoline bed, at the apex of a movement, and at the third movement. This form of report is well-suited for studying actions in sport because (a) it provides access to the action without interfering with performance (Omodéi & McLennan, 1994), (b) it allows interviewers and athletes to view together contextual elements that may have influenced performance (Hauw, et al., 2003), (c) it takes the athletes' subjectivity into account in the modeling of their cognitions and places priority on the intrinsic aspects (D'Arripe-Longueville, et al., 2001), and (d) the postvideo interviews increase the awareness of what the athletes felt and did (Rhea, Mathes, & Hardin, 1997; Tenenbaum, Lloyd, Pretty, & Hanin, 2002).

This study proposed to analyze the actions of elite performers in relation to situations and to differentiate organizing actions as a function of performance level. Course of action theory was used to describe how the streams of actions by elite trampolinists can be differentiated by level of performance. Given the findings of previous studies on trampolining and the extreme accuracy that is required for this sport, we expected to observe in the best performances compared to those at a lower level (a) a greater number of actions of transforming the body position and assessing these transformations and (b) a modification of the location of these different actions in the movement. This organization of activity corresponding to the best performances would provide athletes more possibility to adapt with greater sensitivity to the elements of the unfolding situation.

Method

Participants

Eight trampolinists from the French national team volunteered to participate in the study. Their average age was 24 yr. (range 20–27). Two of them were among the top five trampolinists in the world. They had been participating for more than 10 years in the different stages of the World Cup and had won European and World titles. The four other men were among the top 20 in the world, and the two women were ranked twentieth and thirtieth.

Data Collection

Twenty-seven competition performances from 1999 to 2002 were analyzed. We considered for each athlete between two and four performances in relation to results in competitions. The decision to limit the study to these competitions was based on the theoretical saturation criterion (Strauss & Corbin, 1990); that is, we assumed that any additional data from other competitions would overlap with the information already obtained.

Three types of data were collected: (a) videotapes of the athletes' behaviors during the competitions, (b) field notes and observations, and (c) recorded and transcribed commentaries elicited during self-confrontation interviews. The athletes' performances were videotaped with a stationary camera with a wide-angle view from the gymnasium stands.

A trained researcher was responsible for the field notes and observations. The observations provided documentation for the interviews.

The self-confrontation interviews were held within a week of the competitions. During the interviews, the researcher who took the field notes and each trampolinist viewed the videotape together. The trampolinists were asked to describe and comment upon their own cognitions during the exercise they had performed. The interviewer's prompts were designed to collect three types of information generated as the action unfolded: (a) Objects, e.g., what are you trying to do? What are you thinking about? (b) Representamens, e.g., what is drawing your attention? What do you see? What are you feeling? and (c) Interpretants, e.g., what made you decide to do that at this moment? The prompts asked for descriptions of actions and events as they had been experienced by the trampolinists. Requests for interpretations and generalizations were avoided (Theureau, 1992).

Data Processing

After the interview data were transcribed, three steps were carried out: (a) labeling the elementary units of meaning and their underlying constituents, (b) reformulating the courses of action by labeling the elementary units of meaning-types, and (c) comparing the composition of different courses of action to construct patterns of performance.

Several measures were taken to ensure the reliability of the data. Before processing, we ensured the validity of the data transcripts. The transcripts and video recordings were shown to the participants to make sure their commentaries were accurate and to allow them to make any desired changes. Minor editorial comments were made concerning responses. Then, two experienced investigators, each having conducted previous qualitative research, independently coded the 27 data transcripts into components of triadic signs and elementary units of meaning. The reliability of the coding procedure was assessed using Bellack's agreement rate (Turcotte, 1973). An agreement rate between 78% and 90% was obtained between coders for the different structures (object, representamen, interpretant, and elementary units of meaning).

Labeling the elementary units of meaning and their underlying constituents.—The elementary units of meaning were labeled from verbalizations and videotapes of each trampolinist's behavior, using an action verb followed by a direct object, an adverb, or another complement, e.g., pushing down hard on the trampoline bed, locating oneself in terms of the trampoline center. The labeling reflected responses to a number of questions about the trampolinists' actions, interpretations, and feelings as they appeared in the recordings and self-confrontation data: What are you doing? What are you thinking? What are you feeling?

The underlying components of each elementary unit of meaning were then identified using a set of more specific questions: What is the athlete concerned about in this situation (*Object*)? What element of the situation is the athlete considering, recalling, perceiving, or interpreting (*Representamen*)? What knowledge is the athlete bringing to bear (*Interpretant*)?

Reformulating the course of action by labelling elementary units of meaning-types.—Based on previous research in trampolining (Hauw & Durand, 2001; Hauw, Durand, Cadopi, & Delignières, 2002; Hauw, et al., 2003), each elementary unit of meaning obtained for each of the 27 performances was replaced by one of the five elementary unit of meaning-types representing typical coupling between action and situation. These were labeled as "Getting Ready," "Transforming," "Assessing," "Orienting," and "Waiting." The correspondence between units collected and unit-types was accomplished with a focus on the relationship between the object and representamen. "Getting Ready" consisted of preparing to perform the movement. As the trampolinists prepared for their next movement, they were open to and focused on the elements of the situation directly linked to this concern, e.g., positioning the arms and trunk to orient the takeoff of the following exercise. "Transforming" consisted of modifying the movement. Different types were considered: (a) "Initiating the movement" represented actions in which the trampolinists—with the aim of performing the movement—were open to or focused on elements of the situation linked to initiation, i.e., takeoff; (b) "Attacking the movement" situated the action at the landing on the trampoline bed; (c) "Monitoring the movement" represented actions in which the trampolinists were open to or focused on the elements of the situation linked to controlling the unfolding rotation during flight; and (d) "Extending the movement" represented the focus on elements of the situation leading to the extended angle of the hip at the apex of flight. "Assessing" consisted of evaluating movement. These were actions in which the trampolinists were open to or focused on the elements of the situation linked to judgment of their performance. This was situated in an anticipation of the effect of a transforming action or in the evaluation of the real effect on the movement. "Orienting" consisted of analyzing the current situation as a function of the assessing actions. The trampolinists were open to or focused on the elements of the situation linked to analyzing events in relation to their actions or the ways in which they had to perform the following actions for the rest of the exercise. "Waiting" consisted of the actions in which the athletes did nothing but were open to or focused on the next moment when they would be able to act in order to change something or assess what was happening.

Comparing courses of action to construct patterns of performance.—Comparisons between the overall courses of action were made by the two researchers. First, exercises were assigned to one of three levels of performance, i.e., poor, average, very good, based on the competition results. Score was considered in relation to the rank it normally allowed the athlete to attain in international competition. Eight exercises were considered as poor, i.e., ranked after 20. Ten were rated as average, i.e., ranked between 9 to 19. Nine were assigned as very good, i.e., ranked between 1 to 8. Next, common structures of the courses of action for each level were identified and characterized in relation to (a) the number of elementary unit of meaning-types per movement and (b) their location in the movement.

RESULTS

Three patterns of organizing elementary unit of meaning-types related to performance level were identified (Fig. 1). The first pattern was termed "Racing after-events" and characterized the courses of action in which the athletes had the feeling of trying to catch up to events without ever really managing to control them. It corresponded to exercises labeled as poor. The second pattern, corresponding to exercises labeled as average, was termed "Regulating the situation" and characterized the courses of action in which athletes had the feeling of on-line control of their action despite feeling highly constrained by events. The third pattern was termed "Attentive monitoring" and characterized the courses of action in which athletes closely monitored events and had the feeling of being a bit in advance of their unfolding. It was corresponding to exercises labeled as very good.

Racing After-events

The typical courses of action corresponding to each movement were organized from four elementary units of meaning-types. We distinguished a unit of transforming movement, "Initiating the movement while looking for the most immediate effects of the performance," e.g., turn to land as quickly as possible on one's feet. This was situated at the moment of contact with the trampoline bed. A waiting unit, "Waiting for the action to unfold without knowing exactly how it will end," e.g., let the movement turn to see what will happen, appeared next and was situated from the ascending phase of a movement to the return of visual contact, i.e., in this case, when the body was in the upper third of the descending phase of the movement. An assessment unit, "Trying to know how the action is unfolding," e.g., was the rotation good enough and were there displacements in relation to the center of the trampoline bed, appeared as soon as the trampolinist was able to resume visual contact with the trampoline bed. Last, an orienting unit, "Assessing the situation in terms of what has already happened and what will follow," e.g., I'm too low, I'm very low, I'm going to have a hard time finishing, appeared immediately after the assessing unit. This, arising from an instantaneous observation, defined an interpretation of the unfolding action and thus a new situation.

Regulating the Situation

The second pattern of performance, "Regulating the situation," was characterized by a greater number of elementary unit of meaning-types per movement than the preceding pattern. Three new units were identified. The first was termed "Getting ready to perform the movement." The trampolinists focused on various technical aspects of the movement, in relation to previous movements or typical errors. This defined a modification in the trampolinists' involvement corresponding to the action that preceded it, i.e., orienting unit. It finalized the orientation for the upcoming movement by concentration on the technical order, e.g., raise the arms as high as possible,

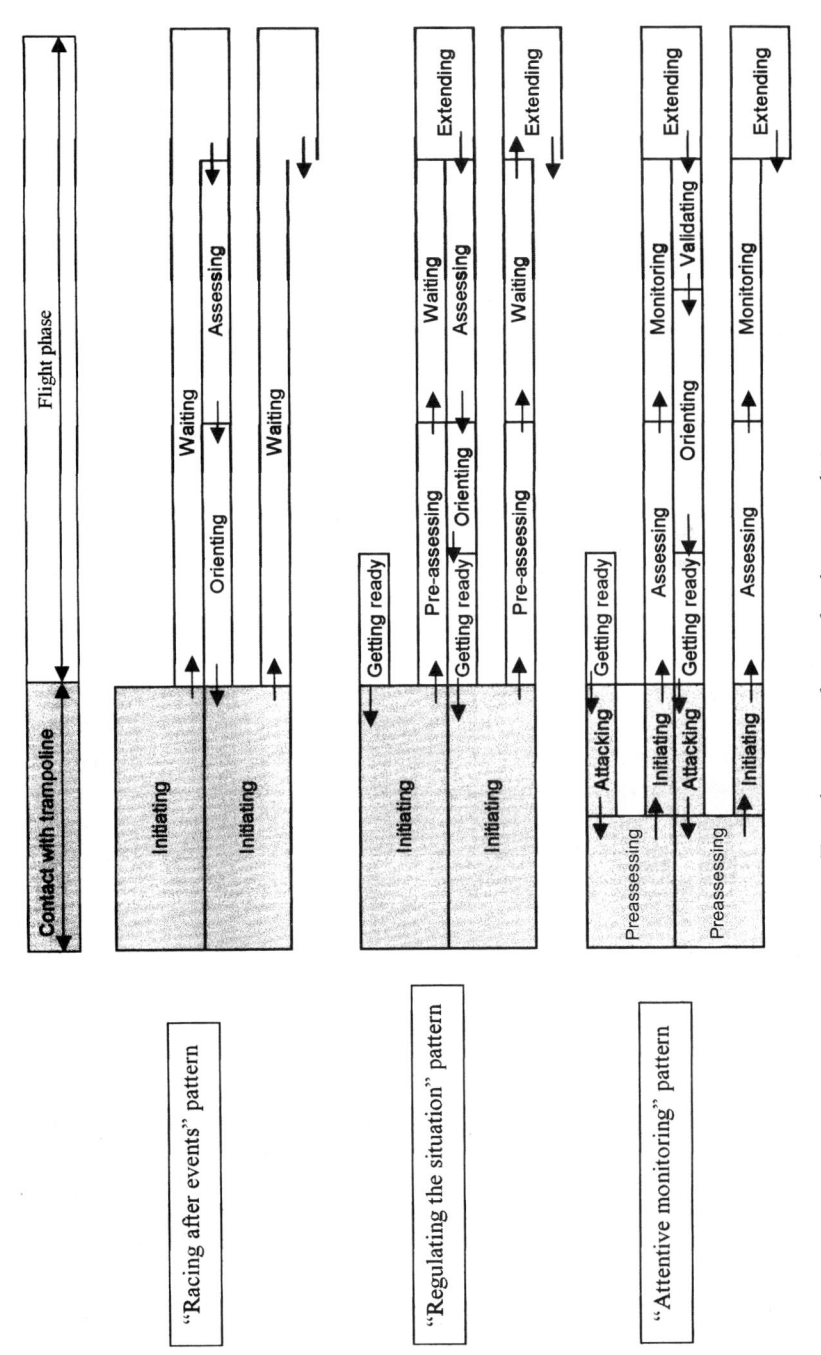

FIG. 1. Typical patterns of action for elite trampolinists

be poised to begin. This unit occurred just before the transformation unit that initiated the next movement. The second unit was termed "Assessing the movement onset." The trampolinists focused on the sensations of coming up off the bed, and thus this unit was situated just after the takeoff. The trampolinists assessed a part of the effects produced by the preceding transforming unit. This pre-assessment concerned the quality of the movement in terms of rotation and height. This modified the assessing unit situated in the descending phase of the movements: at this moment, part of the overall evaluation of the movement had already been made. This second assessment thus concerned the validation of the pre-assessment and the search for information about the displacements. The third new unit-type was a transforming unit termed "Monitoring the movement." The trampolinists focused on certain parts of the body while controlling how the movement was being carried out, e.g., I joined my knees tightly, I'm extended very early. This transforming action, situated at the apex of the movement, principally consisted of regulating the moments of widening the legs–trunk angle to control the rotation speed.

Attentive Monitoring

The organization of these courses of action was characterized by a greater number of elementary units of meaning-types in comparison with the preceding patterns of performance.

The transforming units at the moment of contact with the bed seen in the first two patterns could be decomposed into three new elementary units of meaning-types in this third pattern. The first was a transforming unit concerning the means of coming in contact with the bed termed "Attacking the bed carefully," e.g., I keep my legs behind so I can land on my feet. The second was an assessing unit called "Resisting pushing down too much into the trampoline bed," e.g., I feel very high tension in my back. This characterized a typical concentration oriented toward the body tension during the phase of hitting the bed, and it allowed an evaluation of the quality of the interaction with the trampoline. The trampolinists were thus able to evaluate the way they had deformed the bed. This evaluation was in fact a preassessment for executing the exercise. The third, during the ascending phase, was a transforming unit labeled "Initiating the move for an accurate propulsion." It corresponded to an action adopted by the athletes to initiate the movement, e.g., let oneself be propelled, accentuate the propulsion by pushing, take a forward or backward direction. The rest of the course of action was modified by this new organization. From the moment of takeoff, the trampolinists evaluated the movement. In contrast to the preceding patterns of performance, the trampolinists knew at this moment how the movement had been initiated, i.e., height, rotation, and forward-backward or lateral displacements. A transforming movement unit directly followed this evaluation and was termed "Monitoring the movement." The trampolinists focused on certain parts of the body, using the assessment of how the movement was being carried out. This regulated the movement being executed, e.g., stretch the body to accelerate the rotation, open the arms to slow down the longitudinal rotation, and preceded the transforming unit, i.e., extending action, at the apex of the movement, which was called " Opening the hips to stretch the body." This latter unit placed the athletes in position for the emergence of the next unit-type called "Visually validating the overall assessment," e.g., I'm landing right on the cross, how I thought it would be. At the apex of the movement, the trampolinists could watch the bed again and could use this visual reference point to confirm the assessment they had originally made. For this pattern of performance, the assessing units occurred early in the execution of movements and permitted a validating action.

Discussion

The present research used the course of action theory to describe how elite performance can be characterized by modifications in the stream of action. The three patterns of elementary units of meaning-types describe typical modalities of action corresponding to performance levels. These patterns could be distinguished by (a) an increasing number of elementary units of meaning-types for the same time period and (b) increasingly greater freedom to act by modifying the organization of unit-types for the movement execution.

The first pattern of organization was characterized by a concentration of actions during the descending phase of a movement and at contact with the trampoline bed. The two other patterns differed by allowing the athletes the possibility of extending these actions in time. For the third pattern, new forms of actions were found in both the ascending and descending phases of the movement and at three distinct moments at contact with the bed. The results showed that time was used differently for action. The action of waiting, during which athletes were unable to modify the unfolding of events but rather submitted to them, was replaced by actions of transformation, evaluation or orientation at higher levels of performance, suggesting that these athletes were more able to intervene in the course of events. Although the essential trampoline actions, i.e., those actions that ensured performances within the bounds of the regulations, were concentrated in the vicinity of contact with the trampoline bed, the highest level of performance was associated with an extension and multiplication of actions in time and space. The possibilities of interacting with the context were quantitatively much richer, signifying more modifications in the modes of engagement, i.e., objects, with increasing performance. These results also suggest that the greater number of possibilities with higher performance transformed the time context of action. In the same objective context, action created new situations. The actions of the most elite performer emerged from new modalities of actions in relation to the situation.

The concentration of action at the descending phases and contacts with the trampoline bed, which identified the first pattern of performance, illustrated a strategy of organizing action for the successful completion of a movement (without falling) rather than for excellence. To arrive at the end of the exercise, the trampolinists focused essentially on how to initiate each movement and abandoned the goal of enhancing its quality. The risk inherent in the situation and the requirement of chaining the individual movements weighed heavily on the organization of action. The context was transformed to a situation of examining the possibilities for implementing this requirement. This pattern reflected a necessary reduction in the complexity of action so that a movement could be performed within a wide margin of safety. The patterns corresponding to higher performances reflected an organization of action defined by a new margin of safety, which allowed the development of new actions. To enhance quality, athletes had to be capable of shifting between multiple perspectives that changed the actions and situation. These results suggest that elite performance is characterized by a transformation of the system of actions situated in a given context (Barab & Plucker, 2002; Hauw & Durand, unpublished). Elite performance is defined by a new temporality in which the succession of a great number of actions expresses an enriched sensitivity to the situation and the skill to use it efficiently. This enrichment allows greater adjustment to events.

The comparison of patterns of performance showed evidence of three qualitative and progressive transformations: (a) the disappearance of waiting actions, (b) anticipation of evaluating and orienting actions, and (c) the appearance of validating actions. These three progressive modifications suggested that the transformation in elite performance was characterized by intrinsically differentiated organizing actions. The actions were more diverse in the third pattern and characterized by a reorganization in the chaining of elementary units of meaning and their objects, that is, the modalities of involvement in the situations. For example, contact with the trampoline bed was defined in the first pattern of performance by a transforming action with the goal of initiating the movement, whereas this same time of bed contact was exploited in the third pattern, i.e., corresponding to better performance, for a succession of three actions, i.e., an evaluation at the bottom of the bed surrounded by two distinct transforming actions. Better performance was marked by modifications in action and situation even though the objective context remained the same. Furthermore, although evaluating actions were situated in the descending phases of the movements in the first pattern, anticipation of these evaluations in the other patterns led to the simultaneous emergence of a new validating action. Thus, the action of validation could not exist at the first and the second level of performance and characterized the qualitative transformations of activity.

The results confirmed the hypotheses of the study. As expected, we distinguished more differentiated units of action in these performances, which reflected greater sensitivity to the context on the part of the athletes and thus greater accuracy in making the required adaptations. These results characterized a differentiated form of action related to the athlete's sensitivity to the situation. They concern those activities geared to performing a series of acrobatic actions under intense time pressure and doing so as impressively as possible. The acrobatic component, i.e., numerous rotations, and the context in which these athletes performed, e.g., the size of the trampoline bed and jump height, defined the risky nature of this activity.

The major characteristics of elite performance were found in the modifications of actions and situations defined by the athletes. The development of elite performance can be described as the construction of new spaces for action (Reed, 1993) or as the capacity to exploit events in a highly differentiated manner. Action develops with the deployment of new modalities of interaction with the situation that favor regulation by a much greater mastery of time constraints. From this perspective, elite performance resides neither in the athlete nor in the context. It resides in the modalities of interaction between them.

Research on elite performance could be focused on the highly specific nature of the situated actor-context interaction in different elite sports. This approach could provide a better understanding of the psychological processes underlying such competitive sports and to the development of sport expertise in general. These studies also could help coaches and sport psychologists identify specific and individualized goals to enhance athletes' performance.

REFERENCES

BARAB, S. A., & PLUCKER, J. A. (2002) Smart people or smart contexts? Cognition, ability, and talent development in an age of situated approaches to knowing and learning. *Educational Psychologist*, 37, 165-182.

D'ARRIPE-LONGUEVILLE, F., SAURY, J., FOURNIER, J., & DURAND, M. (2001) Coach-athlete interaction during elite archery competitions: an application of methodological frameworks used in ergonomics research to sport psychology. *Journal of Applied Sport Psychology*, 13, 275-299.

ERICSSON, K. A., & SIMON, H. A. (1993) *Protocol analysis: verbal reports as data.* (Rev. ed.) Cambridge, MA: MIT Press.

HAUW, D., BERTHELOT, C., & DURAND, M. (2003) Enhancing performance in elite athletes through situated-cognition analysis: trampolinists' course of action during competition. *International Journal of Sport Psychology*, 34, 299-321.

HAUW, D., & DURAND, M. (2001) Analysis of the situated cognition of elite trampolinists during competitions for performance enhancement. Paper presented at the 10th World Congress of Sport Psychology, Skiathos, Greece, June.

Hauw, D., & Durand, M. (unpublished) The dynamics of elite trampolinists' actions in a competitive context: a situated analysis.

Hauw, D., Durand, M., Cadopi, M., & Delignières, D. (2002) Situated cognition and expert performance: the variability of trampolinists' courses of action during competition. Poster presented at the meeting of the Association for the Advancement of Applied Sport Psychology, Tucson, AZ, October.

Higgins, J. R., & Spaeth, R. K. (1972) Relationship between consistency of movement and environmental condition. *Quest*, XVII, 61-69.

Kirshner, D., & Whitson, J. A. (1997) *Situated cognition: social, semiotic and psychological perspectives*. Mahwah, NJ: Erlbaum.

Omodéi, M. M., & McLennan, J. (1994) Studying complex decision making in natural setting: using a head oriented video camera to study competitive orienteering. *Perceptual and Motor Skills*, 79, 1411-1425.

Peirce, C. S. (1931–1935) *Collected papers of Charles Sanders Peirce*. Cambridge, MA: Harvard Univer. Press.

Reed, E. S. (1993) The intention to use a specific affordance: a conceptual framework for psychology. In R. Wozniak & K. Fischer (Eds.), *Development in context: acting and thinking in specific environment*. Hillsdale, NJ: Erlbaum. Pp. 45-75.

Rhea, D. J., Mathes, S. A., & Hardin, K. (1997) Video report for analysis of performance by collegiate female tennis players. *Perceptual and Motor Skills*, 85, 1354.

Rosch, E. (1999) Reclaiming concepts. *Journal of Consciousness Studies*, 6(11-12), 61-77.

Saury, J., & Durand, M. (1998) Practical knowledge of expert coaches: on-site study of training in sailing. *Research Quarterly for Exercise and Sport*, 69, 254-266.

Sève, C., Saury, J., Ria, L., & Durand, M. (2003) Structure of expert players' activity during competitive interaction in table tennis. *Research Quarterly for Exercise and Sport*, 74, 71-83.

Sève, C., Saury, J., Theureau, J., & Durand, M. (2002) La construction de connaissances chez les sportifs au cours d'une interaction compétitive [Knowledge construction by athletes during competitive interaction]. *Le Travail Humain*, 65, 159-190.

Strauss, A., & Corbin, J. (1990) *Basics of qualitative research*. London: Sage.

Tenenbaum, G., Lloyd, M., Pretty, G., & Hanin, Y. L. (2002) Congruence of actual and retrospective reports of precompetition emotions in equestrians. *Journal of Sports and Exercise Psychology*, 24, 271-288.

Theureau, J. (1992) *Le cours d'action: analyse sémiologique. Essai d'une anthropologie cognitive située* [*The course of action: semiological analysis: essay on situated cognitive anthropology*]. Berne: Peter Lang.

Theureau, J., & Jeffroy, F. (1994) *Ergonomie des situations informatisées* [*Ergonomics of computerized situations*]. Toulouse: Octares.

Turcotte, C. (1973) La fiabilité des systèmes d'analyse d'enseignement [The reliability of teaching systems]. In G. Dussault, M. Leclerc, J. Brunelle, & C. Turcotte (Eds.), *L'analyse de l'enseignement* [*Teaching analysis*]. Montreal: Presse Universitaire du Quebec. Pp. 189-230.

Von Cranach, M., Kalbermatten, U., Indermühle, K., & Gugler, B. (1982) *Goal-directed action*. London: Academic Press.

Weinberg, R. S., & Gould, D. (1999) *Foundations of sport and exercise psychology*. (2nd ed.) Champaign, IL: Human Kinetics.

Accepted March 30, 2004.

RANDOM NUMBER GENERATION IN NATIVE AND FOREIGN LANGUAGES[1]

HANS STRENGE AND JESSICA BÖHM

University of Kiel, Germany

Summary.—The effects of different levels of language proficiency on random number generation were examined in this study. 16 healthy right-handed students (7 women, 9 men; aged 22 to 25 years, $M = 23.8$, $SD = .83$) attempted to generate a random sequence of the digits 1 to 9 at pacing frequencies of 1, 1.5, and 2 Hz. Randomization was done in German (native language L1), English (first foreign language L2), and French (second foreign language L3). There was a pattern of redundancy and seriation tendencies, increasing with speed of generation for all languages (L1–L3). While using L2 and L3, responses slowed and the number of errors committed increased. Further, there was a peculiar pattern of dissociation in nonrandom performance with an increase of habitual counting in ones and a strong reduction of counting in twos. All effects were most pronounced when subjects used L3 and 2-Hz pacing rates. Slowing and nonrandomness was not correlated with self-assessment parameters regarding language proficiency. We suggest that in a task involving number activation in a nonnative language, lack of proficiency will interfere with random number generation, leading to interruptions and rule breaking, at least when reaching the limits of attentional capacity at higher pacing rates.

In the field of neuropsychology, random number generation has been utilized as a complex executive task which requires sustained attention and involves several simultaneous tasks that make its performance demanding (Jahanshahi & Dirnberger, 1999). When subjects depart from randomness, the nature of the bias is likely to give a clue about the underlying schemata which are determining performance. Many studies of digit generation have shown that there is an avoidance of repetition together with a tendency to produce the digits in counting order (Brugger, Monsch, Salmon, & Butters, 1996; Brugger, 1997; Baddeley, Emslie, Kolodny, & Duncan, 1998; Daniels, Witt, Wolff, Jansen, & Deuschl, 2003).

Both the influence of pacing frequency and number of alternatives have been the subject of a substantial body of research, showing that subjects compensate for difficulties either by decreasing the rate of randomization or increasing the redundancy of the series (Warren & Morin, 1965; Rath, 1966; Slak & Hirsch, 1974; Evans, 1978; Wiegersma, 1984; Daniels, *et al.*, 2003). Although it is estimated that the majority of the people in the world are bilingual (Zeelenberg & Pecher, 2003), there are no experiments so far that

---

[1]Address correspondence to Hans Strenge, Institute of Medical Psychology, University of Kiel, Niemannsweg 147, D-24105 Kiel or e-mail (strenge@med-psych-uni.kiel.de).

have looked at the influence of differential familiarity with the cardinal numbers, if randomization is required in a foreign language. It is well known that numerical abilities of bilingual people can vary extensively, depending on their proficiency (Proios, Weniger, & Willmes, 2002). Thus, it is conceivable that the issue of overload under the conditions mentioned above can easily be extended to the domain of forcign language. The present analysis therefore was designed to examine the patterns of digit responses in native and foreign languages.

METHOD

Participants

Sixteen German university students, 7 women and 9 men, ages 22 to 25 years ($M=23.8$, $SD=.8$), who were studying medicine at the University of Kiel participated in the experiment either voluntarily or for course credit. All participants were native speakers of German. They reported English as their strongest foreign language and had been taught English in secondary school for at least six years ($M=8.4$, $SD=1.0$). All individuals reported French as their second foreign language, with an average training period of 3.9 yr. ($SD=2.6$). The participants were asked to rate their proficiency in English and French on a 5-point Likert-type scale with anchors of 1 = very high and 5 = very low. Their self-assessment scores in English and French were 2.3 ($SD=0.6$) and 3.5 ($SD=0.9$), respectively. All participants were right-handed; the average score on the Handedness Inventory (Oldfield, 1971) was 77.4 ($SD=25.8$). They reported no known neurologic disorders or previous history of neurological or psychiatric illness and were not taking any medication. The participants were naïve about the hypothesis to be tested.

Measures

Three independent behavior patterns have emerged from the human data of random number generation: repetition avoidance, seriation, and cycling (Ginsburg & Karpiuk, 1994; Jahanshahi, Profice, Brown, Ridding, Dirnberger, & Rothwell, 1998; Towse & Neil, 1998). Indices were chosen to reflect these three factors. Repetition score was defined as the number of times the same number was repeated in successive responses (Ginsburg & Karpiuk, 1994, 1995; Brown, Soliveri, & Jahanshahi, 1998; Jahanshahi, *et al.*, 1998). Seriation was assessed using the methods of Spatt and Goldenberg (1993) and considered separate scores calculated for counting forwards and backwards in ones (count score 1) or twos (count score 2) (Brown, *et al.*, 1998; Jahanshahi, *et al.*, 1998; Watkins & Brown, 2002). The run score is the variance of the number of responses in successive ascending runs. The series score is the number of consecutive digrams (e.g., 3, 4, or 8, 7, including the sequences 9, 0 and 0, 9) (Ginsburg & Karpiuk, 1994, 1995). The measure of cycling was provided by the median repetition-gap measure and the coupon score (Ginsburg & Karpiuk, 1994; Brown, *et al.*, 1998; Jahanshahi, *et al.*, 1998). The randomization index is a χ^2-distributed measure that reflects any disproportion of digrams, i.e., adjacent items in a series, in the matrix adjusted for disproportions in the marginal cell frequencies. It varies between 0 = ideal randomness and 1 = perfect predictability (Evans, 1978; Horne, Evans, & Orne, 1982). In addition, two qualitative measures not related to sequential randomness were included, total number of responses per run, reflecting the frequency of skipped beats of the metronome, and total number of errors (Brugger, *et al.*, 1996).

Procedure

Informed consent was obtained from all participants. The experiment was composed of three sessions. Each participant was tested first in German, second in English, and finally in French, with a 2-min break between language changes. Each language session began with an acclimation period when the participants were asked to count forward from 1 to 9 in the given language, three consecutive times, at a rate of 1 Hz indicated by a metronome. Afterwards, participants were required to produce the digits 1 to 9 in random order for 90 trials and to synchronize random number generation with a metronome. The concept of randomness was explained using standard procedures, i.e., instructions based on an analogy of selecting and replacing numbered balls from a hat (Horne, *et al.*, 1982). During one session, each subject performed five runs of random number generation at the following sequence: 1 Hz, 1.5 Hz, 1 Hz, 2 Hz, and 1 Hz. The order of runs did not vary across subjects. The total testing time was approximately 45 min. The numbers were recorded by the experimenter on score sheets and with a video-recorder used for back-up. No feedback was given for correct or incorrect responses.

Data Analysis

The number of responses, error rates, and the randomization measures were calculated from each subject's tape recordings. All data apart from the error rate were distributed normally. Responses with mistakes in the required language were omitted from further data analysis. Analyses of variance with repeated measures were carried out to compare the performances of the subject in each language separately at different frequencies (intrasession) and to compare the German, English, and French responses at certain frequencies (intersession). Error number was analyzed using the Friedman test. In all of the analysis of variance and Friedman tests, if a significant overall effect was found, then student *t* tests and Wilcoxon tests, respectively, were used. In all *post hoc* analyses, Bonferroni corrections for multiple tests were made, leading to a more stringent significance criterion for each of the intrasession ($p = .01$) and intersession comparisons ($p = .02$), respectively. Only such significant results are reported. To investigate the relationship between demographic characteristics, educational self-assessment data, response number, and randomization measures, Spearman correlations were calculated and interpreted with Bonferroni corrections. Two-tailed significance levels were used at $p < .05$.

Results

Although there is no generally accepted way of assessing foreign language proficiency (Zeelenberg & Pecher, 2003), it is fair to say that the participants in the present study were relatively fluent German-English bilinguals with a clearly lower level of proficiency in French.

The duration of each run was timed and the results showed that all individuals were able to synchronize their responses with the pacing metronome during the baseline test and 1-Hz runs in each of the three sessions. Not all subjects, however, followed the pacing signal with high frequencies in the foreign languages. Some subjects tended to pause, especially immediately after incorrect responses, and they seemed to prefer to produce at a lower rate than required. For the 1.5- and 2-Hz pacing conditions, respectively, the actual mean rates of number production were 1.38 Hz ($SD = .13$) and 1.80 Hz ($SD = .17$) in German, 1.38 Hz ($SD = .10$) and 1.73 Hz ($SD = .24$) in English, 1.30 Hz ($SD = .19$) and 1.59 Hz ($SD = .29$) in French.

Concerning the German session, one-way analysis of variance with repeated measures (five runs) on each randomization measure indicated a significant run effect on the randomization index ($F_{4,60} = 9.63$, $p < .001$), series score ($F_{4,60} = 6.75$, $p < .001$), count score ($F_{4,60} = 5.92$, $p < .001$), and run score ($F_{4,60} = 5.71$, $p < .002$). On all seriation measures and the randomization index, *post hoc* analyses showed significant differences between Runs 3 and 4 with higher scores during the fourth run (2 Hz).

For the English session, analysis of variance indicated a significant run effect on the number of responses, count scores 1 and 2, series and run scores, and the randomization index (Table 1). Besides the significant reduction in responses, there were significantly higher count score 1, series, and run scores on the fourth run, and the randomization index was additionally increased during the second run. Moreover, there was a decrease of the count score 2 in the fourth run.

Regarding the French session, analysis of variance showed there was a significant effect on the number of responses and the count scores 1 and 2 and the run score (Table 2). There was no effect on the randomization index. *Post hoc* analyses indicated significant differences between the third and fourth runs, with fewer responses and higher count score 1 and run score and a significant decrease in the count score 2 during the fourth run.

TABLE 1
MEANS, STANDARD DEVIATIONS, AND SIGNIFICANT EFFECTS OF ANALYSIS OF VARIANCE IN
RANDOM NUMBER GENERATION IN STRONGEST FOREIGN LANGUAGE (ENGLISH)

Parameter	1st Run (1 Hz)	2nd Run (1.5 Hz)	3rd Run (1 Hz)	4th Run (2 Hz)	5th Run (1 Hz)	$F_{4,60}$	p
Number of Responses							
M	90.00	84.90	90.60	81.30	89.10	13.43	<.001
SD	3.99	5.45	3.90	9.31	3.21		
Count Score 1							
M	50.30	51.90	39.90	73.31	38.50	8.02	<.001
SD	32.61	27.66	18.90	45.30	23.13		
Count Score 2							
M	26.56	24.25	23.06	20.06	27.50	2.83	.03
SD	10.10	9.20	8.53	9.65	9.55		
Run Score							
M	1.32	1.61	1.27	1.82	1.02	7.05	<.001
SD	0.84	0.86	0.67	0.89	0.50		
Series Score							
M	31.80	33.10	29.90	35.50	28.60	3.75	.009
SD	11.81	9.80	8.37	10.88	9.34		
Randomization Index							
M	0.34	0.37	0.31	0.37	0.32	6.84	<.001
SD	0.06	0.05	0.04	0.06	0.04		

In intersession analyses, i.e., language comparisons of runs at the same pacing rate, analysis of variance showed no effects on the response number at frequencies of 1 Hz ($F_{2,30}=0.39$, $p>.05$) and 1.5 Hz ($F_{2,30}=1.69$, $p>.05$). However, there was an effect ($F_{2,30}=5.25$, $p<.05$) on 2-Hz performances with significantly fewer generated numbers in the 14th (French) than in the second (German) or ninth run (English). Concerning individual randomization measures at 1 Hz, significant effects were found on the series ($F_{2,30}=11.52$, $p<.001$) and run scores ($F_{2,30}=4.83$, $p<.05$) and the randomization index ($F_{2,30}=8.57$, $p<.01$). Post hoc analyses showed significant differences between the third (German) and 13th (French) runs, with higher scores in the latter. Concerning Runs 2, 7, and 12 (1.5-Hz condition), a significant effect was found on the repetition score ($F_{2,30}=5.15$, $p<.05$) and count score 2 ($F_{2,30}=4.57$, $p<.05$). There was a significantly higher repetition score on the seventh than on the second run. The count score 2 was significantly lower in the 12th than in the other two runs. Under 2-Hz conditions, the only significant effect was on the count score 2 ($F_{2,30}=8.31$, $p<.002$), with significant differences between each of the three runs, showing a gradual decrease from the first (German) to the third (French) session.

Correlations showed no significant associations between the randomization measures and any of the parameters concerning demographic data or self-assessment of language acquisition.

tion of number magnitude, consistent with models that assume a semantic representation and activation of numbers on an ordered continuum which is common to all notations (Dehaene, 1992; Brysbaert, 1995; Gobel, Walsh, & Rushworth, 2001). Thus, the present data may extend to the issue of number representation in the brain. Experiments with bilingual random number generation in a systematic, counterbalanced design could provide further insight into this field.

REFERENCES

BADDELEY, A. D., EMSLIE, H., KOLODNY, J., & DUNCAN, J. (1998) Random generation and the executive control of working memory. *The Quarterly Journal of Experimental Psychology*, 51A, 819-852.

BROWN, R. G., SOLIVERI, P., & JAHANSHAHI, M. (1998) Executive processes in Parkinson's disease: random number generation and response suppression. *Neuropsychologia*, 36, 1355-1362.

BRUGGER, P. (1997) Variables that influence the generation of random sequences: an update. *Perceptual and Motor Skills*, 84, 627-661.

BRUGGER, P., MONSCH, A. U., SALMON, D. P., & BUTTERS, N. (1996) Random number generation in dementia of the Alzheimer type: a test of frontal executive functions. *Neuropsychologia*, 34, 97-103.

BRYSBAERT, M. (1995) Arabic number reading: on the nature of the numerical scale and the origin of phonological recoding. *Journal of Experimental Psychology: General*, 124, 434-452.

DANIELS, C., WITT, K., WOLFF, S., JANSEN, O., & DEUSCHL, G. (2003) Rate dependency of the human cortical network subserving executive functions during generation of random number series: a functional magnetic resonance imaging study. *Neuroscience Letters*, 345, 25-28.

DEHAENE, S. (1992) Varieties of numerical abilities. *Cognition*, 44, 1-42.

EVANS, F. J. (1978) Monitoring attention deployment by random number generation: an index to measure subjective randomness. *Bulletin of the Psychonomic Society*, 12, 35-38.

GINSBURG, N., & KARPIUK, P. (1994) Random generation: analysis of the responses. *Perceptual and Motor Skills*, 79, 1059-1067.

GINSBURG, N., & KARPIUK, P. (1995) Simulation of human performance on a random generation task. *Perceptual and Motor Skills*, 81, 1183-1186.

GOBEL, S., WALSH, V., & RUSHWORTH, M. F. (2001) The mental number line and the human angular gyrus. *NeuroImage*, 14, 1278-1289.

HORNE, R. L., EVANS, F. J., & ORNE, M. T. (1982) Random number generation, psychopathology, and therapeutic change. *Archives of General Psychiatry*, 39, 680-683.

JAHANSHAHI, M., & DIRNBERGER, G. (1999) The left dorsolateral prefrontal cortex and random generation of responses: studies with transcranial magnetic stimulation. *Neuropsychologia*, 37, 181-190.

JAHANSHAHI, M., PROFICE, P., BROWN, R. G., RIDDING, M. C., DIRNBERGER, G., & ROTHWELL, J. C. (1998) The effects of transcranial magnetic stimulation over the dorsolateral prefrontal cortex on suppression of habitual counting during random number generation. *Brain*, 121, 1533-1544.

MIYAKE, A., FRIEDMAN, N. P., EMERSON, M. J., WITZKI, A. H., HOWERTER, A., & WAGNER, T. D. (2000) The unity and diversity of executive functions and their contributions to complex "frontal lobe" tasks: a latent variable analysis. *Cognitive Psychology*, 41, 49-100.

OLDFIELD, R. C. (1971) The assessment and analysis of handedness: the Edinburgh inventory. *Neuropsychologia*, 9, 97-113.

PROIOS, H., WENIGER, D., & WILLMES, K. (2002) Number representation deficit: a bilingual case of failure to access written verbal numeral representations. *Neuropsychologia*, 40, 2341-2349.

RATH, G. J. (1966) Randomization by humans. *American Journal of Psychology*, 79, 97-103.

SLAK, S., & HIRSCH, K. A. (1974) Human ability to randomize sequences as a function of information per item. *Bulletin of the Psychonomic Society*, 4, 29-30.

SPATT, J., & GOLDENBERG, G. (1993) Components of random generation by normal subjects and patients with dysexecutive syndrome. *Brain and Cognition*, 23, 231-242.

TOWSE, J. N., & NEIL, D. (1998) Analyzing human random generation behavior: a review of methods used and a computer program for describing performance. *Behavior Research Methods, Instruments and Computers*, 30, 583-591.

WARREN, P. A., & MORIN, R. E. (1965) Random generation: number of symbols to be randomized and time per response. *Perception & Psychophysics*, 14, 337-342.

WATKINS, E., & BROWN, R. G. (2002) Rumination and executive function in depression: an experimental study. *Journal of Neurology, Neurosurgery, and Psychiatry*, 72, 400-402.

WIEGERSMA, S. (1984) High-speed sequential vocal response production. *Perceptual and Motor Skills*, 59, 43-50.

ZEELENBERG, R., & PECHER, D. (2003) Evidence for long-term cross-language repetition priming in conceptual implicit memory task. *Journal of Memory and Language*, 49, 80-94.

Accepted April 1, 2004.

UNDERSTANDING AIR FORCE MEMBERS' INTENTIONS TO PARTICIPATE IN PRO-ENVIRONMENTAL BEHAVIORS: AN APPLICATION OF THE THEORY OF PLANNED BEHAVIOR[1]

MARK S. LAUDENSLAGER

Foreign Military Construction Support
Air Force Materiel Command

DANIEL T. HOLT

Department of Systems and Engineering Management
Air Force Institute of Technology

STEVEN T. LOFGREN

Air Force ROTC Detachment 590
University of North Carolina, Chapel Hill

Summary.—At a single installation, a cross section of 307 active duty Air Force members completed questionnaires to assess whether the theory of planned behavior was useful in explaining the service members' intentions to participate in three environmentally protective behaviors—recycling, carpooling, and energy conservation. While the individual tenets of the theory of planned behavior, i.e., attitude toward the behavior, subjective norms, and perceived control, accounted for differing amounts of variance in intentions, the results indicated that the intentions of these Air Force members to recycle, conserve energy, and carpool were moderately explained by the tenets of the theory of planned behavior collectively when the results of a multiple regression were analyzed.

Recently, the military's leadership has recognized that simply investing fiscal resources and technology does not guarantee the attainment of an array of environmental goals, e.g., to reduce solid waste. Instead, the attainment of many environmental goals may depend on individuals integrating environmentally protective behaviors into their everyday lives. Thus, environmental programs have been instituted in the Department of Defense to attempt to influence the individual's behavior outside of the workplace by encouraging participation in recycling programs, composting programs and carpooling programs. Unfortunately, these programs have had mixed success. For instance, one installation that won a Secretary of Defense environmental award reported that only 60% of the possible household recyclables were actually set out for a curbside recycling program targeted at those living in military family housing (N. A. Carper, personal communication, September 10, 1997). To meet this and other installation goals to reduce solid waste, greater participation is needed. However, research has not offered clear evidence as to what factors influence people's decisions to participate in programs that protect the environment.

---

[1]Address correspondence to Daniel T. Holt, AFIT/ENV, 2950 Hobson Way, Wright-Patterson AFB, OH 45433-7765 or e-mail (daniel.holt@afit.edu).

Many have suggested that one way of understanding participation in pro-environmental programs is to examine attitudes toward the environment. Indeed, empirical data have indicated that those who are sensitive toward environmental issues have a positive attitude toward programs designed to protect the environment (e.g., Dunlap & Scarce, 1991). Yet studies through the decades have found that the relationship between concern for the environment and pro-environmental behaviors is, at best, tenuous (e.g., Scott & Willits, 1994; Unger, 1994; Widegren, 1998). These studies can be summarized simply to say that "most people say they are willing to do a great deal to help curb pollution problems and are fairly emotional about it, but in fact, they actually do very little" (Unger, 1994, p. 288).

We believe one fundamental problem with these studies is that they have no clear theoretical foundation. By applying existing theory to this issue, researchers can better identify the underlying factors that may predict participation in environmentally protective behaviors and guide practitioners as they develop awareness programs that more effectively influence behavior. Accordingly, we applied the concepts prescribed in the theory of planned behavior (Ajzen, 1991), examining intentions to engage in three environmentally protective behaviors—recycling, carpooling, and energy conservation. We focused on these particular behaviors because the agency, a branch of the Department of Defense from which the study's sample was drawn, emphasized the need for its members to do their part in protecting the environment and achieving organizational goals by engaging in these practices.

Theory of Planned Behavior

The theory of planned behavior was designed to help explain people's behavioral choices in specific contexts (Ajzen, 1991). Based on this theory, people's behavioral intentions, rather than their attitudes, are the cognitive precursor to actual behaviors. As a general rule, the stronger the intention to engage in the behavior, the more likely the behavior will actually be performed. Moreover, people's behavioral intentions are shaped by a number of specific attitudes that include their attitude toward the behavior, subjective norms and perceived control. An individual's attitude toward the particular behavior, simply referred to as *attitude* throughout the rest of this manuscript, refers to the way in which a person evaluates the behavior and the extent to which the individual perceives that the behavior will lead to particular outcomes. Subjective norms refer to the extent to which an individual believes that others will approve the behavior that he perceives to be important and significant. Finally, perceived behavioral control refers to the extent to which the individual perceives that he controls the behavior.

The theory of planned behavior has gained considerable empirical support. In health-related research, it has been used to predict successfully a wide array of behaviors to include condom use (e.g., Reinecke, Schmidt, & Ajzen, 1996), breast examinations (e.g., Van Ryn, Lytle, & Kirscht, 1996) and exercise participation (e.g., Van Ryn, *et al.*, 1996). Others have examined students' classroom attendance (Prislin & Kovrlija, 1992) and employees' use of a new information system (Jackson, Chow, & Leitch, 1997). Taken together, the results from these studies have suggested that the underlying factors within the theory of planned behavior are significantly related to one's behavioral intentions (relationships have ranged from .23 to .60), and these intentions have been useful in understanding why one may, or may not, engage in certain behaviors (relationships have ranged from .41 to .61).

Theory of Planned Behavior and the Environment

Little work has explored the predictive validity of the model in an environmental context (cf. Taylor & Todd, 1995; Cheung, Chan, & Wong, 1999). Still, there is considerable literature that supports the application of the theory of planned behavior in order to gain an understanding of people's intentions to participate in an array of environmentally protective behaviors. As noted, the environmental literature has repeatedly found that positive environmental attitudes by themselves share little variance with environmental behaviors (e.g., Scott & Willits, 1994). That indicates that more factors are necessary to predict people's decision to engage in environmentally protective behaviors. In turn, others have concluded that behavioral intentions regarding specific environmental actions were strongly related to actual behaviors. Goldenhar and Connell (1993) found a causal relationship between students' intention to participate in a recycling program and their self-reported behaviors.

Furthermore, research findings have suggested that the other concepts that comprise the theory of planned behavior may be important when trying to understand completely people's behavioral intentions regarding environmental programs. For instance, subjective norms, i.e., the extent to which an individual believes that the behavior will be approved by referent others, seem to play a role in one's decision to recycle based on Bratt's findings (1999) which indicated that people's beliefs concerning their children's, spouses', and neighbors', i.e., referent others', attitudes toward recycling predicted their own attitudes and subsequent recycling behavior. Moreover, Allen and Ferrand (1999) reinforced this idea when they found that a person's perceptions of social desirability were related to self-reported environmentally protective behaviors. Allen and Ferrand's study also suggested the relevance of the perceived behavioral control component of the theory of planned behavior when they reported significant relationships between personal control, conservation behavior and recycling behavior.

In sum, the literature on the environment indicates that the theory of planned behavior may provide a useful framework to help us further understand people's decisions to engage in environmentally protective behaviors. This study further assessed the applicability of the theory of planned behavior to environmentally protective behaviors, namely energy conservation and carpooling in addition to recycling. In other words, we expect the tenets of the theory of planned behavior to be highly correlated with behavioral intentions. In addition, we expected these variables collectively to predict a substantial amount of variance in the subjects' behavioral intentions. By assessing the applicability of the theory of planned behavior to three unique environmentally protective intentions, we could also gain some understanding of the theory's applicability as a framework to understand environmentally protective intentions in general.

Method

Sample

A sample of 307 active duty Air Force members participated. Members were assigned to a large installation in the midwestern USA and were randomly selected to ensure that a wide range of ranks, ages, tenure, and academic backgrounds were represented. Of the mostly male sample ($n = 261$, 85% of the total), 26.3% said that they were enlisted members, and the remaining participants were officers. In addition, 78.2% of the participants indicated that they were less than 35 years old (i.e., 47 participants were 18–25 years old; 186 were 26–35 years old; and 58 were 36–45 years old), with nearly 60% of the participants reporting 10 years or less in the service.

Questionnaire Development and Administration

The questionnaire items were based on those developed by Taylor and Todd (1995) and included items to assess behavioral intentions, tenets of the theory of planned behavior and demographics. Since this questionnaire was an adaptation of one presented by Taylor and Todd, we pretested it twice before administering it. The first pretest focused on the questionnaire's structure, readability and grammar. Results and comments from this pretest indicated that the items were clear and understandable. Next, 26 military officers who were enrolled in a graduate program completed the revised questionnaire to further assess its clarity. In the second pretest, participants had no problems completing the revised questionnaire.

While the participants were randomly selected to participate and participation was voluntary, participants received a letter from the installation commander inviting them to participate and asking them to report to designated classrooms and office areas to complete a questionnaire. Ninety percent of those invited came to the administration site and completed the questionnaire. Prior to the questionnaire's administration, participants were given a brief oral presentation. The presentation explained that the questionnaire's purpose was to capture their true feelings regarding specific environmental programs. The oral review closed with a reminder to participants that all data were to be anonymous. As questionnaires were completed and returned, participants were given an information letter with the researchers' contact information to ensure we could be contacted if they had future questions.

Measures

The items included in the final version and descriptive statistics for each item are presented in Table 1. As noted, the items were an adaptation of scales developed by Taylor and Todd (1995). In our adaptation, participants responded to each item three times with a different environmental action in mind, i.e., recycling, energy conservation, and carpooling.

TABLE 1
QUESTIONNAIRE ITEMS AND ITEM DESCRIPTIVE STATISTICS

Construct and Item	Recycle M	Recycle SD	Conserve Energy M	Conserve Energy SD	Carpool M	Carpool SD
Behavioral Intentions						
I intend to [recycle, conserve energy, or carpool].	4.1	0.9	3.9	0.9	1.7	1.1
Attitude Toward Behaviors						
I like the idea of [recycling, conserving energy, or carpooling].	4.5	0.6	4.4	0.6	2.8	1.3
I have a positive attitude toward [recycling, conserving energy, or carpooling].	4.4	0.7	4.3	0.7	2.8	1.3
Helping the environment by [recycling, conserving energy, or carpooling] is good.	4.5	0.7	4.4	0.7	3.9	1.0
Subjective Norms						
People who influence my decisions think I should [recycle, conserve energy, or carpool].	3.3	0.9	3.4	0.9	2.5	0.9
People who are important to me think I should [recycle, conserve energy, or carpool].	3.3	0.8	3.3	0.8	2.5	0.9
Perceived Control						
Whether or not I [recycle, conserve energy, or carpool] is entirely up to me.	3.9	1.1	3.7	1.1	4.3	1.0
I have complete control over the amount of [recycling, conserving energy, or carpooling] that I do.	3.9	1.1	3.6	1.1	4.1	1.1
My [recycling, conserving energy, or carpooling] will help the environment.	4.3	0.8	4.3	0.7	3.8	1.1

Behavioral intentions.—Behavioral intentions for each of the environmentally protective behaviors were asked with a single item, e.g., "I intend to recycle." Participants indicated the strength of their intentions on a frequency scale with anchors of 1 = seldom and 5 = always.

Tenets of the theory of planned behavior.—Three items measured attitudes toward each behavior, two items measured subjective norms and three items measured perceived behavioral control. Participants responded to each of these items by expressing their agreement on a 5-point Likert-type scale, anchored by 1 = strongly disagree and 5 = strongly agree.

Results

Prior to analyzing the data, we conducted a principal components factor analysis (using SPSS Version 11.5) to determine if the items loaded on the constructs as we had intended. The components were then rotated using varimax rotation. For each of the environmentally protective behaviors, three factors emerged. As hypothesized, the first factor was comprised of the Attitude items, the second factor was made up of the items that tapped Subjective Norms and the third factor tapped the Perceived Behavioral Control. The results suggested that the scales tapped the intended dimensions and could be used in the subsequent analysis.

Descriptive statistics, reliability estimates and correlations between the elements of the theory of planned behavior and the relevant intentions are presented in Table 2. Reliability estimates for each of the multi-item scales were acceptable. That is, coefficients alpha were .86, .81, and .73 for attitudes toward recycling, conserving energy, and carpooling, respectively. In

TABLE 2
Theory of Planned Behavior Variables, Descriptive Statistics, and Relationships With Three Behavioral Intentions ($N = 307$)

Variable	M	SD	α	r: Intention to Recycle	Conserve Energy	Carpool
Recycling						
Attitudes toward recycling	4.5	.6	.86	.54*		
Subjective norms	3.3	.9	.94	.27*		
Perceived control	3.9	1.0	.78	.29*		
Energy Conservation						
Attitudes toward energy conservation	4.3	.6	.81		.48*	
Subjective norms	3.4	.9	.95		.29*	
Perceived control	3.6	1.0	.80		.01	
Carpooling						
Attitudes toward carpooling	3.3	.9	.73			.46*
Subjective norms	2.5	.9	.91			.24*
Perceived control	4.2	1.0	.87			−.18*

*$p < .01$.

addition, coefficients alpha for the subjective norms scales ranged from .91 to .94 and the alphas from the perceived behavioral control scales ranged from .78 to .87. As expected, the mean value for intentions was the highest for recycling ($M = 4.1$, $SD = .9$) and the lowest for carpooling ($M = 1.7$,

$SD = 1.1$), which indicated that the respondents intended to recycle more than they intended to carpool.

In addition, the correlation values were in the hypothesized directions with only one exception. The correlations between intentions to recycle and attitudes toward recycling, subjective norms regarding recycling and perceived behavioral control to recycle ranged from .54 to .29 ($p < .01$), indicating that intentions were related to each tenet of the theory of planned behavior. This general trend seemed to hold true for each of the environmentally protective behaviors except carpooling. In the case of carpooling behaviors, however, the perceived behavioral control was negatively related to intentions, which indicated that Air Force members did not feel that this behavior was within their control.

Multiple regression was used to assess the applicability of the theory of planned behavior for each of the specific pro-environmental behaviors. For example, to predict intention to recycle, an individual's attitude, subjective norm and perceived behavioral control toward recycling were used as predictors. A subsequent regression model was tested for intentions to conserve energy and intentions to carpool. In general, the theory of planned behavior collectively explained a significant portion of the variance in people's intentions to recycle ($R^2 = .35$, $p < .01$), conserve energy ($R^2 = .26$, $p < .01$) and carpool ($R^2 = .21$, $p < .01$).

Discussion

The present study examined the intentions of a sample of military members to participate in pro-environmental behaviors. Whereas most previous research in this domain has focused on the basic relationship between attitude and behavior, we hoped to expand our understanding by using a psychological model, the theory of planned behavior, to explore people's intentions to engage in three specific environmentally protective behaviors—recycling, energy conservation, and carpooling. Essentially, the theory of planned behavior suggests that behaviors are better understood by looking at the attitudes people have toward the behavior, their subjective norms and their perceived behavior control. These beliefs influence their behavior intentions, which in turn influence actual behaviors.

Overall, our results indicated that the theory of planned behavior may be applicable when examining recycling, energy conservation and carpooling behaviors. The relations between the underlying beliefs and the corresponding intentions were as the theory suggested. Taken individually, each of the three tenets of the theory of planned behavior, i.e., attitudes, subjective norms and perceived behavioral control, were related significantly to specific intentions. However, taken together, the three tenets typically explained far more variance in intentions than has been explained by other studies that have explored bivariate relationships between environmental attitudes and environmental behavior. For instance, the constructs of the theory of planned behavior explained 35% of the variance in intentions to recycle as compared to Scott and Willits' study (1994) that explained 10% of the variance in similar behaviors when they measured only general attitudes toward the environment.

Although this study does give us a better understanding of the environmental attitude and environmental behavior relationship, this study is not without limitations. The most significant of these limitations is the absence of objective behavioral measures for the sample. However, this concern is somewhat mitigated given that previous studies in other disciplines have consistently found strong relationships between people's intention and their behavior (e.g., Prislin & Kovrlija, 1992). For instance, studies have indicated that there are consistent relationships between employees' intentions to turnover and actual turnover in organizational settings (e.g., Crampton & Wagner, 1994). Furthermore, the relationship between intention and behavior has been established in the environmental arena as well (cf. Cheung, *et al.*, 1999). Thus, the absence of behavioral measures is an important, but not critical, limitation to this study. Of course, this limitation suggests that the measures used in this study coupled with observations of the actual behaviors provide an opportunity for researchers to test more robustly predictions from the theory of planned behavior in the environmental realm.

Second, the results should be interpreted with the context and sample in mind. These data were collected from a group of active military members. Hence, the generalizability of the findings should be considered. Still, the relevance of the theory of planned behavior should not be overlooked. In addition, these data were collected in a setting where leaders of the organization were encouraging participation. Subsequent studies should explore more diverse samples.

Finally, this study was a simplification of the theory of planned behavior where certain situational elements could be included in subsequent studies to understand further individuals' intentions. It was not surprising, for instance, that the military members viewed carpooling least favorably. In this case, personal control over the situation could be expected to play a role in these perceptions. That is, distance to work, availability of neighbors working in a similar location with similar hours, and requirements at work requiring a vehicle would influence members' intentions regarding this behavior. As with all limitations, this provides an opportunity to extend this research in a way that is consistent with others who have applied the theory of planned behavior in the other arenas (e.g., Prislin & Kovrlija, 1992; Van Ryn, *et al.*, 1996; Allen & Ferrand, 1999).

REFERENCES

AJZEN, I. (1991) The theory of planned behavior. *Organizational Behavior and Human Decision Processes*, 50, 179-211.

ALLEN, J. B., & FERRAND, J. L. (1999) Environmental locus of control, sympathy, and proenvironmental behavior: a test of Geller's actively caring hypothesis. *Environment and Behavior*, 31, 338-353.

BRATT, C. (1999) The impact of norms and assumed consequences on recycling behavior. *Environment and Behavior*, 31, 630-656.

CHEUNG, S. F., CHAN, D. K. S., & WONG, Z. S. Y. (1999) Reexamining the Theory of Planned Behavior in understanding wastepaper recycling. *Environment and Behavior*, 31, 587-612.

CRAMPTON, S. M., & WAGNER, J. A. (1994) Percept-percept inflation in microorganizational research: an investigation of prevalence and effect. *Journal of Applied Psychology*, 79, 67-76.

DUNLAP, R., & SCARCE, R. (1991) The polls-polls trends: environmental problems and protection. *Public Opinion Quarterly*, 55, 651-672.

GOLDENHAR, L. M., & CONNELL, C. M. (1993) Understanding and predicting recycling behavior: an application of the theory of reasoned action. *Journal of Environmental Systems*, 22, 91-103.

JACKSON, C. M., CHOW, S., & LEITCH, R. A. (1997) Toward an understanding of the behavioral intention to use an information system. *Decision Sciences*, 28, 357-389.

PRISLIN, R., & KOVRLIJA, N. (1992) Predicting behavior of high and low self-monitors: an application of the Theory of Planned Behavior. *Psychological Reports*, 70, 1131-1138.

REINECKE, J., SCHMIDT, P., & AJZEN, I. (1996) Application of the Theory of Planned Behavior to adolescents' condom use: a panel study. *Journal of Applied Social Psychology*, 26, 749-772.

SCOTT, D., & WILLITS, F. (1994) Environmental attitudes and behaviors: a Pennsylvania survey. *Environment and Behavior*, 26, 239-260.

TAYLOR, S., & TODD, P. (1995) An integrated model of waste management behavior: a test of household recycling and composting intentions. *Environment and Behavior*, 27, 603-630.

UNGER, S. (1994) Apples and oranges: probing the attitude-behavior relationship for the environment. *Canadian Review of Society and Anthropology*, 31, 288-304.

VAN RYN, M., LYTLE, L. A., & KIRSCHT, J. P. (1996) A test of the Theory of Planned Behavior for two health-related practices *Journal of Applied Social Psychology*, 26, 871-883.

WIDEGREN, O. (1998) The new environmental paradigm and personal norms. *Environment and Behavior*, 30, 75-100.

Accepted April 7, 2004.

DYNAMIC BALANCE IN HIGH LEVEL ATHLETES [1]

CHRISTINA D. DAVLIN

Xavier University

Summary.—The purpose of this study was to investigate dynamic balance performance in highly skilled athletes. Participating athletes were currently competing at the collegiate Division I, professional, elite, or Olympic levels, or their individual coaches believed the athlete performed comparably to these levels. High level male and female gymnasts ($n=57$, M age = 17.3 yr., $SD=4.1$), soccer players ($n=58$, M age = 19.8 yr., $SD=1.6$), swimmers ($n=70$, M age = 17.1 yr., $SD=2.5$), and individuals with no formal competitive sport experience ($n=61$, M age = 16.8 yr., $SD=2.0$) volunteered. Dynamic balance performance was measured on a stabilometer, which requires participants to continuously adjust posture to maintain an unstable platform in the horizontal position for 30 sec. Each participant performed 3 practice trials followed by 7 test trials. Analysis indicated that athletes were superior to nonathletes in balance performance. Gymnasts performed better on the dynamic balance task than all other groups. Soccer players and swimmers performed similarly and were superior to the control subjects. There was no difference between the performance of men and women. Moderate to high negative correlations were found between dynamic balance performance and height and weight.

Balance is a key component of motor skills ranging from maintaining posture to executing complex sport skills. Balance is typically categorized into two types, static and dynamic. When equilibrium is maintained for one stationary body position it is called static balance. Dynamic balance refers to maintaining equilibrium during motion or re-establishing equilibrium through rapid and successively changing positions. Both static and dynamic balance require integrating sensory information from the visual, vestibular, and somatosensory systems (Shupert, Lindblad, & Leibowitz, 1983).

It seems athletes, through years of sport experience, would have superior kinesthetic awareness and body control and would therefore perform better on a test of balance than nonathletes. However, previous studies have not shown a clear relationship between balance performance and athletic participation. Singer (1965), investigating the effects of spectators on balance performance, found that nonathletes performed better than athletes both during practice trials without an audience and during test trials with an audience. Breitenbach (1955) and Ryan (1963) concluded that athletic ability was not significantly related to dynamic balance performance after finding no significant difference between athletes and nonathletes on a balancing

---

[1]Address correspondence to Dr. Christina Davlin, Department of Sport Studies, Xavier University, 3800 Victory Ave., Cincinnati, OH 45207 or e-mail (davlin@xu.edu).

task. Notwithstanding, several studies have shown highly skilled athletes tend to outperform their lowered skilled peers (Mumby, 1953; Gross & Thompson, 1957; Williams & Sissons, 1984). For example, Williams and Sissons (1984) stated that gifted athletes participating in 11 different sports were superior to less skilled people in performing a balance task and in transferring that skill from one task to another.

According to Kioumourtzoglou, Derri, Mertzanidou, and Tzetzis (1997), through experience athletes differ from nonathletes only with regard to specific skills required by their particular sport. This may also apply to athletes participating in different sports. Singer (1970) reported that gymnasts and water skiers were superior on a balance task to nonathletes, as well as football linemen, baseball players, and basketball players. Additionally, Travis (1944) noted that participants who reported previous training in dancing, skiing, gymnastics, and skating tended to perform above normal on dynamic balance measured by a stabilometer.

A few authors have investigated the relationship between balance and sex, height, and weight. There appears to be no clear consensus regarding the possible influence of these variables on balance. Travis (1945) and McLeod and Hansen (1989) found that college-aged women performed better than men on a stabilometer test. Bachman (1961) also stated that women scored higher than men on a stabilometer, but only between the ages of 16 and 21 years. There were no differences between the scores at the ages of 6 to 15 and over the age of 21 years. Conversely, Wapner and Witkin (1950), who tested subjects on a stabilometer under different visual conditions, claimed college-aged men tended to perform better than women.

Travis (1945) found significant negative correlations between balance performance and height and weight measures. Upon further analysis, he concluded that weight was a more significant factor than height in execution of a dynamic balancing task. In a later study with athletes, Singer (1970) noted height and weight were only slightly related to balance performance. However, Espenshade, Dable, and Schoendube (1953), testing adolescent boys between the ages of 12 and 18 years, found that dynamic balance is not related to either their height or weight.

Due to the lack of consistent findings on balance, this study was done to examine dynamic balance performance in high level athletes and nonathletes. Dynamic balance was measured on a stabilometer, which records the amount of time a participant maintains an unstable platform within 5° of horizontal. The primary objectives of this research were to assess whether high level athletes were superior to nonathletes on this dynamic balance task and to examine whether there were differences in specific sport affiliations or by sex. This study also examined a possible association for balance performance with height and weight.

Method

Participants

Top level male and female athletes participating in gymnastics ($n = 57$), soccer ($n = 58$), and swimming ($n = 70$), as well as individuals with no formal competitive sport experience ($n = 61$), volunteered as participants. See Table 1 for specific information regarding the participants. Informed consent was obtained from all subjects in accordance to Xavier University's Institutional Review Board, which also approved the study. High level athletes were chosen for this study if they were currently competing at an elite, collegiate Division I, professional, or Olympic level, or if their individual coaches believed the athletes were performing comparably to these levels (*Note*: some participants had the skill level of a Division I college athlete in their sports but were minors).

TABLE 1
SUBJECTS' CHARACTERISTICS BY SPORT GROUP

Group	n	Height (cm) M	Height (cm) SD	Weight (kg) M	Weight (kg) SD	Shoulder Width (cm) M	Shoulder Width (cm) SD	Age (yr.) M	Age (yr.) SD	Training Time (yr.) M	Training Time (yr.) SD
Gymnasts											
Women	28	151.9	12.0	45.5	10.1	35.2	3.7	13.7	1.7	8.6	3.0
Men	29	169.6	6.5	68.3	4.2	45.1	1.6	20.7	2.5	14.2	4.1
Soccer											
Women	28	167.6	7.0	62.5	7.9	40.9	1.5	19.3	1.0	14.4	1.5
Men	30	176.3	5.9	74.6	6.0	43.8	2.4	20.1	1.8	10.5	2.7
Swimming											
Women	38	169.2	6.0	60.2	6.2	41.6	2.0	17.6	2.1	9.6	2.9
Men	32	174.8	11.2	60.7	18.3	45.3	3.9	16.5	2.7	10.8	3.1
Control											
Women	30	164.6	7.5	60.5	15.4	37.8	2.7	16.8	2.1	0.0	0.0
Men	31	176.8	8.6	80.1	15.0	42.5	3.8	16.7	1.9	0.0	0.0

Procedures

The test session included assessment of (1) age, (2) height, (3) weight, (4) shoulder width (right acromion process to left acromion process), (5) years of sport training, and (6) dynamic balance. Dynamic balance was assessed on a stabilometer (Lafayette Instruments, Inc.). Participants stood with the feet shoulder width apart and with eyes looking straight ahead. Each participant was allowed three practice trials and then performed seven test trials. Each trial lasted 30 sec. Participants were allowed to rest as much as they needed between trials. The stabilometer recorded the amount of time the participant held the platform within 5° of horizontal on either side.

Results

Reliability (Cronbach alpha) for Trials 1 to 7 was .97. The average of all seven test trials was used in the data analysis. The experimental design was a two-way analysis of variance (sex × sport group). The dependent variable was time-on-balance as measured in seconds. There was no interaction between the factors of sex and sports group ($F_{3,238} = .61$, ns). Although there was a main effect for sex ($F_{1,238} = 5.05$, $p = .03$), the effect size as expressed by partial eta squared ($\eta^2 = .02$) was small (Green, Salkind, & Akey, 1997), indicating that only 2% of the variability in the dependent variable (time-on-balance) was explained by sex. *Post hoc* analysis (Tukey's HSD) indicated no significant difference between men and women in overall performance. It further showed that there was no significant difference between the sexes within each sport group.

A significant difference was found between sport groups ($F_{3,238} = 68.74$, $p < .001$). The effect size for sport group was large ($\eta^2 = .46$), indicating that 46% of the variability in the dependent variable was explained by sports group. Gymnasts ($M = 23.1$, $SD = 3.6$) were superior in balance to all other groups. Soccer players ($M = 18.9$, $SD = 3.9$) and swimmers ($M = 17.5$, $SD = 4.3$) did not perform significantly differently from each other but did perform better than the control subjects ($M = 13.1$, $SD = 3.4$), who had the lowest balance scores. Table 2 shows the dynamic balance performance for each sport group by sex.

TABLE 2
Dynamic Balance Performance (Time-on-balance)

Group	M	SD	Range
Gymnastics			
Women	23.2	3.3	17.2–28.2
Men	23.1	3.8	14.2–28.6
Soccer			
Women	19.7	3.6	11.6–25.1
Men	18.1	4.1	12.0–26.7
Swimming			
Women	17.9	3.8	11.6–26.9
Men	17.1	4.8	9.6–27.1
Control			
Women	14.1	3.6	6.3–21.9
Men	12.2	3.2	7.2–20.0

Significant moderate negative correlations were found between balance performance and height ($r = -.43$, $p < .01$) and weight ($r = -.45$, $p < .01$). Further analysis, however, indicated these relationships were not consistent among the groups (Table 3). Moderate to high negative correlations were found only among the female and male swimmers, with regard to balance performance and height. Also, moderate to high negative correlations between balance performance and weight were found for the male swimmers and the women and men in the control group.

TABLE 3
Correlations For Height, Weight, and Balance by Sport Group

Group	Height vs Balance	Weight vs Balance
Gymnastics		
Women	−.40	−.47
Men	.30	−.14
Soccer		
Women	−.34	−.41
Men	−.36	−.17
Swimming		
Women	−.55*	−.36
Men	−.73*	−.48*
Control		
Women	−.20	−.62*
Men	−.08	−.50*

Discussion

If athletes differ from nonathletes only with regards to specific skills required by their particular sport, as suggested by Kioumourtzoglou, *et al.* (1997), then it would therefore be logical that gymnasts, who train to improve their ability to maintain balance as well as recover and regain balance in multiple situations, would outperform the other athletes and nonathletes in this study. This supports Singer's findings (1970) in which athletes who practiced balance skills similar to the one tested on the stabilometer, i.e., water skiers and gymnasts, performed better during the test than both nonathletes and athletes of other sports. Interestingly, despite the different motor requirements of the two sports, soccer players and swimmers performed with similar proficiency on the balance task.

Previous research has suggested that sex, height, and weight may be influential in dynamic balance performance. The results of this study showed that sex was not a significant factor in dynamic balance. Furthermore, although significant moderate negative correlations were found for balance performance with both height and weight, only two of the eight groups showed significant correlations for height and balance performance, and only three groups showed significant correlations for weight and balance performance. It would, therefore, be unwise to conclude that both height and weight are significant factors in dynamic balance.

REFERENCES

BACHMAN, J. (1961) Motor learning and performance as related to age and sex in two measures of balance co-ordination. *Research Quarterly*, 32, 123-137.

BREITENBACH, O. (1955) A study to determine the relationship between athletic ability and dynamic balance. Microcarded master's thesis, Univer. of Wisconsin.

ESPENSHADE, A., DABLE, R., & SCHOENDUBE, R. (1953) Dynamic balance in adolescent boys. *Research Quarterly*, 24, 270-275.

GREEN, S. B., SALKIND, N. J., & AKEY, T. M. (1997) *Using SPSS for Windows: analyzing and understanding data.* Upper Saddle River, NJ: Prentice-Hall.

GROSS, E., & THOMPSON, H. (1957) Relationship of dynamic balance to speed and to ability in swimming. *Research Quarterly*, 28, 342-346.

KIOUMOURTZOGLOU, E., DERRI, V., MERTZANIDOU, O., & TZETZIS, G. (1997) Experience with perceptual and motor skills in rhythmic gymnastics. *Perceptual and Motor Skills*, 84, 1363-1372.

MCLEOD, B., & HANSEN, E. (1989) Effects of the eyerobics visual skills training program on static balance performance of male and female subjects. *Perceptual and Motor Skills*, 69, 1123-1126.

MUMBY, H. (1953) Kinesthetic acuity and balance related to wrestling. *Research Quarterly*, 24, 327-334.

RYAN, E. (1963) Relative academic achievement and stabilometer performance. *Research Quarterly*, 34, 185-190.

SHUPERT, C. L., LINDBLAD, I. M., & LEIBOWITZ, H. W. (1983) Visual testing for competitive diving: a two visual systems approach. Paper presented at the 1983 U.S. Diving Sports Science Seminar, Indianapolis, IN.

SINGER, R. N. (1965) Effect of spectators on athletes and non-athletes performing a gross motor task. *Research Quarterly*, 36, 473-482.

SINGER, R. N. (1970) Balance skill as related to athletics, sex, height, and weight. In G. Kenyon (Ed.), *Contemporary psychology of sport.* Chicago, IL: Athletic Institute. Pp. 645-656.

TRAVIS, R. (1944) A new stabilometer for measuring dynamic equilibrium in a standing position. *Journal of Experimental Psychology*, 34, 418-424.

TRAVIS, R. (1945) Experimental analysis of dynamic and static equilibrium. *Journal of Experimental Psychology*, 35, 216-234.

WAPNER, S., & WITKIN, H. (1950) The role of visual factors in the maintenance of balance. *American Journal of Psychology*, 63, 385-408.

WILLIAMS, L. R. T., & SISSONS, A. C. (1984) Performance, learning and transfer of balance skill in relation to achievement level in sport. *Australian Journal of Science and Medicine in Sport*, 16, 21-23.

Accepted April 5, 2004.

COMMUNICATIVE RESPONSIBILITY AND SEMANTIC TASK IN THE LANGUAGE OF ADULTS WITH DEMENTIA[1]

ROBERT GOLDFARB

Adelphi University

AND

ELMERA GOLDBERG

The Graduate Center, CUNY

Summary.—A probe technique requiring convergent and divergent semantic behavior and representing five levels of communicative responsibility served as the research tool. Stimuli were presented to adults identified as having Alzheimer disease or multi-infarct dementia. Within each group differences were observed on the semantic task (convergent and divergent) and on communicative responsibility. Group characteristics are compared with data previously published in 1994 on aphasic and schizophrenic adults responding to the same stimuli.

Substantial differences have been noted in the language output of adults with Alzheimer disease compared to those with multi-infarct dementia (Bayles & Tomoeda, 1996). With multi-infarct dementia, there may be more varied language changes early on than with Alzheimer disease wherein some functions remain preserved while others are impaired (Chapman, 1997). Language changes tend to progress more slowly with multi-infarct dementia than with Alzheimer disease. Word finding may be less impaired in early multi-infarct dementia than in Alzheimer disease; later, however, the naming impairment in multi-infarct dementia may result in the production of jargon, neologisms, and literal paraphasias, phenomena not usually present in Alzheimer disease (Chapman, 1997). In multi-infarct dementia, speech becomes more concise because of preservation of substantive words. In contrast, speech in Alzheimer disease becomes empty with an increasing loss of substantives. Kontiola, Laaksonen, Sulkava, and Erkinjunnti (1990) found that the most complex linguistic functions, those associated with intellectual and mnestic operations, become impaired in Alzheimer disease. In their study, the Alzheimer disease group had especial difficulty understanding and constructing complex grammatical structures. In contrast, in multi-infarct dementia, it is the more elementary language functions that break down, those functions associated with symbolic aspects such as word recognition, naming, and repetition.

Language use depends on intellectual functioning and memory. Individuals with vascular disease and infarctions in frontal lobes suffer serious intel-

---

[1]This study was supported, in part, by PSC-CUNY and George N. Shuster Foundation grants to the first author. We are grateful for the editorial assistance of anonymous reviewers. Address editorial correspondence to Robert Goldfarb, Ph.D., Department of Communication Sciences & Disorders, Adelphi University, Garden City, NY 11530 or e-mail (Goldfarb2@adelphi.edu).

lectual and memory deficits. The frontal lobes are crucial to normal functioning of working memory that plays a significant role in language comprehension, encoding, activation, and retrieval. Small-vessel ischemic disease, or a frontotemporal form of degeneration, are the most frequent causes of multi-infarct dementia (Grossman, D'Esposito, Hughes, Onishi, Biassou, White-Devine, & Robinson, 1996). Positron emission tomography measurements in normal volunteers, during a graded auditory-verbal memory task, revealed increased memory load correlating with increased regional cerebral blood flow in the cerebellar vermis and hemispheres, thalamus bilaterally, the superior and middle front gyri bilaterally, anterior insular regions bilaterally, anterior cingulate, precuneus, and left and right lateral premotor areas (Grasby, Frith, Friston, Simpson, Fletcher, Frackowiak, & Dolan, 1994, p. 1271).

MacDonald, Almor, Henderson, Kempler, and Andersen (2001) cautioned against assuming that impairments in working memory underlie comprehension deficits. They found vagueness in the term, "working memory", as well as limitations of available working memory tasks. Indeed, they reported that many such tasks bore little relationship to language comprehension. In addition, many tasks were too confusing or difficult for participants with Alzheimer disease. Bayles (2003) also noted a paucity in documentation on how working memory deficits affect communicative functioning. Using five tests of language comprehension and four tests of language expression, Bayles (2003, p. 209) argued that lower scores on language tests resulted primarily from reduced attention span and difficulties focusing attention, encoding, and activating long-term knowledge rather than from loss of linguistic knowledge in her Alzheimer dementia participants.

There are many reports of naming impairment associated with Alzheimer dementia (Huff, Corkin, & Growdon, 1986; Kontiola, et al., 1990; Bayles & Tomoeda, 1996; Chenery, Murdoch, & Ingram, 1996, among others). Chenery, et al. (1996) reported that naming difficulty is evidence of a predominant semantic disruption, the character of which is related to the severity of illness. "As the disease progresses, the integrity of the structural store of semantic memories proceeds to break down" (p. 433). As the semantic function becomes increasingly compromised, the ability to name becomes increasingly restricted. Chenery, et al. (1996) claimed that the severity of the naming deficit can be used to gauge the severity of dementia of an individual. However, there may be a selective impairment in action naming (compared to object naming) among those with multi-infarct dementia, a finding not observed in Alzheimer disease patients (Cappa, Binetti, Pezzini, Padovani, Rozzini, & Trabucchi, 1998). This finding was independent of severity of dementia or of overall language impairment.

Another present concern was the effect of communicative responsibility on the language of our subjects. Communicative responsibility or level of demand for creativity has been thought a factor in stuttering and is an aspect of the "Demands and Capacities" model (Starkweather, Gottwald, & Halfond, 1990), which predicts breakdown "when environmental or self-imposed demands exceed the speaker's cognitive, linguistic, motoric, and/or emotional capacities for responding" (Adams, 1990, pp. 136-137). Communicative breakdowns increase with increased communicative demand. Finally, we examined responses to convergent and divergent semantic tasks. Convergent responses are logical conclusions or logical necessities, and divergent responses are logical alternatives or logical possibilities (Guilford, 1967).

The present study considered effects of communicative responsibility and semantic task on the linguistic performance of two groups of adults, one group with Alzheimer disease and the other with multi-infarct dementia. We hoped the data would facilitate differential diagnosis. Specifically, we hypothesized: (1) more errors would occur on divergent than on convergent semantic tasks, regardless of type of disorder; (2) the number of errors would increase as communicative responsibility increased, regardless of type of disorder; and (3) patterns of errors for the groups would differ from those previously obtained (Goldfarb, Eisenson, Stocker, & DeSanti, 1994) for aphasic and schizophrenic subjects.

Method

Subjects

There were 14 inpatient subjects, all residents of the Terence Cardinal Cooke Health Care Center in New York City. All subjects were diagnosed by attending psychiatrists: 7 were diagnosed with Alzheimer disease, 7 with multi-infarct dementia. They ranged in age from 65 to 92 years. The mean age of the total was 80 yr., the mean of the Alzheimer disease group was 81 yr., and the mean of the multi-infarct dementia group was slightly younger at 79 yr. Education and socioeconomic status were similar among subjects, and none had gross uncorrected auditory or visual impairment. All spoke English as the first language. Each subject was screened with the Mini-Mental State examination (Folstein, Folstein, & McHugh, 1975). A minimum score of 10 (out of a maximum of 30) was required to participate. Scores ranged from 10 to 13 for the subjects with Alzheimer disease ($M = 11.86$) and from 10-20 for the subjects with multi-infarct dementia ($M = 13.86$) (see Table 1). Of the 50 potential subjects originally recruited, 32 were rejected for limited verbal ability, and 4 others (2 Alzheimer disease and 2 multi-infarct dementia) did not achieve the minimum score on the Mini-Mental State examination.

Comparing the experimental groups, no subject in the Alzheimer disease group scored higher than 13 in the Mini-Mental State examination (Folstein, et al., 1975). In contrast, three subjects with multi-infarct dementia

TABLE 1
Characteristics of Subjects With Alzheimer Disease and Multi-infarct Dementia

Diagnosis/Patient	Sex	Age (yr.:mo.)	Mini-Mental State Score
Alzheimer Disease			
DA	Female	78:0	10
FS	Female	87:2	10
MB	Female	86:5	12
DH	Female	73:1	12
VM	Male	83:5	13
AS	Female	79:1	13
AV	Female	79:2	13
Multi-infarct Dementia			
MW	Female	77:5	10
EC	Female	78:4	10
EB	Female	75:4	11
CC	Male	78:1	13
JS	Male	65:0	16
AM	Female	87:0	17
MS	Female	92:0	20

scored above the midpoint of 15: 20, 17, and 16. This suggests that the cognitive impairment of the subjects with Alzheimer disease was greater than that of the multi-infarct group, at least in terms of basic orientation and knowledge-of-world skills.

With respect to orientation, all subjects were impaired, but those with multi-infarct dementia were more aware of place, time of day, and season of year. Writing was more difficult for those with Alzheimer disease; four could not write legibly at all. Reading was also impaired, although those with multi-infarct dementia were less impaired than those with Alzheimer disease. The literacy skills of the oldest subject, age 92 with multi-infarct dementia, were completely spared, and two others in that group showed little reduction in reading.

Probes

Part II (the language portion) of the *Stocker Probe for Fluency and Language* (Stocker & Goldfarb, 1995) was administered to all subjects. The Probe includes five levels of increasing communicative responsibility. These five levels also include three convergent (Levels I, II, and IV) and two divergent (Levels III and V) semantic tasks. There were 10 stimulus items: a lock and key (miniature), nickel, hammer (miniature), postage stamp, candle, shoelace, spoon, whistle, ring, and ruler. Level I is a binary choice task, related to a semantic feature of the stimulus, e.g., "Is it hard or soft?" Level II is a convergent antonym response task, e.g., "What is the opposite of 'loud'?" The associative strength of stimulus words was calculated on the basis of the communality of response which each word received in the Palermo and Jenkins (1964) or the Goldfarb and Halpern (1984) studies. A response of high communality (convergent) was operationally defined as occurring more than 30% of the time on a free-association test. Level III is a divergent antonym response task, e.g., "What is the opposite of 'problem'?" Responses which are low in communality on the basis of associative strength (Palermo & Jenkins, 1964; Goldfarb & Halpern, 1984) are considered to be divergent (Guilford, 1967). A response of low communality was operationally defined as occurring less than 20% of the time in a free-association test. Thus a buffer of 20% to 30% associative frequency separated divergent from convergent tasks. Level IV requires the subject to identify semantic features of the stimulus item ("Tell me everything you know about it."). Level V, "What does this make you think of?" requires paradigmatic and/or syntagmatic associations.

Procedure

Subjects were tested individually by a certified speech-language pathologist familiar to them. The 10 stimulus items were presented, with all five probe levels given per item. Probe questions were ordered pseudorandomly to control for effect of order of presentation. For example, the following Probes relate to the stimulus "hammer." The number in brackets refers to percentage of those antonym responses produced by normal adults on a word-association test: III. What is the opposite of "playing"? (working [14.2%]); II. What is the opposite of "heavy"? (light [42.2%]); V. What does this make you think of; IV. Tell me everything you know about it; I. Is it broken or whole?

Results

Summary of responses are based on a maximum score of 70 (10 probes × 7 subjects) for each probe level in each of the two experimental groups (see Table 2). Level I (an either-or task) was the only one in which both groups provided more correct than incorrect responses. Multi-infarct dementia participants also produced more correct than incorrect responses at Level II. Responses to Levels II and III (convergent and divergent antonyms, respectively) were surprising, as many subjects did not understand what "opposite" meant, and in many cases, supplied synonyms rather than antonyms. Patterns of single-word responses to Levels I, II, and III for participants with Alzheimer disease, and those with multi-infarct dementia were similar to, but lower than those published (Goldfarb, *et al.*, 1994) for aphasic and schizophrenic adults, using the same research tool. Single-word responses by participants with Alzheimer disease were closest to the pattern of responses from adults with Wernicke's aphasia, and the responses of participants with multi-infarct dementia tracked most closely with those of

TABLE 2
Summary of Responses to Five Probe Levels

Group	I	II	III	IV	V
Alzheimer Disease	50	19	7	22	15
Multi-infarct Dementia	50	42	22	29	21

adults with undifferentiated schizophrenia (see Table 3). Either-or responses (to Probe Level I) did not discriminate between the current two experimental groups.

The overall scores of Alzheimer disease participants were lower than those of multi-infarct dementia participants, which was expected in light of the greater severity of impairment among those with Alzheimer disease.

TABLE 3
Means and Standard Deviations of Scores by Level of Communicative Responsibility For Subjects in Current and Previous Studies

Probe Level	Group	n	M	SD
I	Alzheimer Disease	7	7.14	2.34
	Multi-infarct Dementia	7	7.14	2.54
	Broca's Aphasia	13	9.15	1.21
	Wernicke's Aphasia	7	7.00	3.21
	Anomic Aphasia	9	9.78	0.44
	Schizophrenia	26	8.08	2.48
II	Alzheimer Disease	7	2.72	2.81
	Multi-infarct Dementia	7	6.00	4.36
	Broca's Aphasia	13	6.77	2.31
	Wernicke's Aphasia	7	3.71	3.77
	Anomic Aphasia	9	8.78	1.09
	Schizophrenia	26	6.92	2.95
III	Alzheimer Disease	7	1.00	1.29
	Multi-infarct Dementia	7	3.71	3.77
	Broca's Aphasia	13	2.39	2.78
	Wernicke's Aphasia	7	2.00	2.52
	Anomic Aphasia	9	4.89	1.27
	Schizophrenia	26	4.15	3.18
IV	Alzheimer Disease	7	3.14	3.18
	Multi-infarct Dementia	7	4.00	2.45
	Broca's Aphasia	13	5.08	3.28
	Wernicke's Aphasia	7	5.71	4.50
	Anomic Aphasia	9	9.33	0.71
	Schizophrenia	26	7.08	2.70
V	Alzheimer Disease	7	2.14	1.68
	Multi-infarct Dementia	7	3.00	2.58
	Broca's Aphasia	13	6.23	2.80
	Wernicke's Aphasia	7	5.71	4.11
	Anomic Aphasia	9	8.56	1.33
	Schizophrenia	26	3.96	2.88

However, the precipitous decline in the ability of participants with Alzheimer disease to generate antonyms (Levels II and III), compared to those with multi-infarct dementia cannot be explained solely on the basis of severity of impairment. When participants were required to produce multiword responses, as in Level IV ("Tell me everything you know about it.") and Level V ("What does this make you think of?"), patterns of responses emerged which differentiated dementia subjects from those with aphasia, and, to a lesser extent, from those with chronic undifferentiated schizophrenia (see Table 3).

We noted within-group similarities and individual differences. The participants with multi-infarct dementia were all able to produce full sentences, although among them were three who reported being confused by the tasks. One subject exhibited perseverative behavior, and another demonstrated confabulations and literal paraphasias. In contrast, only three of the subjects with Alzheimer disease produced full, meaningful sentences; the others produced truncated utterances, had halting, hesitant speech, or empty syntax.

A one-way between-subjects analysis of variance yielded significant differences ($F_{1,13} = 7.02$, $p < .001$) in responses to the five probe levels. Differences between groups were not significant ($F_{1,12} = 3.43$, $p > .05$), although Alzheimer disease subjects' means were consistently lower for Levels II through V. However, comparisons of means by t ratio were not significant because standard deviations tended to be large (see Table 3). Finally, both groups produced higher mean scores in response to convergent (Levels I, II, and IV) than to divergent (Levels III and V) semantic tasks ($\chi^2 = 4.48$, $p < .05$).

The finding that more errors occurred on divergent than on convergent semantic tasks, regardless of type and severity of disorder, supports our first hypothesis. It is strongly supported by data from normal older individuals as well as those with aphasia and the language of schizophrenia, using the same research tool (Goldfarb, et al., 1994). Tasks requiring logical alternatives or logical possibilities are more difficult for the elderly with dementia than tasks requiring logical conclusions or logical necessities.

The number of errors did not increase as communicative responsibility increased (which did not support our second hypothesis). The greatest number of errors occurred at Level III, a divergent antonym task. We may conclude that the present task was not an accurate measure of communicative responsibility. However, the probes used in the present study have been accurate in determining severity of stuttering (Stocker & Goldfarb, 1995). More likely is the conclusion that increasing demand for creativity, while a robust independent variable for stuttering, is not salient in the language of dementia.

Patterns of errors differentiated responses of participants with Alzheimer disease and multi-infarct dementia independent of severity of impairment. This was especially evident in the greater impairment of participants with Alzheimer disease to produce antonym responses. With regard to multiword responses, both current experimental groups showed more impairment in storytelling (Level V) than feature description (Level IV). Previous data from aphasic adults (Goldfarb, *et al.*, 1994) indicated the opposite tendency, reflecting the word-finding impairment characteristic of aphasia. In addition, responses to Level IV by schizophrenic subjects did not suggest word-finding difficulty to the extent that adults with dementia, and especially those with aphasia, displayed. In summary, participants with Alzheimer and multi-infarct dementia were more impaired for text than for words, although very impaired for both. Those with aphasia were more impaired for words than for text, although very impaired for both, and those with chronic undifferentiated schizophrenia were very impaired at the textual level and much less impaired for words.

Discussion

A comparison of language output in individuals with Alzheimer disease and those with multi-infarct dementia is a difficult enterprise given the variability in the distribution of pathology (infarcts) in individuals with vascular disease. Because the distribution of infarctions and amount of tissue damaged differs markedly among individuals, so also do the behavioral consequences. The lack of information about the extent of pathology in the multi-infarct dementia subjects should be considered a delimitation of the present study. Differentiating between those with Alzheimer disease and those with multi-infarct dementia has consistently been reported to be difficult. Criteria developed for the diagnosis of Alzheimer disease tend to include neuropsychological evaluation, brain imaging, and ultimately postmortem evaluation. A recent review of 56 patients using these criteria (Varma, Snowden, Lloyd, Talbot, Mann, & Neary, 1999) showed good sensitivity in identifying the 30 patients with Alzheimer disease but poor specificity in differentiating them from the 26 patients with frontotemporal dementia. Similarly, traditional aphasia batteries did not distinguish among Alzheimer disease, multi-infarct dementia due to small-vessel ischemic disease, and frontotemporal dementia (Grossman, *et al.*, 1996).

The goal of using the present data to differentiate between those elderly with Alzheimer disease and multi-infarct dementia may be expanded by considering earlier responses to the same research tool (Goldfarb, *et al.*, 1994). Adults with other neurogenic communication disorders, including aphasia (Broca's, Wernicke's, and anomic) and chronic undifferentiated schizophrenia evinced characteristic patterns of responses across Probe levels. All adult groups with neurogenic communication disorders scored best on Level I, with Wernicke's aphasic and dementia subjects producing the lowest scores.

The pattern of responses by multi-infarct dementia participants (as well as the pattern from those with Alzheimer dementia, but at a lower level) tracked most closely with that of undifferentiated schizophrenic subjects. Alzheimer dementia participants were unique in the disproportionately larger number of error responses at all probe levels. Both dementia groups, in contrast to the aphasic subjects, identified semantic features (Level IV) better than they told stories (Level V). This finding was not consistent with many reports describing the naming impairment in Alzheimer dementia and multi-infarct dementia. However, it was consistent with increased impairment associated with more communicative responsibility. Some pragmatic abilities, such as story telling, are relatively preserved in aphasia, but this is not the case in the language of dementia. Finally, the more accurate responses by Alzheimer disease and multi-infarct dementia participants on convergent tasks than on divergent tasks are consistent with the behavior of those adults with aphasia and schizophrenia.

REFERENCES

Adams, M. R. (1990) The demands and capacities model: I. Theoretical elaborations. *Journal of Fluency Disorders*, 15, 135-141.

Bayles, K. A. (2003) Effects of working memory deficits on the communication functioning of Alzheimer's dementia patients. *Journal of Communication Disorders*, 36, 209-219.

Bayles, K. A., & Tomoeda, C. K. (1996) Principles and techniques for managing the memory deficits of persons with mild to moderate dementia. *ASHA Special Interest Division 2: Neurophysiology and Neurogenic Speech and Language Disorders*, October, 21-27.

Cappa, S. F., Binetti, G., Pezzini, A., Padovani, A., Rozzini, L., & Trabucchi, M. (1998) Object and action naming in Alzheimer's disease and frontotemporal dementia. *Neurology*, 50, 351-355.

Chapman, S. B. (1997) Discourse markers of Alzheimer's disease versus normal advanced aging. *ASHA Special Interest Division 2: Neurophysiology and Neurogenic Speech and Language Disorders*, December, 20-26.

Chenery, H. J., Murdoch, B. E., & Ingram, J. C. L. (1996) An investigation of confrontation naming performance in Alzheimer's dementia as a function of disease severity. *Aphasiology*, 10, 423-441.

Folstein, M. F., Folstein, S. E., & McHugh, P. R. (1975) Mini-Mental State: a practical method for grading the mental state of patients for the clinician. *Journal of Psychiatric Research*, 12, 189-198.

Goldfarb, R., Eisenson, J., Stocker, B., & DeSanti, S. (1994) Communicative responsibility and semantic task in aphasia and 'schizophasia'. *Perceptual and Motor Skills*, 79, 1027-1039.

Goldfarb, R., & Halpern, H. (1984) Word association responses in normal adult subjects. *Journal of Psycholinguistic Research*, 24, 37-55.

Grasby, P. M., Frith, C. D., Friston, K. J., Simpson, J., Fletcher, P. C., Frackowiak, R. S., & Dolan, R. J. (1994) A graded task approach to the functional mapping of brain areas implicated in auditory-verbal memory. *Brain*, 117, 1271-1282.

Grossman, M., D'Esposito, M., Hughes, E., Onishi, K., Biassou, N., White-Devine, T., & Robinson, K. (1996) Language comprehension profiles in Alzheimer's disease, multi-infarct dementia, and frontotemporal degeneration. *Neurology*, 48, 183-189.

Guilford, J. P. (1967) *The nature of human intelligence.* New York: McGraw-Hill.

Huff, F. J., Corkin, S., & Growdon, J. H. (1986) Semantic impairment and anomia in Alzheimer's disease. *Brain and Language*, 28, 235-249.

Kontiola, P., Laaksonen, R., Sulkava, R., & Erkinjunnti, T. (1990) Pattern of language impairment is different in Alzheimer's disease and multi-infarct dementia. *Brain and Language*, 38, 364-383.

MacDonald, M. C., Almor, A., Henderson, V. W., Kempler, D., & Andersen, E. S. (2001) Assessing working memory and language comprehension in Alzheimer's disease. *Brain and Language*, 78, 17-42.

Palermo, D., & Jenkins, J. (1964) *Word association norms: grade school through college.* Minneapolis, MN: Univer. of Minnesota Press.

Starkweather, C. W., Gottwald, S. R., & Halfond, M. M. (1990) *Stuttering prevention: a clinical method.* Englewood Cliffs, NJ: Prentice Hall.

Stocker, B., & Goldfarb, R. (1995) *The Stocker probe for fluency and language.* Vero Beach, FL: The Speech Bin.

Varma, A., Snowden, J., Lloyd, J., Talbot, P., Mann, D., & Neary, D. (1999) Evaluation of the NINCDS-ADRDA criteria in the differentiation of Alzheimer's disease and frontotemporal dementia. *Journal of Neurology, Neurosurgery, and Psychiatry*, 66, 184-188.

Accepted April 5, 2004.

EFFECTS OF EXPRESSION AND INHIBITION OF NEGATIVE EMOTIONS ON HEALTH, MOOD STATES, AND SALIVARY SECRETORY IMMUNOGLOBULIN A IN JAPANESE MILDLY DEPRESSED UNDERGRADUATES [1]

SHIZUKA TAKAGI   AND   HIDEKI OHIRA

Kobe College   *Nagoya University*

Summary.—Previous studies have indicated that expression of negative emotions facilitates mental and physical health and inhibition of negative emotions increases susceptibility to illness. This study was conducted to examine whether those findings can be expanded to populations with non-Western cultural backgrounds. Specifically, we explored effects of expression and inhibition of negative emotions on health, mood states, and mucosal immune function in mildly depressed Japanese individuals. 16 depressed and 16 nondepressed female undergraduates were required either to write about their unpleasant experiences and superficial topics or to suppress any emotional responses and thoughts about them. Secretory immunoglobulin A (s-IgA) in saliva and psychological indices were measured at an experimental session and at a follow-up 1 wk. later. Beneficial effects of expression of emotions on subjective health were indicated in the nondepressed group, whereas harmful effects of inhibition on subjective health were shown in the depressed group. Emotional expression by writing improved mood states both in the depressed and nondepressed groups but induced elevation of salivary s-IgA only in the depressed group.

Emotional expression has been considered essential to improved mental and physical health outcomes. For example, recent evidence has suggested that emotional expression may facilitate cognitive changes, such as realistic reappraisal of the situation which might lead to more adaptive behaviors (Greenberg & Safran, 1987). Moreover, it has been associated with a variety of physiological changes, such as cardiovascular reactivity, skin conductance activity and immunological functioning (Pennebaker, Kiecolt-Glaser, & Glaser, 1988). By contrast, inhibition of emotion has been considered deleterious, in being related to increased arousal of the autonomic system (Gross & Levenson, 1993) and to producing unexpected cognitive effects such as increased preoccupation with the inhibited material (Wegner, Shortt, Blake, & Page, 1990).

One method of emotional expression recently investigated is expressive writing. An emotional writing paradigm was introduced in work by Penne-

---

[1]Portions of this study were presented in 13th annual convention of the Japanese Association of Health Psychology, 2000 and in the 27th International Congress of Psychology, Stockholm, 2000. The authors thank Michiko Uetsuka and Ayumi Watanabe for assistance for data collection and Dr. Yutaka Watanabe for measurement of s-IgA. Address correspondence to Hideki Ohira, Department of Psychology, Nagoya University, Furo-cho, Chikusa-ku, Nagoya, Japan 464-8601 or e-mail (ohira@lit.nagoya-u.ac.jp).

baker and his colleagues. Many of studies have used Pennebaker's paradigm in that participants are randomly assigned to write, typically once a day for three or four consecutive days, either about affectively negative experiences or trivial topics. In a study by Pennebaker and Francis (1996) using this paradigm, 72 first-year college students were randomly assigned to write about their thoughts and feelings after coming to college or about superficial topics for three consecutive days. This study suggested that the more the participants used positive emotional words in describing deep thoughts and feelings, the more their subjective health improved. Further, adults who had been laid off from their jobs and wrote about the experiences secured new jobs more quickly (Spera, Buhrfeind, & Pennebaker, 1994). Rachman (1980) proposed that, when individuals become accustomed to unwanted thoughts through repeated exposure, their emotional responses to those thoughts should be reduced and then they should be able to forget them more easily.

Given that writing about emotions regarding previous affectively negative and stressful events was related to improved physical and psychological health, writing should affect an important moderator of physical health, namely, the immune system. Effects of writing on the immune system have been shown by a number of studies. Natural killer (NK) cell activity was elevated after emotional writing (Futterman, Kemeny, Shapiro, Polonsky, & Fahey, 1992), and proliferation reactivity of lymphocytes to a mitogen was facilitated after writing (Knapp, Levy, Giorgi, Black, Fox, & Heeren, 1992). Number of CD4+ helper T cells increased after writing (Petrie, Booth, & Pennebaker, 1998). Furthermore, immune response to a vaccination procedure against Hepatitis B virus were enhanced by emotional writing (Petrie, Booth, Pennebaker, Davison, & Thomas, 1995). On the other hand, inhibition of emotion was followed by lower cell-mediated immune responses (Shea, Burtion, & Girgis, 1993) and induced power NK cell activity (Levy, Herberman, Maluish, Schlien, & Lippman, 1985) and decreased number of CD3+ T cells (Petrie, *et al.*, 1998).

Thus, it has been shown that expression of emotion by writing about negative emotions and stressful events is a profoundly powerful technique that influences subjective and objective well-being. However, to our knowledge, no studies about emotional writing from countries other than Europe and North America have been reported. This raises questions about generalizability of the findings about the writing paradigm. The first aim of the present study was to examine whether emotional writing is beneficial also to Japanese people. The second aim of the present study was to expand the previous findings by examining effects of expression and inhibition of negative emotions on health, mood states, and immune function in mildly depressed persons. As previous studies have focused on normal individuals, we do not know the effects of expression and inhibition of emotion in depressed persons. Some studies have suggested that depressed individuals tend to conceal or not to express significant experiences to others (e.g., Ichiyama, Colbert, Laramore, Heim, Corone, & Schmidt, 1993; Derosa, 2000). Also, depressed individuals have been considered to have chronic negative emotions and lower immune function. Specifically, depressive states were related to decreased NK cell percentage and NK cell activity (Fawzy, Fawzy, Hyun, Elashoff, Guthrie, Fahey, & Morton, 1993) and lower proliferation of lymphocytes (Schleifer, Keller, Bond, Cohen, & Stein, 1989). On the basis of these previous findings, we speculated that one of the critical points concerning problems of physical and mental health in depressed individuals should be a tendency to inhibit their negative emotions. In other words, health, mood states, and even immune functions in depressed individuals might be improved if they could express their negative emotional experiences. To test this hypothesis we examined effects of expression and inhibition of negative emotional events on psychological indexes and immune function in depressed persons using a typical Pennebaker writing paradigm.

In this study, salivary secretory immunoglobulin A (s-IgA) was used as an immunological index. S-IgA is a predominant immunoglobulin in saliva (Hood, Weisman, & Wood, 1978) and is a substance for the main immunological defense in mucosal surfaces (Mestecky, 1993). S-IgA can be measured noninvasively with no discomfort, so it is widely used in studies of stress or emotion in psychological fields. Increase of s-IgA concentration has been consistently found following exposure to acute stressors such as brief but demanding stints at air-traffic control (Zeier, Brauchli, & Joller-Jemelka, 1996), football coaching during a match (Kugler, Reintjes, Tewes, & Schedlowski, 1996), and mental arithmetic tasks (e.g., Ohira, Watanabe, Kobayashi, & Kawai, 1999; Ring, Drayson, Walkey, Dale, & Carroll, 2002). On the other hand, chronic or long lasting stress decreases s-IgA levels (e.g., Deinzer & Schuller, 1999). Negative emotions such as depression, anxiety, guilt, and sadness may be important components for psychoneuroimmunomodulation that accompanies chronic stress. If writing is beneficial also for depressed persons, s-IgA concentration should be predicted to increase after writing of negative emotions compared to after inhibition of those, over a relatively long period of time. If the writing paradigm is effective also for depressed persons, the method would have clinical implications for psychotherapy for depression.

Method

Participants and Experimental Design

The sample consisted of 16 depressed and 16 nondepressed female undergraduates (range of age = 18–22 yr.). The participants were selected on the basis of scores on the Zung Self-rating Depression Scale (Zung, 1965) and the Beck Depression Inventory (Beck, Ward, Mendelson, Mock, & Erbaugh, 1961) administered to 372 female undergraduates. Standard cut-off points for diagnosis of mild depression on the Self-rating Depression Scale and Beck Depression Inventory are 48 and 17, respectively. Following these standards and considering marginal zones, those who scored above 50 on the Self-rating Depression Scale and above 20 on the Beck Depression Inventory were selected as Depressed participants. Those who scored below 45 on the Self-rating Depression Scale and below 5 on the Beck Depression Inventory were selected as Nondepressed participants. The participants were randomly assigned to an Expression group or to an Inhibition group ($n = 8$ for each cell). All participants recalled a negatively emotional topic and a superficial topic in different experimental sessions. Thus, a mixed factorial design of 2 (depressed vs nondepressed) × 2 (expression vs inhibition) × 2 (negative emotion vs superficial topic) was adopted. The first two factors were between subjects and the third was a within-subjects factor. One Depressed participant in the Expression group requested to withdraw from the experiment during the session so the number of subjects in this condition was 7.

Measures

We used a Japanese version of the General Health Questionnaire (Goldberg & Hiller, 1979; Goldberg & Williams, 1988) and Multiple Mood Scale developed by Terasaki, Kishimoto, and Koga (1992) as psychological indices. The General Health Questionnaire is a scale consisted of 60 items developed to measure current subjective health. Reliability and validity have been widely confirmed, and the scale has been extensively used in different settings and different cultures including Japan (Nakagawa & Daibo, 1985; Takeuchi & Kitamura, 1991). In responding to the General Health Questionnaire, the participants were asked to describe their state during "the last week" and they answered on 4-point scales (0 = not at all; 3 = very much). Although there has been controversy about the best method for scoring: bimodal (0-0-1-1) vs Likert (0-1-2-3) styles (Goldberg, Gatter, Sartorius, Ustun, Piccinelli, Gureje, & Rutter, 1997). We adopted the traditional bimodal scoring method following Goldberg and Williams (1988). A high score indicates a subjective deficit in mental health and somatic state.

The Multiple Mood Scale consisted of 40 adjective-items that were arranged in eight dimensions: Depression, Hostility, Pleasure, Comfort, Friendliness, Concentration, Surprise, and Boredom. Reliability and the factor structure of this scale were confirmed, at least in the Japanese population (Terasaki, *et al.*, 1992). Because we focused on state depressive mood of participants, we report here only results on the Depression subscale of 5 items. The participants were asked to describe their mood "right now" using 4-point Likert scales anchored by 1 = not at all and 4 = very much. Further, as an immunological index, concentration of salivary s-IgA was evaluated.

Immunological Assay

Saliva was obtained using a cotton swab. The participants were instructed to place the cotton swab under their tongues to collect saliva passively for a 5-min. period. Saliva was extracted from the cotton by centrifugation at 13×10^2 rpm for 5 min. For each sample, saliva volume was measured by weighing the amount extracted. Then, saliva was frozen for storage at $-20°C$ until time of assay. Using a double-antibody enzyme-linked immunosorbent assay (ELISA), s-IgA concentration (μg/ml) was determined. The antibody for human secretory component (MBL, inc.) diluted in coating buffer to 2 μg/ml was attached to each well of 96-well assay plates and incubated at 37°C for 2 hr. After washing, 100 μl saliva samples and reference standard were entered into the wells of the plates. After incubation at 37°C for 2 hr., the plates were again emptied and washed. The antibody for human IgA conjugated with horseradish peroxidase (Wako-junyaku. Inc.) was introduced into each well. The plates were again incubated at 37°C for 2 hr., then emptied and washed. A final incubation at room temperature for 1 hr. induced color development which was stopped by addition of a 50 μl dilution of 1.25% NaF. The reaction produce was quantified spectrophotometrically at 405 nm by a micro-plate reader (Bio-rad. Inc., Model 3550).

Procedure

The experiment was conducted in a sound-attenuated small chamber. The participants were randomly assigned one of two groups in which they were required either to write about emotional and superficial topics (see below) or to inhibit them. The experiment consisted of an experimental session and a follow-up for each topic. In the first session, the participants wrote or inhibited one of the topics, and they were tested in a follow-up session conducted after 1 wk. After an interval of 1 wk. they participated in another session in which they wrote or inhibited the second topic and the second follow-up was after 1 wk. The order of topics was counterbalanced.

In the emotional topic condition both for the Expression and for the Inhibition groups, the participants were instructed to recall and describe the most unpleasant experiences inside of a month. In the Control (superficial topic) condition they were asked to describe what they do every morning. At this period, the participants were instructed to write only objective facts without mentioning any experienced emotions. For each topic, they wrote for 10 min.

After that, manipulation of expression and inhibition was done. The participants in the Expression groups were asked to think about what they had just recalled and given the following instruction: "For the next 5 min. we want you to write about your thoughts and feelings about the events you recalled and wrote. We want you to focus on your inner feelings and to describe them as accurately as possible. It is strongly important to continue writing for 5 min. Writing the same things repeatedly is allowed." The participants in the Inhibition group were instructed as follows: "For the next 5 min. we want you to try not to think about events you just recalled. You must keep sitting quietly. Otherwise, any inner strategies to suppress your thoughts or feelings about the events are allowed. If at any time you think of any of the things you wrote, please make a check mark on a sheet of paper in front of you."

After the writing or inhibition period, the participants rested for 5 min. After the rest, the same tasks of writing and inhibition were administered again for 5 min. The participants' saliva for immunological assays was collected before the experimental session and after the first and the second writing and inhibition periods. Also, the participants completed the Multiple Mood Scale before and after the session, and completed General Health Questionnaire after the session.

In the follow-up (1 wk. later), the participants came to the experimental chamber again. Their saliva was collected and they completed the two scales.

Results

General Health Questionnaire

The General Health Questionnaire was administered to the participants after the experimental session and at the follow-up (see Table 1). Because distribution of the General Health Questionnaire data was positively skewed, a logarithm translation was performed for analyses. The translated total GHQ scores were subjected to a 2 (Subject: depressed vs nondepressed) × 2 (Task: expression vs inhibition) × 2 (Topic: negative emotion vs superficial topic) × 2 (Time: experimental session vs follow-up) mixed analysis of variance. It yielded statistically significant main effects of subject ($F_{1,27}=41.64$, $p<.001$) and time ($F_{1,27}=22.46$, $p<.001$). Not surprisingly, the scores on the General Health Questionnaire for the Depressed group were generally higher than those for the Nondepressed group. Also, these scores generally decreased from the experimental session to the follow-up. Further, interactions of subject and time ($F_{1,27}=13.58$, $p<.01$) and subject, topic, and time ($F_{1,27}=5.06$, $p<.05$) were significant. Considering the very small number of subjects, we conducted power analyses for the above analysis of variance. Observed powers for the significant main effects of subject and time, and interactions of subject × time and subject × topic × time were above .55, suggesting those effects were relatively large. Powers for main effects and interactions which were not significant were below .08, suggesting such effects were weak and difficult to detect in the present study.

Multiple comparisons using *LSD* tests ($p<.05$) gave results as follows.

TABLE 1
Means and Standard Deviations of General Health Questionnaire Scores

	After Session M	After Session SD	Follow-up M	Follow-up SD
Depressed Group				
Expression				
Negative emotion	29.9	14.5	28.0	17.9
Superficial topic	31.0	15.0	27.8	16.8
Inhibition				
Negative emotion	24.0	12.3	29.3	9.1
Superficial topic	25.8	11.6	19.9	7.9
Nondepressed Group				
Expression				
Negative emotion	15.7	11.4	6.1	7.6
Superficial topic	7.4	5.8	4.9	4.0
Inhibition				
Negative emotion	8.4	5.0	4.4	2.2
Superficial topic	9.1	8.1	5.9	4.7

In the Expression group, the scores on the General Health Questionnaire significantly decreased at the follow-up compared to those at the experimental session only in the condition that the Nondepressed participants wrote about their negative emotions. Writing about superficial topics had no effect on the General Health Questionnaire scores. For the Depressed participants, neither writing about negative emotions nor superficial topics had an effect. On the other hand, inhibition of negative emotions was associated with no change in the General Health Questionnaire scores for the Nondepressed group, whereas in the Depressed group, inhibition of negative emotions induced elevation of the General Health Questionnaire score. Inhibition of superficial topics had no effect in either the Depressed or the Nondepressed group.

Mood of Depression

A 2 (Subject: depressed vs nondepressed) × 2 (Task: expression vs inhibition) × 2 (Topic: negative emotion vs superficial topic) × 3 (Time: before session, after session, follow-up) mixed analysis of variance was performed on the scores of the subscale of Depression of the Multiple Mood Scale. Significant main effects of subject ($F_{1,27}=16.62$, $p<.001$) and time ($F_{2,54}=3.70$, $p<.05$) emerged. A significant interaction between subject, task and topic ($F_{1,27}=3.70$, $p<.05$) was noted. Multiple comparisons using *LSD* tests showed (see Table 2) the scores of Depression were higher in the Depressed group than in the Nondepressed group. In the case of inhibition of negative emotions, there was no change in the Depression scores either in the Depressed or the Nondepressed group. On the other hand, the Depression scores significantly decreased at the follow-up compared to two observation points during the experimental session when the participants wrote about their negative emotions both in the Depressed group and in the Nondepressed group. Changes in scores when they wrote about superficial topics were not significant. Power analysis indicated observed powers for the significant main effects and interaction were above .50, suggesting effects of such factors were relatively robust whereas all observed powers for insignificant main effects and interactions were .05, suggesting effect sizes for such factors were small.

TABLE 2
MEANS AND STANDARD DEVIATIONS FOR SCORES OF DEPRESSION SCALE

	Before Session M	Before Session SD	After Session M	After Session SD	Follow-up M	Follow-up SD
Depressed Group						
Expression						
Negative emotion	13.4	3.5	13.5	4.1	11.9	5.1
Superficial topic	12.9	3.5	12.9	3.4	13.4	4.0
Inhibition						
Negative emotion	15.5	3.7	14.4	3.8	14.1	4.2
Superficial topic	12.8	2.1	11.3	4.0	12.0	2.8
Nondepressed Group						
Expression						
Negative emotion	11.4	3.3	11.7	4.5	9.4	3.6
Superficial topic	10.3	3.7	10.0	3.8	8.1	3.4
Inhibition						
Negative emotion	9.1	3.7	9.3	5.2	7.4	2.1
Superficial topic	8.5	3.7	8.6	3.6	8.1	2.8

s-IgA

Means for s-IgA before the experimental session, during the task (writing or inhibition), after the experimental session, and at the follow-up are shown in Table 3. Data for one Depressive participant and one Nondepressive participant (both in the Expression group) were missing because the amount of collected saliva for them was too little for the assay. The data of s-IgA was subjected to a logarithmic transformation because the distribution was positively skewed, and wide individual differences were then subjected to a 2 (Subject: depressed vs nondepressed) × 2 (Task: Expression vs inhibition) × 2 (Topic: negative emotion vs superficial topic) × 4 (Time: before session, during expression (inhibition), after session, follow-up) mixed analysis of variance. Neither main effects nor interactions attained significance ($F <$ 1.90). Power analyses showed observed powers for main effects and interactions were below .10, suggesting that effect of each experimental manipulation on s-IgA was too small to detect in the present because the number of subjects was so small.

TABLE 3
MEANS AND STANDARD DEVIATIONS FOR CONCENTRATION OF SALIVARY s-IgA (μg/ml)

	Before Session		Task		After Session		Follow-up	
	M	SD	M	SD	M	SD	M	SD
Depressed Group								
Expression								
Negative emotion	207.0	258.7	264.4	410.0	140.0	132.7	344.9	64.3
Superficial topic	200.2	180.5	221.7	196.5	149.5	93.5	228.9	311.6
Inhibition								
Negative emotion	102.4	42.7	128.9	45.4	90.6	34.7	115.5	36.3
Superficial topic	113.7	34.9	122.0	72.6	112.6	26.4	92.9	31.5
Nondepressed Group								
Expression								
Negative emotion	159.9	63.8	213.7	126.6	139.9	59.8	157.0	66.1
Superficial topic	182.5	87.5	190.5	112.1	165.5	110.9	150.5	82.1
Inhibition								
Negative emotion	141.8	108.6	139.0	95.2	164.9	176.4	145.5	112.9
Superficial topic	96.8	28.8	139.0	116.6	140.3	143.2	153.5	128.2

However, for exploratory purposes, we compared levels of s-IgA after the experimental session and the follow-up using LSD tests ($p<.05$) and noted that level of s-IgA was significantly larger at follow-up only when the Depressed participants expressed negative emotions by writing. This requires study with more participants for verification.

DISCUSSION

Scores on the General Health Questionnaire for the Nondepressed group were consistent with findings in previous studies (e.g., Pennebaker & Beall, 1986), suggesting that expression of negative emotions should improve subjective health. Inhibition of negative emotions had no influence on the General Health Questionnaire scores probably because the contents of the negative emotions in the Nondepressed group might not be so serious. On the other hand, subjective health was not improved by writing in the Depressed group but inhibition of negative emotions seemed to be related to lower subjective health. These asymmetrical effects of Expression and Inhibition of negative emotions between the Depressed and Nondepressed groups suggest that, for the Depressed group, the negativity of their emotional states might be more severe and inhibition of their emotions might have a more harmful consequence. We speculated that such more severe negative emotional states in the Depressed group might interfere with expressive writing which was beneficial in the Nondepressed group.

Results of scores on the Depression scale showed effects of expression by writing on depressive mood states over 1 wk. Expression of negative emotions induced reduction of the Depression scores 1 wk. later. This effect of emotional expression was shown both in the Nondepressed and Depressed groups. Thus, writing about negative emotions may have improving effects at least on transient mood states even for depressed persons.

We must conservatively interpret the present results of s-IgA because results of power analyses showed that the effect of each factor manipulated in this study on s-IgA level was small. One of the causes for that is a wide individual difference of s-IgA level. However, it was at least suggested that expression of negative emotions by writing may induce elevation of s-IgA level in the Depressed group. Such elevation of s-IgA level at the follow-up might be immuno-enhancement by writing. However, the Depressed group did not report improvement of their subjective health represented by the General Health Questionnaire scores after writing. Inversely, the Nondepressed showed improvement of subjective health after emotional writing although their s-IgA volume was unchanged. These lags between effects of emotional writing on an immune parameter and on a subjective health rating might be due to the temporal characteristics of both the effects. Presumably any psychological factors including emotional writing might first affect the immune function though some physiological pathways, e.g., autonomic nervous or endocrine systems. This should influence the individual's physical health because the immune function is closely related to resistance to disease. However it might take longer for change in the immune function and its effects on health to be cognitively recognized, because we are not necessarily sensitive to biological states of our bodies. Thus, the relatively short interval (1 wk.) between the writing session and the follow-up in the present study might cause the lags between results of s-IgA and subjective health in the Depressed group. On the other hand, such a cascade of biological and psychological effects of writing might progress faster for the Nondepressed group so responses in s-IgA might be terminated until the follow-up. This issue should be clarified in further study.

On the basis of findings of this study, we consider that previous findings about expression and inhibition of negative emotions can be expanded to Japanese people so those effects might be transcultural. Furthermore, expression and inhibition influence subjective health even in mildly depressed individuals. One problem open to research is related to characteristics of cognition processes in depressed individuals. Beck (1963, 1964, 1967) has argued that depressed individuals have pervasive, systematically negative distortions in both cognitive contents and processes such as arbitrary inferences, selective abstraction, and overgeneralization of specific conceptualizations. It should be critical to examine whether these cognitive distortions might mediate effects of expression and inhibition of emotions on health of depressed individuals.

REFERENCES

Beck, A. T. (1963) Thinking and depression: I. Idiosyncratic content and cognitive distortions. *Archives of General Psychiatry*, 9, 324-333.

Beck, A. T. (1964) Thinking and depression: II. Theory and therapy. *Archives of General Psychiatry*, 10, 561-567.

Beck, A. T. (1967) *Depression: clinical, experimental, and theoretical aspects.* New York: Holder.

Beck, A. T., Ward, C. H., Mendelson, M., Mock, J. E., & Erbaugh, J. K. (1961) An inventory for measuring depression. *Archives of General Psychiatry*, 4, 561-571.

Deinzer, R., & Schuller, N. (1999) Dynamics of stress-related decrease of salivary immunoglobulin A (s-IgA): relationship to symptoms of the common cold and studying behavior. *Behavioral Medicine*, 23, 161-169.

DeRosa, T. (2000) Personality, help-seeking attitudes, and depression in adolescents. *Dissertation Abstracts International: Section B: Science and Engineering*, 61, 3273.

Fawzy, F. I., Fawzy, N. W., Hyun, C. S., Elashoff, R., Guthrie, D., Fahey, J. L., & Morton, D. L. (1993) Malignant melanoma: effects of an early structured psychiatric intervention, coping, and affective state on recurrence and survival six years later. *Archives of General Psychiatry*, 50, 681-689.

Futterman, A. D., Kemeny, M. E., Shapiro, D. P., Polonsky, W., & Fahey, J. L. (1992) Immunological variability associated with experimentally-induced positive and negative affective states. *Psychological Medicine*, 22, 231-238.

Goldberg, D. P., Gatter, R., Sartorius, N., Ustun, T. B., Piccinelli, M., Gureje, O., & Rutter, C. (1997) The validity of two versions of the GHQ in the WHO study of mental illness in general health care. *Psychological Medicine*, 27, 191-197.

Goldberg, D. P., & Hiller, V. F. (1979) A scaled version of the General Health Questionnaire. *Psychological Medicine*, 9, 139-145.

Goldberg, D. P., & Williams, P. (1988) *A user's guide to the General Health Questionnaire.* Windsor, UK: NFER-Nelson.

Greenberg, L. S., & Safran, J. D. (1987) *Emotion in psychotherapy.* New York: Guilford.

Gross, J., & Levenson, R. W. (1993) Emotional suppression: physiology, self-report, and expressive behavior. *Journal of Personality and Social Psychology*, 64, 970-986.

Hood, L. E., Weisman, I. L., & Wood, W. B. (1978) *Immunology.* Menlo Park, CA: Benjamin/Cummings.

Ichiyama, M. A., Colbert, D., Laramore, H., Heim, M., Corone, K., & Schmidt, J. (1993) Self-concealment and correlates of adjustment in college students. *Journal of Student Psychotherapy*, 7, 55-68.

Knapp, P. H., Levy, E. M., Giorgi, R. G., Black, P. H., Fox, B. H., & Heeren, T. C. (1992) Short-term immunological effects of induced emotion. *Psychosomatic Medicine*, 54, 133-148.

Kugler, J., Reintjes, F., Tewes, V., & Schedlowski, M. (1996) Competition stress in soccer coaches increases salivary immunoglobulin A and salivary cortisol concentrations. *The Journal of Sports Medicine and Physical Fitness*, 36, 117-120.

Levy, S. M., Herberman, R. B., Maluish, A. M., Schlien, B., & Lippman, M. (1985) Prognostic risk assessment in primary breast cancer by behavioral and immunological parameters. *Health Psychology*, 4, 99-113.

Mestecky, J. (1993) Saliva as a manifestation of the common mucosal immune system. *Annals of the New York Academy of Sciences*, 694, 189-194.

Nakagawa, Y., & Daibo, I. (1985) [*User's guide to Japanese version of the General Health Questionnaire*]. Tokyo, Japan: Nihon Bunka Kagakusha.

Ohira, H., Watanabe, Y., Kobayashi, K., & Kawai, M. (1999) The type A behavior pattern and immune reactivity to brief stress: change of volume of secretory immunoglobulin A in saliva. *Perceptual and Motor Skills*, 89, 423-430.

Pennebaker, J. W., & Beall, S. K. (1986) Confronting a traumatic event: toward an understanding of inhibition and disease. *Journal of Abnormal Psychology*, 95, 274-281.

Pennebaker, J. W., & Francis, M. E. (1996) Cognitive, emotional, and language processes in disclosure. *Cognition and Emotion*, 10, 601-626.

PENNEBAKER, J. W., KIECOLT-GLASER, J. K., & GLASER, R. (1988) Disclosure of traumas and immune function: health implications for psychotherapy. *Journal of Consulting and Clinical Psychology*, 56, 239-245.

PETRIE, K. J., BOOTH, R. J., & PENNEBAKER, J. W. (1998) The immunological effects of thought suppression. *Journal of Personality and Social Psychology*, 75, 1264-1272.

PETRIE, K. J., BOOTH, R. J., PENNEBAKER, J. W., DAVISON, K. P., & THOMAS, M. G. (1995) Disclosure of trauma and immune response to a hepatitis B vaccination program. *Journal of Consulting and Clinical Psychology*, 63, 787-792.

RACHMAN, S. J. (1980) Emotional processing. *Behavior Research and Therapy*, 18, 51-60.

RING, C., DRAYSON, M., WALKEY, D. G., DALE, S., & CARROLL, D. (2002) Secretory immunoglobulin A reactions to prolonged mental arithmetic stress: inter-session and intra-session reliability. *Biological Psychology*, 59, 1-13.

SCHLEIFER, S. J., KELLER, S. E., BOND, R. N., COHEN, J., & STEIN, M. (1989) Major depressive disorder and immunity: role of age, sex, severity, and hospitalization. *Archives of General Psychiatry*, 61, 81-87.

SHEA, J. D., BURTION, R., & GIRGIS, A. (1993) Negative effect, absorption, and immunity. *Physiological Behavior*, 53, 449-457.

SPERA, S. P., BUHRFEIND, E. D., & PENNEBAKER, J. W. (1994) Expressive writing and coping with job loss. *Academy of Management Journal*, 37, 722-733.

TAKEUCHI, M., & KITAMURA, T. (1991) The factor structure of the General Health Questionnaire in a Japanese high school and university student sample. *The International Journal of Social Psychiatry*, 37, 99-106.

TERASAKI, M., KISHIMOTO, Y., & KOGA, A. (1992) [Construction of a multiple mood scale]. [*Japanese Journal of Psychology*], 62, 350-356. [in Japanese with English abstract]

WEGNER, D. M., SHORTT, J. W., BLAKE, A. W., & PAGE, M. S. (1990) The suppression of exciting thoughts. *Journal of Personality and Social Psychology*, 55, 882-892.

ZEIER, H., BRAUCHLI, P., & JOLLER-JEMELKA, H. I. (1996) Effects of work demands on immunoglobulin A and cortisol in air traffic controllers. *Biological Psychology*, 42, 413-423.

ZUNG, W. W. K. (1965) A self-rating depression scale. *Archives of General Psychiatry*, 12, 63-70.

Accepted April 7, 2004.

LATERAL DIFFERENCE AND INTERHEMISPHERIC TRANSFER ON ARM-POSITIONING MOVEMENT BETWEEN RIGHT AND LEFT HANDERS [1]

MASAKI YAMAUCHI

Faculty of Education
Nagasaki University

KUNIYASU IMANAKA

Graduate School of Science
Tokyo Metropolitan University

MASAO NAKAYAMA AND SHO NISHIZAWA

Faculty of Education
Nagasaki University

Summary.—We investigated the transfer of an arm-positioning movement between the right and left arms of right and left handers. 30 male (15 strong right handers and 15 strong left handers) subjects were asked to perform a constrained criterion movement, 12 cm in length, with right or left arm and a test movement at estimated 6-, 12-, or 24-cm length with the contralateral arm. In the right handers, the constant error of the left arm test movement was near zero, and that of the right arm indicated overshooting. In the left handers, the constant errors of the left arm test movement were farther from zero than those of right arm test movement. Left handers as well as right handers showed manual asymmetry on positioning movement. A plausible explanation for the manual asymmetry on the arm-positioning task is related to interhemispheric transfer of spatial information on positioning movement.

Many investigators have presented explanations for the manual asymmetries for motor performance. These include anatomical asymmetry (Amunts, Schlaug, Schleicher, Steinmetz, Dabringhaus, Roland, & Zilles, 1996; Amunts, Jäncke, Mohlberg, Steinmetz, & Zilles, 2000), innervation of limb muscles (Brinkman & Kuypers, 1972; Todor, Kyprie, & Price, 1982), attention and hemispace (Kinsbourne & Hicks, 1978; Bowers & Heilman, 1980; Bradshaw, Nathan, Nettleton, Wilson, & Pierson, 1987; Barthelemy & Boulinguez, 2001), cognitive strategy (Colley, 1984; Nishizawa, 1987), and directions of interhemispheric transfer (Cook, 1986; Velay & Benoit-Dubrocard, 1999; Velay, Daffaure, Raphael, & Benoit-Dubrocard, 2001). Among these factors, the role of interhemispheric transfer is important for hemispheric asymmetry. Cook (1986) emphasized the role of the corpus callosum for hemispheric functional asymmetries.

In conjunction with the interhemispheric communication, Hatta (1975) investigated hemisphere asymmetries of random forms using the matching

---

[1]Address correspondence to Masaki Yamauchi, Department of Health and Physical Education, Faculty of Education, Nagasaki University, 1-14 Bunkyou-machi, Nagasaki 852-8521, Japan or e-mail (yamauchi@net.nagasaki-u.ac.jp).

judgments method devised by Hatta. The matching method was based on the following: if the right hemisphere is superior to the left hemisphere in the cognition of nonverbal materials (random forms), the right hemisphere, which first receives the standard stimuli (left visual field ahead condition) is more accurate than the left hemisphere (right visual field ahead condition). In subsequent studies, the same author showed that the matching method accurately identified hemisphere laterality for verbal materials (Hatta, 1976a) and nonverbal materials (Hatta, 1976b) in right handers. According to the model proposed by Hatta, one can predict the interhemispheric transfer of spatial information from the right hemisphere to the left is much more effective for processing and transferring spatial information (with much less information-loss) than the transfer from the left hemisphere to the right.

In contrast to the above model, Haude, Morrow-Tlucak, Fox, and Pickard (1987) examined differential visual field-hemispheric transfer of spatial information using a dot-location task (Kimura, 1969). The right-handed subjects in their study showed significant improvement when stimuli were presented to the left visual field of the right hemisphere after practice on the same task presented to the right visual field of the left hemisphere first. No improvement was found when the task was presented to the right visual field of the left hemisphere. They concluded that for right handers, transfer of spatial information to the right hemisphere is facilitated while transfer to the left hemisphere is inhibited, suggesting that the direction of interhemispheric communication is an important factor in lateral differences on spatial task.

A motor-positioning task can be regarded as a spatial localization task with the information processing for execution of the task being generated in the right hemisphere (Roy & MacKenzie, 1978; Grünewald, Grünewald-Zuberbier, Hömberg, & Schuhmacher, 1984; Kurian, Sharma, & Santhakumari, 1989). Roy and MacKenzie (1978) proposed that the right hemisphere may be dominant for spatial discrimination. They, then, examined the laterality of cerebral function with specific reference to lateralization of positioning in space in the kinesthetic modality. The results showed that the left hand was more accurate than the right and suggested that the right hemisphere is dominant for spatial discrimination judgments. Kurian, et al. (1989) also indicated that kinesthetic information arises mainly from changes in the length, tension, and compression, and that such information is probably processed by the right hemisphere of the brain.

Thus, if Hatta's model is applied to an arm-positioning task that demands spatial discrimination judgments, one can assume that when the criterion movement is executed with the left arm, the performance of test movement with right arm will be superior to that with the left because we can interpret that the spatial information in the movement task with the left arm is processed directly by the right hemisphere prior to the left hemisphere. However, this hypothesis disagrees with the prediction of interhemispheric transfer model by Haude, *et al.* (1987), in which the transfer of spatial information to the right hemisphere is facilitated while transfer to the left hemisphere is inhibited. One aim of the present study was to determine the best model, Hatta or Haude, to explain manual asymmetry of arm positioning movement.

The other aim of the present study was to estimate the relationship between handedness and cerebral specialization. Hicks and Kinsbourne (1978) mentioned in their review that hand preference in humans correlates with cerebral specialization for various functions. The interest in handedness lies in the assumption that knowledge of handedness can help us predict something about cerebral organization (Bryden, Bulman-Fleming, & MacDonald, 1996). There is a general agreement that left handedness is somewhat less lateralized than right handedness. Boulinguez, Velay, and Nougier (2001), however, indicated that the relationship between handedness and cerebral functional lateralization is still unclear and claimed that the relations between handedness and hemispheric asymmetries for a variety of perceptual and cognitive-motor processes involved in movement control must be reconsidered.

The purpose of the present study was to examine the following two problems, (1) identify the best of the two models, Hatta or Haude model, to explain manual asymmetry and (2) determine the difference in lateral dominance on arm positioning movement between right-handed and left-handed subjects.

Method

Subjects

Subjects were 30 undergraduate men from Nagasaki University. They ranged in age from 18 to 22 years, and half of them were strongly right handers, and the remaining subjects were strongly left handers. Their handedness was discriminated using H. N. Handedness Inventory (Hatta & Nakatsuka, 1975, 1976). All subjects were volunteers and naive to the purpose of the experiment. The study protocol was performed in accordance with the 2001 Declaration of Helsinki, and verbal consent was obtained from each subject.

Apparatus

The apparatus (cf. Yamauchi, Imanaka, Nakayama, & Matsunaga, 1998) was composed of two boxes (20 cm × 50 cm × 10 cm), each of which opened at the front (subject side) and at the back (experimenter side). The two boxes were fixed on a table side by side on a parallel plane in front of the subject. This allowed the subject to make linear arm positioning movements by moving the handle-plate with either the left or the right hand within the left or right box, respectively. A horizontal linear metal track was mounted inside each box, and a vertical handle-plate was attached on a small carriage that could move freely in a left-to-right direction along the track.

A point 5 cm to the right or left from the midline of the body was the starting position of the arm positioning movement. Both the start and end positions of the linear arm movements were measured to the nearest millimeter using a photosensor attached to the small carriage. Signals from the photosensor were digitized and stored on a personal computer (NEC PC-9801). During the experiment, the subject put on a set of headphones that emitted white noise and tone signals used for indicating either the time for hand placement on the handle-plate, or the time for making a linear movement as a criterion or test trial. The experimental procedure was controlled by the preprogramed personal computer (NEC PC-9801).

Task

A task consisted of a criterion movement, a retention interval, and a test movement. Each subject was required to make a constrained criterion movement of 12 cm in length and asked to make the movement at length of 6, 12, or 24 cm (cf. Yamauchi, *et al.*, 1998). The length of criterion movement was set at 12 cm, so that the distances of test movement (6, 12, 24 cm) would fall within an appropriate movement range. This movement range was reported to be reliable for both cues of distance and location (Roy & Kelso, 1977; Imanaka, Funase, & Yamauchi, 1995). Because the 6-cm and 24-cm test movements were half or double the length of the criterion movement, the information processing needed for the performance of the task should involve complex psychological processes, e.g., inferential thought (Hatta, 1977), which mediate in the imaging of half or double the length of the criterion movement.

A block of six trials randomized, consisting of all probable combinations of the two experimental variables, arm (left and right) and test movement length (6, 12, and 24 cm), was repeated six times. A trial started with the emission of white noise and, 5 sec. later, the subject was ready to perform the criterion movement with a preparatory single beep. Then, after 3 sec., a starting double beep was used. A preparatory single beep for the next test movement was emitted after a 10-sec. retention interval. After 3 sec., a double beep was used to indicate that the test movement should be performed. Ten sec. later, the white noise was eliminated to indicate the completion of the trial sequence. The intertrial interval was 10 sec.

Procedure

The subject was seated in front of the positioning apparatus in a relaxed posture and then was told the purpose and procedure of the experiment. The subject was then asked to put on the headphones and blindfold, and then instructed to keep both hands on the lap. The experimenter set the handle-plate to the left or right by 5 cm from the midline of the subject's body and the stopper to the left or right by 12 cm from the starting position. After that, the experimenter told each subject which of the arms (left or right) must be used for the criterion movement, and after the preparatory single beep, the subject held the handle-plate with the instructed hand.

Following the next double beep, each subject moved the handle-plate away from the body until the stopper blocked it (criterion movement). After completing the criterion movement, the subject returned his hand to the lap. During about 10-sec. retention interval, the experimenter replaced the handle-plate at the original starting position and removed the stopper. Then, the experimenter verbally informed the volunteer to execute the test movement at a length equal to, half, and double the criterion movement as estimated by each subject. On hearing the next preparatory single beep, the subject held the handle-plate with the other arm than the criterion movement, then at the starting double beep signaled 3 sec. later, the test movement started from the midline of the body to the outside. Prior to the experimental trials, a practice session, which consisted of all combinations of the two experimental conditions, was executed to familiarize the subject with the experimental apparatus and procedure.

Experimental Design

We analyzed three independent variables, handedness (left handed and right handed), representing a between-subjects factor, and arms (left and right) and test movement (6, 12, 24 cm), which both represent within-subject factors. Three dependent variables, constant error (CE), variable error (VE), and absolute error (AE), were calculated and recorded. CE is a measure of the deviation of a response from successful test movement, indicating response bias either undershooting (negative CE) or an overshooting (positive CE). VE is a measure of the standard deviation of CE scores (six trials in this study), indicating the response consistency. AE, which is the absolute value of the CE scores, indicates overall accuracy (Schmidt, 1988).

RESULTS

The mean and standard deviation values of CE, VE, and AE scores are presented in Table 1. Each error score was analyzed by 2 handedness groups (left hander, right hander) × 2 arms (left, right) × 3 test movement lengths (6 cm, 12 cm, 24 cm) analysis of variance.

Constant Error

Analysis of variance of the constant error scores showed no significant

TABLE 1
Test Movement Errors For Each Arm of Left Handers and Right Handers ($ns = 15$)

Error	Left Handers				Right Handers			
	Left Arm		Right Arm		Left Arm		Right Arm	
	M	SEM	M	SEM	M	SEM	M	SEM
Constant Error								
Half, 6 cm	7.1	3.4	5.5	2.5	5.5	3.4	15.2	2.7
Same, 12 cm	7.9	3.1	1.0	3.5	1.8	4.6	21.0	4.4
Double, 24 cm	12.0	6.7	1.8	7.4	−.62	7.6	11.8	8.0
Variable Error								
Half, 6 cm	8.2	0.9	6.7	0.6	8.9	0.8	10.0	1.3
Same, 12 cm	14.0	1.8	13.0	1.0	15.0	1.2	15.0	1.2
Double, 24 cm	27.0	2.3	20.0	2.2	22.0	2.8	25.0	2.6
Absolute Error								
Half, 6 cm	13.0	2.1	9.9	1.6	13.0	2.2	17.0	2.4
Same, 12 cm	16.0	1.8	15.0	1.6	19.0	2.4	5.0	3.0
Double, 24 cm	33.0	3.0	30.0	3.5	33.0	2.8	35.0	3.6

main effect for handedness ($F_{1,28} < 1.10$), arm ($F_{1,28} = 2.03$, ns), or test movement lengths ($F_{2,56} < 1.0$). The three-way interaction was significant ($F_{2,56} = 3.71$, $p < .04$). Two-way analysis of variance was then conducted with each handedness group. This analysis showed a significant main effect for the arm side in the right-handed subjects ($F_{1,14} = 13.54$, $p < .01$) but not in the left-handed subjects. There were no significant interactions for both groups (Fig. 1). The mean constant error scores of all test movement lengths (calculated using all data from three test movement-length conditions) of the right and left arms in right-handed subjects were 16.0 mm ($SD = 21.9$) and 0.38 mm ($SD = 21.1$), respectively. This right arm score was significantly different from zero ($t_{44} = 4.85$, $p < .01$), while the left arm score was not significantly different from zero[2] ($t_{44} = 0.11$, $p > .10$). In left-handed subjects, the mean constant error for all movements was 2.78 mm ($SD = 19.21$) and 8.98 mm ($SD = 1.27$) for the right and left arms, respectively. The left arm score was significantly different from zero[2] ($t_{44} = 3.26$, $p < .01$), while the right arm score was not ($t_{44} = 0.97$, ns). These results show that in right-handed subjects, overshooting by the right arm is greater than that by the left arm, and there is a clear overshooting by the preferred arm in left-handed subjects as well as right-handed subjects.

Variable Error

The analysis on variable error yielded a significant three-way interaction ($F_{2,56} = 3.91$, $p < .03$). Two-way analysis of variance was then conducted sepa-

---

[2]This was tested by using the Student t test calculated between the right arm condition and a hypothetical condition in which the mean constant error score was assumed to be 0 mm and the SD was assumed to be the same as that of each arm condition.

rately for the two different handedness groups. The result of analysis in right-handed subjects showed a significant main effect for length of test movements ($F_{2,28} = 27.33$, $p < .001$). In left-handed subjects, there were two significant main effects for arm of test movements ($F_{1,14} = 6.57$, $p < .03$) and length of test movements ($F_{2,28} = 34.12$, $p < .001$). The simple interaction between arm of test movement and length of test movement was not significant ($F_{2,28} = 3.08$, $p = .06$). These results indicate that in left-handed subjects, the variability of right arm test movement is less than that of the left arm, and in both groups, the variability of both arms increased in proportion with the length of test movements.

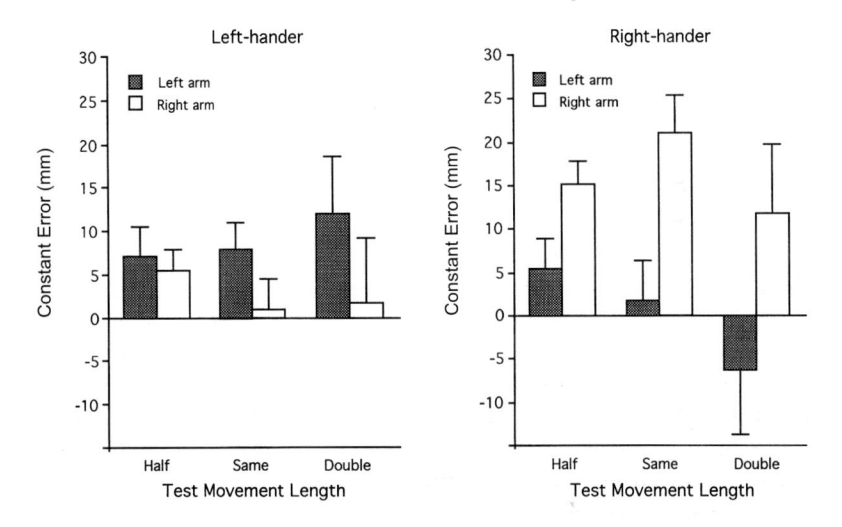

FIG. 1. Mean ± *SEM* of constant error in test movement of each arm in left and right handers

Absolute Error

Three-way analysis of variance on absolute error scores showed a significant main effect for test movement length ($F_{2,56} = 63.54$, $p < .0001$). A *post hoc* test of the main effect was calculated with a Fisher PLSD. There was a significant difference between 6-cm test movement ($M = 13.37$, $SD = 8.56$) and 12-cm test movement ($M = 18.78$, $SD = 9.70$; $p < .03$), 6-cm test movement and 24-cm test movement ($M = 32.81$, $SD = 12.80$; $p < .001$), and 12-cm test movement and 24-cm test movement ($p < .001$). As two-way interaction between arm of test movement and handedness group was significant ($F_{1,28} = 4.97$, $p < .04$), one-way analysis of variance was conducted with each handedness group. In the left-handed subjects, there was no significant difference between left and right arm ($F_{1,45} = 1.85$, ns). In right-handed subjects, significance of the difference between right and left arm was borderline ($F_{1,44} =$

3.77, $p < .06$). These results indicate that the test movements using the left arm tend to be more accurate than those using the right arm of right-handed subjects. However, the results of left-handed subjects indicate that there was no difference in the accuracy of linear movement between the right and left arms.

Discussion

The purpose of the present study was to select the better model, the Hatta or Haude model, that can appropriately explain manual asymmetry on a positioning-movement task and whether the manual asymmetry is different between right-handed and left-handed subjects. Our results showed that in right-handed subjects, the constant error of test movement using the left arm (right arm criterion movement) was close to zero while that using the right arm (left arm criterion movement) showed overshooting. In contrast to right-handed subjects, the constant error of test movement of left-handed subjects using the left arm showed overshooting while the right arm constant error was closer to zero than the left arm. The right arm in the right-handed subjects (the left arm in the left-handed subjects) may consistently overshoot the target because the right hemisphere (the left hemisphere in the left-handed subjects) may actually be overestimating the conditioned distance, providing inaccurate spatial information to the left hemisphere (right hemisphere in the left-handed subjects). It would have been informative to have had subjects estimate conditioned distances with each hand and to compare the performance of each hemisphere when the same hand performs both the criterion and test movements. If those are to be informative, interhemispheric communication through the corpus callosum would be important for cerebral functional asymmetry.

Our results indicate that there is manual asymmetry on the positioning-movement task for right-handed subjects. Further, the results also indicate that the relative position between left arm error score and right arm error score in right-handed subjects is the reverse of that in left-handed subjects, although previous reports indicated that the hand asymmetry in left-handed subjects was weak or absent (Velay & Benoit-Dubrocard, 1999; Civardi, Cavalli, Naldi, Varrasi, & Cantello, 2000; Boulinguez, et al., 2001). According to the assumption by Hatta (1976b), when the left arm for criterion movement was used followed by the use of the right arm for test movement, the performance of test movement with the right arm should be superior to that with the left arm. It is thought that the spatial information processing in left arm-positioning movement makes direct and first input with the right cerebral hemisphere. However, the results of the present study contradicted Hatta's hypothesis.

Our results can be interpreted based on the hypothesis of direction of interhemispheric transformation proposed by Haude, et al. (1987). In right handers, the transfer of spatial information in the right arm criterion movement (in the left hemisphere) to the right hemisphere is facilitated while transfer to the left hemisphere is inhibited. Thus, the left arm test (right arm criterion) movement was superior to the right arm test (left arm criterion) movement. These results suggest that hemispheric functional lateralization for the processing of spatial information in movement task reflects the direction of interhemispheric communication (Cook, 1986; Haude, et al., 1987). The important role of pathways of interhemispheric transfer for visuomotor task has also been demonstrated in a study using positron emission tomography (PET) (Marzi, Perani, Tassinari, Colleluori, Maravita, Miniussi, Paulesu, Scifo, & Fazio, 1999). Furthermore, Velay and Benoit-Dubrocard (1999) also suggested that the transferred information might differ in the two directions, i.e., from the right hemisphere to left hemisphere and from left hemisphere to right hemisphere, which may explain the very asymmetric interhemispheric transfer time of the left-handed subjects.

Another interesting result of the present study was the clear difference of positioning performance between right and left arms in the left-handed subjects as well as in the right-handed subjects. Although several studies have examined the relationship between handedness and functional asymmetry of the cerebral hemisphere, only a few have examined interhemispheric transfer in directed movement (see reviews by Roy, 1996; Velay & Benoit-Dubrocard, 1999). Velay and Benoit-Dubrocard (1999) assumed that manual asymmetry by interhemispheric communication during visuomanual pointing movement is clear for right handers but weaker or absent for left handers. Their results for normal subjects, however, showed no difference between right handers and left handers or between the hands. However, in a partially callosotomized left-handed subject, they found an asymmetry of interhemispheric transfer time with different directions of transfer. The results in left-handed patients suggest the possible existence of different callosal locations for the interhemispheric transfer and may agree with our understanding that the manual asymmetry in a motor-positioning task also occurs in left-handed subjects. However, further studies are needed to explain the relationship between human handedness and asymmetry because it is also reported that left handers showed no asymmetry (Civardi, et al., 2000; Boulinguez, et al., 2001).

In summary, we provided evidence that hemispheric functional asymmetry in positioning-movement task seems to reflect direction of interhemispheric transfer mentioned by Haude, et al. (1987). Furthermore, this manual asymmetry appeared in not only right handers but also left handers.

REFERENCES

Amunts, K., Jäncke, L., Mohlberg, H., Steinmetz, H., & Zilles, K. (2000) Interhemispheric asymmetry of the human motor cortex related to handedness and gender. *Neuropsychologia*, 38, 304-312.
Amunts, K., Schlaug, G., Schleicher, A., Steinmetz, H., Dabringhaus, A., Roland, P. E., & Zilles, K. (1996) Asymmetry in the human motor cortex and handedness. *Neuroimage*, 4, 216-222.
Barthelemy, S., & Boulinguez, P. (2001) Manual reaction time asymmetries in human subjects: the role of movement planning and attention. *Neuroscience Letters*, 315, 41-44.
Boulinguez, P., Velay, J. L., & Nougier, V. (2001) Manual asymmetries in reaching movement control: II. Study of left-handers. *Cortex*, 37, 123-138.
Bowers, D., & Heilman, K. M. (1980) Pseudoneglect: effects of hemispace on a tactile line bisection task. *Neuropsychologia*, 18, 491-498.
Bradshaw, J. L., Nathan, G., Nettleton, N. C., Wilson, L., & Pierson, J. (1987) Why is there a left side underestimation in rod bisection? *Neuropsychologia*, 25, 735-738.
Brinkman, J., & Kuypers, H. G. J. M. (1972) Splitbrain monkeys: cerebral control of ipsilateral and contralateral arm, hand, and finger movements. *Science*, 176, 536-539.
Bryden, M. P., Bulman-Fleming, M. B., & MacDonald, V. (1996) The measurement of handedness and its relation to neuropsychological issues. In D. Elliott & E. A. Roy (Eds.), *Manual asymmetries in motor performance*. Boca Raton, FL: CRC Press. Pp. 57-81.
Civardi, C., Cavalli, A., Naldi, P., Varrasi, C., & Cantello, R. (2000) Hemispheric asymmetry of cortico-cortical connections in human hand motor areas. *Clinical Neurophysiology*, 111, 624-629.
Colley, A. (1984) Spatial location judgements by right and left-handers. *Cortex*, 20, 47-53.
Cook, N. D. (1986) *The brain cord: mechanisms of information transfer and the role of the corpus callosum*. London & New York: Methuen.
Grünewald, G., Grünewald-Zuberbier, E., Hömberg, V., & Schuhmacher, H. (1984) Hemispheric asymmetry of feedback-related slow negative potential shifts in a positioning movement task. *Annals of the New York Academy of Sciences*, 425, 470-476.
Hatta, T. (1975) [Functional hemispheric asymmetry in perception of random forms]. [*The Japanese Journal of Psychology*], 46, 152-161. [English abstract]
Hatta, T. (1976a) Asynchrony of lateral onset as a factor in difference in visual field. *Perceptual and Motor Skills*, 42, 163-166.
Hatta, T. (1976b) Hemisphere asymmetries in the perception and memory of random forms. *Psychologia*, 19, 157-162.
Hatta, T. (1977) Functional hemisphere asymmetries in an inferential thought task. *Psychologia*, 20, 145-150.
Hatta, T., & Nakatsuka, Z. (1975) [The H. N. Inventory]. In S. Ono (Ed.), *Papers in celebration of 63 year birthday of Prof. K. Onishi*. Osaka, Japan: Osaka City Univer. Press. Pp. 224-247. [in Japanese]
Hatta, T., & Nakatsuka, Z. (1976) Note on hand preference of Japanese people. *Perceptual and Motor Skills*, 42, 530.
Haude, R. H., Morrow-Tlucak, M., Fox, D. M., & Pickard, K. B. (1987) Differential visual field-interhemispheric transfer: can it explain sex and handedness differences in lateralization? *Perceptual and Motor Skills*, 65, 423-429.
Hicks, R. E., & Kinsbourne, M. (1978) Human handedness. In M. Kinsbourne (Ed.), *Asymmetrical function of the brain*. New York: Cambridge Univer. Press. Pp. 523-549.
Imanaka, K., Funase, K., & Yamauchi, M. (1995) Behavioral models of motor control and short-term memory. *Bulletin of the Faculty of Liberal Arts, Nagasaki University (Natural Science)*, 35, 95-123.
Kimura, D. (1969) Spatial localization in left and right visual fields. *Canadian Journal of Psychology*, 23, 445-458.
Kinsbourne, M., & Hicks, R. E. (1978) Mapping cerebral functional space: competition and collaboration in human performance. In M. Kinsbourne (Ed.), *Asymmetrical function of the brain*. New York: Cambridge Univer. Press. Pp. 267-273.
Kurian, G., Sharma, N. K., & Santhakumari, K. (1989) Left-arm dominance in active positioning. *Perceptual and Motor Skills*, 68, 1312-1314.

Marzi, C. A., Perani, D., Tassinari, G., Colleluori, A., Maravita, A., Miniussi, C., Paulesu, E., Scifo, P., & Fazio, F. (1999) Pathways of interhemispheric transfer in normals and in a split-brain subject. *Experimental Brain Research*, 126, 451-458.

Nishizawa, S. (1987) Handedness: II. Laterality of spatial and weight discrimination guided by kinesthesis. *Memoria, Seitoku Junior College of Nutrition*, 18, 53-57.

Roy, E. A. (1996) Hand preference, manual asymmetries, and limb apraxia. In D. Elliott & E. A. Roy (Eds.), *Manual asymmetries in motor performance*. Boca Raton, FL: CRC Press. Pp. 215-236.

Roy, E. A., & Kelso, J. A. S. (1977) Movement cues in motor memory: precuing versus postcuing. *Journal of Human Movement Studies*, 3, 232-239.

Roy, E. A., & MacKenzie, C. (1978) Handedness effects in kinesthetic spatial location judgements. *Cortex*, 14, 250-258.

Schmidt, R. A. (1988) *Motor control and learning*. (2nd ed.) Champaign, IL: Human Kinetics.

Todor, J. I., Kyprie, P. M., & Price, H. L. (1982) Lateral asymmetries in arm, wrist and finger movements. *Cortex*, 18, 515-523.

Velay, J-L., & Benoit-Dubrocard, S. (1999) Hemispheric asymmetry and interhemispheric transfer in reaching programming. *Neuropsychologia*, 37, 895-903.

Velay, J-L., Daffaure, V., Raphael, N., & Benoit-Dubrocard, S. (2001) Hemispheric asymmetry and interhemispheric transfer in pointing depend on the spatial components of the movement. *Cortex*, 37, 75-90.

Yamauchi, M., Imanaka, K., Nakayama, M., & Matsunaga, J. (1998) Lateral difference in the reproduction of arm positioning movement: an examination of the hypothesis on the levels of psychological processes. *Applied Human Science: Journal of Physiological Anthropology*, 17, 41-47.

Accepted April 7, 2004.

KNOWLEDGE AND INFORMATION IN PREDICTION OF INTENTION TO PLAY BADMINTON [1]

EVANGELOS BEBETSOS, PANAGIOTIS ANTONIOU,
OLGA KOULI, GEORGIOS TRIKAS

Democritus University of Thrace

Summary.—The aim of this preliminary study was to investigate the contributions of knowledge and information to the prediction of students' intention to play badminton. The sample, 121 students (53 men and 68 women) 18–25 years of age, were beginning students in a semester badminton course. A questionnaire was completed before and after the course (4 mo.). Hierarchical regression analyses showed strong association between the examined variables of the Planned Behavior Questionnaire, specifically signifying that knowledge, information, attitudes, subjective norms, perceived behavioral control, role identity, and attitude strength could account for anticipation of intention towards playing badminton. Overall, systematic access to information and knowledge appeared to accompany relatively greater intentions.

In recent years, many researchers have examined the relation of attitudes to behavior. In the area of sport psychology and exercise, mainstream psychological models have been utilized to predict participants' intentions to become involved in exercise and to increase the understanding of factors in voluntary behavior.

According to the theory of planned behavior, behavior is preceded by an intention. The probability of performing a specific behavior is referred to as 'behavioral intention'. The stronger one's intention the greater the likelihood one will act on that intention (Ajzen & Fishbein, 1980). Intention is determined by a combination of (i) attitude towards the behavior (that is, a positive or negative predisposition towards a specific behavior) and (ii) subjective norms (Ajzen & Fishbein, 1972). These subjective norms are for behavioral beliefs, which reflect attitude towards the behavior, and normative beliefs, which reflect social factors. Each behavioral belief reflects whether important others would approve or disapprove of the behavior (Tesser & Shaffer, 1990). The reasoned action model is effective in examining behaviors over which individuals have high control (Ajzen, 1987).

Additionally, according to theory (Ajzen, 1987, 1988), the execution of behavior does not relate only to the person's intentions. Although behavior can be totally under subjects' control, in most cases various obstacles are present which impinge on the person's decisions to execute a particular be-

---

[1]The authors thank Dr. Marios Goudas, for helpful comments on the manuscript. Address correspondence to Dr. Evangelos Bebetsos, Democritus University, Department of Physical Education and Sport Sciences, Komotini 69100, Hellas or e-mail (empempet@phyed.duth.gr).

havior. Such obstacles can be internal factors, such as agility, knowledge, and planning, or external factors, such as time, opportunity, cooperation with others and so on (Ajzen & Madden, 1986).

Two variables have been added to the main model of planned behavior theory to predict exercise behavior (Theodorakis, 1994). These variables are role identity, a particular social object that represents a dimension of the self, and attitude strength, a variable that expresses how positive, strong and important are the attitudes towards a given behavior. Role identity serves as a link between the individual self and society (Callero, 1985). The concept is based on Burke's identity theory (1980) in which an individual's self-concept is organised into a hierarchy of role identities that correspond to one's position in the social structure. These might include being a parent, a spouse, or an employee (Charng, Piliavin, & Callero, 1988). Ajzen (1985) defined perceived behavioral control as the person's belief as to how easy or difficult the performance of the behavior is likely to be. He suggested that perceived behavioral control is influenced by internal and external factors. External factors include time, opportunity and dependence on other people.

Investigators have already used the theory of planned behavior to predict behaviors in a variety of exercise settings: intention to participate in sports and physical activities (Godin & Shephard, 1986), intention of pregnant women to exercise after giving birth (Godin, Vezina, & Leclerc, 1989), participation in sports and physical activities (Theodorakis, Doganis, Bagiatis, & Goudas, 1991; Theodorakis, 1994) and jogging (Riddle, 1980). Also, studies utilized the theory to understand intention to participate in aerobics (Gatch & Kendzierski, 1990), in sports and physical activity (Dzewaltowski, Noble, & Shaw, 1990) and in team training of young swimmers (Theodorakis, 1992).

It was speculated that the addition of other variables would improve the model. The present preliminary study focused not only on the application of the planned behavior theory to the sport domain but also on the examination of the contribution of knowledge and information to the prediction of intention towards the specific behavior. Research on information and knowledge supports the hypothesis that the consistency between attitudes and behavior will increase as a function of the amount of knowledge and information available (Davidson, Yantis, Norwood, & Montano, 1985; Wilson, Kraft, & Dunn, 1989). Research showed that knowledge about attitude might moderate the effects. The reasons were that knowledgeable people may be more likely to know why they do something, and less knowledgeable people may have inconsistent beliefs about the attitude. Finally, people without knowledge may have weaker attitudes which may change more easily (Fazio, 1986).

Information has often been mentioned as an important factor in understanding attitudes' consistency with behavior (Ajzen & Madden, 1986; Krosnick, Boninger, Chuang, Berent, & Carnot, 1993; Theodorakis, 1994). Limited information and knowledge about the behavior can represent a serious obstacle preventing individuals from carrying out the behavior in question (Theodorakis, 1994). Information is a construct that has not drawn much attention in recent research based on planned behavior theory. Although it is frequently reported as being an important factor in the literature of attitude, few studies provide a clear definition. However, Krosnick and his colleagues (1993) operationalised information, or interest in relevant information as they named it, as 'the extent to which an individual is motivated to gather information about an attitude object' (p. 1133).

Studies have indicated that the variables of planned behavior questionnaire constitute an hierarchical chain. The chain starts with attitudes, and continues with subjective norms, intention, perceived behavioral control, role identity, attitude strength, and knowledge, and ends with information (Theodorakis, 1994; Theodorakis, Bagiatis, & Goudas, 1995). In the present investigation, planned behavior theory was used to investigate the extent to which knowledge and information contributed to the intention to play badminton before and after taking a university course. Badminton is a fairly new and unknown sport for the general public in Greece.

Method

Subjects and Procedure

The sample were 121 students (53 men, 68 women) between the ages of 18 and 25 years ($M = 19.9$, $SD = 1.5$). All subjects completed an anonymous open-ended questionnaire based on Planned Behavior Theory, following the procedure recommended by other studies (Ajzen & Madden, 1986; Theodorakis, 1994; Theodorakis, *et al.*, 1995). The questionnaire was completed on two occasions—before a course at the beginning of the fall semester and after a course at the beginning of the spring semester (see Table 1 below for psychometric characteristics).

Intention was estimated as the mean of the responses to three different questions: "I intend/I will try/I am determined to play badminton regularly next month." Responses to the first question (I intend . . .) were rated on a 7-point scale anchored by 1 = very unlikely and 7 = very likely. A 7-point scale with endpoints with anchors of 1 = definitely no and 7 = definitely yes was used for the other two questions.

Attitudes were estimated as the mean score of responses to the question "For me to play badminton regularly next month is . . ." Responses were rated on a 7-point scale, on six bipolar adjectives (7 = good to 1 = bad, 1 = foolish to 7 = smart, 7 = healthy to 1 = unhealthy, 7 = useful to 1 = unuseful, 7 = nice to 1 = ugly, 7 = pleasant to 1 = unpleasant).

Subjective Norms were estimated as the mean of responses to four questions: "If I play badminton regularly next month, individuals who are important to me . . . ," "Generally, I enjoy doing what some important individuals want me to do," "Some individuals who are important in my life believe that I must play badminton regularly next month," "Generally, I like doing what some important individuals want me to do." Responses were rated on 7-point scales. For Questions 1, 2 and 4 responses were rated using anchors of 1 = will strongly disagree and 7 = will strongly agree and for Question 3 anchors were 1 = very impossible and 7 = very possible.

Perceived Behavioural Control for the specific behavior was estimated as the mean on three questions. Questions were "If I wanted to, I could play badminton regularly next month," "For me to play badminton regularly next month is . . . ," "How much control do you exert over playing badminton regularly next month?" The 7-point scale had anchors of 1 = very unlikely and 7 = very likely, for the first question, 1 = difficult and 7 = easy for the second, and 1 = no control and 7 = complete control for the third, respectively.

Role Identity was measured by four questions: "I consider myself to be able to play badminton regularly next month," "I consider myself a person who will play badminton regularly next month," "It's in my character (temperament) to play badminton regularly next month," and "Generally, I am the type who is going to be playing badminton regularly next month." Responses were rated on 7-point scales using anchors of 1 = strongly disagree and 7 = strongly agree. This scale was adapted from Theodorakis (1994).

Attitude Strength was measured using eight questions (Theodorakis, 1994). The items were "How certain are you that you are going to play badminton regularly next month," "Is it right for you to play badminton regularly next month," "I feel very sure that I will play badminton regularly next month," "Is it important for you personally to play badminton regularly next month," "How interested are you in playing badminton regularly next month," "For me to play badminton regularly next month is . . . ," "With the knowledge I have, I think I will play badminton regularly next-month," and "Do you find it interesting to play badminton regularly next month?" Responses were rated on 7-point scales, for the first item anchors were 1 = very uncertain and 7 = very certain, for the second and sixth items 1 = not at all and 7 = very much so, for the third and seventh items 1 = strongly disagree and 7 = strongly agree, for the fourth item 1 = not important at all and 7 = very important, and for the fifth and eighth items 1 = not at all and 7 = very much.

Knowledge about the specific subject was measured as the mean of ratings on four questions: "Some of us are very well informed about playing badminton regularly, while other individuals aren't. How well informed about playing badminton regularly do you believe that you are," "If someone told you to write anything you know about playing badminton regularly, how much could you write," "In comparison to other students, I believe that I am very well informed on the issue of playing badminton regularly," and "How much do you think that you know on the issue of playing badminton regularly?" The answers were rated on 7-point scales. For the first question anchors were 1 = not informed at all and 7 = very well informed; for the second question anchors were 1 = very little and 7 = a lot; for the third 1 = I strongly disagree and 7 = I strongly agree, and for the last question 1 = no knowledge at all and 7 = a lot of knowledge. This scale was also adapted from Theodorakis (1994).

Information was measured by four questions: "Some individuals told me that they pay attention to different information about playing badminton regularly. How much attention do you pay to different information about playing badminton regularly," "How often do you pay attention to different printed material with information about playing badminton regularly," "I am very interested in any information regarding playing badminton regularly," and "How often do you pay attention to information regarding playing badminton regularly?" Responses were given on 7-point scales, for the first and fourth questions anchors were 1 = I never pay attention and 7 = I very much pay attention; for the second anchors were 1 = never and 7 = very often; for the third they were 1 = I strongly disagree and 7 = I strongly agree, and for the fourth 1 = I never pay attention and 7 = I pay a lot of attention. This scale was adapted from Theodorakis (1994).

Hierarchical regression analysis was performed to indicate the role of the variables knowledge and intention in the prediction of intention of the participants. More specifically, the investigators changed the hierarchical chain of the planned behavior variables (Theodorakis, 1994; Theodorakis, *et al.*, 1995) by entering first the variables of knowledge and information.

RESULTS

Descriptive Statistics

Descriptive statistics were computed for all assessed variables and are presented in Table 1. All scales showed acceptable internal consistency, that is, Cronbach alphas were higher than .79 except the items for Subjective norms so responses to these items were not included in the analyses.

Hierarchical Regression Analyses

Hierarchical regression analysis, as suggested by Ajzen and Madden (1986), was computed to ascertain the best predictor(s) for the intention of participation in the sport of badminton. One set of analyses was performed for the precourse data and one for the postcourse data.

TABLE 1
INTERNAL RELIABILITY AND DESCRIPTIVE CHARACTERISTICS OF ALL VARIABLES

Variable	No. of Items	Precourse M	Precourse SD	Precourse Cronbach α	Postcourse M	Postcourse SD	Postcourse Cronbach α
Attitude	6	5.1	1.1	.86	5.2	1.1	.86
Intention	3	4.2	1.8	.86	4.3	1.8	.87
Subjective Norms	4	3.8	1.3	.62	3.9	1.1	.61
Role Identity	4	4.1	1.5	.82	4.1	1.5	.81
Perceived Behavioral Control	3	4.0	1.5	.79	4.1	1.5	.82
Attitude Strength	8	4.1	1.5	.94	4.1	1.5	.94
Knowledge	4	2.8	1.3	.87	3.2	1.4	.87
Information	4	3.4	1.4	.80	3.5	1.5	.83

Precourse measure.—In the precourse hierarchical analysis, Knowledge and Information were entered at Step 1; Attitude was entered at Step 2; Perceived Behavioral Control was entered at Step 3; and Attitude Strength and Self-identity were entered at Step 4. In Step 1 both variables contributed to the prediction ($\Delta R^2 = .46$, $F_{2,12} = 49.6$, $p < .001$). In Step 2, Attitude significantly contributed to the prediction ($\Delta R^2 = .13$, $F_{1,11} = 38.2$, $p < .001$). In Step 3, Perceived Behavioral Control also contributed to the prediction ($\Delta R^2 = .18$, $F_{1,11} = 93.8$, $p < .001$), and finally in Step 4 only Attitude Strength contributed to the predication ($\Delta R^2 = .02$, $F_{2,12} = 4.2$, $p < .05$) (see Table 2).

Postcourse measure.—The same procedure was followed for the postcourse measure. The variables accounted for 81% of the variance. Knowl-

TABLE 2
PRECOURSE HIERARCHICAL REGRESSION ANALYSIS

Step	Variables Entered Prediction of Intention	B	β	ΔR^2	SE B
1	Knowledge	0.21	.16*		.10
	Information	0.72	.58†	.46	.10
2	Knowledge	0.26	.20		.09
	Information	0.48	.39		.09
	Attitude	0.62	.41†	.13	.10
3	Knowledge	0.12	.09		.07
	Information	0.20	.16		.08
	Attitude	0.37	.24		.08
	Perceived Behavioral Control	0.68	.58†	.18	.07
4	Knowledge	0.09	.07		.07
	Information	0.14	.11		.08
	Attitude	0.25	.16		.09
	Perceived Behavioral Control	0.26	.22		.16
	Attitude Strength	0.42	.36*		.18
	Self-identity	0.14	.12	.02	.010

*$p < .05$. †$p < .001$.

edge and Information were entered at Step 1; Attitude was entered at Step 2; Perceived Behavioral Control was entered at Step 3; and Attitude Strength and Self-identity were entered at Step 4. In Step 1 both variables contributed to the prediction ($\Delta R^2 = .46$, $F_{2,12} = 47.4$, $p < .001$). In Step 2, Attitude significantly contributed to the prediction ($\Delta R^2 = .13$, $F_{1,11} = 33.6$, $p < .001$). In Step 3, Perceived Behavioral Control also contributed to the prediction ($\Delta R^2 = .19$, $F_{1,11} = 88.1$, $p < .001$), and finally in Step 4 both Attitude Strength and Self-identity contributed to the predication ($\Delta R^2 = .04$, $F_{2,11} = 9.8$, $p < .05$) (see Table 3).

TABLE 3
POSTCOURSE HIERARCHICAL REGRESSION ANALYSIS

Step	Variables Entered Prediction of Intention	B	β	ΔR^2	SE B
1	Knowledge	0.37	.47†		.11
	Information	0.57	.29†	.46	.10
2	Knowledge	0.29	.23		.10
	Information	0.32	.26		.10
	Attitude	0.68	.43†	.13	.12
3	Knowledge	0.11	.09		.08
	Information	0.13	.11		.08
	Attitude	0.34	.21		.10
	Perceived Behavioral Control	0.70	.60†	.19	.08
4	Knowledge	0.07	.05		.07
	Information	0.04	.05		.07
	Attitude	0.24	.15		.09
	Perceived Behavioral Control	0.10	.09		.16
	Attitude Strength	0.60	.51†		.16
	Self-identity	0.20	.17*	.04	.20

*$p < .05$. †$p < .001$.

DISCUSSION

The purpose of this preliminary study was to examine the contribution of knowledge and information to the intention of Greek students to play badminton before and after taking a one-semester course in badminton. The analyses supported the validity of the planned behavior model for prediction of intentions. Most importantly, it appears that, when hierarchical chain of the variables was changed and the variables of knowledge and information were entered first in the analyses (Tables 2 and 3), the results indicated that these variables played a very important role on the formation of positive opinion and intentions of the people towards the unknown sport of badminton. Consistent with previous research (Davidson, *et al.*, 1985; Wilson, *et al.*, 1989; Krosnick, *et al.*, 1993; Theodorakis, 1994), the results indicated that the amount of information and knowledge available about an attitude would be a determinant of consistency between attitude and action.

The contribution of knowledge and information to the prediction of intention was the same before and after the course. This indicates that the source of knowledge and information does not necessarily have to be direct experience with the object of attitudes and suggests that this knowledge and information might come from indirect experiences such as media or the opinion of a friend.

Overall, our results showed that the planned behavior variables could account for a significant amount of variance of intention towards badminton. In particular, knowledge, information, attitude, perceived behavioral control, attitude strength and self-identity contributed importantly to explaining variance of intention towards badminton. This study supported findings of previous researchers, who reported that intention significantly predicted the anticipation of participating in physical activity and sports (Dzewaltowski, 1989; Dzewaltowski, *et al.*, 1990).

Possible limitations of the present investigation should be mentioned. Most participants were educated young people who might already have been cognizant of the benefits of getting involved in new sports and whose curiosity might also play an important role.

The present study has implications for individuals who attempt to involve people in unfamiliar sports. Knowledge and information were the main factors that helped the researchers understand the participants' intentions towards their involvement in the sport of badminton. It is possible that these factors can contribute to sport professionals by supporting the challenge they face to modify negative opinions about unfamiliar sports.

REFERENCES

AJZEN, I. (1985) From intentions to actions: a theory of planned behavior. In J. Kuhl & J. Beckman (Eds.), *Action-control: from cognition to behavior*. Heidelberg: Springer. Pp. 11-39.

AJZEN, I. (1987) Attitudes, traits and actions: dispositional prediction of behavior in personality and social psychology. In L. Berkowitz (Ed.), *Advances in experimental social psychology*. New York: Academic Press. Pp. 1-63.

AJZEN, I. (1988) *Attitudes, personality, and behavior*. Bristol, Eng.: Open Univer. Press.

AJZEN, I., & FISHBEIN, M. (1972) Attitudes and normative beliefs as factors influencing behavioral intentions. *Journal of Personality and Social Psychology*, 21, 1-9.

AJZEN, I., & FISHBEIN, M. (1980) *Understanding attitudes and predicting social behavior*. Englewood Cliffs, NJ: Prentice-Hall.

AJZEN, I., & MADDEN, T. J. (1986) Predictions of goal-directed behavior: attitudes, intentions and perceived behavioral control. *Journal of Experimental Social Psychology*, 22, 453-457.

BURKE, P. J. (1980) Measurement requirements from an interactionist perspective. *Social Psychology Quarterly*, 43, 18-29.

CALLERO, P. L. (1985) Role-identity salience. *Social Psychology Quarterly*, 48, 203-215.

CHARNG, H. W., PILIAVIN, J. A., & CALLERO, P. L. (1988) Role identity and reasoned action in the prediction of repeated behavior. *Social Psychology Quarterly*, 51, 303-317.

DAVIDSON, A. R., YANTIS, S., NORWOOD, M., & MONTANO, D. E. (1985) Amount of information about the attitude object and attitude-behavior consistency. *Journal of Personality and Social Psychology*, 49, 1184-1198.

DZEWALTOWSKI, D. A. (1989) Toward a model of exercise motivation. *Journal of Sport and Exercise Psychology*, 11, 251-269.

DZEWALTOWSKI, D. A., NOBLE, J. M., & SHAW, J. M. (1990) Physical activity participation: social cognitive theory versus the theories of reasoned action and planned behavior. *Journal of Sport and Exercise Psychology*, 12, 388-405.

FAZIO, R. H. (1986) How do attitudes guide behavior? In R. M. Sorrentino & E. T. Higgins (Eds.), *The handbook of motivation and cognition: foundations of social behavior.* New York: Pp. 204-243

GATCH, L. C., & KENDZIERSKI, D. (1990) Predicting exercise intentions: the theory of planned behavior. *Research Quarterly for Exercise and Sport*, 61, 100-102.

GODIN, G., & SHEPHARD, R. J. (1986) Psychosocial factors influencing intentions to exercise of young students from Grades 7 to 9. *Research Quarterly for Exercise and Sport*, 57, 44-52.

GODIN, G., VEZINA, L., & LECLERC, O. (1989) Factors influencing intentions of pregnant women to exercise after giving birth. *Public Health Reports*, 104, 188-196.

KROSNICK, J. A., BONINGER, D. S., CHUANG, Y. C., BERENT, M. K., & CARNOT, C. G. (1993) Attitude strength: one construct or many related constructs? *Journal of Personality and Social Psychology*, 65, 1132-1151.

RIDDLE, K. P. (1980) Attitudes, beliefs, behavioral intentions, and behaviors of women and men toward regular jogging. *Research Quarterly for Exercise and Sport*, 51, 663-674.

TESSER, A., & SHAFFER, D. R. (1990) Attitudes and attitude change. *Annual Review of Psychology*, 41, 479-523.

THEODORAKIS, Y. (1992) Prediction of athletic participation: a test of planned behavior theory. *Perceptual and Motor Skills*, 74, 371-379.

THEODORAKIS, Y. (1994) Planned behavior, attitude strength, self-identity, and the prediction of exercise behavior. *The Sport Psychologist*, 8, 149-165.

THEODORAKIS, Y., BAGIATIS, K., & GOUDAS, M. (1995) Attitudes toward teaching individuals with disabilities: application of planned behavior theory. *Adapted Physical Activity Quarterly*, 12, 151-160.

THEODORAKIS, Y., DOGANIS, G., BAGIATIS, K., & GOUDAS, M. (1991) Preliminary study of the ability of reasoned action model in predicting exercise behavior of young children. *Perceptual and Motor Skills*, 72, 51-58.

WILSON, T. D., KRAFT, D., & DUNN, D. S. (1989) The disruptive effects of explaining attitudes: the moderating effect of knowledge about the attitude object. *Journal of Experimental Social Psychology*, 25, 379-400.

Accepted April 7, 2004.

GEOPHYSICAL VARIABLES AND BEHAVIOR: C. INCREASED GEOMAGNETIC ACTIVITY ON DAYS OF COMMERCIAL AIR CRASHES ATTRIBUTED TO COMPUTER OR PILOT ERROR BUT NOT MECHANICAL FAILURE[1]

N. M. FOURNIER AND M. A. PERSINGER

Laurentian University

Summary.—Global geomagnetic activity (aa values) for the days of crashes of airplanes and for each of the three days before and after the crashes were compared for 373 events (years 1940 through 2002) attributed to unknown factors, mechanical errors, electronic/computer failures or pilot errors. Interactions between days and classifications of the crashes were due to the significantly greater geomagnetic activity on the days of crashes attributed to pilot or computer error but not to mechanical or unknown factors. Successive temporal analyses indicated that the elevated activity on the days of crashes attributed to pilot error have not changed over time, but there was an increase in those attributed to electronic errors after 1965. No more than 9% of the variance in geomagnetic activity on the days of the crashes was associated with the type of crash. These results are consistent with our hypothesis that some factor or factors associated with relative increases in geomagnetic activity may affect complex electronic systems composed of either silica (computer) or carbon (brain) aggregates.

Human and nonhuman complex electronic systems are immersed with in the earth's magnetic field. Increased geomagnetic activity is defined as irregular, time-varying alterations within the mHz range with peak-to-peak intensities between 20 nT and several hundreds of nanoTesla. These periods have been moderately correlated (rs between .3 and .5) with increased numbers of neuroelectrical disturbances, such as limbic or temporal lobe seizures, in populations of rats and humans (Michon & Persinger, 1997).

Persinger (1991) reported a moderate strength correlation between the numbers of sudden impulses or rapid changes (primarily increases) in geomagnetic activity and the numbers of air crashes during a 2-yr. period. A more thorough examination by Komarov, Oraevsky, Sizov, Tsiryulnik, Kanonidi, Ushakov, Shalimov, Kimlyk, and Glukhov (1998) of a larger population of air crashes occurring between the years 1989 through 1994 in Russia also demonstrated this relationship. Although Persinger (1991) speculated that increased geomagnetic activity could produce potentially catastrophic effects within onboard computers, the possible effects of these changes on the pilots themselves were mentioned as an alternative or parallel hypothesis.

---

[1]N. M. Fournier now at Department of Psychology, Life Sciences Center, Dalhousie University, Halifax, NS, Canada B3J 4J1. Please send reprint requests to Dr. M. A. Persinger, Behavioral Neuroscience Laboratory, Department of Psychology, Laurentian University, Sudbury, Ontario Canada P3E 2C6 or e-mail (mpersinger@laurentian.ca).

The present study was designed to test the hypotheses that the relationships between numbers of air crashes and increased geomagnetic activity have been related to potential effects upon the pilots' brains as well as on-board computer and electronic systems. If these hypotheses are valid, then the increased geomagnetic activity on the days of air crashes attributed to pilot errors should not have changed over decades. However the intensity of the increased geomagnetic activity over decades for those crashes attributed to computer or electronic errors would have slowly increased statistically, corresponding to the increased complexity (and hence vulnerability) of silicon-based electronic systems.

A total of 373 air crashes between the years 1940 and 2003 were obtained from site[2] with permission of the Master (R. Kebabjian). Only those events for which the source was clearly identified as either known ($n = 102$), mechanical failures (57), electronic or (more recently) computer failures (50), or pilot errors (164) were extracted. The daily global aa (average antipodal) values for geomagnetic activity (in nanoTesla) for the days of the crashes and for each of the three days before and after the crashes were obtained from standard sources.

To test the generalizability of previous observations that air crashes occurred on days when the geomagnetic activity was relatively greater compared to the previous or subsequent days, three two-way analyses of variance with one repeated measure (days) and one between-subject measure (four types of crashes) were completed for the aa values, the log base 10 of the aa values and the day/week ratios of the values. The latter was calculated by dividing the value for each day by the mean for all seven days so that the *relative* activity on the day of the crashes might be enhanced. All analyses involved SPSS software on a VAX computer. *Post hoc* tests included Tukey ($p < .05$) and correlated t tests.

The results of the two-way analyses of variance for the raw and log-transformed data (the latter eliminated the heterogeneity of variance across days) demonstrated a statistically significant difference in geomagnetic activity ($F_{3,369}s = 3.52$, 3.24, $p < .001$, respectively; $\eta^2 = .03$) during the week of the crashes. *Post hoc* analysis indicated that the geomagnetic activity on the days of crashes attributed to pilot errors was significantly greater than for those of the other three categories, although the size of the effect was small.

The interaction between days and types of crashes was not statistically significant for the raw data ($F_{18,2214} = 1.51$, $p < .07$) but was significant statistically for the log-transformed data ($F = 1.72$, $p < .05$; $\eta^2 = .01$) and ratio data ($F = 1.90$, $p = .01$; 2% of variance explained). Again, the effect was very

---

[2](http://www.planecrashinfo.com)

GEOMAGNETIC ACTIVITY AND COMMERCIAL AIR CRASHES 1221

small. The statistically significant difference between days for all three measures ($F_{6,2214}$s = 6.59, 5.55, 4.25, $p < .001$; η^2 about .01) was due, according to *post hoc* tests, to the greater geomagnetic activity on the days of the crashes compared to any of the other six days. As shown in Fig. 1, the source of the interaction between days and type of crash was primarily due to the increased activity on the days of the crashes attributed to electronic or pilot errors relative to mechanical or unknown sources.

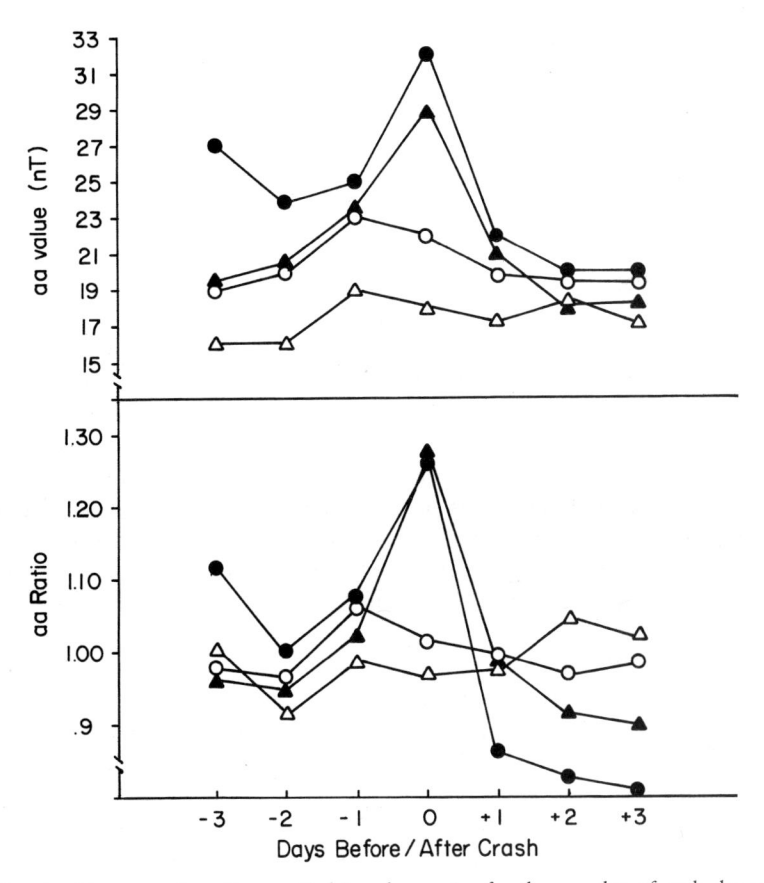

FIG. 1. Mean aa values (in nanoTesla) and aa ratios for the aa value of each day compared to the average for the week for the days before, during, and after four types of air crashes attributed to different sources: unknown (○), electronic (●), mechanical (△), pilot (▲).

The number of crashes within different regions of the world were in North America 107, Central and South America 67, Europe 110, Africa 37, and Asia-Australia 52. Chi-squared analysis ($\chi^2_{12} = 23.97$) indicated a statistically significant ($p = .02$) discordance among the regions for types of crashes. This mild discrepancy ($phi = .32$) was due in large part to the greater proportion of crashes attributed to mechanical failures in North America (24%) compared to Asia-Australia (6%) and the fewer proportions attributed to pilot error in North America (30%) compared to all other regions (46% to 56%). Two-way analysis of variance for the various measures of aa activity or the ratios of activity on the days of the crashes showed no statistically significant interactions ($F_{12,353}s < 1.00$) between types of crashes and locations.

To discern if there were changes over time, numbers of the different types of crashes between 1940 and 1960, 1961 and 1980, and later than 1980 were analyzed for the raw scores for geomagnetic activity on the days of events. Two-way analysis of variance indicated a significant difference ($F_{3,361} = 6.47$, $p < .001$; $\eta^2 = .22$) in geomagnetic activity on the days of the four classes of crashes. There was also an interaction ($F_{6,361} = 2.15$, $p < .05$) between types of crashes and the three bidecades. *Post hoc* analysis indicated that the source of the interaction was primarily due to the increased geomagnetic activity on the days of crashes attributed to electronic errors for the second (1961–1980) and third bidecades (1981–2002) compared to the first (1940–1960) and a decrease in geomagnetic activity on days of crashes attributed to pilot errors during these intervals. The next largest contribution was the inverse relationship between crashes attributed to mechanical errors and unknown causes.

The two-way analysis of variance for the ratio data showed only a statistically significant difference between types of crashes ($F = 5.35$, $p < .01$) with no contribution from either the interaction or the bidecades. *Post hoc* analysis indicated that the ratios were significantly higher on the day of the crashes for those attributed to pilot errors or electronic errors compared to the other two categories. A chi-square analysis for the numbers of events during the three bidecades for the four categories demonstrated a statistically significant discordance ($\chi^2_6 = 28.29$, $p < .0001$; $phi = .27$) due primarily to the reduction (by one-half) of the numbers of crashes attributed to unknown sources and the increases (by a factor of 2 or 3) in the numbers of crashes attributed to mechanical or electronic errors while those attributed to pilots did not change.

To discern the potentially temporal inflection period when the geomagnetic activity became more predominant in the occurrences of the four types of crashes a successive series of one-way analyses of variance were completed for the aa values on the days of the crashes and the ratios for successive 5-yr. periods. The numbers of cases, the means and standard deviations for each increasing aggregate, and the ω^2 estimate (for explained variance) are shown in Table 1. For comparison, the mean and standard deviation for the aa values for the average of the two and three days before the crashes for all

TABLE 1
Means and Standard Errors of Mean For Global aa Values (in nT) For Events Attributed to Unknown Causes, Electrical/Computer Errors, Mechanical Failures or Pilot Errors as a Function of Increasing Aggregates of Years

Years	n	Unknown M	Unknown SEM	Electronic M	Electronic SEM	Mechanical M	Mechanical SEM	Pilot M	Pilot SEM	Omega² %
<1955	74	26	4	23	8	16	3	34	3	9
<1960	116	27	3	23[a]	9	16[a]	3	37[b]	4	8
<1965	160	25	3	27	4	19[a]	3	33[b]	3	6
<1970	196	22[a]	2	30[b]	4	18[a]	3	32[b]	3	6
<1975	223	22[a]	2	30	5	23	3	32[b]	3	4
<1980	252	23[a]	2	31[b]	4	22[a]	3	31[b]	2	3
<1985	273	22[a]	2	32[b]	3	21[a]	3	30[b]	2	4
<1990	304	22[a]	2	32[b]	4	20[a]	3	30[b]	2	4
<1995	336	22[a]	2	32[b]	3	20[a]	3	30[b]	2	4
<2002	373	22[a]	2	32[b]	3	18[a]	3	29[b]	2	5

Note.—n = number of crashes. Omega² estimates (explained variance) are indicated. [a] vs [b] $p < .05$.

cases were 21.0 and 14.0, respectively. The differences between the four types of crashes for this baseline was significant ($F_{3,335} = 2.69$, $p = .05$).

The values for the ratios of geomagnetic activity on the day of the crashes compared to the average of the week are shown in Table 2. For both tables the primary source of the differences was the increased geomagnetic activity on the days of crashes attributed to pilot error. However, the geomagnetic effect for crashes attributed to computer and electronic errors became more evident only when all cases after 1965 were added to the previous aggregate.

These results support our general hypothesis that some factor or factors

TABLE 2
Means and Standard Errors of Mean For Ratios of aa Values on Day of Crash to Mean of Week For Events Attributed to Unknown Causes, Electrical/Computer Errors, Mechanical Failures or Pilot Errors as a Function of Increasing Aggregates of Years

Years	Unknown M	Unknown SEM	Electronic M	Electronic SEM	Mechanical M	Mechanical SEM	Pilot M	Pilot SEM	Omega² %
<1955	1.05	.10	1.00	.26	.93	.10	1.25	.09	9
<1960	1.05	.08	1.07	.17	.88	.09	1.30	.08	7
<1965	1.00[a]	.06	1.09	.14	.95	.08	1.24[b]	.06	5
<1970	.93[a]	.06	1.25	.14	.94[a]	.07	1.24[b]	.06	8
<1975	.97[a]	.06	1.22	.14	.99	.08	1.24[b]	.06	5
<1980	1.00[a]	.06	1.19	.12	1.00	.08	1.25[b]	.06	4
<1985	1.00[a]	.06	1.18	.11	1.00	.07	1.25[b]	.06	4
<1990	1.00[a]	.05	1.21	.11	1.00[a]	.07	1.26[b]	.06	5
<1995	0.99[a]	.05	1.23	.08	1.02[a]	.06	1.28[b]	.06	5
<2002	1.02[a]	.05	1.28[b]	.06	0.98[a]	.06	1.28[b]	.05	4

Note.—Omega² estimates (explained variance) are indicated. [a] vs [b] $p < .05$.

associated with increased geomagnetic activity can disrupt the normal processing of information within complex electronic systems that include human brains (of pilots) and sophisticated computers. We are assuming that the sources responsible for the four categories of crashes were relatively homogeneous. We also appreciate that the validity of the attribution, such as "pilot error," may be questionable. These cases may not be related to intent, negligence, or fatigue but to interactions between machine and pilot of which we are not currently aware.

The effect size was quite small, explaining no more than about 9% of the variance for the differences between types of crashes. Direct causal effects were not likely to be operative for the entire set of crashes. Instead, a unique set of conditions that occurred infrequently and were specific to a subset of crashes may have been produced by increased geomagnetic activity. One analogy would be the marked vulnerability of specific receptors to a particular molecular structure (out of millions of possible structures) that can produce "catastrophic changes" in ion channels. We speculate that intensity *per se* is not the critical variable. Instead there may be intrinsic frequencies or temporally structured patterns (Belisheva, Popov, Petukhova, Pavlova, Osipov, Tkachenko, & Baranova, 1995; O'Connor & Persinger, 1997; Cherry, 2002) associated with specific bands of intensity that may affect the functioning of computerized electronics or even the decision-making processes of the pilots.

REFERENCES

Belisheva, N. K., Popov, A. N., Petukhova, N. V., Pavlova, L. P., Osipov, K. S., Tkachenko, S. E., & Baranova, T. I. (1995) Qualitative and quantitative evaluations of the effect of geomagnetic field variations on the functional state of the human brain. *Biophysics*, 40, 1007-1014.

Cherry, N. (2002) Schumann resonances, a plausible mechanism for the human health effects of solar/geomagnetic activity. *Natural Hazards*, 26, 279-331.

Komarov, F. I., Oraevsky, V. N., Sizov, Y. P., Tsiryulnik, L. N., Kanonidi, Kh. D., Ushakov, I. B., Shalimov, P. M., Kimlyk, M. V., & Glukhov, D. V. (1998) Role of heliogeophysical factors among causes of air incidents. *Biophysics*, 43, 703-706.

Michon, A. L., & Persinger, M. A. (1997) Experimental simulation of the effects of increased geomagnetic activity upon nocturnal seizures in epileptic rats. *Neuroscience Letters*, 224, 53-56.

O'Connor, R. P., & Persinger, M. A. (1997) Geophysical variables and behavior: LXXXII. A strong association between Sudden Infant Death syndrome (SIDs) and increments of global geomagnetic activity—possible support for the melatonin hypothesis. *Perceptual and Motor Skills*, 84, 395-402.

Persinger, M. A. (1991) Geophysical variables and behavior: LXVI. Geomagnetic storm sudden commencements and commercial air crashes. *Perceptual and Motor Skills*, 72, 476-478.

Accepted April 8, 2004.

Perceptual and Motor Skills, 2004, 98, 1225-1233. © Perceptual and Motor Skills 2004

EYE-HAND PREFERENCE IN SCHIZOPHRENIA: SEX DIFFERENCES AND SIGNIFICANCE FOR HAND FUNCTION [1,2]

YI-CHIA LIU AND YEN KUANG YANG

Department of Psychiatry
National Cheng Kung University Medical College and Hospital
Tainan, Taiwan

KEH-CHUNG LIN

Department of Rehabilitation
National Taiwan University Hospital, Taipei, Taiwan
School of Occupational Therapy
National Taiwan University College of Medicine

I HUI LEE

Department of Psychiatry
National Cheng Kung University Medical College and Hospital, Tainan, Taiwan

KEITH J JEFFRIES

National Institute on Deafness and Other Communication Disorders
National Institutes of Health

LI-CHING LEE

Department of Epidemiology
School of Public Health
Johns Hopkins University

Summary.—Hand preference and eye dominance were investigated in 73 (30 women, 43 men) schizophrenic patients and 71 (30 women, 41 men) healthy controls. There were significantly more schizophrenic patients and normal controls who were significantly right-hand dominant. However, schizophrenic patients showed a significant excess of left-eye dominance relative to controls (65.8% vs 29.6%; Odds Ratio = 4.75, $p < .001$). In addition, female schizophrenic patients showed a higher rate of non-right (either left or inconsistent) eye dominance (80%) than male schizophrenic patients (55.8%) and controls (33.3%). Analysis of hand performance on the Purdue Pegboard Test indicated that schizophrenic patients who showed crossed eye-hand dominance scored higher than did patients without crossed eye-hand dominance.

There is evidence for an anomaly in the lateralization process in schizophrenia (Crow, 1990). Left hemispheric dysfunction has been suggested to be related to the disorder (Gur, 1977; Donnelly, 1984; Lobel, Swanda, & Losonczy, 1994). In particular, Crow, Colter, Frith, Johnstone, and Owena (1989) proposed that schizophrenia may be related to an anomaly of the right-shift gene (or cerebral dominance gene), which is thought to control

---

[1]The authors thank Mr. Chih Ming Tsai, Dr. Tzung Lieh Yeh and Dr. Chwen Cheng Chen from the Department of Psychiatry, National Cheng Kung University Medical College and Hospital and Ms. Hsin-mei Chen from School of Occupational Therapy, National Taiwan University College of Medicine for their statistical and editorial assistance in the preparation of this manuscript.
[2]Address correspondence to Dr. Keh-chung Lin, Department of Rehabilitation, National Taiwan University Hospital, 7 Chung-shan South Rd., Taipei, Taiwan or e-mail (kclin@ha.mc.ntu.edu.tw).

cerebral asymmetries. In support of this, some previous reports noted the greater frequency of left-eye dominance among schizophrenic patients than normal people (Oddy & Lobstein, 1972; Piran, Bigler, & Cohen, 1982; Merrin, 1984; Yan, Flor-Henry, Chen, Li, Qi, & Ma, 1985; Gureje, 1988; Cannon, Jones, Murray, & Wadsworth, 1997), although one earlier study also reported an excess of right-eye dominance in a sample of schizophrenic patients (Kameyama, Niwa, Hiramatsu, & Saitoh, 1983). With respect to hand preference, most of the literature strongly supports the view that schizophrenia is either associated with an atypical left shift in the handedness or a higher frequency of mixed-handedness (Carlsson, Hugdahl, Uvebrant, Wiklund, & Wendt, 1992; Cannon, Bryne, Cassidy, Larkin, Horgan, Sheppard, & O'Callaghan, 1995; Orr, Cannon, Gilvarry, Jones, & Murray, 1999; Satz & Green, 1999). However, according to Yan, *et al.*'s report (1985), in which all of the subjects were recruited from the Chinese community, there was a nonsignificant trend toward increasing sinistrality in schizophrenics.

Previous studies have demonstrated there are laterality (hand preference and eye dominance) differences between schizophrenic patients and normal controls. Subjects were tested by handedness and eye-dominance questionnaires (Piran, *et al.*, 1982; Cannon, *et al.*, 1997). Cross-dominance is much more common in male schizophrenic patients (Lobel, *et al.*, 1994), but the results cannot be generalized for all men and women. To understand the discrepancies in previous literature, this study examined: (1) the difference in eye and hand dominance between schizophrenic patients and normal controls, using the Edinburgh Handedness Inventory and the Hole-in-the-Hand technique; (2) the sex effect; and (3) the functional significance of eye-hand preference in schizophrenics using the Purdue Pegboard Test to compare dexterity between individuals with crossed eye-hand dominance, i.e., left eye with right hand, and those with a consistent pattern of eye-hand dominance.

METHOD

Subjects

Seventy-three patients (30 women, 43 men) between the ages of 17 to 59 meeting DSM–IV (American Psychiatric Association, 1994) diagnostic criteria for schizophrenia were recruited for the study. The mean age of the 43 men was 31.9 yr. ($SD = 7.6$) and of 30 women was 32.3 yr. ($SD = 9.2$). Those who had a history of substance abuse, mental retardation, neurological illness, major medical illness that affected brain functions or head injury with loss of consciousness or who had received electroconvulsive therapy in the past two years were excluded given concerns that these factors might confound the results of neuropsychological tests.

Seventy-one healthy volunteers (30 women, 41 men) were also recruited from the community by advertisement and were interviewed by a senior psychiatrist using the Chinese version of the Mini International Neuropsychiatric Interview (Sheehan, Lecrubier, Sheehan, Amorim, Janavs, Weiller, Hergueta, Baker, & Dunbar, 1998) to exclude the possibility of mental illness. All of these individuals were recruited from Taiwan and therefore are ethnic Chinese. Those who had a history of psychiatric illness or substance abuse or a family history of psychiatric illness were excluded from this study. The demographic characteristics of the subjects are shown in Table 1. Before the study began, informed consent was obtained from volunteers themselves and from patients and their key caregivers. The Ethical Committee for Human Research, National Cheng Kung University Medical Center, had approved the study protocol.

TABLE 1
DEMOGRAPHIC AND CLINICAL CHARACTERISTICS OF PATIENTS AND DEMOGRAPHICALLY MATCHED NORMAL CONTROLS

	Schizophrenic Patients				Controls			
	Women		Men		Women		Men	
	M	SD	M	SD	M	SD	M	SD
Age, yr.	32.3	9.2	31.9	7.6	33.7	8.4	35.0	9.5
Education, yr.	12.1	2.9	12.1	2.4	13.0	2.3	13.4	2.7
Age at onset of illness, yr.	24.2	7.1	25.0	7.1				
Duration of illness, yr.	8.9	8.0	6.3	5.2				
Chlorpromazine equivalents, mg	366.31	184.62	403.23	279.56				
Brief Psychiatric Rating Scale Total[a]	13.73	5.00	11.89	6.36				
Handedness score	85.8	18.2	84.9	20.0	86.6	15.4	74.9	24.8
Eye dominance (left or inconsistent), n (%)	24	(80)	24	(55.8)	10	33.3	11	26.8

[a]Overall and Gorham, 1962.

Test Procedure

Patients were examined when they were not in an acute condition. Three functional laterality tests were performed in this study.

Edinburgh Handedness Inventory (Oldfield, 1971).—This is a self-administered questionnaire of hand preference, in which participants are asked to indicate how they perform each of the following 10 tasks: writing, drawing, throwing, using scissors, holding a toothbrush, using a knife, using a spoon, holding a broom, striking a match, and opening a box. The subjects were asked about their preference for the right or left hand, and their scores were recorded as either weak (1 point) or strong (2 points) preference for each task. Laterality Quotients were computed as the total number of right-handed preference minus the total number of left-handed preference divided by the total number of responses, multiplied by 100, as $(R - L/R + L) \cdot 100$.

Hole-in-the-Hand Technique (Robison, Block, Boudreaux, & Flora, 1999).—The dominant eye is defined as the eye whose input is favored in behavioral coordination in which only one eye can be used (Porac & Coren, 1976). In this test, the arms are fully extended, hands placed together with palms facing away, and a small opening about the size of a quarter is made between the junctions of the thumbs and forefingers. The subjects were asked to perform the viewing, through the hole with both eyes open, five times. If the subject used the right hand in all trials, it was recorded as right-eye preference. If the subject used the right or left eye in an inconsistent manner, it was recorded as inconsistent eye preference. If the subject used the left eye in all trials, it was recorded as left eye preference.

Purdue Pegboard Manual Test (Tiffin & Asher, 1948).—The Purdue Pegboard Test consists of a wooden board divided into two rows of 25 holes. Pegs are located in small bins on the extreme right and left sides of the board. Subjects were asked to insert pegs into the holes during a 30-sec. period with the preferred hand and then with the nonpreferred hand.

Statistical Analysis

Data analysis was carried out using the SPSS computer package (SPSS Inc., Chicago, IL). To compare both continuous and dichotomous covariates between the patient and control groups, Mann-Whitney U tests (two-tailed) or chi-square tests were used. Multivariate logistic regression was performed to examine the differences in hand dominance, eye dominance and sex between schizophrenics and controls. Odds Ratios (OR) and 95% Confidence Intervals (95% CI) are presented to indicate the significance of association. Chi-square was calculated to test for a sex effect in cross-dominance. Finally, t test was used to examine the differences of Purdue Pegboard performance between different eye-hand preference (crossed and consistent eye-hand dominance) groups.

Results

Results from bivariate analysis indicated that female schizophrenic patients, male schizophrenic patients, female controls and male controls were not significantly different in age or education (Table 1). There was no sex difference regarding age of onset or duration of schizophrenia in schizophrenic patients. The severity of psychopathology in patients with schizophrenia did not correlate significantly with patients' performance on the tests.

Hand-preference Pattern

On the Edinburgh Handedness Inventory, the schizophrenic group and the control group scored 85.3% and 79.7%, respectively. No significant difference was found in the hand preference patterns between these two groups

($t = 1.60$, ns). Furthermore, there was no significant difference in the handedness scores between male and female schizophrenic patients (male schizophrenic patients: score = 84.9, $SD = 20.0$; female schizophrenic patients: score = 85.8, $SD = 18.2$; $t = .66$, ns); see Table 1.

Eye-preference Pattern

Because the number of left-handers, i.e., those with an Edinburgh Handedness score less than 0 was very small in both the schizophrenic group ($n = 1$) and the control group ($n = 2$), only right-handers were included in the analysis of differences in eye-preference pattern. Results from multivariate logistic regressions are shown in Table 2. Schizophrenic patients had significantly higher handedness mean (OR = 1.01, 95% CI: 1.00–1.03, $p < .01$) and were more likely to be left eyed or inconsistent (OR = 4.75, 95% CI: 2.22–10.12, $p < .001$) after controlling for sex, age and education. Furthermore, the tendency for increased cross dominance, i.e., right hand preference and left/inconsistent eye dominance, in schizophrenia was found in the female group (80%; $\chi^2 = 11.25$, $p < .005$) as well as the male group (55.8%; $\chi^2 = 7.39$, $p < .01$).

TABLE 2
COMPARISON OF SCHIZOPHRENIC PATIENTS AND NORMAL CONTROLS IN CLINICAL CHARACTERISTICS

	Odds Ratio$_{adjusted}$	95% CI
Sex (female)	0.67	0.31, 1.43
Age	0.97	0.93, 1.02
Education	0.82	0.71, 0.95†
Handedness score	1.01	1.00, 1.03
Eye dominance*	4.75	2.22, 10.12‡

*Left or inconsistent. †$p < .01$. ‡$p < .001$.

Functional Significance of Eye-Hand Preference

Data of Purdue Pegboard are only available for 50 schizophrenic patients and 30 healthy controls because the remaining subjects did not participate in the test due to time constraints. Comparison of demographic characteristics between the tested group (included in the analysis) and non-tested group (excluded from the analysis) showed no significant difference. Results of t test showed that the control group was more dexterous than the schizophrenic group (left hand: $F = 27.03$, $p < .01$; right hand: $F = 19.03$, $p < .01$). The performance of participants on the Purdue Pegboard are shown in Table 3. In hand dexterity, the schizophrenic group showed no significant right-hand advantage compared to the control group. Schizophrenics with crossed eye-hand dominance performed significantly better with the right hand than with the left hand on the Purdue Pegboard (see Table 3).

TABLE 3
EYE-HAND PREFERENCE (CROSSED AND CONSISTENT EYE-HAND DOMINANCE) IN RELATION TO PURDUE PEGBOARD PERFORMANCE BY SCHIZOPHRENIC PATIENTS AND NORMAL SUBJECTS

Group and Eye-Hand Dominance	n	Purdue Pegboard Right Hand	Purdue Pegboard Left Hand	t	p
Schizophrenic Group					
Right/Dextral	16	12.19	11.56	1.19	ns
Left or Inconsistent/Dextral	34	12.38	11.00	3.86	<.005
Control Group					
Right/Dextral	19	14.42	14.21	.53	ns
Left or Inconsistent/Dextral	11	15.00	14.36	1.55	ns

DISCUSSION

The findings are consistent with previous studies that report an increased incidence of left eye dominance in schizophrenia (Gur, 1977; Merrin, 1984; Yan, et al., 1985; Gureje, 1988; Cannon, et al., 1997). In a study of 70 schizophrenic patients, no sex difference was found in eye dominance (Oddy & Lobstein, 1972). However, this study also found a higher ratio of nonright eye dominance in the female schizophrenics (80%) than in the males (50%). This result is similar to that of Yan, et al., 1985), who reported that left eye dominance tends to be more common in female schizophrenics (33.7%) than others in a study that included only ethnic Chinese subjects. In general, decrements in the size of temporal lobe structures or the lobe itself and generally associated lateral cerebral ventricular enlargement are more prominent in schizophrenia (Leung & Chue, 2000; Chua, Lam, Tai, Cheung, Tang, Chen, Lee, Chan, Lieh-Mak, & McKenna, 2003). Leung and Chue (2000) suggested that the female brain is more symmetrically organized (less lateralized) than the male brain. Thus, if left hemisphere dysfunction is related to schizophrenia, then eye dominance is directly related to cerebral hemispheric dominance (Kameyama, et al., 1983), and females with schizophrenia might have a greater chance of showing left eye dominance.

Based on Edinburgh Handedness Inventory scores, schizophrenic patients in our study did not show a greater left-handed tendency when compared with healthy controls. This finding is not consistent with those of Western reports (Carlsson, et al., 1992; Orr, et al., 1999; Satz & Green, 1999) but is consistent with a report based on a Chinese sample (Yan, et al., 1985). A model of handedness or lateralization incorporating both genetic and cultural processes has been proposed by Laland, Kumm, Van Horn, and Feldman (1995). Although no genetic variation may underlie variations in handedness, it is possible that variation in handedness or lateralization among humans may be the result of a combination of cultural and developmental factors (Mandal, Harizuka, Bhushan, & Mishra, 2001; Li, Zhu, & Nuttall, 2003). In Eastern societies, children are expected to perform daily activities using the right hand as the dominant side. This cultural pressure causes most individuals to grow up to be right-handed. Hence, the cultural factor may have contributed to the discrepancies in Western versus Eastern findings.

The clinical significance of hand-eye dominance in schizophrenic patients is not clear. With respect to how eye dominance may affect hand performance, results indicate that the individuals with crossed eye-hand dominance showed a tendency for better right hand than left hand performance on the Purdue Pegboard. Individuals with crossed eye-hand dominance may have poorer bilateral cerebral integration than those with consistent eye-hand dominance. Therefore, those with a crossed dominance pattern may show a greater discrepancy between right and left hands in dexterity performance.

Results of this study must be interpreted with caution due to the following limitations. First of all, the power was low in all comparisons, ranging from .18 to .42. Secondly, many confounding factors, such as obstetric complications, deviated sampling (all right handedness as in the current study), and used antipsychotics or other medications, are not adequately controlled. Thirdly, the design of the present study may not be sensitive enough to detect a large effect given the limited sample size. To study a small or moderate effect, one would need a larger sample to have significant findings (Rossi, 1997). Thus, further studies with a larger sample are needed. Finally, syndromatic characteristics may be important factors awaiting elucidation when addressing functional asymmetry in schizophrenia because researchers have argued that it is a heterogeneous syndrome (e.g., Ross, 2000). Gruzelier, Wilson, Liddiard, Peters, and Pusavat (1999) reported that schizophrenic patients with positive syndrome showed a right-sided impairment and negative syndrome showed a left-sided impairment. Further studies exploring the relationship between positive and negative symptoms of schizophrenia and eye and hand dominance are still needed. Additional research is also needed to investigate the effect of the eye/hand dominance pattern on tasks involving visual/manual control in individuals with schizophrenia.

REFERENCES

AMERICAN PSYCHIATRIC ASSOCIATION. (1994) *DSM–IV: diagnostic and statistical manual of mental disorders*. (4th ed.) Washington, DC: American Psychiatric Association.

CANNON, M., BRYNE, M., CASSIDY, B., LARKIN, C., HORGAN, R., SHEPPARD, N. P., & O'CALLAGHAN, E. (1995) Prevalence and correlates of mixed-handedness in schizophrenia. *Psychiatry Research*, 59, 119-125.

CANNON, M., JONES, P., MURRAY, R. M., & WADSWORTH, M. E. (1997) Childhood laterality and later risk of schizophrenia in the 1946 British birth cohort. *Schizophrenia Research*, 26, 117-120.

CARLSSON, C., HUGDAHL, K., UVEBRANT, P., WIKLUND, L. M., & WENDT, L. V. (1992) Pathologi-

cal left-handedness revisited: dichotic listening in children with left vs right congenital hemiplegia. *Neuropsychologia*, 30, 471-481.
CHUA, S. E., LAM, I. W. S., TAI, K-S., CHEUNG, C., TANG, W-N., CHEN, E. Y. H., LEE, P. W. H., CHAN, F-L., LIEH-MAK, F., & MCKENNA, P. J. (2003) Brain morphological abnormality in schizophrenia is independent of country of origin. *Acta Psychiatrica Scandinavica*, 108, 269.
CROW, T. J. (1990) Temporal lobe asymmetries as the key to the etiology of schizophrenia. *Schizophrenia Bulletin*, 16, 433-443.
CROW, T. J., COLTER, N., FRITH, C. D., JOHNSTONE, E. C., & OWENS, D. G. C. (1989) Developmental arrests of cerebral asymmetries in early onset schizophrenia. *Psychiatry Research*, 29, 247-253.
DONNELLY, E. F. (1984) Neuropsychological impairment and associated intellectual functions in schizophrenic and other psychiatric patients. *Biological Psychiatry*, 19, 815-824.
GRUZELIER, J. H., WILSON, L., LIDDIARD, D., PETERS, E., & PUSAVAT, L. (1999) Cognitive asymmetry patterns in schizophrenia: active and withdrawn syndromes and sex differences as moderators. *Schizophrenia Bulletin*, 25, 349-362.
GUR, R. E. (1977) Motoric laterality imbalance in schizophrenia: a possible concomitant of left hemisphere dysfunction. *Archives of General Psychiatry*, 34, 33-37.
GUREJE, O. (1988) Sensorimotor laterality in schizophrenia: which features transcend cultural influences? *Acta Psychiatrica Scandinavica*, 77, 188-193.
KAMEYAMA, T., NIWA, S. I., HIRAMATSU, S. I., & SAITOH, O. (1983) Hand preference and eye dominance patterns in Japanese schizophrenics. In P. Flor-Henry & J. H. Gruzelier (Eds.), *Laterality and psychopathology*. Amsterdam: Elsevier. Pp. 181-194.
LALAND, K. N., KUMM, J., VAN HORN, J. D., & FELDMAN, M. W. (1995) A gene-culture model of human handedness. *Behavior Genetics*, 25, 433-445.
LEUNG, A., & CHUE, P. (2000) Sex differences in schizophrenia: a review of the literature. *Acta Psychiatrica Scandinavica*, 101, 3-38.
LI, C., ZHU, W., & NUTTALL, R. L. (2003) Familial handedness and spatial ability: a study with Chinese students aged 14-24. *Brain and Cognition*, 51, 375-384.
LOBEL, D. S., SWANDA, R. M., & LOSONCZY, M. F. (1994) Lateralized visual-field inattention in schizophrenia. *Perceptual and Motor Skills*, 79, 699-702.
MANDAL, M. K., HARIZUKA, S., BHUSHAN, B., & MISHRA, R. C. (2001) Cultural variation in hemifacial asymmetry of emotion expressions. *British Journal of Social Psychology*, 40, 385-398.
MERRIN, E. (1984) Motor and sighting dominance in schizophrenia and affective disorder. *British Journal of Psychiatry*, 146, 539-544.
ODDY, H. C., & LOBSTEIN, T. J. (1972) Hand and eye dominance in schizophrenia. *British Journal of Psychiatry*, 120, 331-332.
OLDFIELD, R. C. (1971) The assessment and analysis of handedness: the Edinburgh inventory. *Neuropsychologia*, 9, 97-113.
ORR, K. G. D., CANNON, M., GILVARRY, C. M., JONES, P. B., & MURRAY, R. M. (1999) Schizophrenic patients and their first-degree relatives show an excess of mixed-handedness. *Schizophrenia Research*, 39, 167-176.
OVERALL, J. E., & GORHAM, D. R. (1962) The Brief Psychiatric Rating Scale. *Psychological Reports*, 10, 799-812.
PIRAN, N., BIGLER, E. D., & COHEN, D. (1982) Motoric laterality and eye dominance suggest unique pattern of cerebral organization in schizophrenia. *Archives of General Psychiatry*, 39, 1006-1010.
PORAC, C., & COREN, S. (1976) The dominant eye. *Psychological Bulletin*, 83, 880-897.
ROBISON, S. E., BLOCK, S. S., BOUDREAUX, J. D., & FLORA, R. J. (1999) Hand-eye dominance in population with mental handicaps: prevalence and a comparison of methods. *Journal of the American Optometric Association*, 70, 563-570.
ROSS, E. R. (2000) The deficit syndrome and eye tracking disorder may reflect a distinct subtype within the syndrome of schizophrenia. *Schizophrenia Bulletin*, 26, 855-866.
ROSSI, A. (1997) A case study in the failure of psychology as a cumulative science: the spontaneous recovery of verbal learning. In L. L. Harlow, S. A. Mulaik, & J. H. Steiger (Eds.), *What if there were no significance tests?* Mahwah, NJ: Erlbaum. Pp. 175-198.

SATZ, P., & GREEN, M. F. (1999) Atypical handedness in schizophrenia: some methodological and theoretical issues. *Schizophrenia Bulletin*, 25, 63-78.

SHEEHAN, D. V., LECRUBIER, Y., SHEEHAN, K. H., AMORIM, P., JANAVS, J., WEILLER, E., HERGUETA, T., BAKER, R., & DUNBAR, G. C. (1998) The Mini-International Neuropsychiatric Interview (M.I.N.I.): the development and validation of a structured diagnostic psychiatric interview for DSM–IV and ICD–10. *Journal of Clinical Psychiatry*, 59, 22-33.

TIFFIN, J., & ASHER, E. J. (1948) The Purdue Pegboard: norms and studies of reliability and validity. *Journal of Applied Psychology*, 32, 234-247.

YAN, S. M., FLOR-HENRY, P., CHEN, D. Y., LI, T. G., QI, S. G., & MA, Z. X. (1985) Imbalance of hemispheric functions in the major psychoses: a study of handedness in the People's Republic of China. *Biological Psychiatry*, 20, 906-917.

Accepted April 12, 2004.

CONFLICTS, BURNOUT, AND BULLYING IN A FINNISH AND A POLISH COMPANY: A CROSS-NATIONAL COMPARISON [1]

LASSE M. VARHAMA AND KAJ BJÖRKQVIST

Åbo Akademi University

Summary.—The prevalence of conflicts, burnout, and bullying among employees of two similar companies, one situated in Poland ($n=66$) and the other in Finland ($n=330$) was investigated with the Psychosocial Workplace Inventory of Björkqvist and Österman. Both companies were of Finnish ownership and manufacturers in heavy industry. They were similar in most respects, such as organization, production and marketing. Significant differences were found between the two companies. Polish workers had higher scores on conflicts and self-experienced bullying, while Finnish workers reported higher burnout, both self-experienced and observed by others.

Although workplace behavior is a relatively well-researched area, little attention has been given to comparative studies between companies in different countries. The present study investigated the prevalence of conflicts, burnout, and bullying within two similar companies, one in Poland and the other in Finland.

Conflicts are a natural part of today's working-life (Kaufmann & Kaufmann, 1998) and may be defined as a difference of opinions or as a conviction that common goals or objectives cannot be reached (Rubin, Pruitt, & Kim, 1994). Conflicts may arise between groups, inside groups, between individuals or inside an individual (Markham, 1996). Putnam (1988) stressed the positive aspects of conflicts and that they may promote change and development. However, unresolved conflicts often lead to tension, distress, agony, and frustration (DuBrin, 1992). Einarsen, Raknes, Matthiesen, and Hellesöy (1994) found that 38% of Norwegian employees had often experienced conflicts between superiors and subordinates. Vartia and Perkka-Jortikka (1994) found the figure to be 60% in a similar study of Finnish workers. They also reported the frequency of conflicts to increase with company size.

Job stress may have both constructive and destructive consequences. An optimal arousal from mild stress can allow the individual to perform efficiently. On the other hand, excessive stress can result in the individual being unmotivated and too tense (Quick, Quick, Nelson, & Hurell, 1998). Consequences of chronic stress are tiredness, depression, metabolic disturbance and amnesia (Doctare, 2000) and if the exhausting process does not end, it

---

[1]Address correspondence to Lasse Varhama, SVF, Åbo Akademi University, P.O. Box 311, FIN-65101, Vasa, Finland or e-mail (lasse.varhama@abo.fi).

will lead to burnout. According to Maslach and Leiter (1997), the term burnout, coined by Freudenberger (1974), describes a syndrome that constitutes emotional exhaustion, depersonalization, and a decreased sense of personal accomplishment. Maslach and Leiter (1997) have claimed that today's employees typically have to produce too much too fast, i.e., demands and expectations exceed abilities. Kalimo and Toppinen (1997) found in a study of employees in Finland that 50% of their sample ($n = 3,300$) felt some kind of work exhaustion, 20% were very tired due to work, and 7% suffered from severe exhaustion.

Workplace harassment and bullying are used as different terms for the same problem (see Brodsky, 1976; Leymann, 1990; Keashly, Trott, & MacLean, 1994; Einarsen & Skogstad, 1996). According to Vartia (2003, cf. pp. 10-11), the definition of bullying is usually based upon five components: (1) systematic and repeated hostile behavior from the bully, (2) the victim is low in power and therefore unable to defend self in a sufficient way, (3) bullying may occur between individuals or groups and so a bully does not have to be a coworker, but may as well be a client, patient, pupil, or even an organisation, (4) although bullying often is intentional, the bully may at times victimize the other person unknowingly, (5) the negative acts range from social manipulation to physical violence.

According to Einarsen and Skogstad (1996), 17% of 552 employees of a marine engineering and maintenance workshop in Norway reported being bullied at work. Lehto and Sutela (1998) found, in a national study conducted by Statistics Finland, that an average of 16% of 3,800 Finnish employees reported having been exposed to harassment at work. Of the respondents, 40% reported observing bullying among others at their workplace. Björkqvist, Österman, and Hjelt-Bäck (1994) found that 24% of female and 17% of male employees ($n = 338$) at a Finnish university had experienced harassment and being bullied at their workplace. In a review of research in the field, Björkqvist (2001) found that victims of workplace bullying could suffer from a wide range of psychological symptoms, such as depression, sociophobia, and anxiety.

In the present study, workplace bullying, conflicts, and burnout were measured with the Psychosocial Workplace Inventory (Björkqvist & Österman, 1998). It was constructed to get an easy-to-use, still reliable and valid instrument. The rationale behind its development was as follows. Björkqvist (1992), using the Work Harassment Scale (Björkqvist & Österman, 1992), a highly reliable ($\alpha = .95$) 24-item scale, found that workplace harassment or bullying tends to escalate in three distinct stages, or levels: at Level I, the victim is exposed to belittling and degrading comments, rumors, backbiting, and a beginning isolation. At Level II, the degrading behavior becomes more severe and overt, perhaps even public, humiliation occurs. The victim also becomes psychologically isolated from others. At Level III, the isolation is complete, and the victim is "dehumanized" to the extent of being (untruthfully) labeled as crazy or totally impossible, and the colleagues try to force the victim out of the work force. He also found that Level I workplace bullying corresponded well to Work Harassment Scale scores, ranging between 0.25–0.50, Level II bullying corresponded to scores between 0.50–0.75, and Level III to scores >0.75. This finding formed the beginning of the development of the Psychosocial Workplace Inventory, used in the present study. It was developed to create an easy-to-use instrument with fewer items than the Work Harassment Scale.

One prediction of the study was that frequencies of bullying could be higher in Poland than in Finland. Fraczek (1985) conducted a cross-national comparison between Poland and Finland, with respect to the moral acceptance of various aggressive acts, and found that Poles approve of irony to a much greater extent than Finns. Irony is often an effective type of bullying. Fraczek suggested that the high approval of irony may be related to long history of communist rule in Poland, when it was difficult for the people to improve their socioeconomic situation or criticize the authorities. Irony, he suggested, was a way to cope mentally with this problem.

Method

Samples

Two samples were obtained from two similar companies which are parts of multinational cooperatives with headquarters in Finland. They are both manufacturers in the heavy industry, marketing, producing, and selling their own products. They are also part of larger multinational cooperations, albeit different ones. Both white- and blue-collar workers participated. Since both companies wanted to stay anonymous, they are simply referred to as Finnish and Polish samples.

More men than women took part in the study, in both Finland and in Poland ($\chi_1^2 = 4.45$, $p < .05$). In the Finnish sample, the mean age was higher ($t_{394} = 3.78$, $p < .001$). The return percentage was 46% for the Finnish and 60% for the Polish samples. More detailed information about the samples' sex and age distributions is provided in Table 1.

Psychosocial Workplace Inventory

The inventory (Björkqvist & Österman, 1998) investigates all in all five areas important for the psychosocial environment of the workplace. Three areas were chosen, conflicts, burnout, and bullying. Concepts and possible levels, as well as the typical behavior at the various levels, are defined and explained in the instructions provided with the inventory (see below).

In the Psychosocial Workplace Inventory is defined what is meant by

TABLE 1
Sex and Age Distributions in Two Investigated Companies

Company	Sex	n	Age (yr.) M	Age (yr.) SD	% of Total
Poland	Female	23	31	8.2	5
	Male	43	32	7.0	10
	Total	66	32	7.3	15
Finland	Female	78	36	8.4	20
	Male	252	37	8.3	65
	Total	330	37	9.1	85
Total	Female	101	35	8.5	25
	Male	295	36	9.1	75
	Total	396	36	9.0	100

key terms in the inventory, such as bullying, and then the respondent is asked whether he had had experiences of this and to what extent. In that way the questionnaire is kept at a manageable size. A similar strategy was used in Olweus' well-known questionnaire (1978) on bullying in schools.

(1) *Conflicts* were described as: "Interpersonal conflict is a natural phenomenon appearing at all workplaces. If handled objectively and immediately, conflicts are not harmful but may actually improve human relations and working conditions. When not handled at all or wrongly, communication is lost, people get hurt and work performance decreases" (Björkqvist & Österman, 1998, p. 64).

Conflicts were categorized into three levels in the inventory, depending on how resolvable they appeared to be, according to the respondent. The category *no conflict* does not imply a total absence but a feeling that conflicts are manageable. If employees start avoiding each other and quarrel frequently, and if a resolution appears difficult to find, the conflict is categorized as *difficult*. *Extreme conflicts* were defined as those in which people "cannot stand" each other, and there is a total communication breakdown between them.

(2) The definition and explanation of *burnout* provided in the inventory was "People experience being burned out when their working conditions for one reason or another (e.g., a heavy work load, stress, insecurity or conflict) become unbearable. Common symptoms are anxiety, depression, irritability, insomnia or psychosomatic diseases. One or several of these symptoms may appear" (Björkqvist & Österman, 1998, p. 64). The respondents reported if they had experienced or almost experienced a burnout. They also reported whether one or several of their colleagues had experienced a burnout.

(3) *Work harassment*, or workplace bullying, was described as "Work harassment occurs when one or several individuals at the workplace are repeatedly exposed to insulting and infringing behavior, which they, for one

reason or another, cannot defend themselves against. Work harassment is, by its very nature, degrading. Work harassment may occur at three levels, depending on its severity: typical behaviors appearing at *Level I* are belittling and degrading comments, rumors, backbiting and a beginning isolation of the exposed individual. At *Level II*, the degrading behavior becomes more severe, and overt and public humiliation may occur. The exposed individual becomes psychologically isolated from others, who do not want to talk to him or her. It is typical at this level that the exposed individual is described—untruthfully—as having 'difficulties to co-operate'. At *Level III*, the dehumanizing process directed towards the exposed person is brought to a level where she or he is not regarded as having the same human value as others, and it is acceptable to say almost anything about him or her. She or he is now totally isolated, receives suggestions to look for another job and is often regarded—untruthfully—as being mentally disturbed" (Björkqvist & Österman, 1998, p. 65).

RESULTS AND DISCUSSION

The results are presented in Table 2. As the table shows, burnout (both

TABLE 2
NUMBERS OF EMPLOYEES (%) FROM TWO SIMILAR COMPANIES IN POLAND AND FINLAND WITH RESPECT TO CONFLICTS, BURNOUT, AND BULLYING

	Poland	Finland	U	χ^2	η^2	Observed Power	Higher Frequencies
Conflicts							
No conflict	68	74					
Difficult	23	24	10194.0	7.24*	.007	0.39	Poland
Extreme	9	2					
Observed Burnout							
No one	47	34					
One person	19	19	8271.0*	4.67	.013	0.58	Finland
Several persons	34	47					
Self-experienced Burnout							
No	68	66					
Almost	25	32	11396.0	6.17*	.001	0.08	Finland
Yes	7	2					
Observed Bullying							
No	63	65					
Level I	26	25	10674.5	0.52	.001	0.08	
Level II	8	8					
Level III	3	2					
Self-experienced Bullying							
No	76	86					
Level I	20	10					
Level II	1	4	9888.5*	9.72*	.007	0.40	Poland
Level III	3	0					

Note.—Significant differences in numbers of employees estimated with Mann-Whitney's U, χ^2 and observed power ($N=396$). *$p<.05$.

observed and self-experienced) was more frequent in Finland, while conflicts and self-experienced bullying were more prevalent in Poland. Why conflicts and bullying were more common in Poland while burnout was more common in Finland cannot be stated with certainty on the basis of this study. As suggested by Fraczek's study (1985), the fact that Poles generally approve of irony to a much greater extent than Finns may be part of the answer. Irony is a typical form of verbal and indirect bullying (Björkqvist, Lagerspetz, & Kaukiainen, 1992). On the other hand, irony may also be a means of reducing tension, decreasing the risk of succumbing to exhaustion and burnout, something that Finnish employees reported more frequently. Differences in unemployment rates and in salary may also contribute to the finding of more bullying in the Polish sample. Dabkowski (1996) suggested economic and political reasons for bullying among Polish pupils aged 14–16 years. Hard competition on the labor market often results in an unhealthy competition inside companies, too. Insecurity and conflicts may be transformed into bullying (Leymann, 1992).

REFERENCES

BJÖRKQVIST, K. (1992) Trakasserier förekommer bland anställda vid ÅA. *Meddelanden från Åbo Akademi*, 9, 14-15.

BJÖRKQVIST, K. (2001) Social defeat as a stressor in humans. *Psychology and Behavior*, 73, 435-442.

BJÖRKQVIST, K., LAGERSPETZ, K. M. J., & KAUKIAINEN, A. (1992) Do girls manipulate and boys fight? Developmental trends in regard to direct and indirect aggression. *Aggressive Behavior*, 18, 117-127.

BJÖRKQVIST, K., & ÖSTERMAN, K. (1992) *Work Harassment Scale*. Turku, Fin. : Åbo Akademi Univer.

BJÖRKQVIST, K., & ÖSTERMAN, K. (1998) Psychosocial Workplace Inventory. *Pro Facultate*, 4, 63-67.

BJÖRKQVIST, K., ÖSTERMAN, K., & HJELT-BÄCK, M. (1994) Aggression among university employees. *Aggressive Behavior*, 20, 173-184.

BRODSKY, C. M. (1976) *The harassed worker*. Toronto, Canada: Lexington Books, DC Heath.

DABKOWSKI, M. (1996) Bullying: the violence in peer groups. *European Psychiatry*, 11, 230-231.

DOCTARE, C. (2000) *Hjärnstress - Kan det drabba mig?* Hässelby, Sweden: Runa Förlag.

DUBRIN, A. J. (1992) *Human relations for career and personal success*. Englewood Cliffs, NJ: Prentice-Hall.

EINARSEN, S., RAKNES, B. I., MATTHIESEN, S. B., & HELLESÖY, O. H. (1994) *Mobbning og harde personkonflikter. Helsefarlig samspill på arbeidsplassen*. Bergen, Norway: Sigma Förlag.

EINARSEN, S., & SKOGSTAD, A. (1996) Bullying at work: epidemiological findings in public and private organizations. *European Journal of Work and Organizational Psychology*, 5, 185-201.

FRACZEK, A. (1985) Moral approval of aggressive acts: a Polish-Finnish comparative study. *Journal of Cross-Cultural Psychology*, 16, 41-54.

FREUDENBERGER, H. J. (1974) Staff burnout. *Journal of Social Issues*, 30, 159-165.

KALIMO, R., & TOPPINEN, S. (1997) *Työuupumus Suomen työikäisellä väestölla*. Helsinki, Finland: Työterveyslaitos.

KAUFMANN, G., & KAUFMANN, A. (1998) *Psykologi i organisation och ledning*. Lund, Sweden: Studentlitteratur.

KEASHLY, L., TROTT, V., & MACLEAN, L. M. (1994) Abusive behavior in the workplace: a preliminary investigation. *Violence and Victims*, 9, 341-357.

LEHTO, A-M., & SUTELA, H. (1998) *Efficient, more efficient, exhausted: findings of Finnish quality of work life surveys 1977–1997.* Helsinki, Finland: Statistics Finland.

LEYMANN, H. (1990) Mobbing and psychological terror at workplaces. *Violence and Victims*, 5, 119-126.

LEYMANN, H. (1992) *Från mobbning till utslagning i arbetslivet.* Stockholm, Sweden: Publica.

MARKHAM, U. (1996) *Så handskas du med svåra situationer på arbetsplatsen.* Malmö, Sweden: Richters.

MASLACH, C., & LEITER, M. P. (1997) *The truth about burnout.* San Francisco, CA: Jossey-Bass.

OLWEUS, D. (1978) *Aggression in schools: bullies and whipping boys.* Washington, DC: Hemisphere.

PUTNAM, L. L. (1988) Communication and interpersonal conflict in organizations. *Management Communication Quarterly*, 3, 293-301.

QUICK, J. C., QUICK, J. D., NELSON, D. L., & HURELL, J. J. (1998) *Preventive stress management in organisations.* Washington, DC: American Psychological Association.

RUBIN, J., PRUITT, D. G., & KIM, S. H. (1994) *Social conflict: escalation, stalemate, and settlement.* New York: McGraw-Hill.

VARTIA, M. (2003) Workplace bullying: a study on the work environment, well-being and health. *People and Work Research Reports 56.* Finnish Institute of Occupational Health.

VARTIA, M., & PERKKA-JORTIKKA, K. (1994) *Henkinen työväkivalta työpaikoilla: Työyhteisön hyvinvointi ja sen uhat.* Tampere, Finland: Gaudeamus.

Accepted April 13, 2004.

SOCIAL SUPPORT AND SALIVARY SECRETORY IMMUNOGLOBULIN A RESPONSE IN WOMEN TO STRESS OF MAKING A PUBLIC SPEECH[1]

HIDEKI OHIRA

Department of Psychology
Nagoya University

Summary.—Acute experimental stressors transiently increase volume of secretory immunoglobulin A (s-IgA) in saliva. The present study examined buffering effects of social support on response of s-IgA to a brief psychological stress (giving a public speech). 24 women were divided at random into three groups, an emotional support group, an informational support group and a no-support group (control). For each group, s-IgA measures were obtained from each person under baseline conditions, during preparation of a speech when social support or no support was given, immediately after the speech and during a 'recovery' period. Level of s-IgA in the control group significantly elevated during preparation for the speech and just after the speech compared to baseline, suggesting that the speech task stimulated secretory immune function. On the other hand, the subjects in the emotional support group showed increased s-IgA during the preparation period but secretion of s-IgA rapidly returned to the baseline after the speech task. Secretion of s-IgA in the informational social support group was unchanged at any measurement point. These results suggest that social support attenuates the affect of a stressor on somatic state.

A number of epidemiological studies have shown that social support is one of the important factors modulating responses to stressors in the psychological, cardiovascular, endocrine and immune systems. Social support has been generally beneficial for mental and physical health (Coyne & Downey, 1991; Uchino, Cacioppo, & Kiecolt-Glaser, 1996).

Controlled laboratory studies have been conducted to evaluate the mechanisms underlying the effects of social support on physiological responses to several types of stressors. In general, cardiovascular reactions to acute or brief stressors are attenuated by the presence of supportive others (for reviews, see Uchino, *et al.*, 1996; Lepore, 1998). Specifically, the elevation of systolic blood pressure, diastolic blood pressure, heart rate and skin conductance in stress tasks was smaller when subjects performed the tasks with supportive others than when they did them alone (e.g., Kamarck, Manuck, & Jennings, 1990; Lepore, Allen, & Evans, 1993; Gerin, Milner, Chawla, & Pickering, 1995).

---

[1]The author thanks Dr. Yutaka Watanabe and Mrs. Motoko Niimi for their assistance in assay of s-IgA and data collection. Portions of this study were presented at the 24th International Congress of Applied Psychology, July 2002, Singapore. Address correspondence to Hideki Ohira, Ph.D., Department of Psychology, Nagoya University, Furo-cho, Chikusa-ku, Nagoya, 464-8601, Japan or e-mail (ohira@lit.nagoya-u.ac.jp).

On the other hand, findings about linkage of social support and endocrine and immune system function are mixed. Some epidemiological and experimental studies have suggested that social support has potential effects on neuroendocrine and immune functioning. For example, low social support was associated with increased excretion of urinary norepinephrine (Fleming, Baum, Gisriel, & Gatchel, 1982). Response of norepinephrine after watching a violent film was attenuated in subjects with high social support (Arnetz, Edgren, Levi, & Otto, 1985). In a speech task, male subjects provided social support by their girlfriends showed lower salivary cortisol than subjects without social support (Kirschbaum, Klauer, Filipp, & Hellhammer, 1995). Social support was related to greater levels of natural killer cell activity (Levy, Herberman, Whiteside, Sanzo, Lee, & Kirkwood, 1990), proliferation of lymphocytes (Linn, Linn, & Klimas, 1988) and numbers of lymphocytes (Persson, Gullberg, Hanson, Moestrup, & Ostergren, 1994), suggesting enhancement of immune function by social support. However, other studies have reported null effects or only statistically marginal effects of social support on endocrine and immune systems (Schlesinger & Yodfat, 1991; Goodkin, Blaney, Feaster, Fletcher, Baum, Mantero-Atienza, Klimas, Millon, Szapocznik, & Eisdorfer, 1992; Perry, Fishman, Jacobsberg, & Frances, 1992). Furthermore, controlled experimental studies in this research area have been relatively few. Apparently more data are needed.

The aim of the present study is to examine effects of social support on change of secretory immunoglobulin A (s-IgA) in saliva in an experimental setting with a conventional stress task, a public speech. S-IgA is the predominant antibody thought to be a first line of defense against invading organisms in mucosal sites. A decline of the volume of s-IgA has been thought to increase risk for several infectious diseases (Mestecky & McGhee, 1987). Several studies have assayed s-IgA level in saliva as an index of secretory immune functioning in local mucosal sites (Jemmott & Magloire, 1988), although there has been a controversy about whether total volume of s-IgA accurately represents immune system functioning (Stone, Cox, Valdimarsdottir, & Neale, 1987). Numerous studies have reported that chronic stress such as academic examination periods for undergraduates is associated with reductions in levels of s-IgA (Jemmott & Magloire, 1988; Deinzer & Schuller, 1998). In contrast, acute exposure to both naturalistic and laboratory stressors such as air-traffic control (Zeier, Brauchli, & Joller-Jemelka, 1996), a continuous arithmetic task (Ohira, Watanabe, Kobayashi, & Kawai, 1999), mental arithmetic or the cold pressor stimulus (Winzer, Ring, Carroll, Willemsen, Drayson, & Kendall, 1999) reliably produces increases in s-IgA.

Underlying mechanisms in these rapid increases in s-IgA have not been fully explored. Stress-induced activation of the hypothalamic-pituitary-adrenal (HPA) axis modulates immune function. Usually this has been thought to be the main mechanism that mediates chronic stress and reduced immune function. However, there is a time lag before the cortisol-dependent immunological changes are observed (Munck & Guyre, 1991). Thus, the rapid change in s-IgA secretion should be attributed to another mechanism. Some researchers have suggested that activation of the sympathetic nervous system plays a main role in association between acute or brief stressors and changes in the s-IgA immune system (Winzer, et al., 1999). Further, a recent study reported that sympathetic stimulation of the submandibular glands in rats resulted in a six-fold increase in s-IgA secretion (Carpenter, Garrett, Hartley, & Proctor, 1998). Given that sympathetic activation might regulate secretion of s-IgA, based on the previous findings that social support can attenuate sympathetic activation in stressful situations, it was predicted that individuals provided social support would show lower levels of s-IgA elicited by a stress task than those who were provided no support.

Social support has been considered as a multidimensional and multifaceted concept. Some researchers have argued that four types of social support are especially essential, that is, emotional, instrumental, informational and appraisal support (Thoits, 1986; Cohen, 1988; Langford, Bowsher, Maloney, & Lillis, 1997). The second aim of this study was to examine relative importance of two of these four types of social support as argued by Langford, et al. (1997). Specifically this study assessed whether emotional, informational or both types of social support would be more effective in regulating secretory immune responses to a stressor.

In this study effects of social support from a female supporter on another woman's changes in s-IgA level to an experimental stressor were evaluated. Sex differences in effects of social support have been reported. Support provided by women reduced cardiovascular changes in a speech task but support from men did not (Glynn, Christenfeld, & Gerin, 2000). Because this study was to explore these with a relatively small number of subjects, female supporters and female speakers were chosen, as this was expected to be the most effective.

Method

Subjects

Twenty-four undergraduate women (M age = 20.4 yr., SD = 1.0) volunteered to participate in the experiment. All of them reported being right-handed, and none suffered from any chronic and oral illness or took medication or oral contraceptives known to influence immunity. No subjects were excluded based on their menstrual cycle phase. The subjects were instructed to abstain from eating, smoking, drinking any beverages except water, and exercising 2 hr. before the experiment. They were allocated randomly to three experimental groups: Emotional support, Informational support, and Control. Thus in each group were eight subjects.

Salivary s-IgA

To assay concentration of s-IgA, samples of unstimulated saliva were collected using cotton swabs (Salivettes, Sarstedt Ltd.). Two cotton swabs were placed underneath the tongue of each participant for 5 min. After that, the cotton swabs were removed, and saliva was extracted from the cotton by centrifugation at 3.5×10^3 rpm for 10 min. Saliva was stored frozen in capped test tubes at $-20°C$ until assay. S-IgA concentration in saliva was determined by an enzyme-linked immunoabsorbent assay (Kvale & Brandtzaeg, 1986). The thawed saliva aliquots (100 µl) were diluted 1,000 times. Saliva samples were reacted with walls of the wells of 96-well assay plates that labeled the antihuman secretory component (MBL, Inc.). By this procedure, s-IgA was captured on the walls of the wells. After incubation at $37°C$ for 2 hr., the wells were washed twice and reacted with standard antihuman IgA (rabbit IgG / Fab, Wako-junyaku, Inc.) conjugated with horseradish peroxidase. After incubation at room temperature for 2 hr., the wells were washed four times, then enzyme metrical fluid (orthophenylenediamine + 4mM H_2O_2) was added for color development. After incubation at room temperature for 1 hr., the reaction was stopped by addition of NaF. The reaction product was quantified spectrophotometrically at 405 mm with a microplate reader (Bio-rad, Inc., Model 3550).

Self-report Measures

State anxiety was evaluated as a variable related to perceived stress by means of the Japanese version of the State-Trait Anxiety Inventory (Spielberger, Gorsuch, & Lushene, 1970) Form Y-1 (the STAI-State for measurement of state anxiety), which is composed of 20 items, each rated on a 4-point Likert scale.

To validate the manipulation of Emotional and Informational support, the subjects were delivered a questionnaire containing the following items: "Is your impression of the supporter (the confederate) positive," "Did the supporter make you relax," "Was conversation with the supporter helpful to you in composing the contents of your speech?" A Yes or No answer was required to each item by the subjects in the Emotional and Informational support groups.

Procedure

To minimize variation of salivary s-IgA reflecting circadian rhythms, each experimental session was conducted from 10:00 a.m. to noon. After giving written informed consent, subjects were accommodated in a first room where they rested for 15 min. for habituation to the experimental setting (Jennings, Kamarck, Stewart, Eddy, & Johnson, 1992). After that, the first recording of the measures (Baseline) was carried out. The subjects responded to the STAI-State. After washing their mouths, the first samples of their saliva were collected.

Following the baseline recording, an experimenter gave the subjects the following instructions of the speech task: "Your task is to make a persuasive speech on a controversial topic in front of an audience. You have 10 min. to prepare a speech of 3 min. duration on this topic." The experimenter then gave them a paper on which a topic was written: abortion. "You can choose whether to take the pro or con position. Your speech will be evaluated by audiences according to its adequacy, argumentative structure, and speech skills." The need to speak for the entire 3-min. period was strongly emphasized. Making notes for the speech in this preparation period was permitted; however, the subjects were not allowed to use the notes during their speech.

For the first 5 min. the subjects stayed alone, and in the last 5 min. social support was provided to the subjects in the Emotional and Informational support groups. After 5 min. passed from start of the preparation period, the subjects in all groups were told "Another subject in a previous session has just finished her speech task. She will come to this room for her recovery procedure." Then a female confederate serving as another subject entered the room. She was trained to behave in differentiated supportive fashion, depending on the experimental support condition. For the subjects in the Emotional support group, the confederate smiled and wished them good luck. She said that the speech situation she experienced was not difficult and encouraged the subjects with an empathetic attitude. Also, she tried to have some light conversation with the subjects during the remaining preparation period. However, she did not offer any concrete information nor advise specifically about the speech. For the subjects in the Informational support group, the confederate's facial expressions and her attitude to the subjects were neutral; however, she told the subjects concrete situations of the speech, for example, about the room or the audience. Also, she gave the subjects some advice about ways to be relaxed and about contents of the speech. The confederate in the control group just sat silently during the preparation period and showed minimal response to the subjects. The same female undergraduate served as the confederate in all experimental sessions. She left the room at the end of the preparation period. After the manipulation of social support, again subjects responded to the STAI-State, and their saliva was collected for 5 min. (Preparation samples).

When the preparation period finished, the experimenter introduced the subjects to the second room where they would make their speech. The subjects stood in front of five female undergraduates, and a video-recording device was switched on in sight of the subjects to enhance the stressfulness of the situation. The experimenter handed a timer to the subjects to measure 3 min. during the speech, and the subject was then told to start. The audience took notes during the subjects' speeches but did not say anything or express any emotion on their faces. After the 3-min. speech period, the subjects returned to the first room where the third set of measures was conducted (Speech: STAI-State and saliva). The subjects remained seated another 20 min. alone in the room without any stimulation. After this recovery period, the fourth set of measures (Recovery: STAI-State and saliva) was carried out. Subjects were then fully debriefed, and the subjects in the Emotional and Informational support groups filled out a questionnaire as a manipulation check.

Results

Manipulation Check for Social Support

All subjects in the Emotional support group and four of eight subjects in the Informational support group indicated that they had good impressions of the supporter ($\chi_1^2 = 5.33$, $p < .05$). Also, all subjects in the Emotional support group and five of eight subjects in the Informational support group felt that they were relaxed by conversation with the supporter ($\chi_1^2 = 3.69$, $p < .10$). Furthermore, conversation with the supporter was evaluated as helpful by all eight subjects in the Informational support group and by two of eight subjects in the Emotional support group ($\chi_1^2 = 9.6$, $p < .01$). These results suggest that experimental manipulations of two types of social support were effective.

State Anxiety

Table 1 shows changes in the scores of the STAI-State in each group and at each measurement point. A repeated-measure, two-factor analysis of variance (group × measurement point) was conducted on the scores. A main

TABLE 1
Means and Standard Deviations For State Anxiety by Group

Group	Baseline M	Baseline SD	Preparation M	Preparation SD	Speech M	Speech SD	Recovery M	Recovery SD
Emotional support	44.1	5.2	49.3	8.5	36.8	5.4	35.4	7.7
Informational support	44.0	7.3	56.0	6.1	39.8	7.9	32.5	6.3
Control	46.9	6.2	50.6	3.6	43.5	6.6	39.0	7.9

effect of measurement point was significant ($F_{3,60} = 31.28$, $p < .01$). Further analyses using Fisher's *LSD* tests ($p < .05$) indicated that the state anxiety reported was significantly higher at the preparation measure than at the other measurement points. Neither the main effect of group nor the interaction of the two factors was significant ($F_{2,20} = 3.41$; $F_{6,60} = 0.61$).

S-IgA

The s-IgA data of one subject in the control group was excluded from statistical analyses because there was a technical problem in the assay of s-IgA. Changes in concentration of salivary s-IgA are shown in Table 2. A repeated-measure two-factor analysis of variance (group × measurement point) which was conducted for concentration of salivary s-IgA showed a significant main effect of measurement point ($F_{3,57} = 9.90$, $p < .01$) and a significant interaction of group and measurement point ($F_{6,57} = 4.36$, $p < .01$). Results of the Fisher *LSD* tests ($p < .05$) were as follows. At baseline, there was no difference in salivary s-IgA concentration among the three groups. At the preparation testing, concentration of s-IgA significantly increased in the Control group and in the Emotional support group compared to the baseline. Also, concentration of s-IgA was significantly higher in the control group and in the Emotional support group than in the Informational support group. At the speech test, s-IgA in the Control group further significantly increased compared to the values at the preparation testing. The s-IgA value in the Emotional support group returned to baseline. Thus, significant differences in the s-IgA values were shown between the Control group and the other two groups. This pattern of differences was maintained during the recovery period. In the Informational support group, concentration of s-IgA did not change significantly at any later measurement points compared to the baseline.

TABLE 2
MEANS AND STANDARD DEVIATIONS OF CONCENTRATION OF SALIVARY s-IGA BY GROUP

Group	Baseline M	Baseline SD	Preparation M	Preparation SD	Speech M	Speech SD	Recovery M	Recovery SD
Emotional support	76.2	11.5	102.9	24.6	89.4	14.8	84.3	12.8
Informational support	75.7	15.9	80.5	5.9	87.3	13.1	94.5	14.0
Control	81.3	7.3	106.5	10.8	136.2	22.6	131.7	23.5

DISCUSSION

The aim of this study was to examine the effects of different kinds of social support, either emotional or informational support from a confederate pretending to a subject who participated in a prior experiment, on secretion of salivary s-IgA as a response to a social stressor (a speech task). Analysis of subjects' ratings on the manipulation check items indicated that the experimental manipulation of the two types of social support worked well. However, it should be noted that the data of the manipulation check were obtained after the debriefing. Thus, contamination due to demand characteristics cannot be completely ruled out. Still, however, those results seem to show the differentiated influences of the supporter dependent on the condition, suggesting that the manipulation of social support was at least partially valid.

In the Control group, concentration of s-IgA clearly increased during the preparation and speech periods. This result is consistent with previous findings showing rapid increase of s-IgA after acute or brief stressors (Zeier, et al., 1996; Ohira, et al., 1999; Winzer, et al., 1999). Thus, the speech task used in this study can be interpreted as adequately stressful for the subjects. More importantly, the pattern of responses of s-IgA indicated differences between the three experimental conditions. In the Emotional support group, secretion of s-IgA increased as in the control group, but rapidly decreased to near the baseline just after the speech period. In the Informational support group, the response of s-IgA to the stress task had returned to baseline. These results supported the prediction and clarified for the first time that elevation of secretion of s-IgA in saliva as a stress reaction to a brief and social stressor can be attenuated by social support. This finding corresponds to the evidence that social support can reduce the elevation of cardiovascular responses to stressors (Kamarck, et al., 1990; Gerin, Pieper, Levy, & Pickering, 1992; Lepore, et al., 1993; Gerin, et al., 1995). In conclusion, social support can be thought to have buffering effects for affective response to stressors in physiological systems.

Limitations of this study must be recognized. Given the lack of autonomic indices, the relationship of responses in s-IgA and in the sympathetic nervous system could not be evaluated. This study evaluated changes in a limited aspect of the immune system, salivary s-IgA. Clinical implication of the transient and relatively small changes of s-IgA concentration and effects of social support on the changes shown in this study is not clear yet. To conclude whether individuals with social support might truly suffer less infectious disease, influences of social support on many other measures of the immune system must be examined. Another concern about this study is that influence of menstrual cycle phases on s-IgA and self-reported measures was not excluded. No direct evidence has been reported that the cycle phases influence secretion of salivary s-IgA; however, it can affect subjective feelings including anxiety. More studies controlling effects of the cycle phases for women and studies of male subjects are needed.

This study also suggested that, at least for the speech tasks, informational support apparently was more beneficial than emotional support. Informational support nearly eliminated the stress response in mucosal immune function evaluated by s-IgA, whereas emotional support did not reduce anticipatory response in s-IgA while subjects waited to give their speeches. This result might be attributed to a difference in effectiveness of coping with the stressor given the two support types. The public speech is a stressor with which one must actively cope. Concrete information about how one should think, how one can be relaxed, how one should behave and so on might be more important than pure emotional empathy or encouragement in coping with such a stressor. Contrarily, emotional social support might be more effective for different types of stressors such as fearful or aversive situations or negative stress events in everyday life. Such interaction of types of social support and types of stressors must also be clarified by research.

Although social support had clear effects on secretory immune response, it did not have any beneficial influence on perceived stress estimated by state anxiety (STAI-State) scores. Interestingly, such a lack of correspondence between self-reports and physiological measures is typical of social support studies (Kamarck, *et al.*, 1990; Gerin, *et al.*, 1992; Snydersmith & Cacioppo, 1992; Lepore, *et al.*, 1993; Kirschbaum, *et al.*, 1995; Glynn, *et al.*, 2000). Data of this study do not offer the explanations for this difference. One possible speculation is that in individuals who are not psychologically sensitive to social support, the support might work more directly on the person's physiology. However, validity and sensitivity of scales in evaluation of perceived stress and effects of social support must also be considered. Given the small number of subjects in this study, the low statistical power might undermine detection of effects of social support on self-rated state anxiety. Clarification of dissociation between subjective psychological states and somatic states is important for further research on stress and social support.

REFERENCES

Arnetz, B. B., Edgren, B., Levi, L., & Otto, U. (1985) Behavioral and endocrine reactions in boys scoring high on Sennton neurotic scale viewing an exciting and partly violent movie and the importance of social support. *Social Science and Medicine*, 20, 731-736.

Carpenter, G. H., Garrett, J. R., Hartley, R. H., & Proctor, G. B. (1998) The influence of nerves on the secretion of immunoglobulin A into submandibular saliva in rats. *Journal of Physiology*, 512, 567-573.

Cohen, S. (1988) Psychosocial models of the role of social support in the etiology of physical disease. *Health Psychology*, 7, 296-297.

Coyne, J. C., & Downey, G. (1991) Social factors and psychopathology: stress, social support, and coping processes. *Annual Review of Psychology*, 42, 401-425.

Deinzer, R., & Schuller, N. (1998) Dynamics of stress-related decrease of salivary immunoglobulin A (sIgA): relationship to symptoms of the common cold and studying behavior. *Behavioral Medicine*, 23, 161-169.

Fleming, R., Baum, A., Gisriel, M. M., & Gatchel, R. J. (1982) Mediating influences of social support on stress at Three Mile Island. *Journal of Human Stress*, 8, 14-22.

Gerin, W., Milner, D., Chawla, S., & Pickering, T. G. (1995) Social support as a moderator of cardiovascular reactivity in women: a test of the direct effects and buffering hypotheses. *Psychosomatic Medicine*, 57, 16-22.

Gerin, W., Pieper, C., Levy, R., & Pickering, T. G. (1992) Social support in social interaction: a moderator of cardiovascular reactivity. *Psychosomatic Medicine*, 54, 324-336.

Glynn, L. M., Christenfeld, N., & Gerin, W. (2000) Gender, social support, and cardiovascular responses to stress. *Psychosomatic Medicine*, 61, 234-242.

Goodkin, K., Blaney, N. T., Feaster, D., Fletcher, M., Baum, M. K., Mantero-Atienza, E., Klimas, N. G., Millon, C., Szapocznik, J., & Eisdorfer, C. (1992) Active coping style is associated with natural killer cell cytotoxicity in asymptomatic HIV-1 seropositive homosexual men. *Journal of Psychosomatic Research*, 36, 633-650.

Jemmott, J. B. III, & Magloire, K. (1988) Academic stress, social support, and secretory immunoglobulin A. *Journal of Personality and Social Psychology*, 55, 803-810.

Jennings, J. R., Kamarck, T., Stewart, C. H., Eddy, M., & Johnson, P. (1992) Alternate cardiovascular baseline assessment techniques: vanilla or resting baseline. *Psychophysiology*, 29, 742-750.

KAMARCK, T. W., MANUCK, S. B., & JENNINGS, J. R. (1990) Social support reduces cardiovascular reactivity to psychological challenge: a laboratory model. *Psychosomatic Medicine*, 52, 42-58.
KIRSCHBAUM, C., KLAUER, T., FILIPP, S. H., & HELLHAMMER, D. H. (1995) Sex-specific effects of social support on cortisol and subjective responses to acute psychological stress. *Psychosomatic Medicine*, 57, 23-31.
KVALE, D., & BRANDTZAEG, P. (1986) An enzyme-linked immunosorbent assay for differential quantification of secretory immunoglobulins of the A and M isotypes in human serum. *Journal of Immunological Methods*, 86, 107-114.
LANGFORD, C. P., BOWSHER, J., MALONEY, J. P., & LILLIS, P. P. (1997) Social support: a conceptual analysis. *Journal of Advanced Nursing*, 25, 95-100.
LEPORE, S. J. (1998) Problems and prospects for the social support-reactivity hypotheses. *Annual Review of Medicine*, 20, 257-269.
LEPORE, S. J., ALLEN, K. A., & EVANS, G. W. (1993) Work noise annoyance and blood pressure: combined effects with stressful working conditions. *International Archives of Occupational and Environmental Health*, 65, 23-28.
LEVY, S. M., HERBERMAN, R. B., WHITESIDE, T., SANZO, K., LEE, J., & KIRKWOOD, J. (1990) Perceived social support and tumor estrogen/progesterone receptor status as predictors of natural killer cell activity in breast cancer patients. *Psychosomatic Medicine*, 52, 73-85.
LINN, B. S., LINN, M. W., & KLIMAS, N. G. (1988) Effects of psychophysical stress on surgical outcomes. *Psychosomatic Medicine*, 50, 230-244.
MESTECKY, J., & MCGHEE, J. R. (1987) Immunoglobulin A (IgA): molecular and cellular interactions involved in IgA biosynthesis and immune response. *Advances in Immunology*, 40, 153-245.
MUNCK, A., & GUYRE, P. M. (1991) Glucocorticoids and immune function. In R. Ader, D. L. Felton, & N. Cohen (Eds.), *Psychoneuroimmunology*. (2nd ed.) San Diego, CA: Academic Press. Pp. 447-474.
OHIRA, H., WATANABE, Y., KOBAYASHI, K., & KAWAI, M. (1999) The Type A behavioral pattern and immune reactivity to brief stress: changes in volume of secretory immunoglobulin A in saliva. *Perceptual and Motor Skills*, 89, 423-430.
PERRY, S., FISHMAN, B., JACOBSBERG, L., & FRANCES, A. (1992) Relationships over 1 year between lymphocyte subsets and psychosocial variables among adults with infection by human immunodeficiency virus. *Archives of General Psychiatry*, 49, 396-401.
PERSSON, L., GULLBERG, B., HANSON, B. S., MOESTRUP, T., & OSTERGREN, P. O. (1994) HIV infection: social network, social support, and CD4 lymphocyte values in infected homosexual men in Malmo, Sweden. *Journal of Epidemiology and Community Health*, 48, 580-585.
SCHLESINGER, M., & YODFAT, T. (1991) The impact of stressful life events on natural killer cells. *Stress Medicine*, 7, 53-60.
SNYDERSMITH, M. A., & CACIOPPO, J. T. (1992) Parsing complex social factors to determine component effects: I. Autonomic activity and reactivity as a function of human association. *Journal of Social and Clinical Psychology*, 11, 263-278.
SPIELBERGER, C. D., GORSUCH, R. L., & LUSHENE, R. E. (1970) *Manual for the State-Trait Anxiety Inventory*. Palo Alto, CA: Consulting Psychologists Press.
STONE, A. A., COX, D. S., VALDIMARSDOTTIR, H., & NEALE, J. M. (1987) Secretory IgA as a measure of immunocompetence. *Journal of Human Stress*, 13, 136-140.
THOITS, P. A. (1986) Social support as coping assistance. *Journal of Consulting and Clinical Psychology*, 54, 416-423.
UCHINO, B. N., CACIOPPO, J. T., & KIECOLT-GLASER, J. K. (1996) The relationship between social support and physiological processes: a review with emphasis on underlying mechanisms and implications for health. *Psychological Bulletin*, 119, 488-531.
WINZER, A., RING, C., CARROLL, D., WILLEMSEN, G., DRAYSON, M., & KENDALL, M. (1999) Secretory immunoglobulin A and cardiovascular reactions to mental arithmetic, cold pressor, and exercise: effects of beta-adrenergic blockade. *Psychophysiology*, 36, 591-601.
ZEIER, H., BRAUCHLI, P., & JOLLER-JEMELKA, H. I. (1996) Effects of work demands on immunoglobulin A and cortisol in air traffic controllers. *Biological Psychology*, 42, 413-423.

Accepted April 14, 2004.

BODY-SHAPE PERCEPTIONS IN OLDER ADULTS AND MOTIVATIONS FOR EXERCISE [1]

PETRA B. SCHULER, AMANDA BROXON-HUTCHERSON, STEVEN F. PHILIPP, STUART RYAN, ROBERT M. ISOSAARI, AND DESTINI ROBINSON

University of West Florida

Summary.—This study examined the relationships among age, sex, exercise and body-image dissatisfaction in older adults and evaluated the role of body-shape dissatisfaction as a motivation to exercise. A pencil-and-paper questionnaire was administered to 175 older adults (101 women and 74 men) ranging in age from 50 to 98 years ($M = 72$ yr., $SD = 9$) to obtain general information, information regarding exercise participation, motivations for exercise and body-shape perceptions. A body-shape dissatisfaction score was calculated using the difference between the participant's choice for current and ideal body shape from a nine-figure body-silhouette scale. Present study findings suggested that both older adult men and women expressed a desire for a thinner body shape independent of age and current participation in exercise. In addition, the results indicated that body-shape dissatisfaction did not motivate this sample to engage in regular exercise; physical health and physical fitness emerged as the most important motivations to exercise.

While much research has focused on the relationship between exercise and body-shape perception in college students and adolescents (Snyder & Kivlin, 1975; Rossi & Zoccolotti, 1979; Davis & Cowles, 1991; Hallinan, Pierce, Evans, DeGrenier, & Andres, 1991; Salusso-Deonier & Schwartzkopf, 1991; Loland, 2000), few studies have examined this relationship in older adults (Davis & Cowles, 1991; Hallinan & Schuler, 1993; Abadie, Schuler, Hunt, & Lischkoff, 1996; Loland, 2000). Even fewer studies have investigated associations between body-shape perception and exercise motivation in older adults (Davis & Cowles, 1991; Loland, 2000). The present study was designed to examine associations among age, sex, exercise participation and body-shape perception in older adults. In addition, the study assessed to what extent the decision to exercise may be motivated by body-shape perception.

Research on body-shape perception in adolescents and young adults suggests that, while both women and men express dissatisfaction with the current body shape, women tend to be more dissatisfied compared to men (Gray, 1977; Silberstein, Striegel-Moore, Timko, & Rodin, 1988; Demarest & Langer, 1996). Generally, women have body-shape ideals that are signifi-

---

[1]Address correspondence to Petra B. Schuler, Ph.D., Department of Health Leisure and Exercise Science, University of West Florida, 11000 University Parkway, Pensacola, FL 32514 or e-mail (pschuler@uwf.edu).

cantly smaller in size than their perceived current body shapes, whereas men are equally divided between those who want to be bigger in size and those who want to be smaller than their perceived current shape (Drewnowski & Yee, 1987; Silberstein, et al., 1988; Davis & Cowles, 1991). Research on the relationship between exercise participation and body-shape perceptions in adolescents and young adults, although limited, suggests that regular participation in exercise can bring about positive changes in body image and self-concept (Snyder & Kivlin, 1975; Rossi & Zoccolotti, 1979; Salusso-Deonier & Schwartzkopf, 1991). However, body-shape dissatisfaction coupled with excessive exercise and low self-esteem may be indicative of an eating disorder (Keeton, Cash, & Brown, 1990; Beals, 2003). Consequently, even though exercise motivations may vary, past research suggests that the decision to exercise is, in part, motivated by perception of body shape. Both men and women exercise to achieve a preferred body image; generally, young women believe slenderness to be the desirable ideal, whereas young men's ideal body shape is slender and moderately muscular (Grogan, 1999). It remains unclear whether these attitudes are modified by age.

Cross-sectional studies examining body-shape perceptions of various age groups have found that women of all ages (middle school through old age) were less satisfied with their body image than men and that women's dissatisfaction with their body image was surprisingly consistent (Pliner, Chaiken, & Flett, 1990; Lamb, Jackson, Cassiday, & Priest, 1993; Tiggemann & Lynch, 2001). While there is some evidence suggesting that older men were less satisfied with their appearance compared to their younger counterparts (Lamb, et al., 1993; Abadie, et al., 1996), this disparity is nonetheless maintained across the lifespan (Grogan, 1999). Research focusing on the effect of exercise participation on body-shape perceptions in older adults has produced conflicting results. Hallinan and Schuler (1993) assessed the association between regular exercise on body-shape perceptions in older women (60 to 88 years old) and reported that exercising women reported greater body-shape dissatisfaction compared to nonexercising women. A similar study conducted in older men ranging in age between 55 and 90 years (Abadie, et al., 1996) also found the greatest body-shape dissatisfaction in the most active group of older men. On the other hand, McAuley, Blissmer, Katula, Duncan, and Mihalko (2000) as well as Loland (2000) found that for both men and women, perceptions of body appearance were positively related to increased activity.

Only a few studies have investigated body-shape perception as a possible motivation for exercising in older adults (Davis & Cowles, 1991; O'Neill & Reid, 1991; Ransdell, Wells, Manore, Swan, & Corbin, 1998; O'Brien Cousins, 2001). In light of the well-documented age-related changes in body composition and appearance, e.g., loss of muscle mass, increase in body fat and redistribution of body fat (see Spirduso, 1995 for a comprehensive review), it is possible to hypothesize that body dissatisfaction assumes a more significant role as a motivation to exercise in older adults. However, the limited data available in the research literature do not generally support this hypothesis. The most common motivations identified by older adults appear to be improved health and the desire to feel better (Cohen-Mansfield, Marx, & Guralnik, 2003). Other factors include the knowledge that increased physical activity will lead to more successful aging, the experience of the benefits of exercise and increased fitness, and the desire to control body shape and size (O'Brien Cousins, 2001). Even though body-shape dissatisfaction has been consistently identified by the researchers as a motivation to exercise, in neither of these studies was it the focus of the investigation. The present study had three purposes: (1) to assess whether body-shape dissatisfaction occurs among older adult men and women; (2) to examine the relations among age, sex, exercise and body-shape dissatisfaction in older adults and (3) to evaluate the role of body-shape dissatisfaction as a possible motivation to exercise in the selected sample of older adults. Based on previous findings we hypothesized that both older men and women would express a desire for a thinner body shape and that both age as well as participation in regular exercise would be negatively related to body-shape dissatisfaction. We further hypothesized that body-shape dissatisfaction would be a notable motivation to exercise in this population.

Method

Participants

A convenience sample of 175 older adult volunteers (74 men and 101 women) ranging in age from 50 to 98 years ($M=72$, $SD=9$) completed a paper-and-pencil questionnaire. Participants were actively recruited from local fitness centers, community centers and independent living facilities. Once permission was obtained from supervising personnel at these sample sites, researchers visited each site and verbally recruited participants. The majority of respondents were Euro-American ($n=173$); other respondents were African American ($n=2$). Additional descriptive statistics are reported in Table 1 below.

Procedure

A brief overview of the procedures and purpose of the study was provided to all respondents at the beginning of the study. Respondents were then asked to sign an informed consent and complete the questionnaire. At each site, the researchers were present during the completion of the questionnaire to ensure accuracy and completeness of survey responses; participants were encouraged to ask questions when needed. The pencil-and-paper questionnaire took approximately 15 minutes to complete and was composed of four parts: general information; age, sex, height, weight, race, income and education; exercise participation and reasons for exercise participation; body-shape perceptions.

Assessment of Body Shape Perceptions

A variety of methods have been used to assess body-shape perceptions including interviews and questionnaires, picture evaluations or estimations of bodily sizes, using both part body and whole body estimation techniques (see Grogan, 1999, pp. 26-42 for comprehensive review). The current study utilized the silhouette-scale technique. Participants were presented with a nine-figure body silhouette scale designed and validated by Stunkard, Sorenson, and Schulsinger (1983). The figures ranged ordinally from very thin to very heavy; individual figures were assigned a number ranging progressively from 1 = thinnest to 9 = heaviest. Each participant was asked to indicate perceived Current Body Shape (Which body shape looks most like your own?) and Ideal Body Shape (Which body shape do you want to look like?). A Body-shape Dissatisfaction score was calculated using the discrepancy between the participant's choice for Current and Ideal Body Shape. This technique is one of the most widely used quantitative measures of magnitude and direction of Body-shape Dissatisfaction (Grogan, 1999, p. 26).

Assessment of Exercise Participation and Motivation

Participants were asked whether they exercised regularly (Yes/No). Regular exercise was defined as engaging in exercise at least three times a week for a minimum of 30 min. each session. If respondents answered "no," they were asked to give reasons why not; if they answered "yes," they were asked to indicate why they exercised.

Statistical Analysis

Pearson coefficients were used to study associations between selected variables. A 2 (sex: male, female) × 3 (age: 50–65 yr., 66–75 yr. and 76 yr. and older) × 2 (Body Shape: Current, Ideal) analysis of variance was used to judge whether body-shape dissatisfaction occurred in older adult men and women. The relationship between age, sex, exercise and body-shape dissatisfaction in older adults was examined using a 2 (sex: male, female) × 3 (age: 50–65 yr., 66–75 yr. and 76 yr. and older) × 2 (exercise: yes, no) and Body-shape Dissatisfaction (difference between Current – Ideal Body Shape) as the dependent variable. Based on participants' responses, five categories emerged regarding their reasons to exercise: Physical Health, Physical Fitness, Psychological Health, Body-shape Perception and Enjoyment. To establish the role of Body-shape Dissatisfaction as a motivation to exercise, percentages were calculated for each category.

Results

Participants' age and anthropometrics are summarized in Table 1. In addition to these measures, education and socioeconomic status were assessed using the following categories for education: grade school, left high school before graduation, high school graduate, junior college, bachelor's degree, master's or specialist's degree, doctorate and other (rated 1 through 8, respectively). The following income categories were used to examine socioeconomic status: <$20,000 annually; $20–30,000; $31–40,000; $41–50,000 and >$50,000 (rated 1 through 5, respectively). The mean education reported was 4.3 (junior college graduate; $SD=1.3$). The mean income reported was 3.3 ($31,000–40.000; $SD=1.5$). The $2 \times 3 \times 2$ analysis of variance with

TABLE 1
Anthropometric Measures and Age For Women ($n = 101$) and Men ($n = 74$)

Category	Women M	Women SD	Men M	Men SD
Height, cm	162.7	7.7	175.2	10.4
Weight, kg	68.4	1.7	87.1	15.5
Body Mass Index*	25.9	5.5	28.5	5.9
Age, yr.	71.2	9.4	71.2	8.9

*BMI = kg/m².

repeated measures was used to assess whether Body-shape Dissatisfaction occurred in older adult men and women and yielded a significant difference between Current and Ideal Body Shape perceptions ($F_{1,173} = 174.92$, $p < .01$) independent of age and sex. Men and women of all age groups chose a significantly larger body shape for their perceived Current Body Shape (overall $M=4.9$, $SD=1.4$) compared to their perceived Ideal Body Shape (overall $M=3.7$, $SD=0.9$). These findings were in support of our hypothesis that both older men and women expressed a desire for a thinner body shape (see Table 2). A $2 \times 3 \times 2$ analysis of variance investigating the relationship among age, sex, exercise and Body-shape Dissatisfaction (difference between perceived Current – Ideal Body Shape) yielded no significant main effects and no significant interactions (see Table 3). These findings indicated that Body-shape Dissatisfaction did not significantly differ between men and women across age groups and that there was no significant difference in Body-shape Dissatisfaction between those who reported engaging in regular exercise and those who did not. The result of this analysis did not support the hypothesis that both age and participation in regular exercise were negatively related to Body-shape Dissatisfaction.

To determine the importance of Body-shape Dissatisfaction as a possible motivation for exercise, categories were developed based on participants'

TABLE 2
MEAN BODY-SHAPE CHOICES FOR WOMEN ($n = 101$) AND MEN ($n = 74$), CURRENT AND IDEAL BODY SHAPE AND BODY-SHAPE DISSATISFACTION (CURRENT–IDEAL BODY SHAPE)

Sex and Age	Current M	Current SD	Ideal M	Ideal SD	Dissatisfaction M
Women					
50–65	5.1	1.3	3.6	0.8	1.5*
66–75	4.5	1.4	3.4	0.8	1.1*
76+	4.4	1.3	3.3	1.0	1.1*
Men					
50–65	4.9	1.5	3.9	0.8	1.0*
66–75	5.4	1.4	4.2	1.3	1.2*
76+	5.0	1.5	4.1	0.9	0.9*

*Significant difference between Current and Ideal Body Shape, $p < .01$.

responses; participants were allowed to list more than one reason. A total of 80.8% of participants reported engaging in regular exercise (82.2% women and 78.8% men), and 19.3% of participants said they did not engage in regular exercise (17.8% women and 21.2% men). The following five categories emerged as reasons or motivations to engage in regular exercise: Physical Health (39.9%; 40.8% of women and 37.7% of men), Physical Fitness

TABLE 3
SCORES FOR BODY-SHAPE DISSATISFACTION (CURRENT–IDEAL) BY SEX, AGE, AND EXERCISE PARTICIPATION FOR WOMEN ($n = 101$) AND MEN ($n = 74$)

Sex and Age	n	Exercise Participation	Body-shape Dissatisfaction M	SD
Women				
50–65	8	No	2.0	1.0
50–65	21	Yes	1.2	0.8
66–75	6	No	1.5	0.5
66–75	43	Yes	1.0	1.1
76+	4	No	1.0	0.8
76+	19	Yes	1.2	1.0
Men				
50–65	7	No	1.6	1.4
50–65	12	Yes	0.8	0.9
66–75	6	No	0.5	1.9
66–75	27	Yes	1.4	0.9
76+	3	No	0.7	0.5
76+	19	Yes	0.9	1.3

(28.6%; 23.2% of women and 37.9% of men), Enjoyment (11.8%; 13.6% of women and 8.9% of men), Body-shape Perception (10.8%; 15.2% of women and 3.8% of men) and Psychological Health (10.3%; 15.2% of women and 2.5% of men). Of those individuals who did not exercise ($n = 34$; 19.2%) only 10 provided reasons for why they did not exercise: 3

(8.8%) reported they already engaged in enough activity, 2 (5.8%) stated they were too lazy to exercise and 5 (14.2%) participants thought they needed to lose weight before starting an exercise program.

Discussion

The purpose of the present study was to evaluate the relationships among age, sex, exercise and Body-shape Perceptions in older adults and to assess whether Body-shape Dissatisfaction might be a motivation to exercise. Generally, the findings suggested that both older men and women expressed a desire for a thinner body shape which was independent of age and exercise; participants' perceived Ideal Body Shape was consistently one size smaller than their perceived Current Body Shape. Furthermore, even though Body-shape Perception was reported as a motivation for exercise in this population, it only ranked fourth out of five factors identified; the most important motivations reported were Physical Health and Physical Fitness.

In light of the limited literature, the role of sex deserves special consideration when discussing Body-shape Dissatisfaction in older adults. The present findings and previous research indicated that women of all ages expressed a desire for a thinner body shape and that the magnitude of dissatisfaction did not change significantly across the life span (Tiggemann & Lynch, 2001). This is particularly interesting since "a double standard of aging" has been noted, i.e., that aging has more serious social consequences for women than it does for men (Sontag, 1979). According to Sontag (1979), women of all ages are judged more by physical appearance than men, so the diminishing of physical beauty should be more significant for women compared to men. Stevens and Tiggemann (1998) speculated that women shifted their body comparisons to more age-appropriate models as they aged, which explains the consistency of dissatisfaction across the life span. The findings of the present study support their hypothesis: the mean Ideal Body Shape selected from the silhouette scale by the women in this study was 3.4. Studies using the same scale to determine Current and Ideal Body-shape perceptions in young women (Rozin & Fallon, 1988; Tiggemann, 1991) reported Ideal Body Shapes between 2.8 and 3.0, approximately one-half to one size smaller.

Even though men of all ages have been shown to report Body-shape Dissatisfaction, the magnitude and direction of the dissatisfaction is less consistent compared to women. Adolescent and young adult men have been equally divided between those who wanted to lose weight and those who wanted to gain weight (Drewnowski & Yee, 1987; Silberstein, *et al.*, 1988; Davis & Cowles, 1991). With respect to older men, the limited literature suggests that men become more dissatisfied with their appearances as they age and that the direction of the dissatisfaction becomes more consistent in that older men are more likely to want to lose weight (Lamb, et al., 1993; Abadie, et al., 1996). Our results support these findings: older men consistently indicated a desire for a smaller body shape. The mean Current Body Shape chosen by the men in our study was 5.1, whereas the mean Ideal Body Shape was 4.1; this difference was consistent across the age groups included in this study. It is interesting to note that, for both men and women, Body Mass Index was negatively correlated with age ($r_{101} = -.19$, $p < .05$, for women; $r_{74} = -.26$, $p < .01$ for men) implying a decrease in Body Mass Index with advancing age. The correlation between Body-shape Dissatisfaction and age, however, was only significant for women ($r_{101} = -.23$, $p < .01$) and not for men ($r_{74} = -.08$, $p > .05$). This suggests that the decrease in Body Mass Index with advancing age may be associated with less Body-shape Dissatisfaction for women but not for men. We suggest that this apparent lack of association between Body Mass Index and Body-shape Dissatisfaction in men could indicate a more realistic Body-shape Perception for older women than older men.

The second question addressed in the present study was whether Body-image Dissatisfaction in older adults was related to age, sex or exercise. The study findings indicate that age, sex and exercise participation were not significantly related to Body-image Dissatisfaction in the present sample of older adults. Men and women expressed similar levels of Body-shape Dissatisfaction regardless of whether they reported a commitment to regular exercise or not. The results of the present study do not agree with previous findings reporting associations between body-shape perceptions and exercise by older women and men. Hallinan and Schuler (1993) found that older women who were exercising (60–88 years old) reported greater Body-shape Dissatisfaction than nonexercising women in the same age group. Abadie, et al. (1996), in a similar study, found the greatest Body-shape Dissatisfaction in the most active group of older men. The authors hypothesized that a major motivation to exercise for these older men and women was the desire to achieve a certain Body-shape Ideal.

Other findings (Davis & Cowles, 1991; Loland, 2000; McAuley, et al., 2000), however, showed that older men's and older women's perceptions of their Body Shape were positively related to activity levels. Generally, body-image satisfaction increased with increased activity. It is unclear why Body-shape Perceptions did not differ between those individuals who reported to participate in regular exercise and those who did not for the present sample of older adults. Different methods for assessing physical activity and body-shape perceptions, and more important, different age groupings may, in part, explain the discrepancies in findings. Loland (2000) studied adults between the ages of 18 and 67 years, with the oldest group ranging between 45 and 67 years. Davis and Cowles (1991) recruited adults between the ages of

14 and 64, dividing participants into only two groups, young (<25 years) and old (>24 years), whereas McAuley, et al. (2000) studied individuals between the ages of 60 and 75 years. The present study sample was substantially older, with the oldest group ranging between 76 and 98 years. As individuals reach advanced age categories, their decision to exercise may no longer be motivated by a desire to *"look good"* but rather to *"feel good."* Loland (2000): found that Body Mass Index increased linearly with advancing age for the women and men in their study. In the present study, Body Mass Index was negatively correlated with age, suggesting that the importance of body-shape perception as a motivation to exercise may decrease with advancing age.

The final purpose of the present study was to assess the importance of body-shape perception as a potential motivation for exercising in older women and men. It was hypothesized that Body-shape Dissatisfaction may become more important as a motivation to exercise in older adults. However, the limited literature data, as well as the results of the present study, do not support this hypothesis. Physical health (40.8% of women; 37.9% of men) and Physical Fitness (23.2% of women; 37.9% of men) were the most frequently cited exercise motivations in the present sample of older adults. Other motivations mentioned included Psychological Health, Body-shape Perception and Enjoyment. Even though older women and men agreed with respect to the two most important reasons to engage in regular exercise, Physical Health and Physical Fitness, men and women differed with respect to the importance of Body-shape Perception as a reason to exercise. Only 3.8% of the men ($n=3$) compared to 15.2% of the women ($n=19$) listed Body-shape Perception as a motivation to engage in regular exercise. It is interesting to note that only 1 of the 19 women who reported Body-shape Perception as a reason to exercise was in the 76+ age group, whereas two of the three men who reported Body-shape Perception as a motivation to exercise were in the 76+ age group. One might hypothesize that, compared to men, Body-shape Perception becomes less important to women as they reach the extreme end of the aging continuum. However, the small number of individuals per group and the low overall importance rating of Body-shape Perception do not adequately support this conclusion. The findings of the present study agree with the literature, identifying improved health as the most powerful exercise motivation in older adults (Cohen-Mansfield, et al., 2003).

REFERENCES

ABADIE, B., SCHULER, P., HUNT, B., & LISCHKOFF, N. (1996) Perceptions of body shape in elderly white and black men. *Perceptual and Motor Skills*, 83, 449-450.

BEALS, K. A. (2003) Mirror, mirror on the wall, who is the most muscular of all? Disordered eating and body image disturbances in male athletes. *ACSM's Health and Fitness Journal*, 7(2), 6-11.

COHEN-MANSFIELD, J., MARX, M., & GURALNIK, J. M. (2003) Motivators and barriers to exercise

in an older community-dwelling population. *Journal of Aging and Physical Activity*, 11, 242-254.
DAVIS, C., & COWLES, M. (1991) Body image and exercise: a study of relationships and comparisons between physically active men and women. *Sex Roles*, 25, 33-44.
DEMAREST, J., & LANGER, E. (1996) Perception of body shape by underweight, average, and overweight men and women. *Perceptual and Motor Skills*, 83, 569-570.
DREWNOWSKI, A., & YEE, D. K. (1987) Men and body image: are males satisfied with their body weight? *Psychosomatic Medicine*, 49, 626-634.
GRAY, S. (1977) Social aspects of body image: perception of normalcy of weight and affect of college undergraduates. *Perceptual and Motor Skills*, 45, 1035-1040.
GROGAN, S. (1999) *Body image: understanding body dissatisfaction in men, women, and children*. London: Routledge.
HALLINAN, C., & SCHULER, P. (1993) Body-shape perceptions of elderly women exercisers and nonexercisers. *Perceptual and Motor Skills*, 77, 451-456.
HALLINAN, C. J., PIERCE, E. F., EVANS, J. E., DEGRENIER, J. D., & ANDRES, F. F. (1991) Perceptions of current and ideal body shape of athletes and nonathletes. *Perceptual and Motor Skills*, 72, 123-130.
KEETON, P. W., CASH, T. F., & BROWN, T. A. (1990) Body image or body images? Comparative, multidimensional assessment among college students. *Journal of Personality Assessment*, 54, 213-230.
LAMB, C. S., JACKSON, L., CASSIDAY, P., & PRIEST, D. (1993) Body figure preferences of men and women: a comparison of two generations. *Sex Roles*, 28, 345-358.
LOLAND, N. (2000) The aging body: attitudes toward bodily appearance among physically active and inactive women and men of different ages. *Journal of Aging and Physical Activity*, 8, 197-213.
MCAULEY, E., BLISSMER, B., KATULA, J., DUNCAN, T. E., & MIHALKO, S. L. (2000) Physical activity, self-esteem, and self-efficiency relationships in older adults: a randomized controlled trial. *Annuals of Behavioral Medicine*, 22, 131-139.
O'BRIEN COUSINS, S. (2001) Thinking out loud: what older adults say about triggers for physical activity. *Journal of Aging of Behavioral Medicine*, 9, 347-363.
O'NEILL, K., & REID, G. (1991) Perceived barriers to physical activity by older adults. *Canadian Journal of Public Health*, 82, 392-396.
PLINER, P., CHAIKEN, S., & FLETT, G. (1990) Gender differences in concern with body weight and physical appearance over the life span. *Personality and Social Psychology Bulletin*, 16, 263-273.
RANSDELL, L. B., WELLS, C. L., MANORE, M. M., SWAN, P. D., & CORBIN, C. B. (1998) Social physique anxiety in postmenopausal women. *Journal of Women and Aging*, 10(3), 19-39.
ROSSI, B., & ZOCCOLOTTI, P. (1979) Body perception in athletes and nonathletes. *Perceptual and Motor Skills*, 49, 723-726.
ROZIN, P., & FALLON, A. (1988) Body image, attitudes to weight, and misperceptions of figure preferences of the opposite gender: a comparison of men and women in two generations. *Journal of Abnormal Psychology*, 97, 342-345.
SALUSSO-DEONIER, C. J., & SCHWARTZKOPF, R. J. (1991) Sex differences in body-cathexis associated with exercise involvement. *Perceptual and Motor Skills*, 73, 139-145.
SILBERSTEIN, L., STRIEGEL-MOORE, R., TIMKO, C., & RODIN, J. (1988) Behavioral and psychological implications of body dissatisfaction: do men and women differ? *Sex Roles*, 19, 219-232.
SNYDER, E. E., & KIVLIN, J. E. (1975) Development and validation of a test for bulimia. *Journal of Consulting and Clinical Psychology*, 52, 863-872.
SONTAG, S. (1979) The double standard of aging. In J. Williams (Ed.), *Psychology of women*. New York: Academic Press. Pp. 462-478.
SPIRDUSO, W. W. (1995) *Physical dimensions of aging*. Champaign, IL: Human Kinetics.
STEVENS, C., & TIGGEMANN, M. (1998) Women's body figure preferences across the lifespan. *The Journal of Genetic Psychology*, 159, 94-102.
STUNKARD, A. J., SORENSON, T., & SCHULSINGER, F. (1983) Use of the Danish Adoption Register for the study of obesity and thinness. In S. Kety (Ed.), *The genetics of neurological and psychiatric disorders*. New York: Raven. Pp. 115-120.
TIGGEMANN, M. (1991) Body-size dissatisfaction: individual differences in age and gender and relationship with self-esteem. *Personality and Individual Differences*, 13, 39-43.
TIGGEMANN, M., & LYNCH, J. E. (2001) Body image across a life span in adult women: the role of self-objectification. *Developmental Psychology*, 37, 243-253.

Accepted April 13, 2004.

HANDEDNESS DIFFERENCES IN WIDTHS OF RIGHT AND LEFT CRANIOFACIAL REGIONS IN HEALTHY YOUNG ADULTS[1]

ŞENOL DANE, MUSTAFA ERSÖZ, KENAN GÜMÜŞTEKİN, PINAR POLAT, AND ALİ DAŞTAN

Atatürk University

Summary.—In this work, handedness differences in the widths of right and left craniofacial regions were studied in a healthy sample of 39 male and 43 female students, 17 to 23 years old. Width of craniofacial regions was assessed by computerized tomography. Handedness was associated with the left face width especially for women. The left facial region was larger for right-handers than left-handers. The smaller measure for the left face of left-handers might be associated with an advantage of left ear sensitivity.

About two-thirds of humans possess a slightly larger left facial region (Woo, 1931; Burke, 1971). An association of the width of human craniofacial areas and hand preference has been reported previously by Keleş, Diyarbakırlı, Tan, and Tan (1997) and by Dane, Gümüştekin, Polat, Uslu, Akar, and Daştan (2002). In a recent study, Dayı, Güngörmüş, Okuyan, and Tan (2002) reported that the left side of the face was larger than the right side of the face of a sample of left-handers, whereas the right-handers did not show such a right-left difference in facial measurements. They remarked that hand skill and cognitive abilities might be predicted from craniofacial width in right- and left-handed men and women. In the present study handedness differences related to the widths of right and left craniofacial regions in a sample of healthy young adults were reexamined.

METHOD

Subjects were 39 male and 43 female students, 17 to 23 years ($M = 19.7 \pm 1.4$). Hand preference was assessed on the modified version of the Edinburgh Handedness Inventory (Oldfield, 1971; Tan, 1988). Lateral scenograms of the cranium were taken by computerized tomography to measure the linear distances between external openings of the right and left ears and the midline. Then, an axial section passing from top points of both mastoid process and external occipital protuberance was taken for each subject. To define the midline, a line was drawn between the midpoint of foramen magnum (internal occipital crista) and the midpoint of the nasal root. In the last step, the distance between the external openings of each ear and this midline was calculated.

---

[1]Address enquiries to Prof. Dr. Şenol Dane, Department of Physiology, Faculty of Medicine, Atatürk University, Erzurum, Turkey.

The total craniofacial region was calculated as the width of right craniofacial region plus that of the left one. The face asymmetry index was calculated from the formula: 100 (right facial width minus left facial width)/(right facial width plus left facial width). For the statistical evaluation, the two-sample analysis in the SPSS 10.0 for Windows program was applied.

Results and Discussion

In this small sample, there were no handedness differences for right and left facial regions in men. The asymmetry index was negative in right-handers and positive in the left-handers; see Table 1 for means and standard deviations. There was no handedness difference for right facial region of the women, but the left facial region was wider for right-handers than for left-handers ($p < .05$). The asymmetry index was negative for right-handers and positive for left-handers.

TABLE 1
Mean Widths of Right and Left Total Facial Regions and Face Asymmetry Index

Region	Right-handed ($n=22$) M	Right-handed ($n=22$) SD	Left-handed ($n=17$) M	Left-handed ($n=17$) SD	t	p
Men						
Right	69.43	2.44	70.67	3.33	1.34	ns
Left	71.07	2.89	69.53	3.67	1.47	ns
Index	−1.15	.96	.84	1.39	5.26	<.001
Women						
Right	65.22	3.33	64.66	2.41	0.63	ns
Left	66.13	3.55	62.94	2.63	3.33	<.05
Index	− .69	.51	1.35	1.32	6.74	<.001

Dayı, et al. (2002) reported that IQ linearly increased with the index of right minus left face width for left-handers, and was negatively correlated for right-handers. Tan, Tan, Polat, Ceylan, Suma, and Okur (1999) reported that men's IQs correlated with MRI images of the size of the anterior cerebral areas, whereas women's IQs correlated with the size of the posterior cerebral areas. Tan, Okuyan, Bayraktar, and Akgün (2003) reported no sex difference in mental rotation scores using body weight as covariate.

Weinstein and Graves (2001) have shown associations among measures reflecting higher creativity, higher schizotypy and right hemisphere laterality. A study of dichotic listening yielded an association showing better left ear localization with higher creativity scores (Weinstein & Graves, 2002). Bryden, Jey, and Sugarman (1982) reported a left ear advantage for identifying the emotional quality of tonal sequences. McKinnon and Schellenberg (1997) reported a left ear advantage for forced-choice judgements of melodic contour. Mathieson, Sainsbury, and Fitzgerald (1990) found that performance with the left ear was better on nonspeech sounds than the right ear in a dichotic listening paradigm. Emmerich, Harris, Brown, and Springer (1988) stated that the left ears of left-handed subjects showing a dicohtic left ear advantage were slightly, but not significantly, more sensitive than their right ears.

In the present study, handedness was significantly associated with left face width and the face asymmetry index especially for women. The mean left facial region was significantly larger for right-handers than left-handers. Right-handers had negative, but left-handers had positive asymmetry indexes. A smaller craniofacial region has been associated with enhanced middle-ear conduction and a monaural sensitivity advantage (Dane, et al., 2002). The left-handers had a left ear-sensitivity advantage (Dane & Bayırlı, 1998; Dane, et al. 2002; Dane & Gümüştekin, 2003). A smaller craniofacial region on left side or positive asymmetry index for left-handed subjects in this study may be associated with superiority on musical tasks of nonright-handed subjects (Deutsch, 1978) and the higher incidence of left-handedness among musicians (Quinan, 1922; Byrne, 1974; Peterson, 1979). Dane and Erzurumluoğlu (2003) suggested that a high proportion of left-handers among sportsmen and sportswomen (McLean & Ciurczak, 1982; Azemar, Ripoll, Simonet, & Stein, 1983; Annett, 1985) might suggest that left-handers have an intrinsic neurological advantage over right-handers. One may speculate that a smaller left-craniofacial region fuses an advantage for left-handed subjects. This assumption is not consistent, however, with the work of Rushton and Ankney (1995) who claimed that a large brain is associated with better skills. Therefore, their study requires thorough examination and replication with large samples as does the present study.

As a general conclusion, in this sample left-handedness appeared to be significantly associated with the small size of the left side of the face, especially in women. A smaller left face or a positive asymmetry index in left-handers might be indicative of an advantage in left ear (right hemisphere) sensitivity. The association between left-handedness and smaller left face deserves further investigation including more right- and left-handed subjects.

REFERENCES

ANNETT, M. (1985) *Left, right, hand, and brain: right-shift theory.* Hillsdale, NJ: Erlbaum.
AZEMAR, G., RIPOLL, H., SIMONET, P., & STEIN, J. F. (1983) Etude neuropsycologique du comportement des gauschers en escrime. *Cinesiologie,* 22, 7-18.
BRYDEN, M. P., JEY, R. G., & SUGARMAN, J. H. (1982) A left-ear advantage for identifying the emotional quality of tonal sequences. *Neuropsychologia,* 20, 83-87.
BURKE, P. H. (1971) Stereophotogrammetric measurement of normal facial asymmetry in children. *Human Biology,* 43, 536-548.
BYRNE, B. (1974) Handedness and musical ability. *British Journal of Psychology,* 65, 279-281.
DANE, Ş., & BAYIRLI, M. (1998) Correlation between hand preference and duration of hearing for right and left ears in young healthy subjects. *Perceptual and Motor Skills,* 86, 667-672.

DANE, Ş., & ERZURUMLUOĞLU, A. (2003) Sex and handedness differences in eye-hand visual reaction times in handball players. *International Journal of Neuroscience*, 113, 923-929.

DANE, Ş., & GÜMÜŞTEKİN, K. (2003) Sex and handedness differences in hearing durations of the right and left ears in healthy young adults. *International Journal of Neuroscience*, 113, 423-428.

DANE, Ş., GÜMÜŞTEKİN, K., POLAT, P., USLU, C., AKAR, S., & DAŞTAN, A. (2002) Relations among hand preference, craniofacial asymmetry and ear advantage in young subjects. *Perceptual and Motor Skills*, 95, 416-422.

DAYI, E., GÜNGÖRMÜŞ, M., OKUYAN, M., & TAN, Ü. (2002) Predictability of hand skill and cognitive abilities from craniofacial width in right- and left-handed men and women: relation of skeletal structure to cerebral function. *International Journal of Neuroscience*, 112, 383-412.

DEUTSCH, D. (1978) Pitch memory: an advantage for the left-handed. *Science*, 199, 559-560.

EMMERICH, D. S., HARRIS, J., BROWN, W. S., & SPRINGER, S. P. (1988) The relationship between auditory sensitivity and ear asymmetry on a dicohtic listening task. *Neuropsychologia*, 26, 133-143.

KELEŞ, P., DİYARBAKIRLI, S., TAN, M., & TAN, Ü. (1997) Facial asymmetry in right- and left-handed men and women. *International Journal of Neuroscience*, 91, 147-160.

MATHIESON, C. M., SAINSBURY, R. S., & FITZGERALD, L. K. (1990) Attentional set in pure-versus mixed lists in a dichotic listening paradigm. *Brain and Cognition*, 13, 30-45.

MCKINNON, M. C., & SCHELLENBERG, E. G. (1997) A left-ear advantage for forced-choice judgements of melodic contour. *Canadian Journal of Experimental Psychology*, 52, 171-175.

MCLEAN, J. M., & CIURCZAK, F. M. (1982) Bimanual dexterity in major league baseball players: a statistical study. *New England Journal of Medicine*, 307, 1278-1279.

OLDFIELD, R. C. (1971) The assessment and analysis of handedness: the Edinburgh inventory. *Neuropsychologia*, 9, 97-114.

PETERSON, J. M. (1979) Left-handedness: differences between student artists and scientists. *Perceptual and Motor Skills*, 48, 961-962.

QUINAN, C. (1922) A study of sinistrality and muscle coordination in musicians, iron workers and others. *Archives of Neurology and Psychiatry*, 7, 352-360.

RUSHTON, J. P., & ANKNEY, C. D. (1995) Brain size matters: a reply to Peters. *Canadian Journal of Experimental Psychology*, 49, 562-569.

TAN, Ü. (1988) The distribution of hand preference in normal men and women. *International Journal of Neuroscience*, 41, 35-55.

TAN, Ü., OKUYAN, M., BAYRAKTAR, T., & AKGÜN, A. (2003) Covariation of sex differences in mental rotation with body size. *Perceptual and Motor Skills*, 96, 137-144.

TAN, Ü., TAN, M., POLAT, P., CEYLAN, Y., SUMA, S., & OKUR, A. (1999) Magnetic resonance imaging brain size/IQ relations in Turkish university students. *Intelligence*, 27, 83-92.

WEINSTEIN, S., & GRAVES, R. E. (2001) Creativity, schizotypy, and laterality. *Cognitive Neuropsychiatry*, 6, 131-146.

WEINSTEIN, S., & GRAVES, R. E. (2002) Are creativity and schizotypy products a right hemisphere bias? *Brain and Cognition*, 49, 138-151.

WOO, T. L. (1931) On the asymmetry of human skull. *Biometrika*, 22, 324-352.

Accepted April 10, 2004.

ABSTRACTNESS AND EMOTIONALITY VALUES FOR 398 ENGLISH WORDS[1]

GIANLUIGI GUIDO AND MARIA ROSARIA PROVENZANO

University of Lecce

Summary.—This study is aimed to replicate Vikis-Freibergs' classic study (1976) on the values of vividness for French words. Vividness resulted from the concreteness and the emotionality values of words, here defined, respectively, as referring to something that can be experienced through senses and that can arouse pleasant or unpleasant emotions. 398 English words were rated on two different scales, Abstractness and Emotionality, by a group of English native speakers and also by a group of Italian subjects who used English as a second language. Results show a low correlation between the concreteness and emotionality ratings in line with Vikis-Freibergs' previous study of French words (1976). A negative correlation between Abstractness and Emotionality was observed for British data but a slightly positive correlation for the Italian data.

Availability of normative data in different languages allows one to examine whether there are interactions between stimulus attributes, such as those tapping vividness, i.e., abstractness and emotion (cf. Nisbett & Ross, 1980), and the languages of the respondents. The object of such analyses is not the quantitative result as such, but the relationship between the results and the different linguistic and cultural backgrounds of the respondents. These differences imply different cognitive schemata as well as possibly divergent attitudes in people's approach to the words administered.

In a seminal paper, Vikis-Freibergs (1976) compared the values of 398 French words on the two scales of Abstractness and Emotionality, as rated by French-speaking subjects. In this paper, we investigated the Concreteness and the Emotionality values for the English equivalents of these 398 words to provide researchers with material for cross-cultural comparisons between two sets of respondents. In particular, two groups were tested: one of British subjects and the other one of Italian students of English. Taking Vikis-Freibergs' study as a starting-point for the present research, we assessed the ratings of Abstractness and Emotionality for the same set of words to provide a comparison between the effects of different schemata on the approach to the words.

Concreteness was treated normatively in terms of sensory experience and imagery effectiveness, as did Vikis-Freibergs in her study and, prior to

---

[1]Address correspondence to G. Guido, Università di Lecce, Facoltà di Economia, Palazzo Ecotekne, Via per Monteroni, 73100 Lecce, Italy or e-mail (g.guido@economia.unile.it).

that, as had Paivio, Yuille, and Madigan (1968): there concreteness was highly correlated with "imagery," with a "concrete" word easily arousing a complete image of the thing or person referred to. There are several previous cross-cultural studies assessing and comparing the scores for the same set of words by subjects having a different first language.

Campos and Astorga (1986) focused on the "imagery" values of the Spanish equivalents of the 398 words used as stimuli by Vikis-Freibergs. These words were rated by North American, Canadian and Spanish subjects and results indicated consistent differences in the ratings from the three sets of respondents. Similarly, Morris and Reid (1972) presented a cross-cultural study of the imagery ratings for words as rated by Canadian and British subjects; despite words with a North American usage having been excluded from the list, it emerged that the Canadians gave higher ratings than the British.

Emotionality is also approached the way Paivio and associates (1968) and Vikis-Freibergs (1976) did, by referring to the intensity of the emotion. As Vikis-Freibergs pointed out in her study (1976, p. 24), a bipolar scale, with *Unpleasant* and *Pleasant* as the respective anchors and a neutral midpoint gave information about the intensity of the emotional charge. Also, Brown and Ure (1969) provided a useful reference as to the emotionality of English words by providing the results for 650 word-association stimuli.

Method

Two questionnaires were administered to the two groups of English and Italian students: one hundred Italian university students recruited from the Faculty of Economics in Lecce and 45 English students (the 'English' questionnaires were divided into four sections and were completed by different groups of university students). Both groups were asked to rate first the Emotionality value for 398 words on a 7-point scale anchored by 1 = Very Unpleasant and 7 = Very Pleasant, with 4 classified as neutral.

The instructions to the questionnaires were as follows: "We ask for your cooperation in a study aiming to evaluate the emotional charge for 398 English words. You are asked to rate each word on a scale ranging from 'Unpleasant' to 'Pleasant'. We suggest that you follow a three-stage decisional process: first decide whether the word arouses any emotion or is neutral. If the latter is the case, then tick box number 4 for 'neutral'; if the word is emotional, decide whether it is 'pleasant' or 'unpleasant'; finally, rate the word on three category levels corresponding to 'Slightly', 'Fairly', 'Very'."

The questionnaire on concreteness similarly was rated on a 7-point scale ranging from 1 = Very Abstract to 7 = Very Concrete. The instructions were: "We ask for your cooperation in a study aiming to evaluate the abstractness or concreteness for a set of English words. You are asked to rate each word on a 7-point scale. All the words referring to people, substances and things that can be experienced through the senses will receive a 'High' concreteness score; on the contrary, the ones referring to a concept that cannot, will be rated as 'Abstract'. In other words, if a concept can be associated to an image conveying the totality of it, then the word must be rated as 'concrete'. If not, it is to be considered as 'Abstract'. We suggest that you follow a two-stage decisional process: first you should decide whether the word is abstract or concrete; then, evaluate it on the basis of the three standard categories 'Slightly', 'Fairly', 'Very'."

RESULTS AND DISCUSSION

The means and standard deviations for the Concreteness and Emotionality of each word are given in the Appendix which is on file as a supplement to this paper.[2] As for Concreteness, the mean scores are 4.45 and 4.68, respectively, for the Italian and the British respondents; in both cases, the words rated as 'highly concrete' encode personal relationships (*family, woman, mother*) and were rated with a '6' average score. Despite an apparent similarity in the words' evaluation, a t test comparing the ratings for Concreteness from the two samples detected a significant mean difference between them, with the Italians giving slightly higher ratings.

As for Emotionality, *'happiness', 'to love'* and *'peace'* were rated as 'strongly emotional' alongside with the words cited above, whereas *'injustice'* and *'war'* were ranked amid the most unpleasant lexemes.

Correlations between Concreteness and Emotionality as rated by the British and Italian samples were computed; as for the first group, r was on the order of .05, whereas for the Italian sample, the obtained correlation was .26. These data suggest that there is a similarity between the British data and those obtained by Vikis-Freibergs in her study of the French word list (r = .06), implying that the two variables need to be considered as independent. A positive (though slight) correlation was found in the Italian data.

To check the reliability of such correlations, a further check was made by correlating the extreme scores on the scale of Emotionality with those on Concreteness. This computation yielded a negative, significant correlation between the variables with the extremely unpleasant or pleasant words turning out to be less concrete, r = .00 for the British sample and r = .04 for the Italian set of respondents.

On the other hand, correlations on the same construct, i.e., Concreteness, have very positive coefficients (.72 as far as the British-French comparison is concerned; .75 for the Italian-French comparison). For Emotionality,

---

[2]A table of actual values for abstractness and emotionality is in Document APD2004-013 and may be obtained for $15.00 from The Archive for Psychological Data, P.O. Box 7922, Missoula, MT 59807-7922.

$r = .77$ for the British vs French data and .76 for the French vs Italian data. The implication is that the set of words administered has suggested similar choices to the three groups of respondents, regardless of their different mother tongues.

REFERENCES

Brown, W. P., & Ure, D. M. J. (1969) Five rated characteristics of 650 association stimuli. *Journal of Verbal Learning and Verbal Behavior*, 60, 232-249.

Campos, A., & Astorga, V. M. (1986) Spanish, North American, and Canadian ratings of imagery values of words. *Perceptual and Motor Skills*, 63, 889-890.

Morris, P. E., & Reid, R. L. (1972) Canadian and British ratings of the imagery values of words. *British Journal of Psychology*, 63, 163-164.

Nisbett, R. E., & Ross, L. (1980) *Human inference: strategies and shortcomings of social judgement*. Englewood Cliffs, NJ: Prentice-Hall.

Paivio, A., Yuille, J. C., & Madigan, S. A. (1968) Concreteness, imagery, and meaningfulness values for 925 nouns. *Journal of Experimental Psychology*, 76, 41-49.

Vikis-Freibergs, V. (1976) Abstractness and emotionality values for 398 French words. *Canadian Journal of Psychology*, 30, 22-30.

Accepted April 14, 2004.

ROLE OF STRATEGIES AND PRIOR EXPOSURE IN MENTAL ROTATION[1]

ISABELLE D. CHERNEY AND NICOLE L. NEFF

Creighton University

Summary.—The purpose of these two studies was to examine sex differences in strategy use and the effect of prior exposure on the performance on Vandenberg and Kuse's 1978 Mental Rotation Test. A total of 152 participants completed the spatial task and self-reported their strategy use. Consistent with previous studies, men outperformed women. Strategy usage did not account for these differences, although guessing did. Previous exposure to the Mental Rotation Test, American College Test scores and frequent computer or video game play predicted performance on the test. These results suggest that prior exposure to spatial tasks may provide cues to improve participants' performance.

Maccoby and Jacklin's seminal work (1974) on the development of sex differences has served as the impetus for gender research. In their review, they noted that the sexes differed in several aspects of intellectual abilities, namely, in verbal, quantitative and spatial abilities. Although researchers disagree on the magnitude of gender differences (e.g., Hyde, 1981; Feingold, 1988; Hyde & Linn, 1988; Voyer, Voyer, & Bryden, 1995; Bjorklund, 2000; Halpern, 2000), studies show robust cognitive sex differences in mental rotation (Goldstein, Haldane, & Mitchell, 1990; Geary, Gilger, & Elliot-Miller, 1992; Voyer, *et al.*, 1995; Cherney, Jagarlamudi, Lawrence, & Shimabuku, 2003; Cherney & Collaer, submitted) with men generally out-performing women. Mental rotation typically describes the mental manipulation of an entire object to a different position and is considered to be a spatial skill (Halpern, 2000). Spatial ability in general refers to the ability of using nonlinguistic information and includes the recall, transformation, generation and representation of symbolic information (Linn & Petersen, 1985), and it has been shown to be correlated with Scholastic Aptitude Test scores in Mathematics (SAT–M) (Casey, Nuttall, Pezaris, & Benbow, 1995). Scores on the SAT often influence what type of college or major a student might choose to pursue. Currently, women are underrepresented in various fields, with women making up only 14% of those with engineering degrees according to United States Census Bureau statistics (1993). The sex differences in spatial

---

[1]A portion of this study was presented at the 2002 Annual Great Plains Students' Psychology Convention, at the University of Nebraska Kearney, Kearney, NE. We thank Tara Dickey, Judith Flichtbeil and Jordan Winter for their assistance with data collection and coding. Please address correspondence to Isabelle D. Cherney, Department of Psychology, Creighton University, Omaha, NE 68178 or e-mail (cherneyi@creighton.edu).

abilities may therefore place one gender at a disadvantage, for spatial ability, among other skills, is needed in professions such as architecture, engineering, mathematics and the sciences (Scali, Brownlow, & Hicks, 2000). It is therefore crucial to examine empirically the factors involved in these differences and ways in which this gap may be eliminated.

The reasons for these cognitive sex differences are unknown. Several social-psychological factors have been shown to influence performance on Vandenberg and Kuse's Mental Rotation Test (1978). For example, Casey, Nuttall, and Pezaris (1999) found a correlation between participation in spatial activities and spatial ability. They noted that girls with brothers performed better on spatial rotation tasks than girls who did not have any brothers. They assumed that this difference was due to increased playtime with spatial activities, e.g., playing ball, computer games, etc., with their brothers. Other researchers have shown that experience with computer or video games can affect spatial abilities. For example, Greenfield, Brannon, and Lohr (1994) as well as Okagaki and Frensch (1994) stated that long-term expertise with video games predicted performance on a spatial test that required three-dimensional mental manipulation of a two-dimensional stimulus. In addition, Cherney, et al. (2003) reported that a brief exposure to another three-dimensional spatial task improved overall performance on the Mental Rotation Test. Similarly, Lohman and Nichols (1990) showed that extensive training improved speed and accuracy in solving mental rotation problems. Taken together, these findings suggest that prior exposure to spatial activities may increase performance in spatial skills, and specifically, performance on the Mental Rotation Test.

Stereotype threat may be another factor in cognitive sex differences. Stereotype threat refers to one's risk of being viewed negatively due to stereotypes commonly held about one's group (Steele & Aronson, 1995). This self-evaluative threat can result in a decrease in performance to act as a self-fulfilling prophecy. James and Greenberg (1997) found that both men and women regarded spatial ability as a masculine attribute. Because spatial ability is held as a masculine attribute, women's performance may be affected by their unconscious feelings of this negative stereotype. In one study, Sharps, Price, and Williams (1994) manipulated the instructions men and women received prior to completing a mental rotation test. When the spatial nature of the task was emphasized, women performed less well than did men, but there were no differences when the tasks were described as merely cognitive tasks. Women may perform poorly on tests of spatial skills because they believe that they already are at a disadvantage. However, it is possible that prior exposure to spatial tasks might attenuate stereotype threat and so improve performance on spatial tasks. Having previously performed a spatial task might increase women's self-perceptions of efficacy with spatial tasks.

Conversely, doubt about ability may influence the amount of time it takes to complete spatial tasks, thereby leading women to perform more slowly or less accurately when time is an important factor (e.g., Goldstein, et al., 1990). Goldstein, et al. reported that women are more cautious, attempt fewer items and tend to work more slowly. Linn and Petersen (1985) also found that women had a longer response time than men when performing spatial tasks. Similarly, Lohman reported that, although the rate of mental rotation did not differ significantly between the sexes, women tend to be slower. These sex differences in performance factors may be due to strategy choices.

Women may be choosing a slower or less efficient strategy. Collaer and Nelson (2002) reported that men were more likely to use geometrical reference cues, such as using the paper's edge, the tabletop or even mentally imposing an imaginary line when attempting the Judgment of Line Angle and Position Test (based on Benton, Varney, & Hamsher, 1978). This spatial task involves the estimation of the position and angle orientation of target lines by matching each line from a semicircular array of choices (Collaer & Nelson, 2002). Using the same spatial task, Cherney and Collaer (submitted) found that men and women used different strategies. Men tended to report that they determined which line in the comparison array was parallel to the target line whereas women reported more frequently that they imagined a right angle and mentally placed it on the target line(s) for comparison. Additionally, men and women have different response times for different degrees of rotation, suggesting that they are using different strategies (Lohman, 1989; Resnick, 1993). Sex differences in untimed conditions also point to a difference in strategy, for if women were simply slower than men, then no differences would be found when participants are given unlimited time to finish the spatial task (Resnick, 1993; Scali, et al., 2000; Collaer & Nelson, 2002).

Vandenberg and Kuse (1978) developed the Mental Rotation Test based on Shepard and Metzler's stimuli (1971). Each of 20 stimulus arrays features a target object with two distractors and two rotated versions of the target. The target object is a linear 10-block figure that has been bent at three right angles to produce four distinct sections. Participants must identify the two rotated figures that correspond to the target. According to Linn and Petersen (1985), individuals tend to use various strategies to solve these mental rotation problems. For example, some people rotate the figure one section at a time until the entire figure is rotated. Others use a Gestalt-like or "holistic" strategy, rotating the whole integrated figure. Some people check their answers more than once, and some individuals use a part-by-part strategy by continuing to rotate parts of the object to make sure it is the correct answer, even after the other answer choices have been eliminated.

The purpose of the present studies was twofold: First, we wanted to examine whether sex differences on the Mental Rotation Test are in part related to different strategy uses and, second, whether previous exposure to the Mental Rotation Test (even several months earlier) would improve performance on the test. The use of an inefficient or slower strategy may be the reason why women are less likely to finish the test and are less accurate when answering. It was hypothesized that, consistent with previous studies, men would outperform women on the Mental Rotation Test. It was also predicted that men and women would use different strategies, with men using more efficient (less time-consuming) strategies than women. In particular, men were expected to attempt more items within the time allotted and to resort to guessing less frequently than women. Also, it was hypothesized that participants who had previously completed the Mental Rotation Test would have higher accuracy scores than those who had never been exposed to the test. Specifically, women who had previously been exposed to the Mental Rotation Test were expected to score significantly higher than women who had never completed the inventory.

STUDY 1

Method

Participants.—The participants were 20 men and 29 women from a middle-sized private midwestern university. The mean age of the students was 19.5 yr. ($SD = 1.0$). Of these participants 76% were Euro-American, 14% were of Asian descent, 2% were African American and 8% were of Hispanic descent. For their participation, they received extra credit in their psychology classes.

Materials.—Spatial ability was measured using the Vandenberg and Kuse Mental Rotation Test (1978). Each participant was initially exposed to two pages of instructions and three examples of problems. Participants were given as much time as needed to familiarize themselves with the two pages of instructions and examples. The test contains two separate subtests, each with 10 spatial rotation exercises for a total of 20 exercises altogether. Each exercise consists of a drawing of a three-dimensional object composed of blocks (target) and four drawings to the right of the target object. The four drawings show two correctly rotated pictures of the target and two distractors (mirror images). The participants must mentally manipulate the target object and find the two correctly rotated objects. The range of possible scores was between 1 and 40.

Procedure.—Each participant signed a consent form prior to beginning the study. The Mental Rotation Test was administered under timed conditions, with 3.5 min. being allowed for each subtest. If a participant finished the Mental Rotation Test before the allotted time, he had to wait until the time was up to begin the next section. If a participant did not complete the test in the allotted time, he was not allowed to finish. Upon completion of the test, each participant was instructed to write down the answer to the following two questions, "To the best detail possible, please describe exactly how you did the exercise" and "How did you figure out how to answer the questions?"

On a separate page, participants were asked to indicate how often (1 = Used for almost every problem and 5 = Did not use) they used six separate sets of strategies (Linn & Petersen, 1985): (1) I randomly guessed, (2) I imagined the whole object on the left being rotated and then rotated it until it matched one of the answer choices, (3) I rotated each answer choice until one was found that fit the object on the left, (4) I rotated a piece of the object on the left until it matched a piece of one of the answer choices and then rotated a second piece and did so sequentially until all the pieces were matched up, (5) I rotated the answer choices in the manner described in Choice 4 until they matched the choice on the left, and (6) I counted the number of blocks to figure out which matched best. They were also instructed to indicate whether they had previously completed the Mental Rotation Test.

Results

Mental Rotation Test.—The tests were scored using the total numbers of correct choices (2 correct choices per item) with a maximum score of 20. The mean of the total correct items was 10.5 ($SD=4.3$). The test retest correlation r_{47} for the first and second sets of 10 problems each was .61 ($p<.001$). There was no practice effect. A repeated-measures t test showed that scores did not significantly change from the first set of problems ($M=5.6$, $SD=2.5$) to the second set ($M=4.9$, $SD=2.3$; $t_{47}=2.0$, ns).

Sex differences.—Independent t tests yielded a significant difference in the performance of men and women, with men ($M=12.0$, $SD=3.7$) scoring significantly higher than women ($M=9.5$, $SD=4.4$; $t=2.04$, $p=.05$), with a medium effect size ($d=.60$). Although it was hypothesized that women would be less likely to complete the test, no difference was found in the number of problems attempted between men ($M=16.0$, $SD=3.2$) and women ($M=14.8$, $SD=4.1$; $t_{47}=1.07$, ns).

To examine whether previous exposure to the Mental Rotation Test affected scores, an analysis of variance with Mental Rotation Test scores as the dependent variable, sex group, and whether the participant had previously completed the Mental Rotation Test, was performed. The analysis showed that participants (7 men and 8 women) who reported they had previously completed the Mental Rotation Test performed significantly better ($M=13.5$, $SD=4.1$) than those 13 men and 21 women who were taking the test for the first time ($M=9.2$, $SD=3.7$; $F_{1,45}=12.96$, $p=.001$), with a large effect for previous experience ($d=1.15$). There was no significant main effect of sex and no interaction. Previous exposure served as a covariate in the final analyses.

Differences in strategy.—Of the participants 46% reported using mainly one of the strategies, and 54% reported using several strategies. To quantify strategy use, we identified the strategy that each participant reported using most frequently as the main strategy. If one strategy was used infrequently in conjunction with one or more other strategies, then the participant's main strategy was labeled as a mixed strategy. Table 1 lists the participants' primary strategies and the means and standard deviations of their corresponding Mental Rotation Test performance.

TABLE 1
Reported Frequency of Primary Strategy With Means and Standard Deviations in Study 1

Strategy	n	M	SD
Mentally rotate target until it matches the answer choices	13	12.9	4.0
Mentally rotate answer choices until they fit the target	10	10.5	4.0
Sequential rotation of the target	2	8.0	2.8
Sequential rotation of the answer choices	0		
Random guessing	0		
Count the number of blocks	1	15.0	
Mixed strategies	22	9.0	4.3
Total	48	10.5	4.3

Guessing was analyzed in an analysis of variance, with the Mental Rotation Test scores as the dependent variable and sex and guessing as the quasi-independent variables. There was a significant main effect for guessing ($F_{4,43} = 4.11$, $p = .007$; $\eta^2 = .28$). Those who used guessing more often had lower scores on the Mental Rotation Test than those who rarely guessed; however, there was no significant interaction between sex and guessing.

The mental rotation scores were also adjusted for guessing by subtracting one-half the number of wrong items from the number of correct items (50% probability of being correct). A separate repeated-measures analysis on the Mental Rotation Test scores corrected for guessing between the first and second sets of test questions and sex, with previous experience as a covariate, yielded a main effect of sex ($F_{1,46} = 4.55$, $p = .04$; $\eta^2 = .09$). With guessing controlled for, men scored significantly higher ($M = 12.9$, $SD = 3.8$) than women ($M = 10.8$, $SD = 4.2$).

Finally, a 6 (main strategy) × 2 (sex) analysis of covariance with previous Mental Rotation Test experience as the covariate and the total number correct on the Mental Rotation Test as the dependent variable was performed. This analysis showed no significant effects for strategy and main effect for sex which fell short of the desired statistical significance ($F_{1,47} = 4.00$, $p = .05$). There was no interaction between sex and strategy.

Study 2

Participants tended to have difficulty introspecting which strategies they had used to complete the Mental Rotation Test. We therefore developed a more comprehensive and effective way to identify use of strategy and used this questionnaire with a second group of participants. In addition, we collected information on participants' exposure to sports and video or computer games as well as their scores on a standardized test (American College Test or Scholastic Aptitude Test). It was hypothesized that participants who played computer or video games and sports more frequently would score higher on the Mental Rotation Test than those who played less often. In addition, it was predicted that college entrance test scores would predict performance on mental rotation.

Method

Participants.—A total of 103 undergraduate students (30 men and 73 women) with a mean age of 20.1 yr. ($SD = 1.7$) from the same university participated. Seventy-eight percent were of Euro-American descent, 7% were Asian American, 5% African American, 1% Hispanic, and 7% were considered from Other ethnic backgrounds. Students received credit toward their psychology classes for their participation.

Materials and procedure.—Consistent with Study 1, participants were first given Vandenberg and Kuse's Mental Rotation Test (1978) in two timed sessions. Second, they were asked to complete a strategy questionnaire. Participants first answered the open-ended question, "Please describe the strategy that you used to find the matching targets on the test" and whether they had changed their strategy after the first set of 10 Mental Rotation Test questions. On a separate page, the participants were presented a set of six strategies and were asked to identify the most effective strategy to solve the test items. We also collected demographic information as well as students' SAT and ACT scores and their weekly involvement in sports and video or computer game play. Finally, each participant completed the same strategy questionnaire used in the first study. Students were encouraged to report why they used guessing to solve the Mental Rotation Test.

Results

Overall, 19% (10 men and 10 women) of the sample had taken the Mental Rotation Test previously, 49% of the participants completed the test in the allotted 7 min., and 33% reported that they randomly guessed as they were running out of time. Furthermore, 45% of them noted that they changed strategy after the first session of the Mental Rotation Test.

Mental Rotation Test.—The mean total correct items was 9.8 ($SD = 1.7$). A repeated-measures t test on the first and second set of problems indicated that scores changed significantly from the first 10 problems ($M = 5.2$, $SD =$

2.8) to the second 10 ($M = 4.6$, $SD = 2.6$; $t_{102} = 2.6$, $p = .01$), with mean scores decreasing.

Sex differences.—Consistent with the hypothesis, independent sample t tests on the number of correct scores yielded a significant sex difference ($t_{101} = 4.7$, $p = .001$), with men ($M = 13.0$, $SD = 4.3$) outperforming women ($M = 8.4$, $SD = 4.5$) with a large effect size ($d = 1.06$). An independent sample t test on the number of attempted items further confirmed that, congruent with our hypothesis, women attempted significantly fewer items ($M = 17.4$, $SD = 3.5$) than men ($M = 18.8$, $SD = 2.0$; $t_{101} = 2.1$, $p = .03$).

An analysis of variance with Mental Rotation Test scores as the dependent variable, and sex and whether participants had previously completed the Mental Rotation Test, was performed. The findings showed a main effect of sex ($F_{1,97} = 15.5$, $p = .001$; $\eta^2 = .14$), but the main effect of previous exposure fell short of statistical significance ($F_{1,97} = 3.5$, $p = .06$; $\eta^2 = .04$). Those who had previously completed the Mental Rotation Test ($M = 12.3$, $SD = 4.5$) somewhat outperformed those who had never completed it previously ($M = 10.1$, $SD = 4.5$). There was no interaction. To test whether women who had previously been exposed to the test would score higher than those who had never completed the Mental Rotation Test, an independent sample t test was performed. The results were not significant ($t_{71} < 1.00$, ns).

Differences in strategies.—Responses to the open-ended questions were coded by three independent individuals. Interrater reliability was 95%. Responses were placed into six categories: participant rotated the target and matched it to the other images (men = 12, women = 27), participant rotated the four images and matched them to the target (men = 3, women = 17), part rotation ($n = 3$), angle comparison ($n = 9$), counted boxes ($n = 5$) and guessed ($n = 4$). A chi-square test on these categories and sex was not significant ($\chi^2_5 = 6.9$, ns). There was a significant sex difference among participants who reported rotating the target and then matching it to the other images ($t_{37} = 3.3$, $p = .002$), with men ($M = 13.1$, $SD = 3.6$) scoring higher than women ($M = 8.19$, $SD = 4.5$). Comparison with participants who reported rotating the four images to match the target fell short of statistical significance ($t_{18} = 1.9$, $p = .06$).

The strategy participants judged as most effective were analyzed using separate t tests for each of the six proposed strategies. Table 2 lists t ratios, mean scores and standard deviations by sex group and strategy.

A 2 (sex) × 2 (whether participant used guessing) analysis of variance on the Mental Rotation Test scores showed significant main effects of sex ($F_{1,99} = 10.8$, $p = .001$) and guessing ($F_{1,99} = 4.1$, $p = .04$), but no interaction. On the average, participants who admitted guessing scored significantly lower ($M = 8.9$, $SD = 3.7$) than those who did not guess ($M = 11.4$, $SD = 5.1$). Separately by sex, analyses showed a significant main effect of guessing only for

TABLE 2
MEANS AND STANDARD DEVIATIONS FOR EACH STRATEGY MEN AND WOMEN CONSIDERED MOST EFFICIENT IN STUDY 2

Strategy	Sex	n	M	SD	t	p
Rotating a piece of the object on the left until it matches a piece of one of the answer choices and then rotating a second piece sequentially until all the pieces are matched up.	Male	4	13.7	2.9		
	Female	10	5.3	2.9	4.2	.001
Rotating each answer choice until one is found that fits the object on the left.	Male	4	15.5	3.0	4.4	.001
	Female	9	6.1	3.1		
Random guessing.	Male	0				
	Female	0				
Imagining the whole object on the left being rotated and then rotating it until it matches one of the answer choices.	Male	14	11.6	4.9		
	Female	38	8.5	4.3	1.4	ns
Rotating the answer choices in the manner described in choice 4 until they match the choice on the left.	Male	6	12.3	3.6		
	Female	13	12.1	4.5	–.07	ns
Counting the number of blocks to figure out which matches best.	Male	1				
	Female	2				

women ($t_{71} = -2.1$, $p = .04$). Furthermore, regression analyses by sex on the mental rotation scores with strategies as the predictors showed that for women, random guessing was predictive ($F_{6,65} = 2.2$, $p = .05$; $b = 1.4$) of their lower mental rotation scores.

Background information.—The Scholastic Aptitude Test scores, American College Test scores, the number of hours of sports and the number of hours on computer or video games participants reported playing were correlated with the total mental rotation scores. There were significant positive correlations for mental rotation scores with ACT scores ($r_{85} = .27$, $p = .01$) and video or computer game play ($r_{103} = .22$, $p = .02$). On the average, men reported playing sports ($t_{101} = 3.1$, $p = .002$) and video or computer games ($t_{101} = 4.0$, $p = .001$) more frequently than women. Men also reported significantly higher ACT scores ($t_{83} = 2.5$, $p = .01$). An analysis of covariance with ACT scores, sports activity and computer hours as covariates and sex as a between-subject variable still produced a main effect of sex ($F_{1,80} = 8.4$, $p = .005$). On the average, men identified 12.7 items correctly ($SD = 4.3$) and women 8 items ($SD = 4.5$).

Finally, a stepwise regression analysis with mental rotation scores as the criterion and (a) strategy use, (b) ACT scores, (c) hours of video or computer game play, and (d) sex as the predictors was performed to investigate contributions of each score to total variance. The total regression and R^2 were significant ($R^2 = .19$; $F_{1,81} = 19.4$, $p = .001$). Guessing alone accounted for 19% of the variance. ACT scores added another 6% to variance ($R^2_{change} = .06$; $F_{change} = 6.5$, $p = .013$), video or computer game hours added another

5% ($R^2_{change} = .05$; $F_{change} = 5.9$, $p = .02$) and sex no significant contribution, 3% ($R^2_{change} = .03$; $F_{change} = 3.3$, $p = .07$). In total, these variables accounted for 33% of the proportion of variance of the mental rotation scores.

Discussion

The results of both studies are consistent with previous research that has shown overall sex differences on various mental rotation tests (e.g., Goldstein, et al., 1990; Geary, et al., 1992; Resnick, 1993; Casey, et al., 1995; Voyer, et al., 1995; Nordvik & Amponsah, 1998; Scali, et al., 2000; Cherney, et al., 2003; Cherney & Collaer, submitted) on which men outperformed women. Several studies suggest that procedural factors affect the magnitude of sex differences on the Mental Rotation Test (Vandenberg & Kuse, 1978). For example, Goldstein, et al. (1990), Linn and Petersen (1985), as well as Lohman and Nichols (1990) reported that women tended to be slower and more careful in completing the Mental Rotation Test. One consequence of this is that women attempt fewer items than men. Congruent with these findings, the second study yielded sex differences in the number of items attempted, or women attempted fewer questions than men. This finding suggests that it takes women longer to complete the mental rotations. Voyer (1997) proposed that speed of processing may be one factor affecting performance on the Mental Rotation Test. He found that there were no sex differences in an untimed administration of the Mental Rotation Test. Although the results of the first study yielded no sex difference in attempted items, the pattern of the second study suggests that women were more prone to guess under time pressure. They were more likely than men to report that they used guessing when they were running out of time. In addition, guessing was the best predictor of the (lower) scores on the mental rotation test.

The reason why women in these samples were less accurate on the Mental Rotation Test than the men was probably due, in part, to their differential guessing but not necessarily to differential strategy use. In general, men and women did not differ in their judgment of what the most effective strategy would be. With the exception of guessing (presumably due to time constraints), they tended to use the same strategies. Thus, the hypothesis that women may be more likely to use a less efficient strategy was not supported. Linn and Petersen (1985) described many of the different strategies presently investigated, and, while the strategies were all used to some extent, men did not use one strategy more frequently than women and vice versa. These findings suggest that average differences between men and women on mental rotations are not simply due to women using a less efficient problem-solving strategy.

In a study examining strategy use for the Judgment of Line Angle and Position Test, Cherney and Collaer (submitted) reported that men and women tended to use different strategies, with men making use of parallel lines and women using superimposition of lines more frequently. Although participants who used the parallel strategy had overall higher scores on the Line Angle and Position Test, when strategy use was statistically controlled, sex was the only significant predictor of performance. In the present study, using one strategy rather than another did not significantly affect participants' performance, except when guessing. Participants who used random guessing to complete the Mental Rotation Test (Vandenberg & Kuse, 1978) tended to have lower scores than those who did not guess. In addition, the results showed that men scored significantly higher than women even when controlling for guessing. Taken together, these findings suggest that sex differences were not eliminated even when the Mental Rotation Test scores are controlled for guessing.

One reason why there were no differences between strategy use and overall Mental Rotation Test scores may be the difficulty participants had in correctly identifying what strategy they used. From the open-ended responses, we were able to ascertain that participants had difficulties describing complex mental processes in words. The participants may not have been very descriptive simply because they were unsure how to identify the mental processes they used to complete the Mental Rotation Test (Vandenberg & Kuse, 1978). Collaer and Nelson's (2002) research brings up another possible explanation. They found that men were more likely to use geometrical reference cues when completing the Judgment of Line Angle and Position Test, but the men were not aware that they were doing so. It is possible that participants rely on these or other cues, but that they are unaware that they are using them.

The results of the first study showed that prior exposure to the mental rotation test tended to increase participants' subsequent performance on the test. There was a practice effect with both men and women benefitting from having completed the Mental Rotation Test previously. These findings suggest that performance on the test is influenced by familiarization with the task. In the second study, previous exposure to the test was not as beneficial as in the first study, although in absolute numbers, both men and women improved their performance. However, exposure to another spatial task, i.e., video or computer play, was significantly related to the higher scores on the Mental Rotation Test. In general, training studies have been beneficial for both men and women (e.g., Baenninger & Newcombe, 1989; Cherney, et al., 2003) depending on the tasks and duration of the training. Baenninger and Newcombe (1989) performed a meta-analysis on the role of experience in spatial test performance. They confirmed that both men and women benefit from certain experiences. Training studies using computer games have shown significant improvements on mental rotation tasks (e.g., Greenfield, et *al.*, 1994; Okagaki & Frensch, 1994; Subrahmanyam & Greenfield, 1994). Studies have also shown that a brief exposure to another spatial task before testing is enough to produce significant changes. For example, when men and women were exposed for 2 min. to another pencil-and-paper rotation task (Cube Rotation Test), the sex differences on the Mental Rotation Test disappeared (Cherney, *et al.*, 2003). However, the time-course of these improvements is unclear. Furthermore, few studies have investigated whether the improvements transfer to other spatial skills. Taken together, these findings indicate that simple practice and training may influence performance on mental rotation. Thus, it is important to investigate further the effects of practice and training not only to improve spatial ability but also to eliminate sex differences.

The results of Study 2 further suggest that ACT scores are predictive of performance on the Mental Rotation Test (Vandenberg & Kuse, 1978). Casey, Nuttall, and Pezaris (1997) found that scores on a mental rotation task significantly predicted women's performance on the SAT–M subsection. Given the high correlation between Scholastic Aptitude Test and American College Test standardized scores, it is not surprising that the latter scores are predictive of mental rotation as well. The majority of the current students completed the American College Test and not the Scholastic Aptitude Test. Presumably, latter scores would also be predictive of mental rotation scores with a larger sample.

Overall, the results suggest that there is a robust sex difference in mental rotation. However, several factors that have been shown to eliminate the differences were not considered. For example, Tan, Okuyan, Albayrak, and Akgun (2003) showed that height and weight are significantly related to mental rotation. Their results indicated that, when using weight, height and testosterone levels as covariates, performance on mental rotation tests reversed, with women scoring higher than men. In another study Tan, Okuyan, Bayraktar, and Akgun (2003) also found that heavier women tended to score higher than light men. Similarly, Silverman and Phillips (1993) found that estrogen levels influenced women's performance on the Mental Rotation Test. During low estrogen levels, mean mental rotation scores were the highest.

The homogeneity and size of the sample precludes generalization of the results. Furthermore, some of the strategies were used more frequently than others. This imbalance created unequal cell sizes which, coupled with this relatively small sample size, lowered the power of the analyses. A more comprehensive and thorough study of strategy should be performed, for the self-report questionnaire was limited in its effectiveness. For example, the Mental Rotation Test could be administered individually, with the participant being interviewed immediately after completion and the session videotaped.

This interview could probe into the participant's general explanation of how he completed the exercise. The interviewer could also explain the most common types of strategies in greater detail than was given on this present study's self-report questionnaire to gauge how often the participant may have used these strategies. By administering the test to each participant individually, the time to complete the exercise could also be noted.

In sum, given the relationship between occupational choices, sex and spatial skills, it is important to investigate further not only the bases of these sex differences, but also the ways in which these discrepancies might be eliminated. At any rate, reliable differences between men and women across many investigations can guide our understanding of the etiology of sex differences and the nature of the inferential brain-behavior relationships.

REFERENCES

BAENNINGER, M., & NEWCOMBE, N. (1989) The role of experience in spatial test performance: a meta-analysis. *Sex Roles*, 20, 327-344.

BENTON, A. L., VARNEY, N. R., & HAMSHER, K. (1978) Visuospatial judgment: a clinical test. *Archives of Neurology*, 35, 364-367.

BJORKLUND, D. F. (2000) *Children's thinking: developmental function and individual differences.* (3rd ed.) Belmont, CA: Wadsworth/Thomson Learning.

CASEY, M. B., NUTTALL, R. L., & PEZARIS, E. (1997) Mediators of gender differences in mathematics college entrance test scores: a comparison of spatial skills with internalized beliefs and anxieties. *Developmental Psychology*, 33, 669-680.

CASEY, M. B., NUTTALL, R. L., & PEZARIS, E. (1999) Evidence in support of a model that predicts how biological and environmental factors interact to influence spatial skills. *Developmental Psychology*, 35, 1237-1247.

CASEY, M. B., NUTTALL, R. L., PEZARIS, E., & BENBOW, C. P. (1995) The influence of spatial ability on gender differences in mathematics college entrance test scores across diverse samples. *Developmental Psychology*, 31, 697-705.

CHERNEY, I. D., & COLLAER, M. (submitted) Sex differences in line judgment: relationship to mental rotation, academic preparation and strategy use.

CHERNEY, I. D., JAGARLAMUDI, K., LAWRENCE, E., & SHIMABUKU, N. (2003) Experiential factors on sex differences in mental rotation. *Perceptual and Motor Skills*, 96, 1062-1070.

COLLAER, M. L., & NELSON, J. D. (2002) Large visuospatial sex difference in line judgment: possible role of attentional factors. *Brain and Cognition*, 41, 1-12.

FEINGOLD, A. (1988) Cognitive gender differences are disappearing. *American Psychologist*, 43, 95-103.

GEARY, D. C., GILGER, J. W., & ELIOTT-MILLER, B. (1992) Gender differences in three-dimensional rotation: a replication. *The Journal of Genetic Psychology*, 153, 115-117.

GOLDSTEIN, D., HALDANE, D., & MITCHELL, C. (1990) Sex differences in visual-spatial ability: the role of performance factors. *Memory & Cognition*, 183, 546-550.

GREENFIELD, P. M., BRANNON, C., & LOHR, D. (1994) Two-dimensional representation of movement through three-dimensional space: the role of video game expertise. *Journal of Applied Developmental Psychology*, 15, 87-103.

HALPERN, D. F. (2000) *Sex differences in cognitive abilities.* (3rd ed.) Hillsdale, NJ: Erlbaum.

HYDE, J. S. (1981) How large are cognitive gender differences? A meta-analysis using ω^2 and d. *American Psychologist*, 36, 292-301.

HYDE, J. S., & LINN, M. C. (1988) Gender differences in verbal ability: a meta-analysis. *Psychological Bulletin*, 104, 53-69.

JAMES, K., & GREENBERG, J. (1997) Beliefs about self and about gender groups: interactive effects on the spatial performance of women. *Basic and Applied Social Psychology*, 19, 411-425.

LINN, M. A., & PETERSEN, A. C. (1985) Emergence and characterization of sex differences in spatial ability: a meta-analysis. *Child Development*, 56, 1479-1498.

LOHMAN, D. F. (1989) The effect of speed-accuracy tradeoff on sex differences in mental rotation. *Perception & Psychophysics*, 39, 433-436.

LOHMAN, D. F., & NICHOLS, P. D. (1990) Training spatial abilities: effects of practice on rotation and synthesis tasks. *Learning and Individual Differences*, 2, 67-93.

MACCOBY, E. E., & JACKLIN, C. N. (1974) *The psychology of sex differences.* Stanford, CA: Stanford Univer, Press

NORDVIK, H., & AMPONSAH, B. (1998) Gender differences in spatial abilities and spatial activity among university students in an egalitarian education system. *Sex Roles*, 38, 1009-1023.

OKAGAKI, L., & FRENSCH, P. A. (1994) Effects of video game playing on measures of spatial performance: gender effects in late adolescence. *Journal of Applied Developmental Psychology*, 15, 33-58.

RESNICK, S. M. (1993) Sex differences in mental rotations: an effect of time limits? *Brain and Cognition*, 21, 71-79.

SCALI, R. M., BROWNLOW, S., & HICKS, J. L. (2000) Gender differences in spatial task performance as a function of speed or accuracy orientation. *Sex Roles*, 43, 359-376.

SHARPS, M. J., PRICE, J. L., & WILLIAMS, J. K. (1994) Spatial cognition and gender: instructional and stimulus influences on mental image rotation performance. *Psychology of Women Quarterly*, 18, 413-425.

SHEPARD, R. N., & METZLER, J. (1971) Mental rotation of three-dimensional objects. *Science*, 171, 701-703.

SILVERMAN, I., & PHILLIPS, K. (1993) Effects of estrogen changes during the menstrual cycle on spatial performance. *Ethology and Sociobiology*, 14, 257-269.

STEELE, C. M., & ARONSON, J. (1995) Stereotype threat and the intellectual test performance of African Americans. *Journal of Personality and Social Psychology*, 69, 797-811.

SUBRAHMANYAM, K., & GREENFIELD, P. M. (1994) Effect of video game practice on spatial skills in girls and boys. *Journal of Applied Developmental Psychology*, 15, 13-32.

TAN, Ü., OKUYAN, M., ALBAYRAK, T., & AKGUN, A. (2003) Sex differences in verbal and spatial ability reconsidered in relation to body size, lunch volume, and sex hormones. *Perceptual and Motor Skills*, 96, 1347-1360.

TAN, Ü., OKUYAN, M., BAYRAKTAR, T., & AKGUN, A. (2003) Covariation of sex differences in mental rotation with body size. *Perceptual and Motor Skills*, 96, 137-144.

UNITED STATES BUREAU OF THE CENSUS. (1993) *Highest degree and field of degree, by sex, race, Hispanic origin, and age, with persons with post-secondary degrees.* Washington, DC: Author.

VANDENBERG, S., & KUSE, A. R. (1978) Mental rotations: a group test of three dimensional spatial visualization. *Perceptual and Motor Skills*, 47, 599-604.

VOYER, D. (1997) Scoring procedure, performance factors, and magnitude of sex differences in spatial performance. *American Journal of Psychology*, 110, 259-276.

VOYER, D., VOYER, S., & BRYDEN, M. P. (1995) Magnitude of sex differences in spatial abilities: a meta-analysis and consideration of critical variables. *Psychological Bulletin*, 117, 250-270.

Accepted April 15, 2004.

MASTERY OF NUMBER CONSERVATION BY A MAN WITH SEVERE COGNITIVE DISABILITIES [1]

JESSICA LYNN CAMPBELL, K. MARINKA GADZICHOWSKI, AND ROBERT PASNAK

George Mason University

Summary.—An autistic 21-yr.-old with a mental age of four years was taught number conservation. Mastery of this concept requires concrete operational thought and has not been thought to be possible for persons with severe disabilities. A learning set of 105 problems was used to promote generalization, and a "fade-out" procedure was used to make mastery of the problems as easy as possible. Combination of these techniques produced the first recorded success in teaching number conservation to a person with severe disabilities. This demonstration that one individual can perform at this cognitive level opens the door to research to determine the generality and limits of the potential of other individuals with severe cognitive disabilities.

Inhelder's comprehensive research (1968) indicated that individuals who had severe disabilities did not develop the abstract thought necessary for concrete operations. To date, there have been no published instances of individuals who have severe mental disabilities mastering even early concrete operations such as number conservation.

Nearly all teaching involves helping persons apply thinking abilities they already possess in new ways to new types of problems or contexts. This is the idea of the "zone of proximal development" or "readiness." Many methods can work well. However, to teach anyone to think at a higher level of abstraction than they currently possess, that is, beyond their "zone of potential development," is extraordinarily difficult—or impossible, according to Inhelder and Piaget (1959/1964). Special methods are essential to produce significant progress.

Two such methods were used in this research. One was the learning-set approach (Harlow, 1949; Gagné, 1968), in which an abstract principle is represented concretely in numerous problems that vary widely in perceptual characteristics. After mastering enough problems that differ sufficiently in appearance and details, the learner internalizes and applies that principle easily to any new problem. The other was a "fade-out" procedure, i.e., using extra cues to make the correct response so obvious that *no* learning is required. The extra cues are gradually reduced, until the learner solves the problem without them.

Participant.—An autistic 21-yr.-old African American with Full Scale scores of 40 on both the TONI and WISC–III participated.

---

[1]Address enquiries to R. Pasnak, Ph.D., Psychology 3f5, George Mason University, 4400 University Drive, Fairfax, VA 22030.

Procedure.—A multiple baseline was planned. He scored zero on a 12-problem number conservation pretest and 6 on a 10-problem transitivity test. (His score on the latter did not differ significantly from a chance score of five.) For the next 12 weeks, he was taught number conservation for 15 min. five mornings a week.

First the terms "more," "less," and "same," written in large letters, were placed next to a row of items. On random trials one item was added to or subtracted from the row, or nothing was done, and he was asked, "How many are there now?" A spotlight was projected onto the correct term for 20 such problems and gradually dimmed until he answered correctly without it. Perceptual transformations were then introduced by also compressing or expanding the row, or only touching it, in random order. The fade-out procedure guided him through 30 problems until it was not needed.

Next, his name was printed below one row of items and the teacher's name above another row. An item was added to or subtracted from one row, and he was asked "Who has more (or less)?" The fade-out procedure was used for 20 problems until he pointed to the correct name consistently. Then he was asked "Do you (or the teacher) have more (or less or the same)?" After 15 problems he was consistently correct without the spotlight. Perceptual transformations of the rows were added, and the fade-out procedure used until after 20 problems he no longer needed it.

Results.—He scored 11/12 correct when retested on conservation, a significant gain ($z = 3.53$, $p < .01$). Thus, he accurately generalized the concept across many different test items not used in the instruction. His transitivity posttest score was 4—still equivalent to random guessing and not significantly different from his pretest score.

Discussion and conclusions.—Training on transitivity was planned to complete the multiple baseline, however, the research was terminated, and instruction on transitivity was not attempted. Whether the experimental procedures would have produced mastery of this somewhat more advanced concept remains unknown. The research does show that even an individual with very severe disabilities can be helped to function at the level of abstraction demanded by number conservation problems. Perhaps such individuals can be taught to function at more abstract levels in many more domains and thereby improve their achievement and independence.

REFERENCES

GAGNÉ, R. M. (1968) Contributions of learning to human development. *Psychological Review*, 75, 177-191.
HARLOW, H. H. (1949) The formation of learning sets. *Psychological Review*, 56, 51-65.
INHELDER, B. (1968) *The diagnosis of reasoning in the mentally retarded.* New York: Day.
INHELDER, B., & PIAGET, J. (1959/1964) *The early growth of logic in the child: classification and seriation.* (E. A. Lunzer & D. Papert, Transl.) London: Routledge & Kegan Paul.

Accepted April 12, 2004.

ANCHORING PROCEDURES IN RELIABILITY OF RATINGS OF PERCEIVED EXERTION DURING RESISTANCE EXERCISE [1]

KRISTEN M. LAGALLY AND ELIZABETH M. COSTIGAN

Illinois State University

Summary.—Although the validity of perceived exertion as a method of monitoring the intensity of resistance exercise has been established, little is known about the test-retest reliability of ratings of perceived exertion during resistance exercise. Specifically, it is unknown whether the use of different anchoring procedures influences the reliability of ratings of perceived exertion. 30 men were assigned to an Exercise, Memory, or combined Exercise and Memory anchoring group. Participants completed an assessment of maximal leg-extension strength and were introduced to the Borg 15-category rating of perceived exertion scale through anchoring procedures that varied across groups. During two sessions of resistance exercise, participants rated active muscle perceived exertion after performing one repetition of the leg-extension exercise at 40%, 50%, 60%, 70%, 80% and 90% of the one-repetition maximum. A three-factor (Group × Intensity × Session) analysis of variance was performed to examine the perceived exertion data. Perceived exertion increased significantly ($p<.01$) with increasing exercise intensity in all groups and in both sessions. Mean ratings did not differ significantly among groups. Reliability was assessed for each group. Intraclass correlation coefficients ranged from .07 to .80 and percent agreement ranged from 60% to 90%. The results indicate that the reliability of ratings of perceived exertion during resistance exercise is acceptable regardless of the type of anchoring procedures used.

Ratings of perceived exertion (RPE) have been shown to increase as certain indices of the intensity of dynamic resistance exercise increase. These indices include the percentage of the one-repetition maximum lifted (Suminski, Robertson, Arslanian, Kang, Utter, DaSilva, Goss, & Metz, 1997; Gearhart, Goss, Lagally, Jakicic, Gallagher, Gallagher, & Robertson, 2002; Lagally, Robertson, Gallagher, Gearhart, & Goss, 2002), total weight lifted (Robertson, Goss, Rutkowski, Lenz, Dixon, Timmer, Frazee, Dube, & Andreacci, 2003), blood lactic acid concentration (Pierce, Rozenek, & Stone, 1993; Garbutt, Boocock, Reilly, & Troup, 1994; Suminski, *et al.*, 1997), and muscle activity (Lagally, Robertson, Gallagher, Goss, Jakicic, Lephart, McCaw, & Goodpaster, 2002). The relation between ratings of perceived exertion and these variables has established the validity of perceived exertion as a method of assessing intensity during a single bout of resistance exercise. The repeatability of ratings of perceived exertion, on the other hand, has

---

[1]Address correspondence to Kristen M. Lagally, School of Kinesiology and Recreation, Illinois State University, Horton Fieldhouse, Campus Box 5120, Normal, IL 61790 or e-mail (kmlagal@ilstu.edu).

not been examined during resistance exercise. Thus, it is unknown whether ratings of perceived exertion remain consistent at a given intensity of resistance exercise over the course of training.

To promote consistency in rating, researchers and practitioners often perform scaling and anchoring procedures to educate participants on how to use the perceived exertion scale correctly during exercise, i.e., scaling, and to familiarize participants with the range of sensations that they may experience during exercise, i.e., anchoring. Scaling is achieved by reading a set of instructions to participants prior to exercise, while anchoring can be achieved in one of several ways. Noble and Robertson (1996) suggested that a scale can be anchored through definition, i.e., memory anchoring, or through experience, i.e., exercise anchoring. With memory anchoring for resistance exercise, the feelings of exertion associated with a 7 on the Borg 15-category RPE scale would be defined as lifting a "very light resistance" and the feelings of exertion associated with a 19 on the RPE scale would be defined as lifting the "heaviest resistance imaginable." With exercise anchoring, participants perform an activity that elicits the feelings of exertion associated with a 7 and a 19 on the scale. Exercise anchoring is accomplished for resistance exercise by having a participant assign the feelings of exertion during an unweighted repetition a scale rating of 7 and the feelings of exertion during a maximal repetition a scale rating of 19. Thus, exercise anchoring for resistance exercise requires one-repetition maximum testing in order to establish the maximal repetition.

Scaling and anchoring procedures specifically designed for resistance exercise were recently validated (Gearhart, Goss, Lagally, Jakicic, Gallagher, & Robertson, 2001). These procedures include both exercise and memory anchoring components. Participants perform exercise anchoring during an initial one-repetition maximum testing session and are reminded of these feelings of exertion through memory anchoring in all subsequent exercise sessions. Because exercise anchoring requires one-repetition maximum testing, memory anchoring alone may be preferable, particularly in health clubs, schools and rehabilitation settings. However, a concern with using memory anchoring alone is that many individuals may be unfamiliar with the feelings of exertion associated with maximal resistance exercise. For these individuals, the experience of maximal sensations of exertion, i.e., exercise anchoring, sometime prior to exercise may promote better reliability of ratings of perceived exertion than memory anchoring, with which participants are asked to imagine or recall the feelings of exertion associated with maximal resistance exercise. Thus, this investigation included exercise anchoring as part of the Borg RPE scale familiarization procedures. This is hypothesized to result in more reliable ratings of perceived exertion than memory anchoring alone.

METHOD

Participants

Thirty recreationally trained male volunteers participated. These participants were divided equally into three groups including an Exercise-anchoring group, a combined Exercise and Memory-anchoring group and a Memory-anchoring group. With an effect size of .80 and alpha = .05, power was assessed to be .80 with 10 subjects per group. Descriptive data for the participants are shown in Table 1. Age, height, mass, percent body fat, and maximal leg strength did not differ significantly among the three groups. Participants were recruited from introductory kinesiology classes at Illinois State University and reported being moderately trained, recreational weightlifters, i.e., lifting weights two to three times per week for at least three months prior to testing, who had not previously participated in any structured maximal lifting and who were unfamiliar with the Borg RPE scale.

TABLE 1
PARTICIPANTS' CHARACTERISTICS

Group	Age (yr.) M	Age (yr.) SD	Height (in.) M	Height (in.) SD	Mass (kg) M	Mass (kg) SD	Body Fat (%) M	Body Fat (%) SD	Maximal Strength (kg) M	Maximal Strength (kg) SD
Exercise	20.7	1.3	70.1	1.9	81.2	14.1	12.4	5.0	64.7	6.7
Exercise-Memory	21.3	1.5	70.9	3.5	81.8	9.3	11.3	4.3	70.9	12.9
Memory	21.7	3.1	71.9	3.3	85.5	12.6	13.0	3.7	63.0	9.2

Procedure

During the course of testing, participants were instructed to refrain from any nonexperimental anaerobic or resistance exercise, maintain normal dietary habits, and abstain from alcohol, caffeine and nicotine for at least 24 hours prior to the testing sessions. Participants were tested at the same time of day during each experimental session. Each completed a medical history questionnaire and provided written informed consent before participating. The questionnaire was immediately reviewed by the primary investigator who is an American College of Sports Medicine (ACSM) certified exercise specialist. Any individual who was assessed to be at moderate or high risk for a cardiac event during exercise or who had any skeletal muscle, cardiovascular or endocrine disorders that would preclude exercise testing was excluded from the investigation. The Institutional Review Board of Illinois State University approved all procedures used.

Assessment session.—The investigation was conducted over three to four sessions, depending upon group assignment. Exercise and Exercise-Memory group participants attended three sessions, and Memory group participants attended four sessions total. The first session provided an orientation to the testing procedures. Descriptive information for each participant was also obtained. This included measurement of height and weight and the estimation of body density via skinfolds, with percent body fat predicted from three sites according to the procedures of Jackson and Pollock (1985). For participants in the Exercise and Exercise-Memory groups, a one-repetition maximum assessment was determined for the leg-extension exercise using the methods of Lombardi (1989). For participants in the Memory group, a 10-repetition maximum assessment was performed by adapting the methods of Lombardi (1989) to accommodate 10 repetitions. The assessments were performed on a Nautilus™ leg-extension machine. Only the dominant lower extremity was tested. Lower extremity dominance was determined by asking the participants with which leg they would kick a ball. The one-repetition maximum and 10-repetition maximum values were used to set the 40, 50, 60, 70, 80 and 90% intensities that were presented in the two experimental sessions. Participants were not informed of the results of the assessments and were not aware of the intensities used during the experimental sessions until after they had completed their participation.

Experimental sessions.—Each participant took part in two experimental sessions, the first of which was performed one week after the assessment session. During these sessions, participants performed a warm-up that consisted of two sets of 10 repetitions at 20% of their maximal strength and then performed one repetition of the leg-extension exercise using the dominant leg at 40%, 50%, 60%, 70%, 80% and 90% of their maximal strength. Although exact percentages were impossible to achieve in all cases, 5- and 2½-lb. plates were used to obtain a resistance as close to the desired percentage as possible. Resistance was rounded up when necessary. Active muscle, i.e., specific to the quadriceps muscle group, ratings of perceived exertion were collected using the Borg 15-category RPE scale immediately after the repetition at each intensity. The order of the intensities was randomly assigned. This was done separately for the two experimental sessions so that the intensities were performed in a different order each time. Repetition speed was paced by a metronome set at 70 beats · min.$^{-1}$ during both experimental sessions. Participants were asked to perform each repetition in a two count up, two count down pattern. Therefore, one repetition was performed for every four beats of the metronome. At this pace, each repetition lasted for approximately three and one-half seconds. Participants rested for 2 min. between intensities. The weight stack of the leg-extension machine was completely covered so that participants were unaware of the weights that they were lifting. Experimental Session 2 was a repeat of Experimental Session 1 and was used to assess the test-retest reliability of ratings from the Borg RPE scale. The experimental sessions were performed one week apart.

Scaling instructions.—All participants were provided scaling instructions and anchoring procedures during all sessions. The scaling instructions for all groups defined perceived exertion and explained the nature and use of the scale, differentiated ratings and the correctness of responses. The instructions also included statements that explained the range of sensations corresponding to the Borg RPE scale (Noble & Robertson, 1996). These statements were based on the type of anchoring that each group experienced. For the Exercise and combined Exercise-Memory groups, participants were instructed to use the feelings of exertion experienced when performing the unweighted and maximal repetitions during the one-repetition maximum assessment as a reference point when rating perceived exertion during exercise. For the Memory anchoring group, participants were instructed to recall previous feelings of exertion associated with light and heavy exercise and use those feelings as a reference point when rating perceived exertion during exercise. All participants were provided with an opportunity to ask questions regarding the scale and its use. The scaling instructions were read to the participants by the investigators during the assessment session. Participants read the instructions to themselves during the experimental sessions.

Anchoring procedures.—Participants in the Exercise anchoring group performed exercise anchoring in all three sessions (one assessment and two experimental sessions). After the scaling instructions were administered, each participant performed an unweighted repetition and a maximal repetition. The participant was instructed to assign the feelings of exertion during the unweighted repetition a scale rating of 7 and the feelings of exertion during the maximal repetition a scale rating of 19. These anchors were performed as part of the one-repetition maximum testing during the assessment session and were performed at the beginning of the experimental sessions.

Participants in the Exercise-Memory group performed exercise anchoring as described for the Exercise group, but only during the assessment session as part of the one-repetition maximum assessment. In both experimental sessions, Exercise-Memory group participants were memory anchored by reading the scaling instructions as described above. The Exercise-Memory group procedures exactly followed those recommended by Gearhart, *et al.* (2001).

Participants in the Memory group did not perform any exercise anchoring but were memory anchored in all three sessions. During the assessment session, they were read instructions which asked them to recall previous feelings of exertion that corresponded to the lowest resistance imaginable and the heaviest resistance imaginable and associate these feelings with a 7 and a 19 on the Borg scale, respectively. The participants reread these instructions to themselves prior to both experimental sessions. With memory anchoring, it is assumed that all people have, at some time in their lives, experienced very light and very hard lifting-type exercise, and therefore already possess a reference for those sensations of exertion. For this reason, the Memory group performed a 10-repetition maximum instead of a one-repetition maximum during the assessment session to avoid the experience of a maximal repetition immediately prior to the experimental sessions. To ensure that the 10-repetition maximum assessment was an accurate predictor of maximal strength, Memory group participants attended a fourth session to perform a one-repetition maximum assessment. Predictions of maximal strength from the 10-repetition maximum assessments were 98% of actual maximal strength or higher for all 10 participants.

Statistical analysis.—The ratings of perceived exertion data for each group at each intensity were evaluated with a three-factor Group (Exercise, Exercise-Memory, Memory) × Intensity (40, 50, 60, 70, 80, 90% maximal strength) × Session (Experimental Session 1, Experimental Session 2) analysis of variance, with repeated measures on the Intensity and Session factors. Dependent t tests were performed to examine significant effects. An alpha level of $p<.05$ was used to established statistical significance. Intraclass correlation coefficients were calculated from a two-way analysis of variance model to assess test-retest reliability. Intraclass correlation coefficients were chosen to examine reliability because there has been some concern over the use of bivariate correlations as a method of assessing agreement between repeated measures (Lamb, Eston, & Corns, 1999). Several previous studies have used intraclass correlation coefficients to examine the reliability of ratings of perceived exertion (Lamb, 1995; Lamb, *et al.*, 1999; Leung, Chung, & Leung, 2002). The analysis of variance and intraclass correlation coefficient analyses were performed using the Statistical Package for the Social Sciences (SPSS). Percent agreement was also calculated by hand to assess the percentage of participants that provided ratings from session to session that were either exactly the same or within one category, i.e., number, on the RPE scale.

Results

Results of the three-factor analysis of variance indicated that there were no three-way or two-way interactions, and no significant Group or Session main effects. The analysis of variance did indicate a significant ($p<.01$) main effect of Intensity. Dependent t tests with the alpha adjusted using the Bonferroni procedure ($.05/5 = .01$) indicated that ratings of perceived exertion were significantly ($p<.01$) different at all intensities in each group with the exception of 50% and 60% in the first estimation session for the Memory group. Means and standard deviations for active muscle ratings of perceived exertion at the six intensities in both estimation sessions are presented in Table 2. The range of intraclass correlation coefficients for the Exercise

TABLE 2
MEANS, STANDARD DEVIATIONS, AND INTRACLASS CORRELATION COEFFICIENTS (ICC) FOR ACTIVE MUSCLE RATINGS OF PERCEIVED EXERTION AT SIX RESISTANCE EXERCISE INTENSITIES ($ns = 10$)

Group	Session	40% M	40% SD	50% M	50% SD	60% M	60% SD	70% M	70% SD	80% M	80% SD	90% M	90% SD
Exercise	1	7.9	1.1	9.8	1.3	11.8	1.9	14.3	1.3	16.1	1.9	18.0	1.7
	2	8.3	1.3	10.8	1.6	12.6	2.1	14.3	1.5	16.3	1.5	18.2	1.0
	ICC	0.57		0.07		0.63		0.50		0.46		0.47	
Exercise-Memory	1	8.2	1.4	10.1	1.5	12.3	1.2	14.1	1.4	16.1	1.6	18.4	.84
	2	8.4	1.4	10.4	2.1	12.1	1.6	13.9	1.9	16.0	2.1	18.6	1.4
	ICC	0.73		0.46		0.74		0.53		0.75		0.51	
Memory	1	8.0	1.2	10.6[a]	1.5	11.2[a]	1.7	13.6	1.7	15.6	1.5	17.8	1.6
	2	7.9	1.3	10.2	1.3	12.0	1.6	13.3	.96	15.5	2.4	17.2	2.2
	ICC	0.40		0.28		0.80		0.64		0.57		0.69	
All	ICC	0.57		0.25		0.70		0.56		0.60		0.61	

Note.—Within a group, means with the same superscript are not significantly different at $p < .01$. Within an intensity, means are not significantly different among groups or between sessions.

group was .07 to .63, for the Exercise-Memory group was .46 to .75, and for the Memory group was .28 to .80. The intraclass correlation coefficients for each intensity and group are also presented in Table 2. Percent agreement ranged from 60% to 90%. The percentages for all groups and intensities are shown in Table 3.

TABLE 3
Percentage of Subjects Who Rated Within One Category on Borg Scale Between Sessions (ns = 10)

Group	Intensity (Percentage of One-repetition Maximum)					
	40%	50%	60%	70%	80%	90%
Exercise	80	60	70	80	60	70
Exercise-Memory	90	60	90	60	70	80
Memory	80	70	80	80	70	80

Discussion

The results of this investigation suggest that the reliability of ratings of perceived exertion during resistance exercise is acceptable across a wide range of exercise intensities. Contrary to our hypothesis, the results indicate that the inclusion of exercise anchoring procedures does not necessarily promote better understanding of the use of the perceived exertion scale and does not improve reliability over other types of anchoring procedures. Ratings of perceived exertion were similar at a given exercise intensity regardless of the type of anchoring procedures administered, and RPE increased with increasing exercise intensity. This suggests that all three types of anchoring procedures are valid for use during resistance exercise.

To our knowledge, no other investigations have examined reliability of ratings of perceived exertion during resistance exercise, although several articles have been published on the reliability of estimated ratings of perceived exertion from the Borg RPE scale during dynamic aerobic exercise (Skinner, Hutsler, Bergsteinova, & Buskirk, 1973; Stamford, 1976; Lamb, 1995; Lamb, et al., 1999; Leung, et al., 2002). Previous investigations examining reliability using intraclass correlations found coefficients for cycle ergometer exercise performed at four exercise intensities ranging from .43 to .95 (Lamb, 1995) and .52 to .90 (Leung, et al., 2002) and for treadmill exercise performed at four exercise intensities ranging from .75 to .82 (Lamb, et al., 1999). The participants in these investigations seem to have been anchored using memory procedures.

As mentioned above, intraclass correlation coefficients are considered to be an appropriate method of examining reliability in perceived exertion investigations (Lamb, 1995; Lamb, et al., 1999; Leung, et al., 2002). However, these coefficients are reduced when there is limited between-subject variance

(Deneger & Ball, 1993; Lamb, 1995). We believe this to have been a challenge to our analyses, primarily because we asked all participants to provide ratings at the same relative exercise intensity. Many of our participants selected the same or similar ratings at a given relative exercise intensity, which resulted in limited between-subject variance. The previous investigations assessed ratings of perceived exertion during aerobic exercise at absolute workloads, which likely resulted in greater between-subject variance and higher intraclass correlations than in the present investigation. Another potential explanation for the lower coefficients in the present investigation is that in the previous investigations (Lamb, 1995; Lamb, et al., 1999; Leung, et al., 2002), exercise intensities were performed progressively and in the same order in both experimental sessions. In the present investigation, intensities were performed in a different order during each experimental session.

To provide a clearer picture of reliability, percent agreement was calculated. The results of these calculations indicate that in all cases, the majority rated their perceived exertion during Experimental Session 2 within one category of their previous rating, which represents acceptable, if not excellent, reliability. Out of 180 possible pairs of ratings (30 participants × 6 intensities in each session), only 27 (15%) were two categories apart, and only 16 (9%) were greater than two categories apart on the Borg scale. At a given exercise intensity, even a two-category difference in ratings from the Borg scale is reasonable, given that there may have been some natural variations in maximal strength, motivation and fatigue between sessions, and fatigue due to order effects within sessions. Although we instructed participants to avoid exercise prior to testing, it is possible that some forgot these instructions on one of the testing days, resulting in higher ratings on that day. In spite of these potential limitations, the information in Table 3 suggests that the reliability of ratings of perceived exertion in this investigation was good. Certainly, further investigation of reliability during resistance exercise is warranted. What was examined in the present investigation was the stability of ratings over time during a single effort at six relative exercise intensities. Further investigations should examine the reliability of ratings of perceived exertion during resistance exercise performed at absolute workloads. It would be of interest to know whether individuals can use ratings of perceived exertion to select a given resistance consistently across training sessions.

It was hypothesized that the inclusion of exercise-anchoring procedures would result in more reliable ratings of perceived exertion than would memory-anchoring procedures alone. The rationale for this was based on a potential lack of familiarity among participants with the feelings of exertion associated with maximal lifting. The results indicate that performing repeated exercise-anchoring did not consistently produce more reliable ratings than exercise-memory-anchoring or memory-anchoring alone. Thus, repeated exercise-anchoring procedures as performed here would not be recommended because they appear not to offer any benefit over the others and require more time and effort. Memory-anchoring alone may be the preferred choice in most situations, particularly when performing a one-repetition maximum would be impractical or unsafe. However, it is important to note that, although our participants had not participated in structured maximal lifting, they did have some experience with lifting. Therefore, the results of this investigation may not necessarily apply to novice lifters. It is possible that for novice lifters, exercise-anchoring may result in more reliable ratings of perceived exertion than memory-anchoring.

In all three groups, ratings of perceived exertion increased as the intensity of resistance exercise increased from 40% to 90% of the one-repetition maximum. These results indicate that ratings of perceived exertion during resistance exercise are related to percentage of the one-repetition maximum lifted. These findings agree with those of Suminski, et al. (1997), Gearhart, et al. (2002) and Lagally, Robertson, Gallagher, Gearhart, and Goss (2002). The only ratings that were not significantly different were 50% and 60% from the first estimation session in the Memory group. The importance of this may be minimal, primarily because the rating at 60% of the one-repetition maximum was significantly higher than the rating at 50% of the one-repetition maximum during the second estimation in this group. Mean ratings of perceived exertion were not significantly different among groups at any of the six resistance exercise intensities in either experimental session. Thus, ratings of perceived exertion provide information about the intensity of resistance exercise regardless of the type of anchoring procedures administered.

In conclusion, the results of this investigation suggest that ratings of perceived exertion from the Borg RPE scale are valid and reliable during resistance exercise. The choice of which anchoring procedures are most appropriate to use may be based upon the setting, the fitness of the participant and the amount of resistance exercise experience that the participant has. However, our results support the use of memory-anchoring for experienced weight lifters in most settings given its ease of administration.

REFERENCES

DENEGER, C. R., & BALL, D. W. (1993) Assessing reliability and precision of measurement: an introduction to intraclass correlation and standard error of measurement. *Journal of Sport Rehabilitation*, 2, 35-42.

GARBUTT, G., BOOCOCK, M. G., REILLY, T., & TROUP, J. D. G. (1994) Physiological and spinal responses to circuit weight training. *Ergonomics*, 37, 117-125.

GEARHART, R. F., GOSS, F. L., LAGALLY, K. M., JAKICIC, J. M., GALLAGHER, J., GALLAGHER, K. I., & ROBERTSON, R. J. (2002) Ratings of perceived exertion in active muscle during high-intensity and low-intensity resistance exercise. *Journal of Strength and Conditioning Research*, 16, 87-91.

GEARHART, R. F., GOSS, F. L., LAGALLY, K. M., JAKICIC, J. M., GALLAGHER, J., & ROBERTSON, R. J.

(2001) Standardized scaling procedures for rating perceived exertion during resistance exercise. *Journal of Strength and Conditioning Research*, 15, 320-325 .

JACKSON, A. S., & POLLOCK, M. L. (1985) Practical assessment of body composition. *The Physician and Sportsmedicine*, 13, 76-90.

LAGALLY, K. M., ROBERTSON, R. J., GALLAGHER, K. I., GEARHART, R. F., & GOSS, F. L. (2002) Ratings of perceived exertion during low- and high-intensity resistance exercise by young adults. *Perceptual and Motor Skills*, 94, 723-731.

LAGALLY, K. M., ROBERTSON, R. J., GALLAGHER, K. I., GOSS, F. L., JAKICIC, J. M., LEPHART, S. M., MCCAW, S. T., & GOODPASTER, B. (2002) Perceived exertion, electromyography, and blood lactate during acute bouts of resistance exercise. *Medicine and Science in Sports and Exercise*, 34, 552-559.

LAMB, K. L. (1995) Children's ratings of effort during cycle ergometry: an examination of the validity of two effort rating scales. *Pediatric Exercise Science*, 7, 407-421.

LAMB, K. L., ESTON, R. G., & CORNS, D. (1999) Reliability of ratings of perceived exertion during progressive treadmill exercise. *British Journal of Sports Medicine*, 33, 336-339.

LEUNG, M-L, CHUNG, P-K., & LEUNG, R. W. (2002) An assessment of the validity and reliability of two perceived exertion rating scales among Hong Kong children. *Perceptual and Motor Skills*, 95, 1047-1062.

LOMBARDI, V. P. (1989) Safe maximum testing. In A. Lockhart & J. Mott (Eds.), *Beginning weight training*. Dubuque, IA: Brown. Pp. 197-204.

NOBLE, B. J., & ROBERTSON, R. J. (1996) *Perceived exertion*. Champaign, IL: Human Kinetics.

PIERCE, K., ROZENEK, R., & STONE, M. H. (1993) Effects of high volume weight training on lactate, heart rate, and perceived exertion. *Journal of Strength and Conditioning Research*, 7, 211-215.

ROBERTSON, R. J., GOSS, F. L., RUTKOWSKI, J., LENZ, B., DIXON, C., TIMMER, J., FRAZEE, K., DUBE, J., & ANDREACCI, J. (2003) Concurrent validation of the OMNI Perceived Exertion Scale for resistance exercise. *Medicine and Science in Sports and Exercise*, 35, 333-341.

SKINNER, J. S., HUTSLER, R., BERGSTEINOVA, V., & BUSKIRK, E. R. (1973) The validity and reliability of a rating scale of perceived exertion. *Medicine and Science in Sports and Exercise*, 5, 94-96.

STAMFORD, B. A. (1976) Validity and reliability of subjective ratings of perceived exertion during work. *Ergonomics*, 19, 53-60.

SUMINSKI, R. R., ROBERTSON, R. J., ARSLANIAN, S., KANG, J., UTTER, A. C., DASILVA, S. G., GOSS, F. L., & METZ, K. F. (1997) Perceived effort during resistance exercise. *Journal of Strength and Conditioning Research*, 11, 261-265.

Accepted April 13, 2004.

EFFECTS OF RANDOM OUTCOMES ON CHOICE BEHAVIOR[1]

ELIZABETH KUDADJIE-GYAMFI

Long Island University

Summary.—Decision-making researchers have shown that making optimal decisions is aided by the detection of information salient to the task. When the task involves random events, humans tend to perceive these events as contingent. In this study, outcomes were grouped together with choices to identify some of the conditions under which random events are correctly perceived. Of the two groups ($ns = 40$) only one was provided information regarding the relationship between choice and outcome. This provision did not improve the detection of the relationship between random events any more than direct contact with the underlying contingencies. Findings are discussed in terms of experiential contact with and sensitivity to underlying contingency.

A fundamental aspect of decision-making is correctly identifying the relations between one's choices and their outcomes. To predict an event correctly, one must first perceive the relationship between the antecedent of the event and the event itself. Also, correct detection of the relation between the event and its consequence will facilitate choice for the event (if the unfolding of the event is under one's control). Previous studies (Lander, 1997; Kimbrough, Wright, & Shea, 2001) have shown that it is possible to improve the saliency of such relationships so they are better perceived. Such improvements in saliency and subsequently in detection make decisions more optimal (Lander, 1997).

In a series of studies (Kudadjie-Gyamfi & Rachlin, 1996, 2002) choices and outcomes were grouped in triads per trial, i.e., groups of three choices and consequent outcomes, with an intertrial interval of 30 sec. Participants in this condition made more optimal choices than participants in control groups in which choices and outcomes were not grouped. Grouping the choices and outcomes into triads had the effect of imposing a pattern on choice behavior; this significantly improved the saliency of the dependent relationship between choice and outcome.

An important question based on these findings is whether individuals detect the random relationship between unrelated events when the events are presented in triads as mentioned above. Previous research has shown

---

[1]I am grateful to Howard Rachlin, a professor of psychology at SUNY Stony Brook, who provided mentoring and to William Guethlin, a microcomputer applications specialist, who wrote the computer program for the experiment. I am also grateful to the reviewers who provided helpful comments on the previous draft. Address correspondence to Elizabeth Kudadjie-Gyamfi, Department of Psychology, Long Island University, 1 University Plaza, Brooklyn, NY 11201 or e-mail (kudadjie@liu.edu).

that, when choices and outcomes are independent of one another, i.e., random, human subjects tend to perceive a nonrandom relation when there are long runs of choices and outcomes with symmetry (Lopes & Oden, 1987) or when such choice and outcome pairs are contiguous (Matute, 1994). This, in turn, leads to an increased likelihood of engagement in superstitious behavior (Hake & Hyman, 1953; Niness & Niness, 1998; Rudski, Lischner, & Albert, 1999).

Such behavior derives from the perception that at least two unrelated events have a nonrandom relationship (Pisacreta, 1998). For example, pigeons that engaged in terminal behavior before free reinforcements were received exhibited more of these behaviors, especially when such reinforcement was on a fixed time schedule (Skinner, 1948). Human athletes have been documented to engage in behaviors such as ice-bathing before a game, using lucky charms and repeating secret phrases under the belief that such acts improve performance (Bleak & Frederick, 1998). Conditions, such as absence of explicit instructions, richer schedules of reinforcements and accuracy of rules (Matute, 1994; Rudski, et al., 1999; Dixon, Hayes, & Aban, 2000) increase engagement in superstitious behavior. Also, when past behavior is allowed to influence predictions of later occurrences of random events, such random events are more likely to be perceived as nonrandom (Hake & Hyman, 1953), resulting in superstitious behavior.

However, factors such as feedback on one's performance and experience with random processes tend to reduce the formation of such nonrandom relations between events (Lopes & Oden, 1987). These factors may have this effect because they provide more accessible information about the nature of the relations. Yet, feedback and formal training have been shown to have less effect in everyday situations experienced outside the laboratory for the reason that the characteristics of randomness emphasized in the laboratory are unimportant in everyday life. The kind of experience that comes from role-playing (Resnick & Wilensky, 1998) and frequent interaction with random processes (Doerr, 2001) is more likely to transfer to real-life situations. It appears that grouping of trials in triads allows more frequent contact with the true and contingent nature of the relationship (Kudadjie-Gyamfi & Rachlin, 1996). Furthermore, behavior established without explicit instructions but with such triads is more sensitive to changes in the implicit contingencies than behavior generated by explicit rules (Kudadjie-Gyamfi & Rachlin, 2002). This suggests that, when individuals make experiential contact with nonexplicit underlying rules, they are more sensitive to subsequent changes in implicit rules. It is possible that experiential contact will enhance the detection of the random relationship between events in which explicit instructions are absent, i.e., situations that more closely mimic real-life events, thereby reducing superstitious behavior.

This study investigated whether instructions about the relationship between random choices and their outcomes would facilitate detection of the relationship better than experiential contact. In light of the above findings that individuals perceive random events as nonrandom and also that contingency-generated behavior (through experiential contact) is more resistant to change than rule-generated behavior (through instruction following), it was hypothesized that under random relation conditions, experiential contact with underlying contingencies would provide more information than explicit instructions, thereby facilitating detection. This study therefore seeks to extend the findings that experiential contact with underlying contingencies is more informative in decision-making than explicit rules (Kudadjie-Gyamfi & Rachlin, 2002) in situations in which contingencies are random.

To do this, a paradigm was instituted in which the outcomes of a participant's behavior were partly independent of the behavior. That is, a random relation was established between a participant's behavior and its supposed outcome. The questions of interest are (1) what kind of a relationship would be perceived between these two events when information is limited; (2) how would perception of a possible relationship between behavior and outcome affect subsequent choices; and (3) how would unsignaled changes in underlying contingencies be handled when a noncontingent relation holds between behavior (choice) and outcome?

Method

Participants

Eighty students (M age = 19.3 yr., SD = 3.8) enrolled in an undergraduate psychology course at the State University of New York at Stony Brook served as participants. Their participation was a course requirement and was in accordance with guidelines of the American Psychological Association. The participants were randomly divided into two groups of 40.

Material

The experimental conditions had been written as a computer program and installed on a computer to which was attached a small metal box, 7 × 8 × 5.5 inches. There were two buttons on the upper elevated side of this box.

Procedure

The procedure used here is a variation of that used by Kudadjie-Gyamfi and Rachlin (1996, 2002). Participants chose between a more favorable overall alternative (A) and a more favorable local alternative (B) by pressing one of two buttons. Each choice was followed by a delay and rewarded with a single point (the outcome). The alternatives differed only in the prereward delay after a choice had been made. When a total delay time of 650 sec. had elapsed, the experiment ended.

The prereward delay imposed after each choice followed these rules: The delay after choosing B was N sec.; that after choosing A was N+3 sec., where N equaled the number of B choices made by the participant in the previous 10 trials. Thus, if there were 5 B choices in the set of 10 prior choices (as was the case for each subject when the experiment began), the current delay after choosing B was 5 sec., while that after choosing A was 8 sec. Hence, a subject who chose B under these conditions would have chosen the less delayed reward (more favorable local choice) for the trial. However, the choice of B on that trial would increase N by 1 sec. for the next 10 trials. The gain of 3 sec. on that particular trial would be more than offset by the loss of 1 sec. on each of the next 10 trials, resulting in a net loss of 7 sec. for each B choice (except for the last few choices of the session).

In this experiment, the set of 10 previous trials was modified such that the first nine choices made by the participant were replaced with random choices made by the computer. Hence, the current outcome of a subject's choice was determined mostly by random choices made by the computer. Only the subject's *current choice* (which was subsequently replaced by the computer's random choice) was taken into account in determining prereward delay before point allocation (payout). Random selection by the computer was such that there were no more than four consecutive choices of the same alternative.

To parallel previous experiments, choice and outcomes were grouped in triads with an intertrial interval of 30 sec. This was done in order to impose a patterning effect, to improve saliency and to allow for the study of such an effect on noncontingent choice-outcome sets (Kudadjie-Gyamfi & Rachlin, 1996, 2002). Total delay time was maintained at 650 sec.

Also, a nonverbalized change in the underlying contingencies, introduced in a previous experiment, was maintained (Kudadjie-Gyamfi & Rachlin, 2002). The nonverbalized change in the underlying contingencies occurred halfway through the experiment and affected prereward delay in the following way: choice outcomes made after $t=325$ sec. no longer followed the prereward delay rules above. Instead, the delay was fixed at the number of As and Bs in the last 10 trials preceding time $t=325$. If at time $t=325$ sec. a participant had four As and six Bs in the previous set of 10 trials, the delay was fixed at 6 sec. for a choice of B and 9 sec. for a choice of A. Thus, the payout after time $t=325$ sec. was no longer contingent on the previous 10 trials for a given choice but was based on the previous 10 trials at time $t=325$ sec. Payout was fixed and the more optimal behavior would be exclusive choice of B.

There were two conditions, No Hint/random and Hint/random. In the No Hint/random condition, there were noncontingent outcomes as stated above and Instruction Sheet 1 (cf. Appendix, p. 1304) which provided no hints. In the Hint/random condition, there were noncontingent outcomes and instructions which provided information (hereafter referred to as a Hint) regarding the effect of *A* choices on outcomes for *B*. The following phrase replaced "Your job is to figure out the combination of left and right choices that will give you the highest point total and that will enable you to make the best use of the time" (cf. Appendix, p. 1304): "The left side button and the right side button will each give you the same amount when you press one of them. However, the rate at which you earn these points depends on your previous combination of left and right choices. As you will see, the left button is always faster than the right. But if you press the left button too much, the future rate for both buttons will decrease. Your job is to make a combination of right and left choices that will give you as fast a rate as possible overall." This provision was only partly accurate, since actually in the first 325 sec., the computer's choices were used to determine outcome in subsequent trials.

Participants faced the computer screen with easy access to the buttons and keyboard. On the computer screen was information about the delay time remaining, the number of points they had earned and the button they had just pressed. Each participant was tested individually and spent about 30 minutes on the experiment. All participants were asked to make a series of choices by pressing button *A* or button *B*. Each press added one point to a counter. At the end of the experiment participants were paid 10 cents for each point earned.

Results and Discussion

Table 1 shows mean total choices (which also reflect points) and percent *A* choices within the first block of 325 sec., before the instituted change in underlying contingencies, and within the second block after the change, respectively, for the two groups. A 50% choice of *A* indicates behavior based on a perception that neither *A* nor *B* affects choice outcome differently. A one-sample test was conducted to determine whether the behavior of either group resembled that of random behavior. In both blocks, group No Hint/random made choices in a nonrandom manner ($t_{39} = -2.81$, $p < .05$; $t_{39} = -4.24$, $p < .005$, two-tailed, respectively). The Hint/random group behaved randomly on Block 1 ($t_{39} = -1.001$, ns) but nonrandomly on Block 2 ($t_{39} = -4.88$, $p < .005$). Thus, under conditions in which information was derived mostly from experiential contact, participants tended to behave as though there was a contingent relationship.

A repeated-measures analysis of variance yielded nonsignificant differences between the two groups on type of instruction ($F_{1,78} = 1.57$, ns), but a significant difference within groups due to change in contingencies ($F_{1,78} =$

TABLE 1
Means and Standard Deviations of Choices Made in the
No Hint/random and Hint/random Groups

Group	"A" Choices (%)				Total Choices			
	Block 1		Block 2		Block 1		Block 2	
	M	SD	M	SD	M	SD	M	SD
No Hint/random	42	17*	31	28*	53.1	2.4	50.0	7.2
Hint/random	47	18†	38	17†	52.5	3.1	49.2	5.6

Note.—Statistical analysis was conducted only on percent A choices. Significant differences noted within each group between choices made before (Block 1) and after (Block 2) the nonsignaled and nonverbalized change in contingency. *$p<.05$. †$p<.005$.

25.33, $p<.005$). There were no interactions between change in contingencies and instructions ($F_{1,78}=0.01$, ns). Planned-comparison tests indicate that in each group, there were significantly fewer A choices after the nonsignaled and nonverbalized change in contingencies (No Hint/random: $t_{39}=2.98$; Hint/random: $t_{39}=4.86$, $p<.05$). In each case, this suggests sensitivity to the change in the experimental condition.

Participants in the Hint/random group appeared to be as sensitive to the nonverbalized changes as were participants in the No Hint/random group. Indeed, the participants in the Hint/random condition did not appear to be influenced differently by the hints and behaved as their counterparts in the No Hint condition who had to rely on only experiential contact with the underlying contingencies. This contrasts with expectations and also with findings that subjects follow rules regardless of accuracy and in spite of contrary contingencies (Newman, Buffington, & Hemmes, 1995; Dixon, *et al.*, 2000). If participants in the Hint/random group had followed rules regardless of accuracy (accuracy is detected only through experiencing the underlying contingencies), they would have chosen significantly more As in each block and disregarded the nonverbalized and nonsignaled change.

This raises the possibility that the Hint/random participants may have simply ignored the rules after testing them (they started with more A choices). Alternatively, participants in the No Hint/random condition may have generated self-rules (Vyse, 1991) that were similar to the rules provided to the Hint/random group (Dixon, *et al.*, 2000). (Anecdotal information obtained during debriefing suggested that, although self-rules were generated, they were not as specific as given in the hints.) These findings also suggest that perhaps in the presence of information which is only partly accurate, the imposition of a patterning effect in random conditions (in this instance, that provided by the presentation of choices and outcomes in groups of three in both conditions) may enhance sensitivity to the underlying contingencies, thus moderating the effect of the inaccurate rules (Kudadjie-Gyamfi & Rachlin, 2002). This possible effect needs to be explicitly and extensively tested.

Previous studies have shown that behavior patterns established by contingencies are more effective in maintaining self-control behavior than behavior established by instructions when unexpected changes are encountered (Catania, Matthews, & Shimoff, 1982, 1989, 1990; Hayes, Brownstein, Zettle, Rosenfarb, & Korn, 1986; Shimoff, Matthews, & Catania, 1986; Kudadjie-Gyamfi & Rachlin, 2002). However, this study suggests that this may not be the case for all events. Under the random conditions tested here, accuracy of the instructions may be significant in detecting such underlying contingencies. Perhaps, grouping choices and outcomes into triads provided all the information that was needed. Additional instruction then, regardless of accuracy, would be useless.

In summary, the above findings imply that under conditions in which participants had to rely on experience alone, they behaved as though a contingent relation was in effect. By relying on experience, they detected the instituted change in the underlying contingencies and changed their behavior accordingly, reflecting more optimal decision-making. Additional information (in this case, partly accurate) regarding the relations did not improve performance.

Further research is needed to examine the interactive effects of imposed patterning and nonrandom relations and to establish more specific conditions under which the saliency of choice-outcome relations may be enhanced to enable differentiation of random from nonrandom contingencies within the same paradigm. Furthermore, data on concurrent verbal behavior as participants engage in such nonverbal tasks may yield clues to the generation of self-rules about how random events affect each other. This would clarify how and when explicit rules and nonverbalized contingencies affect choice behavior.

Perhaps in this way, individuals with a tendency to impose a nonrandom relation on random events would be better equipped to make a finer differentiation and well-informed decisions.

REFERENCES

BLEAK, J. L., & FREDERICK, C. M. (1998) Superstitious behavior in sports: levels of effectiveness and determinants of use in three collegiate sports. *Journal of Sport Behavior*, 21, 1-15.

CATANIA, A. C., MATTHEWS, B. A., & SHIMOFF, E. (1982) Instructed versus shaped human verbal behavior: interactions with non-verbal responding. *Journal of the Experimental Analysis of Behavior*, 38, 233-248.

CATANIA, A. C., MATTHEWS, B. A., & SHIMOFF, E. (1989) An experimental analysis of rule-governed behavior. In S. C. Hayes (Ed.), *Rule-governed behavior: cognition, contingencies, and instructional control.* New York: Plenum. Pp. 119-150.

CATANIA, A. C., MATTHEWS, B. A., & SHIMOFF, E. (1990) Properties of rule-governed behavior and their implications. In D. E. Blackman & H. Lejeune (Eds.), *Behavior and analysis in theory and practice.* London, UK: Erlbaum. Pp. 215-230.

DIXON, M. R., HAYES, L. R., & ABAN, I. B. (2000) Examining the roles of rule following, reinforcement, and preexperimental histories on risk-taking behavior. *The Psychological Record*, 50, 687-704.

DOERR, H. M. (2001) How can I find a pattern in this random data? The convergence of multiplicative and probabilistic reasoning. *Journal of Mathematical Behavior*, 18, 431-454.

HAKE, W., & HYMAN, R. (1953) Perception of the statistical structure of a random series of binary symbols. *Journal of Experimental Psychology*, 45, 64-74.

HAYES, S. C., BROWNSTEIN, A. J., ZETTLE, R. D., ROSENFARB, I., & KORN, Z. (1986) Rule-governed behavior and sensitivity to changing consequences of responding. *Journal of the Experimental Analysis of Behavior*, 45, 237-256.

KIMBROUGH, S. K., WRIGHT, D. L., & SHEA, C. H. (2001) Reducing the saliency of intentional stimuli results in greater contextual-dependent performance. *Memory*, 9, 133-143.

KUDADJIE-GYAMFI, E., & RACHLIN, H. (1996) Temporal patterning in choice among delayed outcomes. *Organizational Behavior and Human Decision Processes*, 65, 61-67.

KUDADJIE-GYAMFI, E., & RACHLIN, H. (2002) Rule-governed versus contingency-governed behavior in self-control task: effects of changes in contingencies. *Behavioural Processes*, 57, 29-35.

LANDER, J. (1997) Strategies to improve clinical judgments about pain. *Perceptual and Motor Skills*, 84, 573-574.

LOPES, L. L., & ODEN, G. C. (1987) Distinguishing between random and nonrandom events. *Journal of Experimental Psychology*, 13, 392-400.

MATUTE, H. (1994) Learned helplessness and superstitious behavior as opposite effects of uncontrollable reinforcement in humans. *Learning and Motivation*, 25, 216-232.

NEWMAN, B., BUFFINGTON, D. M., & HEMMES, N. S. (1995) The effects of schedules of reinforcement on instruction following. *The Psychological Record*, 45, 463-476.

NINESS, H. A. C., & NINESS, S. A. (1998) Superstitious math performance: interactions between rules and schedules contingencies. *The Psychological Record*, 48, 45-62.

PISACRETA, R. (1998) Superstitious behavior and response stereotypy prevent the emergence of efficient rule-governed behavior in humans. *The Psychological Record*, 48, 251-274.

RESNICK, M., & WILENSKY, U. (1998) Diving into complexity: developing probabilistic decentralized thinking through role-playing activities. *Journal of the Learning Sciences*, 7, 153-172.

RUDSKI, J. M., LISCHNER, M. I., & ALBERT, L. M. (1999) Superstitious rule generation is affected by probability and type of outcome. *The Psychological Record*, 49, 245-260.

SHIMOFF, E., MATTHEWS, B. A., & CATANIA, A. C. (1986) Human operant: sensitivity and pseudosensitivity to contingencies. *Journal of the Experimental Analysis of Behavior*, 46, 149-157.

SKINNER, B. F. (1948) Superstition in the pigeon. *Journal of Experimental Psychology*, 38, 168-172.

VYSE, S. A. (1991) Behavioral variability and rule generation: general, restricted, and superstitious contingency statements. *The Psychological Record*, 41, 487-506.

Accepted April 14, 2004.

APPENDIX

Instruction Sheet 1

Hi! Welcome to the 'dime-a-point' game. Today we would like you to play our computer game and earn some money.

The way to make money is to get as many points as possible in our game. You have 650 sec. within which to do this. A 'dime-a-point' is how much we'll pay you when you are through. It may not sound like much, but an expert can make as many as 100 points and can win up to $10.00 in a short time.

The rules of the game are easy. On the computer screen in front of you is a sample game set up with 10 choices for you to make. Read the rest of the instructions, and then you can practice on this sample game. All of your choices will be made with the button box attached to the computer. The left side button is one alternative and the right side button is the other.

You can see that there is one box in the middle of the screen labeled 'choice'. Any choice that you make during the session will count towards your final total. The nice thing about our game is that, at any period in the experiment, you are informed of the total number of points you have made. The left side button and the right side button will each give you the same amounts when you press one of them.

Also on the screen is a timer indicating at any time how much time you have left within which to make your points. Your job is to figure out the combination of left and right choices that will give you the highest point total and that will enable you to make the best use of the time.

After you are done with the practice game, follow the instructions on the screen, and you will play for real, making as many choices as you can within the time indicated on the screen.

If you have any questions about these instructions or how to use the button box, please ask the experimenter.

SLEEP DEPRIVATION AND HEMISPHERIC ASYMMETRY FOR FACIAL RECOGNITION REACTION TIME AND ACCURACY [1]

STÅLE PALLESEN, BJØRN HELGE JOHNSEN

Department of Psychosocial Science
University of Bergen
Royal Norwegian Naval Academy

ANITA HANSEN, JARLE EID

Royal Norwegian Naval Academy

JULIAN F. THAYER

National Institute on Aging
Baltimore, Maryland, USA

TROND OLSEN

Royal Norwegian Naval Academy

KENNETH HUGDAHL

Department of Biological and Medical Psychology
University of Bergen

Summary.—We investigated the processing of emotional stimuli during a non-sleep-deprived state and following sleep deprivation in 36 right-handed men. Using the visual half-field technique, cartoon line drawings of emotional facial expressions were flashed on a computer screen for 250 msec. The participants were instructed to remember the content of the picture seen and to recognize it among nine alternatives shown immediately after the display of a single picture. Compared to the nondeprived condition, response latencies increased and accuracy decreased in sleep deprivation. Moreover, response latencies indicated that the performance of the right hemisphere deteriorated more following sleep deprivation than did the performance of the left hemisphere. The results also showed that hemispheric preference (for response latencies and response accuracy) tended to favour the left hemisphere when the participants were tested during sleep deprivation.

Sleep deprivation has consistently been associated with impairments in human performance (Pilcher & Huffcutt, 1996), and lack of adequate sleep has even been assumed to be responsible for catastrophic accidents like the Three Mile Island incident (Mitler, Carskadon, Czeisler, Dement, Dinges, & Graeber, 1988). Sleep deprivation in general impairs performance on a wide range of cognitive tasks and sensory functions such as mental arithmetic, selective attention, divergent thinking, logical reasoning, memory, reaction time, and vigilance (Williams, Lubin, & Goodnow, 1959; Donnell, 1969; Hockey, 1970; Opstad, Ekanger, Nummestad, & Raabe, 1978; Haslam, 1985; Horne, 1988; Jha, 1988; Smith & Maben, 1993; Blagrove, Alexander, & Horne, 1995; Harrison & Horne, 2000; Blagrove & Akehurst, 2001). Studies have also demonstrated that metacognition is negatively influenced by sleep deprivation (Blagrove & Akehurst, 2000). Lately, research has also demon-

---

[1]Address correspondence to Ståle Pallesen, Ph.D., Department of Psychosocial Science, University of Bergen, Christiesgt. 12, 5015 Bergen, Norway or e-mail (staale.pallesen@psysp. uib.no).

strated that tasks dependent on the prefrontal cortex are particularly sensitive to loss of sleep (Harrison, Horne, & Rothwell, 2000), providing a neuroanatomical localization of the impairments. Research studies of hemispheric asymmetry have indicated reduced right hemispheric arousal during sleep deprivation (Johnsen, Laberg, Eid, & Brun, 1999; Kim, Lee, Kim, Park, Go, Kim, Lee, Chae, & Lee, 2001; Johnsen, Laberg, Eid, & Hugdahl, 2002), pointing to possible effects on emotional functioning (Murray, 1965; Pilcher & Huffcutt, 1996). Because the right hemisphere is assumed to be superior in recognizing facial emotional expressions (Milner, 1974; Etcoff, 1989; Tucker & Frederick, 1989), impaired processing of facial expression during sleep deprivation could be indicated by reduced right hemispheric arousal during sleep deprivation.

We studied the effects of sleep deprivation on perception of facial emotional expressions. If sleep deprivation causes detrimental effects on recognition for facial expressions, longer reaction times and lower performance would be expected during a sleep-deprived condition as compared to a nonsleep-deprived condition. The second aim of this study was to explore whether sleep deprivation affects hemispheric function differentially. It was expected that right hemisphere function would be more impaired by the sleep deprivation than the left hemisphere's function. For this reason, we presented the pictures of facial emotional expressions either in the right or left visual half-field, a technique ensuring unilateral hemispheric stimulus presentation.

METHOD

Participants

The initial sample consisted of 59 male volunteers, all students at the Royal Norwegian Naval Academy. Eight volunteers were excluded due to technical problems with the equipment, and eight participants were excluded because they were left-handed on a questionnaire. Also, seven subjects were excluded because, during the nonsleep-deprived condition, they reacted faster to the pictures presented on right visual half-field than to the pictures on the left visual half-field. This was done to ensure that the included subjects constituted a homogeneous group as facial expressions presented in the right visual half-field (which travel to the left hemisphere) are assumed to be processed slower than facial expressions presented in the left visual half-field (which travel to the right hemisphere) in subjects with normal hemispheric dominance for facial recognition. Hence, the final sample constituted 36 right-handed men (M age = 25.6 yr., SD = 4.0, range = 20.6–37.6 years) who during the nonsleep-deprived state demonstrated right hemispheric processing superiority according to reaction times.

Materials

Computer task.—The stimuli were nine different facial expressions as cartoon line-drawings (see Fig. 1). Facial expressions varied on two dimensions: eyebrow position (pointing upwards, horizontal or downwards) and lip direction: (pointing upwards, horizontal or downwards; see Hugdahl,

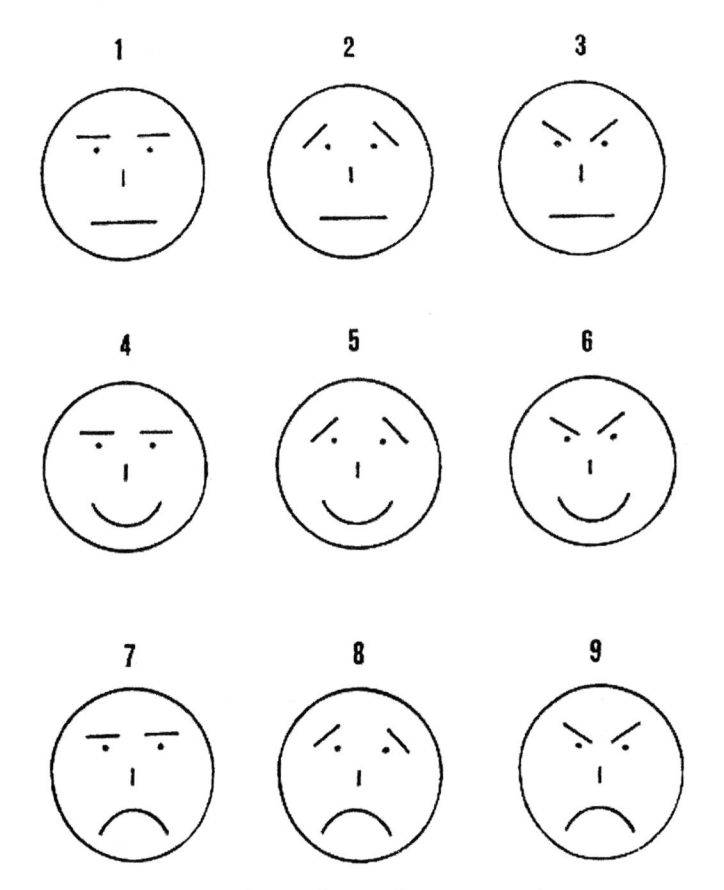

FIG. 1. The nine faces in the computer task

Iversen, & Johnsen, 1993). With this simple manipulation of the eyebrow and lip line positions, it is possible to create nine different facial expressions, including negative, positive, neutral and ambivalent emotions. Each cartoon (4.0 × 4.5 cm) was presented for 250 msec. using the visual half-field technique. This technique allows unilateral stimulation of one hemisphere (McKeever, 1986). Eyes are fixated on a point in the middle of the visual field while visual stimuli are briefly flashed either to the right or left of the midpoint fixation, in this case 3.5 cm to the left or right from the fixation point. This technique ensures that only the contralateral hemisphere initially is stimulated, provided that the stimulus duration is sufficiently brief to prevent eye movement (≤ 250 msec.). The cartoons were presented in black and white on a computer screen (23 × 17.5 cm), and the whole experiment was controlled by a computer program written on the MEL-2 programming platform (Schneider, 1988). After each cartoon presentation, a new picture (9.0 × 11 cm) presented in the middle of the screen immediately emerged, containing all the nine facial expressions, numbered from 1 to 9. The picture with nine faces stayed on for 3000 msec. or until a response was made. The participant's task was to identify from the nine facial expressions, as fast as possible, the specific facial expression that was flashed on the previous trial, then press the corresponding response key on the computer keyboard. The vertical viewing angle was 90°, and the subjects were seated in a distance of 50 cm from the computer screen. Reaction time and response accuracy were the main dependent variables. In all, there were 54 trials, with the different facial expressions presented in a randomized order. Of the 54 trials, 27 were presented in the left visual half-field, and 27 trials were presented in the right visual half-field.

Stanford Sleepiness Scale.—The Stanford Sleepiness Scale is a one-item scale, where the participant is instructed to rate the current degree of sleepiness on a 7-point scale ranging from 1 = Feeling active, vital, alert or wide awake to 7 = No longer fighting sleep, sleep onset soon, having dream-like thoughts. Higher scores indicate greater sleepiness (Hoddes, Zarcone, Smythe, Phillips, & Dement, 1973). The scale is widely used as a state measure of subjective sleepiness and it has consistently been shown to be sensitive to acute sleep deprivation (Mitler, Carskadon, & Hirshkowitz, 2000), although scores do not always correlate with objective measures of sleepiness such as the Multiple Sleep Latency Test and pupillography (Danker-Hopfe, Kraemer, Dorn, Schmidt, Ehlert, & Herrmann, 2001).

Handedness questionnaire.—This had 17 items related to manual preference, on which the respondent indicates the preferred hand from common manual items like writing, drawing, use of tooth brush, scissors, etc. The responses to the items in the questionnaire have been validated against actual performance of individual performance tests (Raczkowski, Kalat, & Nebes, 1974). The handedness questionnaire was completed by the participants in the nonsleep-deprived condition. The criterion for inclusion in the experiment was at least 11 out of 17 item responses with right-hand scores.

Design and Procedure

All 36 participants were tested twice. Both testing occasions (computer task and Stanford Sleepiness Scale) took place between 10 a.m. and 12 noon under similar testing conditions. Half of the participants were tested first during sleep deprivation, which took place during a military exercise at the Royal Norwegian Naval Academy lasting 5 days, then under a nonsleep-deprived condition. A counterbalanced design was employed in which the order of presentation was reversed for the other half of the participants. The nonsleep-deprived testing took place one day after termination of the sleep-deprivation period, following one recovery night where the subjects were free to sleep for at least 12 hours for half of the participants, and two days before the sleep-deprivation period for the other half. The sleep-deprivation condition included sleep deprivation of 72 to 120 hours. After completion of the exercise, the participants estimated the total sleep obtained (M duration = 4 hr., 18 min., SD = 1 hr., 47 min., range = 1 hr., 30 min. to 8 hours). These self-reports were validated against observation by external raters who followed each platoon during the exercise and rated the amount of sleep each participant obtained. They estimated the mean duration of the participant's sleep during the same period to be 5 hr., 6 min. (range = 3 to 7 hours).

Statistical Analysis

The data were analyzed using the STATISTICA software, Version 6.0 (StatSoft, Inc., 2001). A 2 × 2 analysis of variance design was employed in the data analysis for the computer test. The first factor, State, had two levels, nonsleep-deprived and sleep-deprived. The second factor, Half-field, had two levels, left visual half-field and right visual half-field. Fisher exact probability test was used to detect changes in hemispheric processing superiority between the sleep-deprived and nonsleep-deprived states.

Results

The results from the Stanford Sleepiness Scale showed a higher score during the sleep-deprived condition than during the nonsleep-deprived condition (t_{35} = 9.21, p < .01). Mean scores during sleep deprivation were 4.06 and 1.53 in the nonsleep-deprived condition. The analysis of reaction times showed a main effect of State ($F_{1,35}$ = 6.70, p < .02) indicating overall longer reaction times in the sleep-deprived compared to the nonsleep-deprived condition (see Table 1). A significant main effect of Half-field was also observed ($F_{1,35}$ = 64.02, p < .001), reflecting longer reaction times for stimuli presented in the right compared to the left visual half-field. A significant interaction (State × Half-field) was also observed ($F_{1,35}$ = 8.71, p < .01), reflecting that mean reaction time to stimuli targeted in the left visual half-field during sleep deprivation compared to the nonsleep-deprived condition was relatively longer than the mean reaction time for the right visual half-field. All 36 participants showed faster responses for the right hemisphere during the nonsleep-deprived state, while 11 showed faster reaction time for the left

TABLE 1
Mean Reaction Times (msec.) and Standard Deviations on Computer Task During Nonsleep-deprived State and Sleep Deprivation

	Right Visual Half-field		Left Visual Half-field	
	M	SD	M	SD
Nonsleep-deprived	3189	573	2838	527
Sleep-deprived	3320	517	3162	581

hemisphere during sleep deprivation. According to Fisher's exact probability test, this difference was statistically significant (Fisher, $p < .001$).

For response accuracy (number of correctly identified facial expressions), a main effect of State was observed ($F_{1,35} = 16.7$, $p < .01$), reflecting higher accuracy during the nonsleep-deprived state than during sleep deprivation (see Table 2). However, the main effect of Half-field and the interaction effect (State × Half-field) were not statistically significant. In terms of accuracy, 21 participants showed a right hemisphere and seven participants showed a left hemisphere preference, while eight participants did not show any preference during the nonsleep-deprived state. The corresponding numbers for the sleep-deprived state were 12, 18 and 6, respectively. According to Fisher's exact probability test, this difference was statistically significant (Fisher, $p < .003$).

TABLE 2
Mean Response Accuracy Scores and Standard Deviations on Computer Task During Nonsleep-deprived State and Sleep Deprivation

	Right Visual Half-field		Left Visual Half-field	
	M	SD	M	SD
Nonsleep-deprived	24.36	2.60	23.78	2.29
Sleep-deprived	22.58	3.24	22.17	3.43

Discussion

The results showed that the scores on the Stanford Sleepiness Scale were significantly higher during sleep deprivation. This finding indicates that the participants experienced more subjective sleepiness when tested during sleep deprivation, validating the experimental manipulation.

In general, the reaction times were longer during sleep deprivation than in the nonsleep-deprived state. This finding is supported by previous studies showing that reaction time increases as a function of sleep loss (Koslowsky & Babkoff, 1992) and is generally in line with the lapse hypothesis. According to this hypothesis, sleep deprivation causes lapses (periods where the subject is nonresponsive). With length of sleep deprivation, the lapses increase in frequency and duration, during which microsleep is assumed to occur (Williams, *et al.*, 1959). Our finding is also compatible with the view of Kjellberg (1977), who suggested that sleep deprivation, in addition to lapses, causes a general deterioration of all reaction times.

A significant main effect of half-field was also observed, reflecting longer reaction time for stimuli presented in the right compared to the left visual half-field. As visual stimuli presented in the left visual half-field travel to the right hemisphere and stimuli presented in the right visual half-field travel to the left hemisphere, the findings are in line with the assumption that the right hemisphere is quicker in processing facial expressions (Etcoff, 1989).

Furthermore, we found that reaction times for the left visual half-field during sleep deprivation compared to the nonsleep-deprived condition were relatively longer than corresponding reaction times for the right visual half-field. Also, all 36 participants showed a right hemisphere preference in the nonsleep-deprived state in terms of reaction time, while 11 of these changed to a left hemisphere preference in the sleep-deprived state. This may indicate that the right hemisphere was more negatively influenced by sleep deprivation than the left hemisphere.

Analyzing the data based on response accuracy showed that accuracy was higher in the nonsleep-deprived state compared to the sleep-deprived state. This finding was expected, as several previous studies have shown deterioration of performance during sleep deprivation (Pilcher & Huffcutt, 1996). In contrast to the results for reaction time, no significant interaction (State × Half-field) effect was found for response accuracy. However, relatively more participants showed preference for stimuli presented in the right visual half-field during the sleep-deprived state in terms of accuracy compared to the nonsleep-deprived state. Thus, there seems to be some manifestation of hemispheric effect of sleep deprivation in terms of performance accuracy.

One explanation for the findings may be that, during sleep deprivation, participants may change their hemispheric mode of processing the stimuli from a visuospatial/emotional mode to a verbal mode, e.g., the left face in row one in Fig. 1 could be coded as "eyebrows horizontal, lip downwards." Thus, an advantage of left hemisphere over the right hemisphere could be expected in the sleep-deprived state (Bryden, 1982). Our findings are consistent overall with the hypothesis that sleep deprivation particularly causes impairments in right hemisphere function. Still, it is not clear why the capacity of the right hemisphere would be more negatively affected by sleep deprivation than the left. It may be speculated that it is the consequence of a change in alertness or arousal which involves the noradrenergic pathways. These pathways are more strongly lateralized to the right than the left hemisphere (Posner & Petersen, 1990). Studies have shown reduced sensitivity to norepinephrine after prolonged release, as in a state of lengthened arousal.

Because the locus coeruleus, from which the noradrenergic pathways project, is inactive during rapid eye movement (REM) sleep, it is suggested that REM sleep helps restore the brain's sensitivity to norepinephrine and the ability to keep us alert (Steriade & McCarley, 1990). Thus, according to this line of reasoning, we would expect the right hemisphere to be more negatively affected by sleep deprivation. The findings could also be interpreted in terms of the white matter hypothesis for nonverbal learning disabilities. According to this hypothesis, the functions of the right hemisphere are more dependent upon intact and functional association and projection fibres within the hemisphere than the functions of the left hemisphere (Rourke, 1995). Hence, if sleep deprivation causes dysfunction in the white matter of the brain, the right hemisphere would be expected to be more negatively affected than the left hemisphere, and our data are compatible with such a presumption. The negative effects of sleep deprivation may also be indicative of a temporary and reversible state of neglect. The neglect phenomenon is normally due to damage to the right hemisphere and causes the person to neglect information presented contralaterally to the side of the damage (Jeannerod, 1987).

When it comes to limitations of the present study, it should be noted that the subjects who might process visuospatial information in the left cerebral hemisphere were deselected. Thus, the results of this investigation might, therefore, not generalize to such individuals. Another potential limitation is that half of the subjects were tested in the nonsleep-deprived condition after just one recovery night following the sleep-deprivation period. This may represent a problem as studies have shown that recovery from sleep deprivation may take several days (Bonnet, 2000). Thus, the subjects tested in the nonsleep-deprived state following the recovery night might still have been under the influence of sleep deprivation. However, we will argue that this fact actually worked in favour of the conclusions drawn from this study, as this implies that the lateralization effect was obtained with a relatively small one-night manipulation (one recovery night) for half of the participating subjects.

We suggest that the issue of the lateralized effects of sleep deprivation should be pursued in subsequent studies, which should include more varied kinds of tasks. Such studies should also aim to explore how long a sleep-deprivation period has to last for asymmetric hemispheric effects to become manifest. Research should also aim at identifying possible factors mediating the lateralized effects of sleep deprivation, e.g., age, personality, etc. Studies using functional magnetic resonance imaging (fMRI) and other brain-imaging techniques should also be conducted to investigate the issue of hemispheric asymmetric responses to sleep deprivation.

REFERENCES

Blagrove, M., & Akehurst, L. (2000) Effects of sleep loss on confidence-accuracy relationships for reasoning and eyewitness memory. *Journal of Experimental Psychology: Applied*, 6, 59-73.

Blagrove, M., & Akehurst, L. (2001) Personality and the modulation of effects of sleep loss on mood and cognition. *Personality and Individual Differences*, 30, 819-828.

Blagrove, M., Alexander, C., & Horne, J. A. (1995) The effects of chronic sleep reduction on the performance of cognitive tasks sensitive to sleep deprivation. *Applied Cognitive Psychology*, 9, 21-40.

Bonnet, M. H. (2000) Sleep deprivation. In M. H. Kryger, T. Roth, & W. C. Dement (Eds.), *Principles and practice of sleep medicine*. (3rd ed.) Philadelphia, PA: Saunders. Pp. 53-71.

Bryden, M. P. (1982) *Laterality: functional asymmetry in the intact brain*. New York: Academic Press.

Danker-Hopfe, H., Kraemer, S., Dorn, H., Schmidt, A., Ehlert, I., & Herrmann, W. M. (2001) Time-of-day variations in different measures of sleepiness (MSLT, pupillography, and SSS) and their interrelations. *Psychophysiology*, 38, 828-835.

Donnell, J. M. (1969) Performance decrement as a function of total sleep loss and task duration. *Perceptual and Motor Skills*, 29, 711-714.

Etcoff, N. L. (1989) Asymmetries in recognition of emotion. In F. Boller & J. Grafman (Eds.), *Handbook of neuropsychology: 3*. Amsterdam: Elsevier. Pp. 363-402.

Harrison, Y., & Horne, J. A. (2000) Sleep loss and temporal memory. *The Quarterly Journal of Experimental Psychology*, 53A, 271-279.

Harrison, Y., Horne, J. A., & Rothwell, A. (2000) Prefrontal neuropsychological effects of sleep deprivation in young adults: a model for healthy aging? *Sleep*, 23, 1067-1073.

Haslam, D. R. (1985) Sustained operations and military performance. *Behavior Research Methods, Instruments, & Computers*, 17, 90-95.

Hockey, G. R. (1970) Changes in attention allocation in a multi-component task under loss of sleep. *British Journal of Psychology*, 61, 473-480.

Hoddes, E., Zarcone, V., Smythe, H., Phillips, R., & Dement, W. C. (1973) Quantification of sleepiness: a new approach. *Psychophysiology*, 10, 431-436.

Horne, J. A. (1988) Sleep loss and "divergent" thinking ability. *Sleep*, 11, 528-536.

Hugdahl, K., Iversen, P. M., & Johnsen, B. H. (1993) Laterality for facial expressions: does the sex of the subject interact with the sex of the stimulus face? *Cortex*, 29, 325-331.

Jeannerod, M. (Ed.) (1987) *Neurophysiological and neuropsychological aspects of spatial neglect*. Amsterdam: North Holland.

Jha, S. S. (1988) Personality and vigilance during sleep deprivation. *Indian Psychologist*, 5, 49-54.

Johnsen, B. H., Laberg, J. C., Eid, J., & Brun, W. (1999) Sleep deprivation: effects on the right hemisphere of the brain. In P. Napoli, S. Cardini, & F. Russo (Eds.), *35 Simposio internazionale di psicologia militare applicata*. Firenze: Ministero della Difesa. Pp. 167-171.

Johnsen, B. H., Laberg, J. C., Eid, J., & Hugdahl, K. (2002) Dichotic listening and sleep deprivation: vigilance effects. *Scandinavian Journal of Psychology*, 43, 413-418.

Kim, D-J., Lee, H-P., Kim, M. S., Park, Y-J., Go, H-J., Kim, K-S., Lee, S-P., Chae, J-H., & Lee, C. T. (2001) The effect of total sleep deprivation on cognitive functions in normal adult male subjects. *International Journal of Neuroscience*, 109, 127-137.

Kjellberg, A. (1977) Sleep deprivation and some aspects of performance: II. Lapses and other attentional effects. *Waking and Sleeping*, 1, 145-148.

Koslowsky, M., & Babkoff, H. (1992) Meta-analysis of the relationship between total sleep deprivation and performance. *Chronobiology International*, 9, 132-136.

McKeever, W. F. (1986) Tachistoscopic methods in neuropsychology. In J. F. Hannay (Ed.), *Experimental techniques in human neuropsychology*. New York: Oxford Univer. Press. Pp. 167-211.

Milner, B. (1974) Hemispheric specialization: scope and limits. In F. O. Schmitt & F. G. Wordens (Eds.), *The neurosciences: third study program*. Cambridge, MA: MIT Press. Pp. 75-89.

Mitler, M. M., Carskadon, M. A., Czeisler, C. A., Dement, W. C., Dinges, D. F., & Graeber, R. C. (1988) Catastrophes, sleep, and public policy: consensus report. *Sleep*, 11, 100-109.

MITLER, M. M., CARSKADON, M. A., & HIRSHKOWITZ, M. (2000) Evaluating sleepiness. In M. E. Kryger, T. Roth, & W. C. Dement (Eds.), *Principles and practice of sleep medicine*. (3rd ed.) Philadelphia, PA: Saunders. Pp. 1251-1257.

MURRAY, E. J. (1965) *Sleep, dreams, and arousal*. New York: Appleton-Century-Crofts.

OPSTAD, P. K., EKANGER, R., NUMMESTAD, M., & RAABE, N. (1978) Performance, mood, and clinical symptoms in men exposed to prolonged, severe physical work and sleep deprivation. *Aviation, Space, and Environmental Medicine*, 49, 1065-1073.

PILCHER, J. J., & HUFFCUTT, A. I. (1996) Effects of sleep deprivation of performance: a meta-analysis. *Sleep*, 19, 318-326.

POSNER, M. I., & PETERSEN, S. E. (1990) The attention system of the human brain. *Annual Review of Neuroscience*, 13, 25-42.

RACZKOWSKI, D., KALAT, J. W., & NEBES, R. D. (1974) Reliability and validity of some handedness questionnaires. *Neuropsychologia*, 12, 43-47.

ROURKE, B. P. (Ed.) (1995) *Syndrome of nonverbal learning disabilities: neurodevelopmental manifestations*. New York: Guilford.

SCHNEIDER, W. (1988) Micro-experimental laboratory: an integrated system for IBM PC compatibles. *Behavior Research Methods, Instruments, & Computers*, 20, 643-661.

SMITH, A., & MABEN, A. (1993) Effects of sleep deprivation, lunch, and personality on performance, mood, and cardiovascular function. *Physiology and Behavior*, 54, 967-972.

STATSOFT, INC. (2001) STATISTICA for Windows, Version 6.0. [Computer program manual] Tulsa, OK: StatSoft, Inc.

STERIADE, M., & MCCARLEY, R. W. (1990) *Brainstem control of wakefulness and sleep*. New York: Plenum.

TUCKER, D. M., & FREDERICK, S. L. (1989) Emotion and brain lateralization. In H. Wagner & A. Manstead (Eds.), *Handbook of social psychophysiology*. Chichester, UK: Wiley. Pp. 27-70.

WILLIAMS, H. L., LUBIN, A., & GOODNOW, J. J. (1959) Impaired performance with acute sleep loss. *Psychological Monographs*, 73 (Whole No. 484).

Accepted April 14, 2004.

CANCEL AND RETHINK IN THE WASON SELECTION TASK: FURTHER EVIDENCE FOR THE HEURISTIC-ANALYTIC DUAL PROCESS THEORY [1]

KAZUSHIGE WADA

Osaka University

HIROSHI NITTONO

Hiroshima University, Higashi-Hiroshima

Summary.—The reasoning process in the Wason selection task was examined by measuring card inspection times in the letter-number and drinking-age problems. 24 students were asked to solve the problems presented on a computer screen. Only the card touched with a mouse pointer was visible, and the total exposure time of each card was measured. Participants were allowed to cancel their previous selections at any time. Although rethinking was encouraged, the cards once selected were rarely cancelled (10% of the total selections). Moreover, most of the cancelled cards were reselected (89% of the total cancellations). Consistent with previous findings, inspection times were longer for selected cards than for nonselected cards. These results suggest that card selections are determined largely by initial heuristic processes and rarely reversed by subsequent analytic processes. The present study gives further support for the heuristic-analytic dual process theory.

The Wason selection task has been an important investigative tool to assess conditional reasoning (Wason, 1966; Evans, 1998b; Roberts & Newton, 2001). In the original letter-number problem, four cards, each with a number on one side and a letter on the other side, were presented with a conditional rule, "if there is a vowel on one side of the card, then there is an even number on the other side," which has the form "if p then q." The four cards show "A" (p card; true antecedent), "D" (not-p card; false antecedent), "4" (q card; true consequent), and "7" (not-q-card; false consequent). The participants' task is to select the card(s) they must turn over to determine whether the rule is true or false. Logically, participants should select the p and not-q cards. However, in this task, people tend to select the p and q cards or only the p card. Typically, less than 10% of participants make the logical response (Wason, 1966).

Although the tendency toward illogical responses is quite robust, it remains unclear what conscious or unconscious processes people use to reach the final decision in the selection task. Evans has proposed the *heuristic-analytic theory*, which suggests that reasoning is a dual process (Evans, 1984, 1995, 1996; Evans & Over, 1996). According to Evans, heuristic processes are preconscious (or implicit) processes focusing attention on relevant parts

---

[1]Address correspondence to Kazushige Wada, Department of General Psychology, Faculty of Human Sciences, Osaka University, 1-2 Yamadaoka, Suita 565-0871, JAPAN or e-mail (wada@hus.osaka-u.ac.jp).

of a problem, whereas analytic processes are conscious (or explicit) processes dealing only with the information obtained through the heuristic processes. For the selection task, Evans (1996, 1998a; Evans & Over, 1996) suggested that heuristic processes led a person to illogical responses, and analytic processes only rationalized the selection of cards made in heuristic processes. In a series of experiments by Evans (1996), participants were asked to solve a computer-presented version of the selection task. The four cards were presented simultaneously on a computer screen. Participants were required to touch a card with a mouse pointer while they were thinking about the card and to click on the card when they decided to select it. The total duration that the pointer was on each card was calculated cumulatively and termed *inspection time*. Evans assumed that, if participants additionally applied analytic processes to the cards selected by heuristic processes, inspection times would be longer for selected than for nonselected cards, regardless of card contents (true antecedent, false antecedent, true consequent, and false consequent). Conversely, if there were only one stage (either heuristic or analytic), no systematic differences in inspection time would be expected among the cards. The results showed that inspection times were longer for selected than for nonselected cards and appeared to support the heuristic-analytic dual process theory.

Roberts (1998a, 1998b) questioned the validity of the mouse-pointing methodology of Evans (1996) as a source of evidence for initial heuristic processes. In Evans' experiments (1996), all cards were visible at the same time and the click was required only for selections. Roberts (1998b) and Roberts and Newton (2001) pointed out two potential problems in this procedure. First, participants may forget to move the mouse pointer on a thinking card because all cards were visible all the time even without pointing. Second, participants may pause before making an active decision, i.e., selecting a card by a mouse click. The latter possibility could lead to the bias toward longer inspection times for selected cards, although irrelevant to the reasoning processes. Roberts (1998b) examined these two possibilities in a series of experiments. After replicating the findings of Evans (1996) using the original procedure (Exp. 1), the task was modified so that only the card pointed to was visible (Exp. 2) or so that an active response was required both for selection and for nonselection (Exp. 3). Both experiments produced results similar to that of Evans (1996) in that inspection times were longer for selected than for nonselected cards, although the effect size was reduced. However, when both modifications were applied at the same time, inspection times did not differ between selected and nonselected cards (Exp. 4). Moreover, when participants were asked to "deselect" the cards that were not necessarily turned over, the relationship between selection and inspection time was reversed (Exp. 5). Roberts (1998b) concluded that the effect of inspection time reported by Evans (1996) was based on an artifact and did not provide satisfactory evidence for the existence of initial heuristic processes. In a recent study, however, Roberts and Newton (2001) used a new task called "change" task to dissociate card selection from the act of response. They found that the relationship between card selection and inspection time occurred independently of the relationship between the act of response and inspection time. Furthermore, they suggested that, when rapid responses were required, participants tended to select the cards matching the rule. These data were generally consistent with the heuristic-analytic framework.

In the present study, we examined the reasoning process in the selection task from a different point of view. None of the previous studies using an inspection-time measure allowed participants to cancel their selections. This irreversibleness may lead to longer inspection times for selected cards because inspection times are affected by the tendency to hesitate before making a final response (Roberts, 1998b; Roberts & Newton, 2001). In the present study, we allowed participants to cancel their previous selections at any time and encouraged them to think for as long as they wished. According to the heuristic-analytic dual process theory, three predictions can be made. First, if card selection is determined by initial heuristic processes, the cards once selected will be rarely cancelled even when the participants are encouraged to rethink. Second, if the analytic processes only rationalize the initial heuristic selection, cancelled cards will tend to be reselected later. Third, if the analytic processes are applied selectively on the cards identified by the heuristic processes, inspection times will be longer for selected than for nonselected cards regardless of card contents, which is consistent with the previous findings. We adopted the procedure of Roberts (1998b, Exp. 2), hiding the cards except for the one pointed to, and added the cancel option. Two versions of the selection task were used: the original letter-number problem and the drinking-age problem. The latter problem is known to strongly facilitate logical responses (e.g., Griggs & Cox, 1982; Cheng & Holyoak, 1985). The effects of the order of problems on correct response rate and card inspection pattern were also examined.

Method

Participants

Twenty-four student volunteers participated in the experiment (7 men and 17 women, 19–24 years old, $M = 21.0$ yr.). We matched the number of participants to the number of patterns of laying four cards out on the selection screen ($4! = 24$). All of them were undergraduate or graduate students at Osaka University. Each participant received a payment equivalent to about 200 yen (approximately US$ 1.50) for participation. None had prior knowledge of the selection task.

Materials

Two problems with different thematic contents were used. The following instructions appeared on the first screen (the original was in Japanese).

The letter-number problem.—"On the next screen, four cards are presented. Each card has a capital letter on one side and has a single figure number on the other side. All cards are covered with a black curtain. When you move the mouse pointer onto a covered card, you can see only one side of the card. Now, you need to find out whether these cards conform to the following rule: If a card has a vowel on one side, then it has an even number on the other side. Which of the four cards do you need to turn over to confirm whether these cards conform to the rule? Please select the card(s) you need to turn over by clicking on the card(s). Note that more than one card may need to be selected."

The drinking-age problem.—"Imagine that you are a police officer on duty. It is your job to ensure that people conform to a certain rule. On the next screen, four cards are presented. Each card has information about a person sitting in a bar. On one side of a card is a person's age, and on the other side of the card is what the person was drinking. All cards are covered with a black curtain. When you move the mouse pointer onto a covered card, you can see only one side of the card. The law is as follows: If a person is drinking alcohol, then the person must be over 20 years of age. Which of the four cards do you need to turn over in order to confirm whether these four people violate the law? Please select the card(s) that you need to turn over by clicking on the card(s). Note that more than one card may need to be selected."

The four cards in the letter-number problem were "A" (true antecedent), "D" (false antecedent), "4" (true consequent), and "7" (false consequent). Those in the drinking-age problem were "Beer" (true antecedent), "Cola" (false antecedent), "22 years old" (true consequent), and "16 years old" (false consequent). The layout of these cards on the screen was counterbalanced across participants. Task presentation and response measurement were operated by NEC PC-9821Xp personal computer with a 17-in. cathode-ray tube display. Fig. 1 shows an example of the card selection screen. There were four cards at each corner, a conditional sentence at the center, and an "End" button below the sentence.

Procedure

Participants were tested individually in front of the computer. Half of the participants did the letter-number problem first, whereas the other half did the drinking-age problem first. Before the experimental trials, they performed a practice trial to get familiarized with the mouse actions used in the

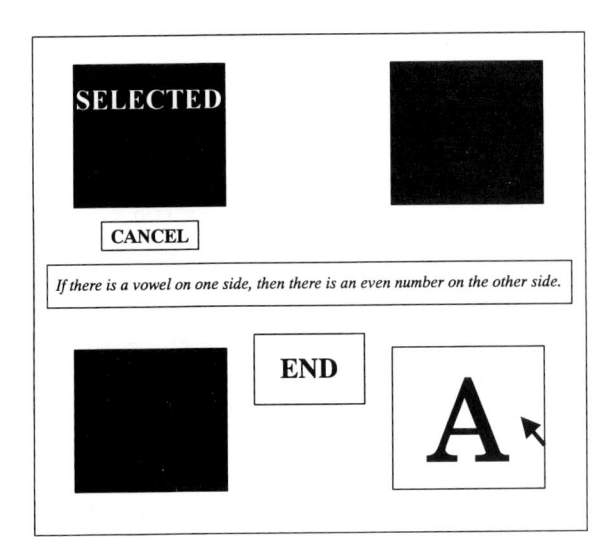

FIG. 1. An example of the card selection screen. Only the card touched by the mouse pointer was visible. The total card exposure time was measured as inspection time for each card. Selected cards could be cancelled by clicking on the CANCEL button at any time.

experiment, i.e., seeing, selecting, and canceling a card. The card-selection screen on the practice trial was the same as that on the experimental trials except for problem and card contents. On the experimental trials, instructions were presented on the display first. After the experimenter confirmed that the participant understood what to do, the card-selection screen was presented. Participants were able to see only one card content at a time by moving a mouse pointer onto it. They had to keep pointing to the card while inspecting it. When they wanted to select a card, they clicked on the card. When a card was selected, the indicator "Selected" appeared on the card, and the "Cancel" button was presented below the card. Once selected, the card content was not seen by mouse pointing. By clicking on the "Cancel" button, the selection of the card was cancelled, and the card content could be seen by mouse pointing again. Inspection time for each card (equivalent to the time for which a specific card was exposed by pointing) was calculated cumulatively. The task was finished when the participant clicked on the "End" button. The time between the appearance of the card selection screen, and the click on the "End" button was measured as solution time. Participants were encouraged to think for as long as they wished.

Statistical Analysis

First, the numbers of selections, cancellations, and reselections were counted and analyzed with nonparametric binominal tests. Second, the data for solution time were analyzed after logarithmic transformation by a two-way analysis of variance with factors of order (letter-number first vs drinking-age first; between participants) and task contents (letter-number vs drinking-age; within participants). Finally, the data for inspection time were analyzed after logarithmic transformation by a 2 × 2 × 2 mixed analysis of variance with factors of order, task contents, and selection (selected vs nonselected; within participants) and a 2 × 2 × 4 mixed analysis of variance with factors of order, task contents, and card (true antecedent, false antecedent, true consequent, and false consequent; within participants). Tukey's *HSD* test was used for *post hoc* comparison. The alpha level was set at .05. Effect sizes were reported in terms of partial η^2, i.e., the explained proportion of the total variance from which the variance due to the other main effects and interactions were partialled out.

Results

Card Selection and Cancellation

Table 1 shows the numbers of selections, cancellations, and reselections as well as the number of participants who responded correctly. Only few participants (2 out of 24, 8.3%) were correct in the letter-number problem, whereas most participants (20 out of 24, 83.3%) were correct in the drinking-age problem. Among 92 selections, cancellation occurred only nine times (9.8%; significantly different from 50% in the binominal test, $p < .01$). Moreover, 8 of 9 cancelled cards were selected again (88.9%, $p < .05$ in the binominal test). Overall, there was only one case out of 48 trials in which the initial selection was finally changed.

TABLE 1
Numbers of Selections, Cancellations, Reselections, and Correct Answers (*N* = 24)

	Cards				Correct
	Antecedent		Consequent		
	True	False	True	False	
Letter-number					2 (0, 2)
Selected	20 (9, 11)	4 (3, 1)	15 (6, 9)	8 (4, 4)	
Cancelled	1 (0, 1)	0 (0, 0)	2 (1, 1)	3 (1, 2)	
Reselected	1 (0, 1)	0 (0, 0)	1 (1, 0)	3 (1, 2)	
Drinking-age					
Selected	24 (12, 12)	0 (0, 0)	1 (1, 0)	20 (9, 11)	20 (9, 11)
Cancelled	1 (0, 1)	0 (0, 0)	0 (0, 0)	2 (0, 2)	
Reselected	1 (0, 1)	0 (0, 0)	0 (0, 0)	2 (0, 2)	

Note.—The first and second values in parentheses show the numbers for the group presented the letter-number problem first (*n* = 12) and for the group presented the drinking-age problem first (*n* = 12), respectively.

Solution Time

Table 2 shows the mean solution times. On average, the letter-number problem had a longer solution time than the drinking-age problem ($F_{1,22} = 5.02$, $p < .05$, $\eta^2 = .19$). The main effect of order was also significant ($F_{1,22} = 13.10$, $p < .005$, $\eta^2 = .37$). The interaction between order and task contents was significant ($F_{1,22} = 20.00$, $p < .0005$, $\eta^2 = .48$), so tests for simple effects were performed. When participants experienced the drinking-age problem first, the solution time of the letter-number was shortened ($F_{1,44} = 28.78$, $p < .005$, $\eta^2 = .40$). In contrast, the solution time of the drinking-age problem was not affected by the order of problem ($F < 1.00$, $\eta^2 = .02$).

TABLE 2
MEAN SOLUTION TIME (SEC.) FOR EACH PROBLEM IN EACH ORDER (ns = 12)

Order	Letter-number M	Letter-number SD	Drinking-age M	Drinking-age SD
Letter-number first	71.1[a]	23.4	38.1[b]	13.2
Drinking-age first	27.1[b]	13.8	34.2[b]	19.3

Note.—Different superscripts indicate significant differences between the means both down columns and across rows.

Card Inspection Time

Table 3 shows card-inspection times by selection and nonselection for each problem. The mixed analysis of variance performed on the log-transformed data showed that the order of problem did not interact with the

TABLE 3
MEAN INSPECTION TIMES (SEC.) FOR SELECTED VS NONSELECTED CARDS (ns = 12)

Order	Letter-number M	Letter-number SD	Drinking-age M	Drinking-age SD
Letter-number first				
Selected	11.5	4.1	8.7	3.2
Nonselected	7.5	4.4	4.6	2.2
Drinking-age first				
Selected	3.8	1.6	6.2	3.6
Nonselected	3.7	3.2	4.7	2.5
Total ($N = 24$)				
Selected	7.7[a]	5.0	7.4[a]	3.7
Nonselected	5.6[b]	4.3	4.6[b]	2.3

Note.—Different superscripts indicate significant differences between means both down columns and across rows.

other variables. Selected cards were inspected longer than nonselected cards ($F_{1,22} = 9.45$, $p < .01$, $\eta^2 = .30$). This tendency appeared regardless of task contents (Task Contents × Selection interaction, $F < 1.00$, $\eta^2 = .03$).

Table 4 shows the inspection times by card for each problem. The mixed analysis of variance performed on the log-transformed data showed a significant main effect of order and a significant interaction between order and task contents ($F_{1,22} = 8.64$, $p < .01$, $\eta^2 = .28$; $F_{3,66} = 9.11$, $p < .01$, $\eta^2 = .29$, respectively). These results mirrored the effect of order on solution time. No interaction between order and card was found, which suggests that inspection pattern among cards did not differ significantly with the order of problems. The main effect of card was significant ($F_{1,22} = 8.64$, $p < .01$, $\eta^2 = .18$). Although the interaction between card and task contents was not significant ($F_{3,66} = 2.39$, $p = .076$, $\eta^2 = .10$), we performed separate one-way analyses of variance for both task contents. A significant effect of card was obtained for the drinking-age problem alone ($F_{3,69} = 6.03$, $p < .005$, $\eta^2 = .21$). Post hoc test showed that inspection times were significantly larger for true antecedent and false consequent cards than for a false antecedent card ($p < .05$). For the letter-number problem, the main effect of card was not significant ($F < 1.00$, $\eta^2 = .04$).

TABLE 4
MEAN INSPECTION TIMES (SEC.) FOR FOUR CARDS IN EACH PROBLEM (ns = 12)

Order	Letter-number M	Letter-number SD	Drinking-age M	Drinking-age SD
Letter-number first				
True antecedent	10.7	5.8	7.8	3.7
False antecedent	8.4	6.0	3.7	2.1
True consequent	12.5	7.8	5.6	3.1
False consequent	8.7	5.0	8.7	5.2
Drinking-age first				
True antecedent	3.1	1.1	6.9	6.6
False antecedent	4.4	3.9	3.6	2.3
True consequent	3.7	2.2	5.7	3.8
False consequent	5.1	4.0	5.5	2.5
Total ($N = 24$)				
True antecedent	6.9	5.6	7.4[a]	5.4
False antecedent	6.4	5.4	3.6[b]	2.3
True consequent	8.1	7.3	5.6	3.5
False consequent	6.9	4.9	7.1[a]	4.4

Note.—Different superscripts indicate significant differences among the means for the four card types.

DISCUSSION

The present study examined the problem-solving behavior in the selection task when participants were allowed to cancel their previous selections at any time. In agreement with the predictions, three main findings were obtained: (1) once the cards were selected they were rarely cancelled, (2) cancelled cards tended to be reselected, and (3) inspection times were longer for finally selected cards than for nonselected cards, regardless of card contents. The order of problem affected the solution time of the letter-number problem.

One of the criticisms of the inspection time effect reported by Evans (1996) was that the extended inspection time for selected cards might be due to the response processes instead of the initial heuristic processes (Roberts, 1998b). Roberts and Newton (2001) used a special version of the selection task and successfully dissociated the effect of selection and the effect of active response, which were independent of each other. In the present study, we used a classical version of the selection task and reduced the participants' tendency of response hesitation by allowing them to cancel their selections at any time. The results showed that, even when the participants were given a chance to rethink, they rarely changed their initial selections. The data are consistent with the heuristic-analytic framework, suggesting that the cards finally selected are determined by initial heuristic processes and the selections are not reversed by subsequent analytic processes.

The finding that selected cards were inspected longer than nonselected cards is consistent with most of the previous experiments (Evans, 1996; Roberts, 1998b, Exp. 1, 2, 3). Significant differences in inspection time among cards (true antecedent, false antecedent, true consequent, and false consequent) were found for the drinking-age problem but not for the letter-number problem. In the drinking-age problem, pragmatic cues based on daily experiences, i.e., drinking beer is not allowed for a person under 20 years old, were used at the heuristic stage (Evans, Over, & Manktelow, 1993; Evans, 1996; Evans & Over, 1996), so that the same cards ("beer" and "16 years old") were commonly inspected by most participants. In the letter-number problem, however, the cards were inspected differently across participants probably because pragmatic cues were lacking. Nevertheless, finally selected cards were inspected longer than nonselected cards in both problems independent of card contents. The overall pattern of the results is consistent with the dual process theory. In the heuristic stage, some cues lead a person to focus attention on a subset of the cards. The initial selection of cards at this stage depends on the thematic contents of the problem. In the analytic stage, then, additional inspections were operated on these selected cards. Consequently, inspection times became longer for these cards independent of their contents.

The solution time of the letter-number problem was decreased when it was preceded by the drinking-age problem. The order of problem did not affect the solution time of the drinking-age problem. These results suggest that two types of difficulties can be distinguished in the selection task: the difficulty of understanding the task contents and the difficulty of logical reasoning *per se*. Participants who encountered the letter-number problem first appeared to be uncertain about what they should do. When they experienced the drinking-age problem first, this type of uncertainty was lowered, which was reflected in the decrease in solution time. Nevertheless, neither the correct response rate nor the pattern of card inspection was affected by the order of problem. This result agrees with previous findings that the transfer of logical response from a thematic problem to an abstract problem is difficult (e.g., Cheng, Holyoak, Nisbett, & Oliver, 1986; Price & Driscoll, 1997) and suggests that initial heuristic processes were critical for the correct response in the selections task.

Although the present study shows the importance of heuristic processes, it does not mean that analytic processes do not operate at all in the Wason selection task. To conceptualize the relation between heuristic and analytic processes, the mental models theory (Johnson-Laird & Byrne, 1991) may serve as a useful framework applicable to various reasoning tasks such as conditional reasoning (e.g., Johnson-Laird & Byrne, 2002) and syllogistic reasoning (e.g., Cardaci, Gangemi, Pendolino, & di Nuovo, 1996). According to this theory, participants first construct an incomplete mental representation of the task and then attempt to flesh it out to a more complete model so that they can make a decision. Heuristic processes probably play an important role in the initial construction of a mental model, whereas analytic processes serve to elaborate the model. The implication of the heuristic-analytic dual process theory here is that, when the initial representation is inadequate, the reasoning person cannot reach a logically correct answer however much analysis is done. It appears difficult for analytic processes to revise a wrong initial representation. Further research will be required to examine what factors determine the heuristic selection (e.g., Yama, 2001) and how the analytic processes work under constraints posed by the heuristic processes (e.g., Schroyens, Schaeken, Fias, & d'Ydewalle, 2000).

In conclusion, the present study gives further support for the heuristic-analytic dual process of reasoning in the Wason selection task. Although the findings cannot be considered conclusive because a relatively small number of participants and trials were involved, they suggest that analytic processes rarely reverse the initial heuristic selections even when there is a chance of correction. Recently, Ball, Lucas, Miles, and Gale (2003) criticized the use of the mouse-pointing method as a measure of thinking time and proposed a more precise method like eye-movement tracking. Despite the methodological flaw of using the mouse-pointing method, the procedure introduced in the present study, where participants are encouraged to cancel and rethink, may help investigate the characteristics of analytic processes.

REFERENCES

BALL, L. J., LUCAS, E. J., MILES, J. N. V., & GALE, A. G. (2003) Inspection times and selection task: what do eye-movements reveal about relevance effects? *Quarterly Journal of Experimental Psychology*, 56A, 1053-1077.

CARDACI, M., GANGEMI, A., PENDOLINO, G., & DI NUOVO, S. (1996) Mental models vs integrated models: explanations of syllogistic reasoning. *Perceptual and Motor Skills*, 82, 1377-1378.

CHENG, P. W., & HOLYOAK, K. J. (1985) Pragmatic reasoning schemas. *Cognitive Psychology*, 17, 391-416.

CHENG, P. W., HOLYOAK, K. J., NISBETT, R. E., & OLIVER, L. M. (1986) Pragmatic versus syntactic approaches to training deductive reasoning. *Cognitive Psychology*, 18, 293-328.

EVANS, J. ST. B. T. (1984) Heuristic and analytic processes in reasoning. *British Journal of Psychology*, 75, 451-468.

EVANS, J. ST. B. T. (1995) Relevance and reasoning. In S. E. Newstead & J. St. B. T. Evans (Eds.), *Perspectives on thinking and reasoning: essays in honour of Peter Wason.* Hove, UK: Erlbaum. Pp. 147-172.

EVANS, J. ST. B. T. (1996) Deciding before you think: relevance and reasoning in the selection task. *British Journal of Psychology*, 87, 223-240.

EVANS, J. ST. B. T. (1998a) Inspection times, relevance, and reasoning: a reply to Roberts. *Quarterly Journal of Experimental Psychology*, 51A, 811-814.

EVANS, J. ST. B. T. (1998b) Matching bias in conditional reasoning: do we understand it after 25 years? *Thinking and Reasoning*, 4, 45-82.

EVANS, J. ST. B. T., & OVER, D. E. (1996) *Rationality and reasoning.* Hove, UK: Psychological Press.

EVANS, J. ST. B. T., OVER, D. E., & MANKTELOW, K. I. (1993) Reasoning, decision making and rationality. *Cognition*, 49, 165-187.

GRIGGS, R. A., & COX, J. R. (1982) The elusive thematic-materials effect in Wason's selection task. *British Journal of Psychology*, 73, 405-420.

JOHNSON-LAIRD, P. N., & BYRNE, R. M. J. (1991) *Deduction.* Hove, UK: Erlbaum.

JOHNSON-LAIRD, P. N., & BYRNE, R. M. J. (2002) Conditionals: a theory of meaning, pragmatics, and inference. *Psychological Review*, 109, 646-678.

PRICE, E. A., & DRISCOLL, M. P. (1997) An inquiry into the spontaneous transfer of problem-solving skill. *Contemporary Educational Psychology*, 22, 472-494.

ROBERTS, M. J. (1998a) How should relevance be defined? What does inspection time measure? A reply to Evans. *Quarterly Journal of Experimental Psychology*, 51A, 815-817.

ROBERTS, M. J. (1998b) Inspection times and the selection task: are they relevant? *Quarterly Journal of Experimental Psychology*, 51A, 781-810.

ROBERTS, M. J., & NEWTON, E. J. (2001) Inspection times, the change task, and the rapid-response selection task. *Quarterly Journal of Experimental Psychology*, 54A, 1031-1048.

SCHROYENS, W., SCHAEKEN, W., FIAS, W., & D'YDEWALLE, G. (2000) Heuristic and analytic processes in prepositional reasoning with negatives. *Journal of Experimental Psychology: Learning, Memory, and Cognition*, 26, 1713-1734.

WASON, P. C. (1966) Reasoning. In B. M. Foss (Ed.), *New horizons in psychology: 1.* Harmondsworth, UK: Penguin. Pp. 135-151.

YAMA, H. (2001) Matching versus optimal data selection in the Wason selection task. *Thinking and Reasoning*, 7, 295-311.

Accepted April 14, 2004.

THE FRAGMENTED SELF[1]

DAVID LESTER

The Richard Stockton College of New Jersey

Summary—For a sample of 182 undergraduates analysis of responses to a 10-item scale to measure the plurality of the self yielded three orthogonal factors and only moderate reliability.

Altrocchi (1999; McReynolds, Altrocchi, & House, 2000) devised a 10-item yes/no scale to measure the plurality of the self, that is, does the person feel that he is one coherent self or many selves? The present study was designed to conduct an item analysis of this scale.

The 10-item plural self scale ($M=5.52$, $SD=2.24$) was administered to 48 male and 134 female undergraduate students enrolled in social science courses ($M_{age}=22.0$ yr., $SD=4.4$). The data were subjected to a principal components extraction and a varimax rotation using SPSS (Windows Version 11.0). Three eigenvalues were greater than 1.00, so three orthogonal (independent) factors were extracted. The first factor (Items 5, 6, 7, and 8, accounting for 26.0% of the variance) concerned feeling and appearing to be the same, e.g., "People who know me say that my behavior changes from situation to situation," scored negatively. The second factor (Items 3, 4, 9, and 10, accounting for 12.4% of the variance) concerned acting and feeling differently at various times, e.g., "I sometimes have conflicts over whether to be one kind of person or a different kind." The third factor (Items 1 and 2, accounting for 10.7% of the variance) concerned being predictable, e.g., "People who know me well would say I'm pretty predictable." Cronbach alpha was .64, indicating moderate reliability.

For a brief scale of 10 items, whose face content appears to measure only one dimension of personality, the scale was factorially complex and had only moderate reliability in this sample.

REFERENCES

ALTROCCHI, J. (1999) Individual difference in pluralism. In J. Rowan & M. Cooper (Eds.), *The plural self*. London, UK: Sage. Pp. 168-182.

MCREYNOLDS, P., ALTROCCHI, J., & HOUSE, C. (2000) Self-pluralism. *Journal of Personality*, 68, 347-381.

Accepted April 30, 2004.

---

[1]Address enquiries to David Lester, Ph.D., Psychology Program, The Richard Stockton College of New Jersey, P.O. Box 195, Jimmie Leeds Road, Pomona, NJ 08240-0195.

A MOBILE DEVICE FOR MEASURING SENSORIMOTOR TIMING IN SYNCHRONIZED TAPPING [1]

TOSHITERU HATAYAMA

Tohoku University

MISAKO HATAYAMA AND NAOKO KIKUCHI

Miyagi Gakuin Women's University

Summary.—This paper describes the design of a mobile device for examining sensorimotor timing. Control software installed in this device has facilities for storing time series data of interstimulus onset intervals, intertap onset intervals, and response duration in a comma-delimited file of ASCII text format as well as for running an experiment on synchronization tapping. The device provides a highly convenient way to allow collecting such timing data even in real situations like a kindergarten or a day care center for elderly people, given its mobile property and ease of use.

The present report describes a notebook PC-based device for measuring the timing of synchronization tapping responses to enable collection of data not only from university students in psychology laboratories, but also from subjects in real situations like kindergartens or day care centers for elderly people.

One of the most important applications of synchronization tapping techniques is probably to the field of evaluating psychological disorders. The measurement of synchronization tapping could be particularly useful for understanding clearly how children and elderly people with various difficulties can regulate their timing of tapping movements. Further, the temporal analyses of synchronization tapping, as Cousins, Corrow, Finn, and Salamone (1998) suggested, can be seen as useful to identify subtle motor impairments observed in extrapyramidal disorders like Parkinsonism. However, we do not always have definite dependent variables adequate for assessing temporal aspects of such behavior. In addition, there is a problem with space for a measuring system. Since the system needed for the specified measurement of synchronization tapping contains a set of independent elements such as stimulus presentation, tap detection, and data-processing, the space used for making the system available is not so small as to carry it easily from the research laboratory. By overcoming these technical problems, such a synchro-

---

[1]This study was supported in part by a Grant-in-Aid for Scientific Research, Japan Society for the Promotion of Science, No. 12610073. Address correspondence to Dr. Toshiteru Hatayama, Department of Psychology, Tohoku University, Kawauchi, Aoba-ku, Sendai 980-8576, Japan or e-mail (hatayama@sal.tohoku.ac.jp).

nization tapping device would be useful for elaborating on studies of finger motor control in clinical settings as well as in daily life situations.

Response measures used in most synchronization tapping basically reflect temporal aspects of movement. Wing (1980) pointed out that the timing of movement in skills is an indispensable component in defining the coordination of different phases of movement. It is particularly an important element in studying temporal patterning of repetitive fine movements involved in synchronization tasks. These require subjects to press a key at a given rate synchronous with the presentation of pacing signal. Studies using such a task have a fairly long history over more than 100 years (Aschersleben, 2002). Although the ease of use has broadened a range of applications of psychological studies, temporal analysis of the dependent variables in finger-tapping tasks has been made only for overall response rate (number of taps divided by time). Cousins, et al. (1998) suggested that there has been little empirical attention paid to other temporal parameters of responding such as intertap onset intervals and duration of key-depletion. Recently, more emphasis has been placed on the importance of treating tapping responses as time series data (Ding, Chen, & Kelso, 2002). An application software for this kind of data processing requires a computer system with fast throughput. Fortunately, recent personal computers are powerful enough to meet the basic requirements. In addition, with laptops or notebook PCs, smaller and lighter with the power of a desktop model, the problems of the device's size and portability can be solved.

The method of synchronization tapping appears to have an important advantage over the procedure of simple tapping (in which the subject is required to depress a key with the fingers as rapidly as possible or at a speed convenient to him) in that the method can produce differential patterns of continuous stimulus-response relations among different subjects. The analysis of synchronization tapping might give a major step for analyzing the control mechanism underlying cognitive processes. Some cognition researchers have found this method useful for understanding the mechanism of sensorimotor functions. There are many examples of testing different models to account for synchronization error (taps preceding signals by several tens of milliseconds) (Aschersleben, 2002), investigating principles underlying synchronizing taps (Repp, 2001a, 2001b), estimating model parameters for synchronization tapping (Wing & Kristofferson, 1973a, 1973b; Schulze & Vorberg, 2002), and searching for the underlying mechanisms of perceptual-motor coordination (Lutz, Specht, Shah, & Jäncke, 2000; Ding, et al., 2002). These studies suggest that evaluating synchronization tapping might be a useful method for examining the timing control processes of behavior.

We have devised a compact data-processing system for analyzing temporal parameters of synchronization tapping using a notebook PC. In designing the device by utilizing such a PC, its main requirements based on our previous study (Hatayama, 2002) were that it can generate as a click stimulus a pure tone of a 1,000 Hz with 100 msec. duration or less; can regulate interstimulus onset intervals, with the shortest being 250 msec., the longest 1,000 msec.; can set a trial length of time less than 1-min. long; can set up a push-button for tapping about 1 m away from a notebook PC; and can execute all of the fundamental data processing from data input through storage to display.

Fig. 1 shows the structure of a measurement device for measuring the timing of synchronization tapping. The device is composed of a notebook PC[2] and an external response-key box. The signal-processing system is operated by a PC program called PTA[3]. The program has facilities for creation of stimulus file, data registration, and graphic output of the data obtained, consisting of the following three main functional units.

PTA control unit.—The PTA program allows the user to specify the stimulus tone conditions by choosing "production of stimulus sequence" from the Set menu on a Menu bar and to store all necessary stimulus sequences as stimulus files on the hard disk (WAV is the file extension). Stimulus sequences consisted of tones separated by pauses, the types of which stimulus sequences can be selected from the following (Appendix 1, p. 1332) isochronous, fast-to-slow, slow-to-fast, and random sequences. The stimulus parameters you can define in advance are (a) stimulus patterns, (b) wave form of sine wave or square one, (c) tone duration, and (d) tone frequency. The interstimulus onset intervals (ISIs) can be varied from 200 to 2,000 msec. in any type of stimulus sequences. This device has two kinds of waveforms (sine and square waves) that can be set up between 50 and 1,000 msec. in duration and between 500 and 4,000 Hz in frequency. The produced files also can be edited manually about the ISIs. In conducting an experiment, the stimulus conditions are set by choosing one of the files on the hard disk and entering the subject information before beginning trials.

Data processing unit.—A push-button switch with a square-shaped key (11 × 11 mm) mounted in a response-key box (150 × 80 × 30 mm) was used as an input device connected to an I/O PC card (PCMCIA) to record the tapping performance. Then, PTA was used to ensure the elimination of sources of input error resulting from mechanical switch bouncing. The mea-

---

[2] Here a notebook computer, Dell Inspiron 2500, was used: Intel Mobile Celeron™ processor at 700MHz, 128MB SDRAM, 20GB hard drive, and MS Windows 2000 professional for OS.
[3] PTA (Paced TApping) program is a PC control software, available for any PC running Windows 98SE or higher, that has been developed to manage a synchronization tapping experiment as well as its response measures. The software has been written in MS Visual C++ Language. PTA is commercially available from TESCO Co. in Sendai, Japan. Contact the e-mail address, chida@tescomed.co.jp, for more information.

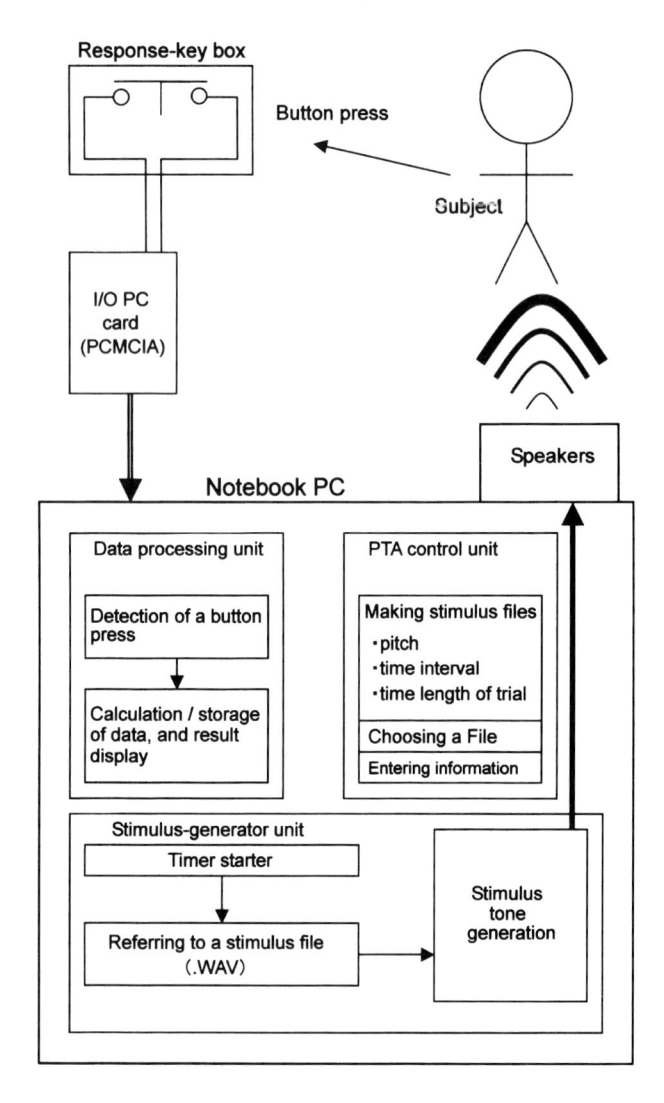

FIG. 1. Structure of a measuring device for synchronization tapping, in which major control functions are represented as the three units inside a PC: the PTA control unit, data-processing unit, and stimulus-generator unit. These functional units enable production of stimulus sequences, organize an experiment on tapping performance, and store the collected data for further analyses on the hard disk.

surements of synchronization tapping are made on the order of a measurement precision of 1 msec. at any stimulus sequence chosen. An experimental trial can be interrupted or modified at any time. With its completion, the time series data on ISIs and intertrial intervals (ITIs) are stored on the hard drive by the PTA program, new Windows folders that were created when PTA was installed. In the PTA folder, two kinds of data files are created with the file extensions of .PTA and .CSV.[4] The former is mainly used for graphic output of accumulated intertap onset and interstimulus onset intervals, while the latter for further analyses of collected data and for drawing graphs researchers need.

Stimulus-generator unit.—Based on a given stimulus file, ISIs produced by a PC timer define the exact timing of stimulus tone generation. The internal digital audio system of the PC was used as a stimulus generator.

It has been found during experiments conducted in our laboratory, which are reported in detail elsewhere, that this system is suitable for recording subjects' timing of tapping responses. An example of data from a 4-yr.-old girl (Fig. 2) was obtained from an experiment at a kindergarten in Sendai. Its mobility and ease of use recommend it for a wide variety of psychological research on timing behavior.

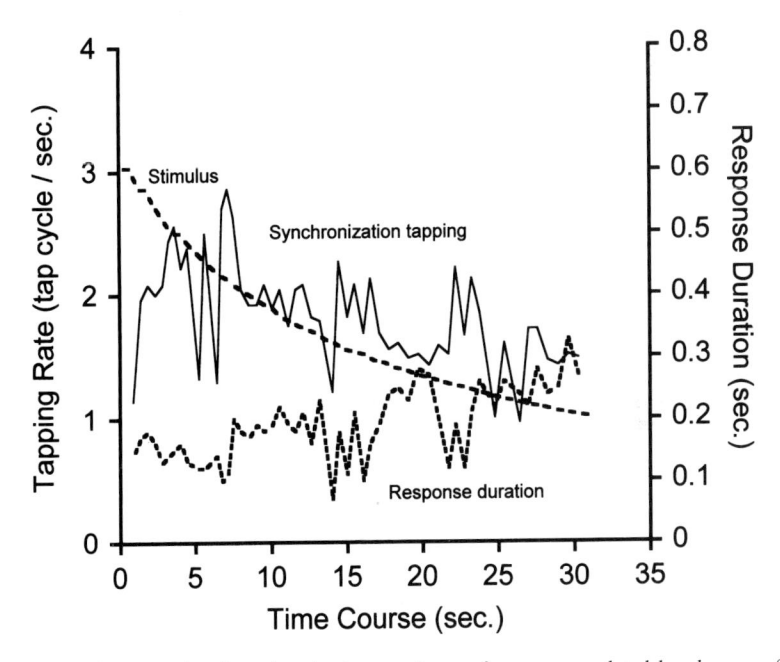

FIG. 2. An example of synchronization tapping performance regulated by changes of interstimulus onset intervals with gradually decreased frequency from 3 to 1 Hz by a 4-yr.-old girl. Here she was required to use her right index finger to press a button. Response duration showed the tendency to increase as the tapping rates were gradually decreased.

---

[4]CSV indicates a Comma-delimited file, which is a file in ASCII or plain text format with the fields separated by commas.

REFERENCES

ASCHERSLEBEN, G. (2002) Temporal control of movements in sensorimotor synchronization. *Brain and Cognition*, 48, 66-79.

COUSINS, M. S., CORROW, C., FINN, M., & SALAMONE, J. D. (1998) Temporal measures of human finger tapping: effects of age. *Pharmacology Biochemistry and Behavior*, 59, 445-449.

DING, M., CHEN, Y., & KELSO, J. A. S. (2002) Statistical analysis of timing errors. *Brain and Cognition*, 48, 98-106.

HATAYAMA, M. (2002) [A follow-up study of the regulation of paced tapping performance in young children.] [*Journal of Developmental Science (Miyagi Gakuin Women's College)*], 2, 75-79. [in Japanese]

LUTZ, K., SPECHT, K., SHAH, N. J., & JÄNCKE, L. (2000) Tapping movements according to regular and irregular visual timing signals investigated with fMRI. *NeuroReport*, 11, 1301-1306.

REPP, B. H. (2001a) Phase correction, phase resetting, and phase shifts after subliminal timing perturbations in sensorimotor synchronization. *Journal of Experimental Psychology: Human Perception and Performance*, 27, 600-621.

REPP, B. H. (2001b) Process underlying adaptation to tempo changes in sensorimotor synchronization. *Human Movement Science*, 20, 277-312.

SCHULZE, H., & VORBERG, G. (2002) Linear phase correction models for synchronization: parameter identification and estimation of parameters. *Brain and Cognition*, 48, 80-97.

WING, A. M. (1980) The long and short of timing in response sequences. In G. E. Stelmach & J. Requin (Eds.), *Tutorials in motor behavior*. Amsterdam: North-Holland. Pp. 469-486.

WING, A. M., & KRISTOFFERSON, A. B. (1973a) Response delays and the timing of discrete motor response. *Perception & Psychophysics*, 14, 5-12.

WING, A. M., & KRISTOFFERSON, A. B. (1973b) The timing of interresponse intervals. *Perception & Psychophysics*, 13, 455-460.

Accepted April 14, 2004.

APPENDIX 1

How to make interstimulus onset intervals ($200 \leq ISI \leq 2{,}000$ msec.):

(A) *Fast to slow*. Let x = the first ISI in msec., let y = the last ISI in msec., and let l = the length of stimulus sequence in msec. ($30{,}000 \leq l \leq 90{,}000$ msec.). The initial ISI is 0 msec. and the nth ISI is calculated according to the following: N^{th} ISI $(n) = x + \Sigma ISI \ (n-1) \times (y-x)/l$.

(B) *Slow to fast*. Let x = the first ISI in msec., let y = the last ISI in msec., and let l = length of stimulus sequence in msec. ($30{,}000 \leq l \leq 90{,}000$ msec.) The initial ISI is 0 msec. and the nth ISI is calculated according to the following: N^{th} ISI $(n) = x + \Sigma ISI \ (n-1) \times (y-x)/l$.

(C) *Random*. Let x = the first ISI in msec., let y = the last ISI in msec., and let R = a random number. The initial ISI is 0 msec. and the nth interval is calculated by substituting a random number obtained from the rand() function of the C Language in: N^{th} ISI $(n) = (x-y) \times R + y$.

DIFFERENCES IN AFRICAN-AMERICAN AND EURO-AMERICAN ATHLETES' PERCEPTIONS OF TREATMENT BY COACHES[1]

STEVEN F. PHILIPP AND PETRA B. SCHULER

University of West Florida

Summary.—Analysis of responses from 418 respondents from southern USA (198 African-American, 220 Euro-American adults) in 53 different locations at 4 colleges and universities showed that African-American and Euro-American high school and college athletes differed significantly in agreement on 4 of 12 statements representing their treatment by coaches. African-American athletes rated their coaches significantly more negatively on these items. Implications for coaches lie in planning, design and evaluation of coaching behaviors by African-American athletes.

Many studies have explored expectation-performance interaction in sport environments to explain athletes' perceptions and performance (2, 4, 7). Most have focused theoretically on the "self-fulfilling prophecy" effect, which suggests that a coach forms expectations based upon both personal, e.g., sex, age, and performance, e.g., effort, past performance, cues (3). These personal and performance-based expectations can influence coaching attitudes and behavior. When coaches' perceptions are consistently communicated and understood by the athlete, athletes may alter their behavior to conform to the coach's original expectation (6). If so, then the self-fulfilling prophecy cycle continues. There is little research, however, on the association of ethnicity and coaches' expectations in sport environments (5). Anshel and Sailes (1) found that African-American athletes trusted Euro-American coaches less than did Euro-American athletes and were significantly less responsive to negative comments from Euro-American coaches than their Euro-American teammates. Solomon (5) argued for differential athletic feedback patterns and management styles based upon coaches' and athletes' ethnicity. To understand the role of ethnicity in sports environments in the present study racial differences in former or current adult athletes' perceptions of coaches' decisions were explored.

METHOD

A sample of 479 adult respondents from the southern USA were asked to complete a paper-and-pencil questionnaire in 53 different sample locations at four college or university study sites. Locations were chosen from a wide range of college or university areas, e.g., library, cafeteria, fitness cen-

---

[1]Address correspondence to Dr. Steven F. Philipp, Division of Health, Leisure and Exercise Science, University of West Florida, 11000 University Parkway, Pensacola, FL 32514.

ter, science building, arts building, administration buildings, walkways, etc., to increase the likelihood of selecting a representative group of students.

Questionnaires were given to respondents by graduate students in each location during 3 wk. in March, 2003. These graduate students were trained in survey administration techniques to minimize interviewer bias. All respondents who entered the site during the survey time and answered "yes" to "did you play sports in high school or college" were asked to complete the questionnaire. Of the 418 respondents who completed the questionnaire (87% response rate) 47% were African American, 53% Euro-American; 49% were women, 51% men. Twenty-four percent were 18 to 19 yr. old, 28% were 20 to 21 yr. old, 27% were 22 to 24 yr. old, 12% were 25 to 29 yr. old, and 9% were 30 yr. old or more. Fifteen percent had played sports as part of a school team for 1 to 2 yr., 31% for 3 to 4 yr., 23% for 5 to 6 yr., 17% for 7 to 8 yr., and 12% for 9 yr. or longer. Seventy-three percent played most of the time on the team(s), 24% played some of the time, and 3% did not usually play.

A two-page questionnaire was developed. A panel of 20 graduate students with extensive experience in sports or coaching compiled a list of 107 different coaching evaluation factors from the sports and coaching literature which might be influenced by race. Of these factors 12 were selected as "most important" by this expert panel. Respondents rated the 12 factors to reflect: "Consider your sports career, then think about how your coaches treated you. Now, rate the following statements on how they match your overall feelings about coaches." Each statement was marked on a 6-point Likert-type scale on which anchors were 1 = Disagree and 6 = Agree, with no labeling of the other categories. Information on sex, race, age, where lived while growing up, how many years played sports, how much playing time on the team(s), and what main reason for playing sports was requested.

Results

Table 1 presents mean scores and t ratios by ethnic group on athletes' recalled treatment by coaches. Statistical analysis utilized two-tailed t tests, with an F (folded) statistic to test for equality of the two variances. This analysis showed four of 12 statements (33%) were rated significantly differently ($p < .01$) by the two groups. These significant differences remained when other effects or other factors were statistically controlled. The negatively rated four statements concerned removed me from play before other team members, disciplined for mistakes more than others, understood the different cultural backgrounds of all team members, and expected me to work harder than others.

That no significant difference was found for "coaches treated all racial groups the same," suggests the African-American athletes did not feel the

TABLE 1
Mean Ratings and *t* Ratios For Recalled Treatment by Coaches by Two Groups

Treatment by Coaches	African-American Group M	African-American Group SD	Euro-American Group M	Euro-American Group SD	t	p
Coaches expected me to work harder than other team members.	4.1	1.6	3.5	1.6	3.38	.001
Coaches gave me less playing time than members of similar skill.	2.5	1.6	2.3	1.4	1.18	
Coaches helped me as much as other team members.	4.4	1.3	4.7	1.2	−2.01	
Coaches valued me as a person.	4.7	1.3	4.9	1.3	−1.37	
Coaches praised me as often as other team members for similar accomplishments.	4.3	1.3	4.1	1.4	−1.23	
Coaches blamed me for fouls/penalties more than other players.	2.4	1.4	2.3	1.3	0.90	
Coaches removed me from play before other team members.	2.5	1.5	2.2	1.3	2.61	.01
Coaches disciplined me for mistakes more than other team members.	2.9	1.6	2.4	1.4	3.52	.001
Coaches understood the different cultural backgrounds of all team members.	3.9	1.6	4.3	1.5	−2.82	.01
Coaches expected me to maintain the same academic standards as other team members.	4.6	1.4	4.9	1.3	−2.23	
Coaches punished me more severely than others for breaking team rules.	2.6	1.6	2.3	1.4	2.02	
Coaches treated all racial groups the same.	4.6	1.4	4.7	1.4	−0.88	

coach was making decisions solely based on race or overt prejudice but on cultural factors. In support of this interpretation, the African-American athletes agreed significantly less than Euro-American athletes with the statement "coaches understood the different cultural backgrounds of all team members." Perhaps the African-American athletes come from cultural backgrounds in which they react more negatively to some coaching decisions or treatments. This would support Anshel and Sailes (1) who reported that African-American athletes were significantly less responsive to negative comments from Euro-American coaches than their Euro-American teammates.

In summary, the two groups of athletes showed different perceptions of coaching decisions and treatments in several areas, which may reflect cultural factors more than perceived prejudice, discrimination, or racism. This finding suggests increased opportunities for coaches' comments to be made in more culturally sensitive ways to African-American athletes. Solomon (5) suggested that coaches may have differential athletic feedback patterns and management styles based on the race/ethnicity of athletes. The present study was exploratory and has many limitations, including the sample and statements about coaches, plus no control for subtle response biases. Researchers must clarify present data by testing larger and more representative samples with appropriate statements and corroborative measures.

REFERENCES

1. ANSHEL, M. H., & SAILES, G. (1990) Discrepant attitudes of intercollegiate athletes as a function of race. *Journal of Sport Behavior*, 13, 87-102.
2. EVANS, V. (1978) A study of perceptions held by high school athletes towards coaches. *International Review of Sport Sociology*, 13, 47-53.
3. HORN, T. S., LOX, C., & LABRADOR, F. (1998) The self-fulfilling prophecy theory: when coaches' expectations become reality. In J. M. Williams (Ed.), *Applied sport psychology: personal to peak performance*. Mountain View, CA: Mayfield. Pp. 74-91.
4. SINCLAIR, D. A., & VEALEY, R. S. (1989) Effects of coaches' expectations and feedback on the self-perception of athletes. *Journal of Sport Behavior*, 12, 77-91.
5. SOLOMON, G. B. (1999) Ethnic identity and coach feedback: implications for effective coaching. *The Journal of Physical Education, Recreation, and Dance*, 70, 75-78.
6. SOLOMON, G. B., DIMARCO, A. M., OHLSON, C. J., & REECE, S. D. (1998) Expectations and coaching experience: is more better? *Journal of Sport Behavior*, 21, 444-455.
7. SOLOMON, G. B., GOLDEN, A. J., CIAPPONI, T. M., & MARTIN, A. D. (1998) Coach expectations and differential feedback: perceptual flexibility revisited. *Journal of Sport Behavior*, 21, 298-310.

Accepted April 15, 2004.

EFFECTS OF STRATEGY USE ON ACQUISITION OF A MOTOR TASK DURING VARIOUS STAGES OF LEARNING [1]

L. KEITH TENNANT	NICHOLAS P. MURRAY	LAURIE M. TENNANT
University of Kansas	*East Carolina University*	*University of Kansas*

Summary.—To specify the optimal point for introducing a learning strategy, 50 participants were randomly assigned into five groups based on the timing of strategy introduction while learning a badminton serve. Groups were instructed in the use of Singer's Five-step Strategy either prior to starting their acquisition trials (100% group) or following acquisition Trial Blocks 1 (83% group), 3 (50% group), 5 (17% group) or were assigned to a control (0% group) group). Participants were asked to complete six acquisition trial blocks of 10 serves each, followed by a break and then two retention trial blocks. Scores were obtained by hitting shuttles into a scoring grid, which served as the dependent measure. Data were analyzed using a mixed-model analysis of variance with a group × trial blocks design, which yielded significant main effects for both factors during acquisition. Introduction of a learning strategy may be more efficient once participants have become familiar with the task. No significant differences were observed between groups who received the strategy early and the control group. Thus, it appears that learning strategies should be introduced later in the learning process and may distract if provided too early.

The search for a means to enhance learning and performance has always maintained a high priority among teachers, coaches, sport psychologists, and researchers. One fruitful area has been the use of cognitive learning strategies both in learning and during performance. Researchers who have examined the effectiveness of strategies have reported positive outcomes for learning and performance in both the cognitive (Dansereau, Brooks, Holley, & Collins, 1983; Pressley, Johnson, Symons, McGoldrick, & Kurita, 1989) and the psychomotor domains (Zervas & Kakkos, 1995; Lidor, Tennant, & Singer, 1996; Radlo, Hyllegard, & Karg, 2000) for various types of strategies. In sport, strategies have included self-talk or statements about self-efficacy (Mahoney, 1984; Weinberg, Grove, & Jackson, 1992), self-evaluating (Kirschenbaum, 1987), readying for performance (Singer, 1988), attentional focusing (Takai, 1998), and imagery or mental practice (Bohan, Pharmer, & Stokes, 1999) to mention a few.

The general paradigm in research on learning strategies introduces a strategy either concurrently with the onset of early instruction or shortly after the acquisition of a skill has begun, the rationale being that an earlier use of the strategy leads to quicker and more effective skill improvement. However, this tends to disregard two important possible aspects. First, the strat-

---

[1]Send correspondence to Nicholas P. Murray, 383 Ward Sports Medicine Building, East Carolina University, Greenville, NC 27858 or e-mail (murrayni@mail.ecu.edu).

egy may actually serve as a distractor to the student in an early stage of learning where focusing on more relevant cues for successful learning (Singer, Cauraugh, Tennant, Murphey, Chen, & Lidor, 1991) may be more critical to learning than trying to master or apply a strategy. Second, the effective use of some strategies requires a basic understanding of the skills being performed, and the novice may not yet have acquired those skills, negating any value of early introduction of a strategy.

Based on the potential distraction of introducing a strategy in early learning as described above, a somewhat later introduction and utilization of the learning strategy may prove as or more effective than a strategy introduced to the learner initially while learning a new task. One earlier study (Singer, Flora, & Abourezk, 1989) examined a similar scenario but reported that the early strategy-use group performed better than the control and other treatment groups given the strategy later in learning. This unexpected result may have been due to the nature of the task (a tapping task with little complexity) and the appropriateness of the strategy used for this type of task (Singer Five-step Strategy).

To test the timing of strategy introduction, Singer's Five-step Strategy (1988) was utilized. This strategy is a metacognitive one best suited for self-paced activities. The components of this strategy are (a) readying, (b) imaging, (c) focusing, (d) executing and (e) evaluating. Readying refers to the ability to prepare mentally and physically for an upcoming task by attempting to attain an optimal emotional and attitudinal state of mind prior to task initiation. An individual should assume a comfortable position, relax, think positively and motivate self by establishing reasonable goals. Imaging is creating or recreating a mental picture of self performing the task successfully and feeling the movements that should be executed. Focusing allows the individual to disregard irrelevant cues and thoughts that may inhibit task performance and, if distracted, to refocus on the task. Ideally, an individual should direct their attention to one relevant aspect of a task. Executing is simply the performance of the task, while remaining focused, without thinking about the movement or the final performance outcome. Evaluating, the final step, requires an individual assess task performance through the use of available sensory feedback or feedback from an external source.

There is growing support for the Five-step Strategy (Kim, Singer, & Radlo, 1996) as an effective strategy for improved performance on self-paced motor skills in both laboratory and ecologically valid situations. Examples of the strategy being used with laboratory tasks have included a modified table tennis serve and seated underhand dart throw (Singer, DeFrancesco, & Randall, 1989), underhand dart throwing (Singer & Suwanthada, 1986), and a stylus-to-target timing task (Singer, Flora, & Abourezk, 1989). Racquetball skills (Tennant, 2000), gun shooting (Kim, Chen, Singer, Tennant, & Chung,

1993; Kim & Tennant, 1993), and a tennis serve (Bouchard & Singer, 1998) are examples of actual sports in which the strategy has been used. More recent research has also demonstrated that the Five-step Strategy is an effective way to aid older adults in the acquisition of self-paced motor tasks (Steinberg & Glass, 2001) as well as improvement of acquisition and retention of motor task for children with disabilities (Yang & Porretta, 1999).

However, as stated above few researchers have examined the optimal point of timing for the introduction of a learning strategy during skill acquisition. The potential implication is that instructional and practice time may be more effectively used during class. Therefore, the purpose of this study was to examine the effects of introducing a strategy during learning while acquiring and performing a new self-timed motor skill, i.e., a badminton serve. Based on the evidence presented above, it was hypothesized that groups using the Five-step Strategy in later learning (groups who received learning strategy after 50% and 83% of the learning trials) would perform better during both learning and retention trials than participants using the strategy 100% or 17% of the time and than participants who received no strategy.

Method

Participants

Participants ($N = 50$) were comprised of men ($n = 42$) and women ($n = 8$) novice badminton players from a southern university. Players were initially asked to execute 10 serves for screening purposes, and all were novices since they were unable to perform the serve correctly. They then read and signed their informed consent before proceeding with the study. Participants ($n = 10$) were randomly assigned into one of five treatment conditions based upon the number of acquisition trials which remained to be completed: (1) all trial blocks (100% group), (2) after 1 trial block (83% group), (3) after 3 trial blocks (50% group), (4) after 5 trial blocks (17% group), or (5) a control (0% group) with no strategy.

Apparatus and Task

The study was conducted on a regulation indoor badminton court, and participants were provided standard badminton racquets and shuttlecocks. Players were asked to perform a series of high, deep underhand badminton serves into the back section of the service receiving area located diagonally on the opposite side of the net. The target area, measuring 4.72 m × 5.18 m, was subdivided into six equal scoring zones with the highest score adjacent to the baseline. Thus, zones and scores ranged from 1 (low score; zone nearest to the net) to 6 (high score; the area nearest the baseline) in which a score was given if the shuttlecock landed in a particular zone (if it landed in

Zone 1, one point was awarded, if it landed in Zone 2, two points were awarded, etc.), and any shuttlecocks that landed outside of the target area were assigned a score of zero, as were serves that did not clear the net. Participants were told that in badminton a good underhand serve is one that lands just inside the baseline whereas a poor underhand serve would land near the net (in the service receiving area). Serves were required to clear the net and an upright standard (2.44 m) positioned at the mid-court region of the receiving area. The purpose of the standard was to simulate an opponent's position in the opposite court and to force the server to maintain a high service trajectory. The dependent variable was the mean number of points scored for the badminton serve for each trial block.

Conditions

The learning strategy utilized in this study was based upon the Five-step Strategy (Singer, 1988). This strategy is a global one and is applicable to many different self-paced sport skills. This strategy and a control condition served as the treatment for the experimental groups and the control group, respectively.

Experimental groups.—Each of the experimental groups received the same instructions on utilization of the Five-step Strategy, but the timing for introduction of the strategy varied for each experimental group. The timing for introduction ranged from 100% to 17% of the total trials remaining for each participant. Specific information on the timing for strategy introduction is provided in the Procedure.

At the designated time while learning the skill, each participant in an experimental group was introduced to the Five-step Strategy. This introduction took place in an isolated room via taped instructions without the experimenter present. The taped instructions lasted for 12 min. and began with general information about how to use the strategy with self-paced sport skills. Subsequent information contained a description of each of the five steps (readying, imaging, focusing, executing, and evaluating) as they related to this specific badminton serve and accompanying practice activities after each step. Participants received an initial explanation for each respective step, a talk-through practice trial with an unrelated sport skill activity, and then were instructed to repeat without prompting three similar trials related to this task. Upon completion of the instructional tape, each participant was provided an opportunity to ask questions. Once the experimenter addressed questions, participants then returned to the badminton court and utilized the strategy to execute their remaining skill trials.

Control group.—The time spent and conditions for the control group were similar to those experienced by the experimental groups but with the exception that no strategy was provided. Rather, the control group listened to a 12-min. tape describing the various aspects of the sport of badminton including history, scoring, equipment and other general information. This condition was initiated to provide a similar experience. After completion of the tape, participants were allowed to ask questions and then proceeded to the badminton court to execute their serves.

Procedure

Once novice participants were identified and the informed consent form was read and signed, each participant was given directions and instructed on how to make the appropriate serve, then executed four practice trials. Then each participant received the respective treatment at the appropriate time and performed the service on an indoor regulation badminton court. After the practice trials and during the acquisition phase, participants served 60 attempts arranged in 6 blocks of 10 trials with 2-min. intervals between trial blocks. No skill correction or instruction was provided once the acquisition phase began. Each participant received the Five-step Strategy at their respective treatment group's designated time during the acquisition phase. Participants in the 100% group received the strategy prior to the start of any acquisition trials and could make use of the strategy for the entire study. The 83% group was instructed in strategy use following completion of Trial Block 1 and then could make use of the strategy during the remaining five trial blocks. Those participants in the 50% group received their strategy at the 50% mark upon completion of Trial Block 3. Players in the 17% group were administered the strategy following the execution of Trial Block 5 and used it for the remaining trial block. During acquisition, once the strategy had been received, the treatment groups were reminded every two trial blocks to use their strategy. The control group (0% group) and experimental groups, prior to obtaining their strategy introduction, were encouraged to "do their best."

Upon completion of the acquisition phase prior to the retention phase, all participants were asked to complete a simple 30-item arithmetic calculation test during this 10-min. interval to distract their thoughts from the task and treatment. At the end of this rest, participants executed the retention phase, which consisted of two trial blocks of 10 trials with a 2-min. interval between trial blocks. During retention, no mention was made regarding strategy use and no group was encouraged. At the end of the testing period, the experimental groups were assessed on a short questionnaire to examine the extent that the Five-step Strategy was utilized during the acquisition and retention phases of the study whereas the control group was questioned about strategy use.

RESULTS

Data for the acquisition phase were analyzed with a 5 (Group) × 6

(Trial Blocks) mixed-model analysis of variance with repeated measures on the last factor. Data for the retention phase were analyzed using a 5 (Group) × 2 (Trial Blocks) mixed-model analysis of variance with repeated measures on the last factor. Also, a 5 (Group) × 2 (Trial Blocks) mixed-model analysis of variance with repeated measures on the last factor was calculated to analyze Trial Block 6 of the acquisition phase and the first retention trial block. Alpha level was set at $p < .05$ and a Tukey *HSD* test was employed to follow-up significant main effects whereas simple effects tests were conducted as follow-up analyses for significant interactions.

Acquisition Phase

The results yielded a significant group main effect ($F_{4,45} = 2.95$, $p < .05$). Players in the 50% group performed significantly better serves than players in the 83%, 17% or 0% groups (see Table 1). However, no significant difference was found between the 100% group and the 50% group or the 0%

TABLE 1
MEANS AND STANDARD DEVIATIONS FOR GROUPS IN ACQUISITION PHASE

Group	M	SD
0%	2.73	.76
17%	2.87	.74
50%	3.15	.49
83%	2.87	.65
100%	2.95	.80

group. A significant Trial Block main effect ($F_{5,225} = 10.01$, $p < .05$) was found (see Table 2). Trial Block 6 was significantly higher than Trial Blocks 1, 2 and 3. Trial Blocks 4 and 5 were significantly higher than Trial Blocks 1 and 2. No significant Group × Trial Block interaction was obtained.

TABLE 2
MEANS AND STANDARD DEVIATIONS FOR TRIAL BLOCKS IN ACQUISITION PHASE

Trial Block	M	SD
1	2.52	.73
2	2.60	.70
3	2.81	.54
4	3.14	.69
5	3.16	.74
6	3.25	.65

Retention Phase

Analysis yielded a lack of significant findings for the retention phase. Furthermore, no significance was found when Trial Block 6 (acquisition phase) and Trial Block 1 (retention phase) were analyzed.

Strategy Follow-up Questionnaire

Analysis of the data obtained from the strategy follow-up questionnaire indicated that participants in the four experimental groups used the Five-step Strategy approximately 94% of the time after the strategy was made available. This was found for both the acquisition and retention phases.

Discussion

As expected, the 50% group made significantly better badminton serves than the 0% group and the 17% group. In addition, the 50% group performed better than the 83% but unexpectedly did not outperform the 100% group. The 100% group, while not significant, did perform better than the 0% group (which had the worst performance of all groups). This suggests that overall performance may decline in the absence of a strategy or if a strategy is provided at a point-in-time that is too late for learners to benefit from using that strategy. Furthermore, the 100% group was not significantly different from the 50% group, possibly indicating that introduction of a strategy should be incorporated with the learning of a skill or after the participant has become familiar with the skill.

Although very little research has been done, this finding is contradictory to what other researchers have found. As stated in the introduction, Singer, Flora, and Abourezk (1989) reported that the earlier a strategy is introduced to a learner the better the performance will be on a novel motor task of a low skill complexity. Perhaps the optimal point of time for introducing a strategy depends upon the type of task, the skill of the learner, and the type of strategy employed (Tennant, 2000).

Lastly, mean scores increased for all five groups during acquisition indicating that there was learning. Lack of significant differences between the acquisition and retention trials was an indication that performance gains made during the acquisition phase were true and not just performance artifacts (Magill, 1998). One may infer that learning occurred during acquisition and was maintained during retention.

The findings of this investigation appear to support the hypothesis that later strategy introduction is more effective than introduction of the strategy earlier in the acquisition process for a real world task. This finding suggests it may be more effective for students to acquire a basic understanding of the task first and then receive the learning strategy. If strategy benefits are unlikely to occur until after an individual becomes familiar with the task, then perhaps early strategy use is not the most efficient use of time for either the students or teacher. However, these later points need further examination in complex tasks to be generalized to different levels of skill and population types.

REFERENCES

BOHAN, M., PHARMER, J. A., & STOKES, A. F. (1999) When does imagery practice enhance performance on a motor task? *Perceptual and Motor Skills*, 88, 651-658.

BOUCHARD, L. J., & SINGER, R. N. (1998) Effects of the Five-step Strategy with videotape modeling on performance of the tennis serve. *Perceptual and Motor Skills*, 86, 739-746.

DANSEREAU, D. F., BROOKS, L. W., HOLLEY, C. D., & COLLINS, K. W. (1983) Learning strategies training: effects of sequencing. *Journal of Experimental Education*, 51, 102-108.

KIM, J., CHEN, D., SINGER, R N., TENNANT, L. K., & CHUNG, S. (1993) The Five-step Strategy and air gun shooting performance of expert versus novice shooter. *Journal of Exercise and Sport Psychology*, 15(Suppl.), S46.

KIM, J., SINGER, R. N., & RADLO, S. J. (1996) Degree of cognitive demands in psychomotor tasks and the effects of the Five-step Strategy on achievement. *Human Performance*, 9, 155-169.

KIM, J., & TENNANT, L. K. (1993) Effects of visualization and Danjeon breathing on target shooting with an air pistol. *Perceptual and Motor Skills*, 77, 1083-1087.

KIRSCHENBAUM, D. S. (1987) Self-regulation of sport performance. *Medicine and Science in Sports and Exercise*, 19, S106-S113.

LIDOR, R., TENNANT, L. K., & SINGER, R. N. (1996) The generalizability effect of three learning strategies across motor task performances. *International Journal of Sport Psychology*, 27, 23-36.

MAGILL, R. A. (1998) *Motor learning: concepts and applications*. (5th ed.) Boston, MA: McGraw-Hill.

MAHONEY, M. J. (1984) Cognitive skills and athletic performance. In W. F. Straub & J. M. Williams (Eds.), *Cognitive sport psychology*. Lansing, NY: Sport Science Associates. Pp. 11-27.

PRESSLEY, M., JOHNSON, C. J., SYMONS, S., MCGOLDRICK, J. A., & KURITA, J. A. (1989) Strategies that improve children's memory and comprehension of text. *The Elementary School Journal*, 90, 3-32.

RADLO, S. J., HYLLEGARD, R., & KARG, J. A. (2000) Combating competitive stress: an evaluation of a 16-week comprehensive stress management program. *Journal of Sport and Exercise Psychology*, 22, S88.

SINGER, R. N. (1988) Strategies and metastrategies in learning and performing self-paced athletic skills. *The Sport Psychologist*, 2, 49-68.

SINGER, R. N., CAURAUGH, J. H., TENNANT, L. K., MURPHEY, M., CHEN, D., & LIDOR, R. (1991) Attention and distractors: considerations for enhancing sport performance. *International Journal of Sport Psychology*, 22, 95-114.

SINGER, R. N., DEFRANCESCO, C., & RANDALL, L. E. (1989) Effectiveness of a global learning strategy practiced in different contexts on primary and transfer self-paced motor tasks. *Journal of Sport and Exercise Psychology*, 11, 290-303.

SINGER, R. N., FLORA, L. A., & ABOUREZK, T. L. (1989) The effect of a five-step cognitive learning strategy on the acquisition of a complex motor task. *Applied Sport Psychology*, 1, 98-108.

SINGER, R. N., & SUWANTHADA, S. (1986) The generalizability effectiveness of a learning strategy on achievement in related closed motor skills. *Research Quarterly for Exercise and Sport*, 57, 205-214.

STEINBERG, G. M., & GLASS, B. (2001) Can the Five-step Strategy enhance the learning of motor skills in older adults? *Journal of Aging and Physical Activity*, 9, 1-10.

TAKAI, K. (1998) Cognitive strategies and recall of pace by long-distance runners. *Perceptual and Motor Skills*, 86, 763-770.

TENNANT, L. M. (2000) Cognitive learning strategies: their effectiveness in acquiring racquetball skill. *Perceptual and Motor Skills*, 90, 867-874.

WEINBERG, R., GROVE, R., & JACKSON, A. (1992) Strategies for building self-efficacy in tennis players: a comparative analysis of Australian and American coaches. *The Sport Psychologist*, 6, 3-13.

YANG, J. J., & PORRETTA, D. L. (1999) Sport/leisure skill learning by adolescents with mild mental retardation: a four-step strategy. *Adapted Physical Activity Quarterly*, 16, 300-315.

ZERVAS, Y., & KAKKOS, V. (1995) The effect of visuomotor behavior rehearsal on shooting performance of beginning archers. *International Journal of Sport Psychology*, 26, 337-347.

Accepted April 16, 2004.

STUDENTS' PERCEPTIONS OF DANGEROUSNESS TO PUBLIC SAFETY OF PARAPHRASES FROM THE KORAN, NEW TESTAMENT, BOOK OF MORMON, TIBETAN BOOK OF THE DEAD, AND EGYPTIAN BOOK OF THE DEAD PRESENTED AS PATIENTS' BELIEFS[1]

M. A. PERSINGER

Laurentian University

Summary.—In one experiment 40 first-year psychology students were asked to judge dangerousness to society of 10 fictitious patients who professed beliefs about an "alien." The statements were actually paraphrases primarily concerning death and killing from the New Testament, the Koran, the Book of Mormon, the Egyptian Book of the Dead and the Tibetan Book of the Dead. In a second experiment 39 first-year psychology students were asked to rate the dangerousness of the verbatim statements with their sources identified. In the first experiment, statements from the Koran, which involved accessing a positive afterlife by killing nonbelievers in the name of a deity, were ranked as more dangerous. The differences between the sources accommodated 33% of the variance in the rankings for dangerousness. The group of students who were given the original statements and their actual sources ranked the statements from the New Testament and the Koran as significantly less dangerous than those who were told the statements were from patients. These results suggest that statements about killing and death may be rated as less dangerous if the person believes the source was a "sacred text."

The primary theme of religious beliefs involves death and the survival of death through affiliation with an omnipotent, omniscient and eternal Being. All religions emphasize one of three anxiolytic solutions to the cognitive sequence "I will die" that can be considered a semantic form of conditioned suppression (Persinger, 1985). Challenge of the absolute truth of these beliefs threatens the person's anticipation that some component of the self survives.

One response by groups of *Homo sapiens* who endorse the same religious belief has been to marginalize or even to kill those who do not believe similarly. The simple existence of these "others" potentially indicts the validity of the group's one "true" deity and all of the assumptions associated with it (Persinger, 1987). Although some scholars may attribute this behavior to secondary factors such as poverty, restrictive religious environments, or the intrinsic discrimination by human perception, the propensity to kill

---

[1]Address correspondence to Dr. M. A. Persinger, Behavioral Neuroscience Laboratory, Department of Psychology, Laurentian University, Sudbury, ON Canada P3E 2C6 or e-mail mpersinger@laurentian.ca).

others who "do not believe" may be encouraged by reading statements that are believed to be the words of Yahweh, Allah or some God-equivalent.

Beliefs encourage the reflexive acceptance of the meaning of statements attributed to deities or to cultural traditions if they are coupled with the person's definition of self or the self's survival of death. A phrase such as "belief requires faith rather than logic or proof" is a common example. However, this mentality may be dangerous. About 7% of a sample of university students reported they would kill in God's name if He told them to do so (Persinger, 1997). This percentage increased to 45% if the person was male, displayed elevated complex partial epileptic-like signs, reported a religious experience as a child, and attended church regularly (Buckman, 2002).

Some religious texts, such as the Koran, contain statements that promise greater access to a positive afterlife (Paradise) if the believer kills others or is killed in the process of killing others, particularly nonbelievers, in the deity's (Allah's) name. The purpose of the present study was to discern if beliefs about killing or death, extracted from five scriptural traditions, would be judged by a sample of university students as differentially dangerous to society. To remove the religious association with these statements, the names of the deities were changed in one experiment to "The Alien," and words that might identify the source were paraphrased.

Method

Subjects

In Exp. I (2001-2002) a total of 13 men and 27 women and in Exp. II (2002-2003) 15 men and 24 women who were enrolled in first-year psychology courses were recruited as subjects. Their ages ranged between 19 and 35 years of age. About 60% of the subjects indicated they were Roman Catholic, 25% reported they were some variation of Protestant, and 15% indicated they were not affiliated, agnostic or atheists.

Procedure

In a single sitting in March (2002 and 2003) during the last hour of a regular 3-hr. class period students were asked to read the following information under the title "Clinical Rating Exercise." The subjects had been exposed to about six hours of lecture material regarding abnormal psychology and had read multiple examples of letters from individuals who were diagnosed with different pathologies. All of the students who attended the lectures completed the task that required about 20 min.

In Exp. I (March 2002) the instructions were "Read the following comments of delusional patients about their reports of receiving special information during alien abductions." [The specific names of "the entity" have been changed simply to "alien."] Your task is to determine which of these patients are most dangerous to society because of their beliefs about their own immortality or definitions of self with respect to dissolution of the self, i.e., death. Your job is to protect the public from "dangerous offenders." The subjects were then given a Likert-type scale with anchors of 1 (not dangerous) and 4 (ambiguous) and 7 (very dangerous). The instructions below the scale stated "Read each patient's comments and then rank the risk of killing others due to the 'logic' of the delusion by assigning a number from 1 through 7."

The "patients" were identified only by letters A to J. The comments for the 10 patients were paraphrased from five sources of scriptures (2 per source) that included the New Testament (Jehovah Witness translation: New World Translation of the Holy Scriptures, 1984), the Egyptian Book of the Dead (Budge, 1967), the Tibetan Book of the Dead (Evans-Wentz, 1960), the Koran (Dawwood, 1956) and the Book of Mormon (1981). The two paraphrases were comments concerning killing, dying/destruction, or creation/survival that had been selected randomly from a list of statements and page numbers (from the author's notes when the documents were read several years ago) containing these words. The specific paraphrases that the subjects read, and the actual sources (indicated in parentheses) are listed below.

A. I saw the dead, the great and the small, standing before the Alien. The books were opened; it was the book of life. The dead were judged according to what was reported in the books. These things indicted the behavior of the dead when they were living. Those names not found in the book will be thrown into a lake of fire (Bible, Revelations 20:12-14).

B. When you die, you experience illusions. Along the bright light path there are hallucinations of fear, awe, and terror. The forces of anger protect us in the front and in the back. If we are lucky, we are saved from passing through the narrow and fearful passage and enter into a state with the Alien (Tibetan Book of the Dead; Budge, 1967).

C. If you should die or be killed in the cause of the Alien, the Alien's forgiveness and mercy would be surely better than all the riches. If you die or be killed, you will be taken by the Alien into his midst (the Koran, the Imrans; Dawwood, 1956, p. 410).

D. The Alien created the universe. The Alien made human beings. The Alien is merciful to those who embrace his existence. If you think about him, he knows this. If you admit the Alien is there he knows you and he will protect you (the Egyptian Book of the Dead; Budge, 1967, p. xciii).

E. The Alien became flesh like a person. He died for all people so that all people might be helped by the Alien. All humans must die. To fulfill the plan of the Creator of the Universe there must be the phenomenon of surviving death. Death occurred because people engaged in nonoptimal behav-

TABLE 1
Means and Standard Deviations For Ranks of Dangerousness Given Statements From Religious Books Masked as Comments From Delusional Patients (Exp. I) or Stated Verbatim With Sources Identified (Exp. II) and Means and Standard Deviations For Various Questionnaire Data and Percentages For Information Items

Variable	Exp. I (n=40) Masked Paraphrase M	SD	Exp. II (n=39) Actual Quote M	SD	ω^2_{est}, %
Dangerousness Ratings					
New Testament (Bible)	4.0	1.3	2.6	1.5	20
Koran	5.4	1.1	4.5	1.9	8
Book of Mormon	4.1	1.5	4.9	1.7	7
Tibetan Book of the Dead	3.1	1.3	2.9	1.6	ns
Egyptian Book of the Dead	4.3	1.1	3.4	2.1	ns
Questionnaire Data					
Tobacyk Religious Subscale	4.2	1.8	4.0	1.6	ns
Dissociative Experiences	16.2	10.7	17.7	10.9	ns
Rotton's Paralogic	8.1	2.1	7.8	2.0	ns
Coopersmith Self-esteem	67.7	14.9	63.5	15.2	ns
Wilson-Barber Imaginings	22.9	8.7	22.0	7.0	ns
Personal Philosophy Inventory					
Religious Beliefs	32	30	30	18	ns
Exotic Beliefs	54	26	51	25	ns
Temporal Lobe Scale	42	18	40	17	ns
Religious Extreme Beliefs	15	19	14	23	ns
Forbidden Knowledge	47	27	48	25	ns
History of Sensed Presence	20	26	33	31	10
Prose/Poetry Meaningfulness	39	31	41	31	ns
Vestibular Effects	43	34	38	27	ns
Parapsychological Experiment	37	25	29	25	ns
Single Item Responses (%)					
Believe in God	73		68		
Attend Church Once/Month	20		13		
Had a religious experience	29		19		

Experiment I ("Delusional Statements")

Three-way analysis of variance as a function of the five sources (scriptures) for the paraphrases and the rater's endorsement of religious beliefs (lower third, middle third, upper third of the scores for Tobacyk's scale) and sex demonstrated no statistically significant differences in the overall ranking of perceived dangerousness of the "patients" as a function of the intensity of endorsement of religious beliefs ($F_{2,31} = 2.14$, ns) or sex ($F_{1,31} = 2.62$, ns). The interaction between sex and religious beliefs was not significant ($F_{2,31} = .18$, ns).

However there was a significant difference ($F_{4,124} = 17.62$, $p < .001$; $\eta^2 = .33$) between the ranks of dangerousness for the "patients" representing the five scriptures. *Post hoc* analysis (correlated t tests) indicated that the patients whose paraphrases were derived from the Koran were ranked as significantly ($p<.01$) more dangerous to society than patients whose paraphrases were from the Tibetan Book of the Dead, Book of Mormon, or the New Testament. The scores for the Egyptian Book of the Dead occupied intermediate positions.

To accommodate individual differences the z scores for the person's ranks for each of the five sources were calculated by subtracting the raw score for each source from the mean for all five sources and then dividing by the standard deviation of the scores for all five sources. The differences among the five sources of paraphrases were statistically significant ($F_{4,124}=16.89$, $p<.001$; variance explained = 32%).

The only statistically significant correlations (all *rho*s) between the scores for each of the five sources and the five different questionnaires and the nine different clusters from the Personal Philosophy Inventory given 5 mo. earlier were between a History of a sensed presence, Extreme religious beliefs, Parapsychological experiences, and Forbidden knowledge, and scores on the items derived from the Koran. The ranking of dangerousness for Patients C ($rho=-.30$) and F ($rho=-.33$) whose statements were paraphrases from the Koran were significantly ($p<.05$) correlated with the students' scores for extreme religious beliefs. Their scores for forbidden knowledge ($rho=-.33$) were associated with ranking for Patient C while a history of sensed presence was associated ($rho=-.35$) with the ranking for Patient F.

Exp. II: Direct Sources Identified

Three-way analysis of variance with one within-subject level (sources) and two between-subject levels (trichotomy of subject's scores for Tobacyk's scale and sex) indicated a statistically significant difference between the overall ratings of dangerousness ($F_{1,33}=5.09$, $p<.05$). *Post hoc* analysis indicated that the individuals with the highest scores (above 4.8) for religious belief rated all statements as more dangerous ($M=4.5$, $SD=1.2$) than those with the intermediate scores (2.8 through 4.7; dangerousness $M=3.2$, $SD=1.0$). There were no statistically significant sex differences or interaction between sex and religious belief.

The differences in ratings of dangerousness between sources was statistically significant ($F_{4,160}=11.32$, $p<.001$; $\eta^2=29\%$). This effect size did not change appreciably when the z scores, standardized for within-subject variance, were analyzed separately. The two two-way interactions and the three-way interaction were not statistically significant. *Post hoc* t tests for the original scores indicated that statements from the Koran, Book of Mormon, and Egyptian Book of the Dead were ranked as more dangerous than the statements from the New Testament and the Tibetan Book of the Dead.

Correlations (Spearman *rho*s) between the scores for dangerousness and those on each of the 14 scales were statistically significant between the ratings of dangerousness for the quotes from the New Testament and the religious belief cluster from the Personal Philosophy Inventory (.36), the religious belief scale from Tobacyk (.50), and the experience of meaningfulness while reading prose and poetry (–.40). The only other source that was significantly ($p < .05$) correlated with the psychometric variables was the Tibetan Book of the Dead. Ratings of dangerous were negatively correlated with complex partial signs (–.46), and histories of sensed presences (–.40), vestibular-auditory experiences (–.45), and parapsychological experiences (–.30).

To investigate the potential source for the positive correlation ($r = .44$, $p < .01$) between the ratings of dangerousness for the scriptures from the New Testament and the magnitude of religious belief, partial correlations with each of the 14 scales were completed (all $dfs = 38$). Removal of the shared variance with these variables did not appreciably alter the strength of the correlation between dangerousness and the intensity of religious belief that remained between .40 and .44.

Both Groups Compared

According to a two-way analysis of variance with one between- and one within-subject level (source: Bible, Koran, Mormon, Egyptian, and Tibetan) the students who knew the actual sources of the statements rated them as significantly less dangerous ($F_{1,77} = 4.71$, $p < .05$; $\eta^2 = 6\%$) than those who did not. However, there was a significant interaction between the specific source and the two groups ($F_{4,308} = 26.62$, $p < .001$; $\eta^2 = 25\%$).

Post hoc analysis with one-way analysis of variance (all $dfs = 1,77$) indicated that the group who were given the exact quote and their sources rated the statements from the New Testament as significantly less dangerous ($F = 19.40$, $p < .001$) than those who read the paraphrases as originating from delusional patients. Statements from the Koran were judged as less dangerous by the group who knew the original source ($F = 6.71$, $p < .01$) while the statements from the Book of Mormon were rated as more dangerous ($F = 5.97$, $p < .01$). There were no statistically significant differences between the groups for their ratings of the statements from the Tibetan and Egyptian books of the dead. There were no statistically significant differences between the two groups on any of the 14 scales indicated in Table 1.

DISCUSSION

The major themes of religious texts are: (1) there is an implicit organizing force in the universe (the largest conceptual set for space), (2) there is meaning to existence and (3) a component of the self is eternal or infinite (the largest conceptual set for time). Religious texts refer frequently to death and its most common precipitant: killing. Considering the role of religious beliefs as possible neurocognitive processes that reduce death anxiety by principles of operant conditioning (Persinger, 1985), these themes would be expected.

However, many of these texts, such as the Bible and the Koran, contain many references to death by killing. Often the killing of other groups of people (even in their own habitat) is considered justified because members of the reference group assumed they were "the chosen people" by the "only" God. Frequently there are statements, attributed to God, that condone the execution of nonbelievers because they are "less than human," dangerous or even the defined manifestation of the cultural symbol for the most intense aversive stimuli ("evil").

The results of the first study indicated that the statements referring to death or killing from the Koran (even though the subject did not know this was the source) were ranked as more dangerous than statements from other religious texts. The primary source of this dangerousness was the theme that to access the maximum benefits of eternal life (the maximum reduction of death anxiety) the believer must kill nonbelievers. Even when these statements were disguised as comments from delusional patients, the comments were ranked as more dangerous to society by these first-year university students. The mean of the ranks for the paraphrases from the Koran was the only value within the range of "dangerous to society" along the Likert-type scale.

Students who ranked the statements from the Koran as less dangerous scored higher on clusters of items that reflect that some knowledge is forbidden and extreme religious beliefs (such as "if God told me to kill, I would in His Name"). Those who ranked the statements from the Koran as less dangerous were also more likely to have reported the experience of a sensed presence. Clearly, the variables that encourage an experience of a sensed presence to be associated with the perceived permission to kill others in the presence's name must be discerned.

An association between the beliefs that killing is endorsed by the believer's deity and that access to specific areas of knowledge by scientific inquiry should be restricted has serious cultural implications. Scientific examination of *all* knowledge, including the genetic definition of human life, might enhance anxiety because the results could repudiate the validity of the belief and hence the person's immortality. Such avoidance might be a normal cognitive process which prevents a conclusion whose consequences could be devastating to the person's sense of self.

The results of Exp. II, completed 1 yr. later, also showed significant differences between the rankings of dangerousness of statements from the five sources even when they were clearly identified for the subjects. The statements from the Koran and the Book of Mormon were ranked as significantly more dangerous than those from the Tibetan Book of the Dead, the Egyptian Book of the Dead, or the New Testament.

When data of both studies were compared, rankings of dangerousness were significantly less when the group was told the sources of the statements. Even the dangerousness of the statements from the Koran was ranked lower when the source was identified at the time of the ranking. However, the most powerful result was the marked reduction, by a standard deviation, in the judged dangerousness of statements from the New Testament when the subjects knew the source. This predominately Christian sample rated the statements as effectively not dangerous.

A significant positive correlation ($rho = .50$) was noted between the rating of dangerousness for the statements from the New Testament and the magnitude of the endorsement of religious beliefs for the subjects who knew the sources. Partial correlation analyses with scores for dissociation, temporal lobe signs, imaginings, self-esteem, logical solutions, and other measures did not significantly alter the strength of this association. Unless this correlation is an artifact of the restricted range of the score, this relationship suggests that respondents who are more religious within the Christian tradition actively rank the statements as more dangerous. Whether they are unaware of this implication or their belief increases their sensitivity to dangerousness, even when derived from the New Testament, remains to be tested.

The differences in ratings between the two groups might be an artifact of two different classes tested in two different years. However if these striking differences are not spurious, then the role of attribution and source in the rankings of dangerousness of verbal sequences could be more important than previously assumed. It is possible that the emphasis in Canada upon "multiculturalism," "coerced political correctness," and the "concern about hurting people's feelings" may have contributed to the lower scores for the dangerousness of statements from the Koran when the subjects knew it was the source. The role of duplicity or learned avoidance of decisions which could be judged as confrontational rather than cooperative must still be evaluated.

The limitation of this study is clearly related to the phrases that were selected from the various religious scriptures and to testing by questionnaires. The results do not necessarily suggest that Islamic believers who endorse the Koran are any more or less extreme than the primarily Roman Catholic students who were subjects in this study. Islamic believers were not tested. However, if the denotative and connotative properties of the semantic and syntactic organizations of a person's language affect personal behavior, then the numbers of repetitions of phrases referring to killing others might become associated with the probability of these responses. This argument has been invoked, although without empirical causal evidence to "protect the public," to restrict or deny access to television programs, movies, Web sites, and even printed material.

REFERENCES

BERNSTEIN, E. M., & PUTNAM, F. W. (1986) Development, reliability, and validity of dissociation scale. *Journal of Nervous and Mental Disease*, 184, 727-734.

The Book of Mormon. (1981) Salt Lake City, UT: Corporation of the President of the Church of Jesus Christ and the Latter-day Saints.

BUCKMAN, R. (2002) *Can we be good without God?* New York: Prometheus.

BUDGE, E. A. W. (Transl.) (1967) *The Egyptian book of the dead.* New York: Dover.

DAWWOOD, N. J. (Transl.) (1956) *The Koran.* New York: Penguin.

EVANS-WENTZ, W. Y. (Transl.) (1960) *The Tibetan book of the dead.* London: Oxford.

New world translation of the Holy Scriptures. (1984) Brooklyn, NY: Watchtower Bible & Tract Society of New York.

PERSINGER, M. A. (1985) Death anxiety as a semantic conditioned suppression paradigm. *Perceptual and Motor Skills*, 60, 827-830.

PERSINGER, M. A. (1987) *Neuropsychological bases of god beliefs.* New York: Praeger.

PERSINGER, M. A. (1992) Criterion validity for Rotton's paralogic test: beliefs of forbidden knowledge may negatively affect inferential problem solving. *Perceptual and Motor Skills*, 74, 1027-1030.

PERSINGER, M. A. (1997) I would kill in God's name: role of sex, weekly church attendance, report of a religious experience, and limbic lability. *Perceptual and Motor Skills*, 85, 128-130.

PERSINGER, M. A., & MAKAREC, K. (1993) Complex partial epileptic signs as a continuum from normals to epileptics. *Journal of Clinical Psychology*, 49, 33-43.

TOBACYK, J. (1985) Paranormal beliefs, alienation, and anomie in college students. *Psychological Reports*, 57, 844-846.

WILSON, S. C., & BARBER, T. X. (1984) The fantasy-prone personality: implications for understanding imagery, hypnosis, and parapsychological phenomena. In A. A. Sheikh (Ed.), *Imagery: current theory, research and application.* New York: Wiley. Pp. 340-387.

Accepted April 15, 2004.

MOCK JURORS' PERCEPTIONS OF FACIAL HAIR ON CRIMINAL OFFENDERS [1]

RICHARD P. CONTI

College of Saint Elizabeth
Montclair State University

MELANIE A. CONTI

College of Saint Elizabeth

Summary.—Two studies were conducted to measure whether mock jurors would stereotype criminal offenders as having facial hair. In Study 1, participants were asked which photograph belonged to a defendant in a rape case and which photograph belonged to a plaintiff in a head-injury case after they were "accidentally" dropped. The photographs were similar in appearance except one had facial hair. 78% of 63 participants (or 49) identified the photograph with facial hair as being involved in the rape case. In Study 2, 371 participants were asked to sketch the face of a criminal offender. 82% of the sketches (or 249) contained some form of facial hair. Results are consistent with the hypothesis that criminal defendants are perceived as having facial hair.

It is a well-known practice among attorneys to advise their clients to shave prior to trial (Bailey & Rothblatt, 1987), however, no empirical research was found for the effectiveness of this practice or how a jury might respond. Historically, fictional characters portrayed as "villains" in movies, comics, and in books tend to have some form of facial hair, e.g., Brutus from Popeye, Blackbeard the infamous pirate, bandits of the old West, while the "hero" is usually clean-shaven, e.g., superheroes, James Bond. Even the devil, who is considered the most evil of all, has facial hair. Based on the above examples, it seems that in the media, "bad guys" are stereotyped as having facial hair. In reality, many leaders of nations who have been considered in the United States at one point in time unfriendly have facial hair. Some examples include Castro, Stalin, Lenin, Hitler, Saddam Hussein, and more recently, Osama Bin Laden. In contrast, few U.S. politicians, especially former presidents, have facial hair. In one criminal trial, the prosecution struck two jurors because they were the only two who had facial hair. According to the prosecutor, the mustaches and the beards looked suspicious (*Purkett v. Elem*, 1995). Even Disneyland employees are prohibited from wearing beards; the company recently lifted a 45-yr.-old ban prohibiting all facial hair on employees (a neatly trimmed mustache is allowed). The company stated that it receives daily feedback from its guests and wants to be a role model for young children (Disney, 2000).

---

[1]Address correspondence to Richard P. Conti, Department of Psychology, College of Saint Elizabeth, 2 Convent Road, Morristown, NJ 07960-6989 or e-mail (mconti@cse.edu).

Research on facial hair has shown that men with beards tend to be perceived as more aggressive, dominant, powerful (Addison, 1989), emotionally distant (Freedman, 1969; Addison, 1989), masculine (Freedman, 1969; Roll & Verinis, 1971; Kenny & Fletcher, 1973; Pellegrini, 1973; Feinman & Gill, 1977; Pancer & Meindl, 1978; Addison, 1989; Cunningham, Barbee, & Pike, 1990), dirtier, extroverted (Roll & Verinis, 1971; Kenny & Fletcher, 1973), stronger (Roll & Verinis, 1971; Kenny & Fletcher, 1973; Pancer & Meindl, 1978; Addison, 1989), outgoing, reckless, younger (Pancer & Meindl, 1978), and less competent (Terry & Krantz, 1993). Mustachioed men are seen as unkind and bad (Roll & Verinis, 1971). From the above descriptions, men with facial hair seem to be perceived as "hypermasculine" or somewhat threatening. Shakespeare once remarked, "He that hath no beard is less than a man". Conversely, men who are clean-shaven are perceived as more attractive, sociable (Wogalter & Hosie, 1991), kind, clean, and good (Roll & Verinis, 1971), and babyish (Cunningham, et al., 1990). Physically attractive defendants tend to gain the sympathy of the jury, be found not guilty, and receive lighter sentences (Downs & Lyons, 1991; Wuensch, Castellow, & Moore, 1991; Mazzella & Feingold, 1994; DeSantis & Kayson, 1997). Research has also shown that criminal offenders are perceived as less physically attractive than controls (Raine, 1993).

Based upon the above review of effects related to facial hair, two studies were conducted to measure stereotypes of criminal defendants with facial hair. It was hypothesized that mock jurors would identify criminal offenders (or defendants perceived as offenders prior to trial) as having some sort of facial hair.

In Study 1, college students between the ages of 18 and 25 years were individually seen in each author's office during scheduled office hours for an unrelated issue. As the students were leaving, a fictional case file was "accidentally" dropped in the presence of each participant. As the folder dropped, two black and white photographs of similar looking men, one clean-shaven the other bearded, fell to the ground. The experimenter retrieved the file with the two photographs and remarked, "one of these is a defendant in a rape case and the other is a plaintiff in a head injury case. I cannot remember which is which." If any participant responded by saying "this one looks like...", the response was recorded. The folder was dropped on 72 occasions. Nine participants had no opinion of which photograph belonged to which crime. Of those who responded ($N=63$), 78% (49) felt the photograph of the bearded man belonged with the rape case, while only 22% (14) felt the clean shaven man belonged with the rape case.

In the second study, adults eligible for jury duty ($N=371$) between the ages of 19 and 63 were asked to sketch the face of a criminal offender. A recall method rather than a recognition method was used to avoid priming.

The sketches were then examined for facial hair. The tally was obtained: 67% (249) of the drawings had a beard or facial hair other than a moustache; 15% (54) had just a moustache. The proportion of sketches with facial hair was 82% (303).

These two studies assessed whether there is a greater likelihood of jurors to believe defendants have facial hair. Previous research has indicated that men with facial hair are perceived in ways which one could easily associate with the stereotypical criminal offender. As Cunningham, et al. (1990) pointed out, "the presence of a beard may cause a face that already appears mature to look too dominant and, thus, threatening" (p. 63). The results of both studies indicate that jurors may stereotype criminal offenders as having some type of facial hair. Thus, the advice given by attorneys to appear in court clean-shaven seems to be sensible and may even be an asset to one's case.

REFERENCES

Addison, W. E. (1989) Beardedness as a factor in perceived masculinity. *Perceptual and Motor Skills*, 68, 921-922.

Bailey, F. L., & Rothblatt, H. B. (1987) *Successful techniques for criminal trials*. (2nd ed.) Rochester, NY: Lawyers Cooperative.

Cunningham, M. R., Barbee, A. P., & Pike, C. L. (1990) What do women want? Facial metric assessment of multiple motives in the perception of male facial physical attractiveness. *Journal of Personality and Social Psychology*, 59, 61-72.

DeSantis, A., & Kayson, W. A. (1997) Defendants' characteristics of attractiveness, race, and sex and sentencing decisions. *Psychological Reports*, 81, 679-683.

Disney shaves facial hair ban. (2000) *Workforce*, 79, 26-27.

Downs, A. C., & Lyons, P. M. (1991) Natural observations of the links between attractiveness and initial legal judgments. *Personality and Social Psychology Bulletin*, 17, 541-547.

Feinman, S., & Gill, G. W. (1977) Females' response to males' beardedness. *Perceptual and Motor Skills* 44, 533-534.

Freedman, D. G. (1969) The survival value of the beard. *Psychology Today*, 3(10), 36-39.

Kenny, C. T., & Fletcher, D. (1973) Effects of beardedness on person perception. *Perceptual and Motor Skills* 37, 413-414.

Mazzella, R., & Feingold, A. (1994) The effects of physical attractiveness, race, socioeconomic status, and gender of defendants and victims on judgments of mock jurors: a meta-analysis. *Journal of Applied Social Psychology*, 24, 1315-1344.

Pancer, S. M., & Meindl, J. R. (1978) Length of hair and beardedness as determinants of personality impressions. *Perceptual and Motor Skills*, 46, 1328-1330.

Pellegrini, R. J. (1973) Impressions of the male personality as a function of beardness. *Psychology: A Journal of Human Behavior*, 10, 29-33.

Raine, A. R. (1993) *The psychopathology of crime: criminal behavior as a clinical disorder*. San Diego, CA: Academic Press.

Roll, S., & Verinis, J. S. (1971) Stereotypes of scalp and facial hair as measured by the semantic differential. *Psychological Reports*, 28, 975-980.

Terry, R. L., & Krantz, J. H. (1993) Dimensions of trait attributions associated with eyeglasses, men's facial hair, and women's hair length. *Journal of Applied Social Psychology*, 23, 1757-1769.

Wogalter, M. S., & Hosie, J. A. (1991) Effects of cranial and facial hair on perceptions of age and person. *The Journal of Social Psychology*, 131, 589-591.

Wuensch, K. L., Castellow, W. A., & Moore, C. H. (1991) Effects of defendant attractiveness and type of crime on juridic judgment. *Journal of Social Behavior and Personality*, 6, 713-724.

Accepted April 29, 2004.

DEMENTIA AND IDENTIFICATION OF WORDS AND SENTENCES PRODUCED BY NATIVE AND NONNATIVE ENGLISH SPEAKERS [1]

ANGELA N. BURDA, CARLIN F. HAGEMAN,
KELLY T. BROUSARD, AND ANDREA L. MILLER

University of Northern Iowa

Summary.—The accurate identification of 30 words and 15 sentences spoken by native English, Taiwanese, and Spanish speakers was compared for 16 persons with and 16 persons without dementia. Statistically significant differences for words and sentences occurred between groups of listeners.

Dementia is a growing problem in the USA (Hybels & Blazer, 2002), but the need to communicate with others, both native and nonnative speakers of English, does not diminish in the presence of dementia. Dementia, when caused by Alzheimer disease or vascular disease, is a progressive disease with the key feature being severe memory loss for recent events and information (Hopper & Bayles, 2001). In dementia, reduced memory leads to inaccurate processing during listening and inappropriate responses to the communicating partner, contributing to a breakdown in communication. Individuals with dementia may act out, withdraw, or become agitated (Santo Pietro & Ostuni, 2003). Written supplements may reduce working memory and improve communication (Bourgeois, 1992). To that end, the following hypotheses were tested: that dementia affects accurate identification of words and sentences spoken by native and nonnative speakers of English, and that the native language of the speaker affects the accuracy of identification of words and sentences in persons with and without dementia.

METHOD

Participants

Participants, all volunteers, were 32 English-speaking residents in assisted living facilities from small Midwest communities. Sixteen had early to middle stage dementia (3 men, 13 women) due to either Alzheimer disease or vascular disease according to their medical charts (ages 63 to 97 years, $M = 85.1$, $SD = 8.2$). The other sixteen served as neurologically intact controls (3 men, 13 women; ages 58 to 93 years, $M = 83.5$, $SD = 8.6$). All had finished high school or more, passed a hearing screening, and completed the Mini-Mental State Examination (Folstein, Folstein, & McHugh, 1975) with a

---

[1]Address correspondence to Angela N. Burda, Ph.D., Department of Communicative Disorders, University of Northern Iowa, 230 Communication Arts Center, Cedar Falls, IA 50614-0356 or e-mail (angela.burda@uni.edu).

mean score of 19.1 ($SD=4.95$) for those with dementia and 27.4 ($SD=1.6$) for those without dementia.

Stimuli

Three native female speakers of English, Taiwanese, and Spanish produced the words and sentences in English. Nonnative speakers were judged by two expert raters to have moderate accents. Thirty words and 15 sentences ranging in length from 6 to 10 words were taken from the Assessment of Intelligibility of Dysarthric Speech (Yorkston & Beukelman, 1984). A blocked random sample of spoken words was chosen based on sounds problematic for nonnative speakers of English, e.g., /r/, th/. Stimuli were digitized onto a compact disc at 21,000 samples per second and matched for intensity within 1 dB using the Cool Edit Pro audio editing program.

Procedure

Stimuli were presented in a quiet room at conversational intensity (60–65 dB) measured by a sound level meter (Qwest, Model No. 1400) located where listeners sat. Presentation of words and sentences was counterbalanced. Using 48-point Times New Roman font, written words (3 foils and one correct) and sentences (one foil and one correct) were given to participants (see Appendix, p. 1362). Listeners heard each stimulus word once and were instructed to point to the item they heard.

Results

Overall mean accuracy of identification of the correct words and sentences was obtained for both groups of participants across the three speakers (see Table 1). A series of two-by-three analyses of variance tested for statistically significant differences across groups and speakers. Statistically significant differences occurred between listener groups for words ($F_{1,90}=8.8$, $p<.005$) and sentences ($F_{1,90}=9.5$, $p<.005$), and across speakers for words ($F_{2,90}=4.0$, $p<.05$). Post hoc testing indicated that words produced by the native English speaker were more accurately recognized than those spoken by the native Spanish speaker (Tukey value = 1.3, $p<.01$) but not by the Taiwanese speaker (Tukey value = .63, $p>.33$). No statistically significant differences were obtained across speakers for the sentences ($F_{2,90}=.6$, $p>.05$). Interaction effects were not significant for words ($F_{2,90}=.6$, $p>.05$) or sentences ($F_{2,90}=.2$, $p>.05$).

Effect size (d) was estimated and interpreted using Cohen (1988) where 0.2 is a small effect size, 0.5 is a medium effect size, and 0.8 is a large effect size (Table 1). The effect size for differences between demented and nondemented listeners was medium or large across all speakers (range .4 to .9). The largest effect sizes occurred between the native Spanish and Taiwanese speakers.

TABLE 1
MEANS FOR CORRECT IDENTIFICATION OF WORDS AND SENTENCES

Task	Total Possible	Dementia M	SD	No Dementia M	SD	Effect Size	Power
Words							
Overall	30	22.1	5.1	24.7	5.5	0.5	0.7
English	10	8.4	2.1	9.0	1.1	0.4	0.8
Taiwanese	10	7.6	2.0	8.6	1.4	0.6	0.7
Spanish	10	6.7	1.9	8.6	2.4	0.9	0.3
Sentences							
Overall	15	13.5	3.0	14.9	0.3	0.7	0.6
English	5	4.6	1.1	5.0	0.0	0.5	0.7
Taiwanese	5	4.6	0.7	5.0	0.0	0.8	0.4
Spanish	5	4.3	1.3	4.9	0.3	0.6	0.6

Note.—Effect size (Cohen, 1988) and power (Howell, 2004) were calculated using $p < .05$.

In summary, the presence of dementia resulted in a statistically significant decrement in performance by the demented listeners compared to the nondemented listeners. All listeners, regardless of their mental status, found the native Spanish speaker most difficult to understand. There were no interactions of speaker with words or sentences.

DISCUSSION

Persons with dementia have considerable difficulty with recent memory, making it difficult to process what is spoken to them. Findings from this study suggest that presence of dementia makes verbal recognition tasks more difficult and so does the presence of a speaker's accent for words. These preliminary data raise several issues concerning how best to facilitate communication with demented persons residing in health care centers. Further study of accented speech in the daily care of this population is indicated. Likewise, the length and complexity of stimuli presented to listeners with dementia are also in need of further study using male and female speakers and a variety of accents, with and without written supplements to aid comprehension. In summary, this investigation showed large effects for persons showing the presence or absence of dementia for listening tasks which required recognition of printed responses. However, the influence of a speaker's accent requires further study.

REFERENCES

BOURGEOIS, M. S. (1992) Evaluating memory wallets in conversation with persons with dementia. *Journal of Speech and Hearing Research*, 35, 1344-1357.
COHEN, J. (1988) *Statistical power analysis for the behavioral sciences.* (2nd ed.) Hillsdale, NJ: Erlbaum.
FOLSTEIN, M. F., FOLSTEIN, S. E., & MCHUGH, P. R. (1975) Mini-Mental State. *Journal of Psychiatric Research*, 12, 189-198.
HOPPER, T., & BAYLES, K. A. (2001) Management of neurogenic communication disorders asso-

ciated with dementia. In R. Chapey (Ed.), *Language intervention strategies in aphasia and related neurogenic communication disorders*. (4th ed.) Baltimore, MD: Lippincott, Williams & Wilkins. Pp. 829-846.

HOWELL, D. C. (2004) *Fundamental statistics for the behavioral sciences*. (5th ed.) Belmont, CA: Duxbury.

HYBELS, C. F., & BLAZER, D. G. (2002) Epidemiology and geriatric psychiatry. In M. T. Tsuang & M. Tohen (Eds.), *Textbook in psychiatric epidemiology*. (2nd ed.) New York: Wiley-Liss. Pp. 603-628.

SANTO PIETRO, M. J., & OSTUNI, E. (2003) *Successful communication with Alzheimer's Disease patients: an in-service manual*. (2nd ed.) Newton, MA: Butterworth-Heinemann.

YORKSTON, K. M., & BEUKELMAN, D. R. (1984) *Assessment of intelligibility of dysarthric speech*. Austin, TX: Pro-Ed.

Accepted April 24, 2004.

APPENDIX

SAMPLES OF WORDS AND SENTENCES

Words:
Seat	Sea*	Beast	Reef
Best	Dread	Rest*	Said
Paste	Pace	Spade	Spray*

Sentences: I think we'll be lucky with this one.
He rode horseback through the woods.
The book has a red cover.*

Even my sister didn't get to see it.*
Just don't fill them too full.*
The train approached the depot slowly.

*Indicates the correct item.

EFFECTS OF AUTOMATICALLY DELIVERED STIMULATION ON PERSONS WITH MULTIPLE DISABILITIES DURING THEIR USE OF A STATIONARY BICYCLE[1]

G. E. LANCIONI	N. N. SINGH	M. F. O'REILLY
University of Leiden	*ONE Research Institute*	*University of Texas at Austin*

F. CAMPODONICO, D. OLIVA	J. GROENEWEG
Lega F. D'Oro Research Center	*University of Leiden*

Summary.—We assessed the effects of automatically delivered favorite stimulation on engagement and indices of happiness of two adults with multiple disabilities during their use of a stationary bicycle. The participants typically received four 5-min. sessions per day over a period of about 3.5 mo. Analysis showed that one participant had a significant increase in both those measures while the other participant had a significant increase in engagement during the intervention phases of the study (when the stimulation was present) as opposed to the baseline periods (when the stimulation did not occur). Implications of the findings are discussed.

Persons with profound and multiple disabilities tend to have low levels of physical activity with consequent problems of physical fitness, such as low muscle strength and loss of bone mineral density (Center, Beange, & McElduff, 1998; Wagemans, Fiolet, van der Linden, & Menheere, 1998). Two main types of programs of mild physical activity, i.e., easily acceptable for these persons, have been reported as efforts to curb these problems of fitness. They consist of the use of (a) simple occupational tasks involving ambulation to different places (Lancioni, Gigante, O'Reilly, Oliva, & Montironi, 2000) and (b) basic exercise tools such as a stationary bicycle and a stepper (Caouette & Reid, 1991; Lancioni, Singh, O'Reilly, Oliva, Campodonico, & Groeneweg, 2003).

The second approach may be considered easier to implement, i.e., less time consuming, than the first within education and home settings. It can also be easily combined with the use of favorite stimuli contingent on the persons' engagement in exercise (Lancioni, *et al.*, 2003). Although only limited data are available, this combination seems suitable to help people with profound and multiple disabilities improve exercise performance and general mood (indices of happiness) (Lancioni, *et al.*, 2003). The practical relevance of these data is obvious, and new research seems warranted to specify their generality (Richards, Taylor, Ramasamy, & Richards, 1999).

---

[1]Please address correspondence to G. E. Lancioni, Department of Psychology, University of Bari, Via Quintino Sella 268, 70100 Bari, Italy or e-mail (g.lancioni@psico.uniba.it).

This study was to extend the research in this area and involved two participants (women) with multiple disabilities who used a stationary bicycle that was combined with favorite stimulation. A positive outcome of this new study would represent encouraging evidence in support of the applicability of this approach and the generality of the data previously obtained (Richards, *et al.*, 1999).

Method

Participants

The participants (Emma and Lori) were 37 and 36 yr. old and attended a center for persons with multiple disabilities. They were blind but had normal hearing. Although no IQ scores were available, psychological reports rated them in the profound disability range. They could carry out simple activities such as assembling and sorting familiar objects. Their age equivalents for daily living skills were about 2.5 yr. on the Vineland Adaptive Behavior Scales (Sparrow, Balla, & Cicchetti, 1984). Given a concern about their physical fitness, e.g., body strength and bone mineral density, efforts had been made to introduce some form of exercise into their daily program. Families and staff personnel had consented to this study.

Equipment and Favorite Stimuli

The equipment consisted of an electronic control device (the same as in Lancioni, *et al.*, 2003) linked to a stationary bicycle and a variety of favorite stimuli (see description below). The battery-powered control device served for activating the favorite stimuli in concomitance with the participants' engagement. During the intervention, each half-pedaling cycle produced the activation of one or more stimuli for 3 or 4 sec. A new half-pedaling cycle, occurring when the stimuli following the previous half-pedaling cycle were still on, reset a timer, restarting a 3- to 4-sec. stimulation period. Five or six favorite stimuli were selected for each participant at the beginning of the study through a stimulus-preference screening procedure (Crawford & Schuster, 1993). The stimuli included, among others, recordings of music and songs, excited messages of encouragement and hand clapping, air blowing, and multiple forms of vibratory input. The screening procedure was repeated two more times during the study (at intervals of 4 or 5 wk.) to recruit new stimuli or variations of those already available, such as different music and noise, to reduce risks of satiation.

Sessions, Measures, and Data Collection

Exercise sessions were set to last 5 min. on the advice of staff. Participants typically received four sessions a day, four to six days a week. Measures included half-pedaling cycles and indices of happiness. The first measure was recorded automatically via the electronic control device. Indices of happiness, i.e., smiling, laughing, excited head and trunk movement or excited vocalizations (Green & Reid, 1996), were recorded from the videotapes of the sessions. This was done with a partial-interval procedure in which each 10-sec. observation was followed by a 5-sec. recording. Percentages of interrater agreement on indices of happiness (checked in 16% of the sessions) were within the 80–100 range, with means exceeding 95.

Experimental Conditions

Each participant was exposed to an ABAB design in which A indicated the baseline and B the intervention phases.

Baseline.—During baseline sessions, the electronic control device would record the participants' half-pedaling cycles without activating the favorite stimuli contingent on them. Verbal prompts were available at the end of each minute if the participants were inactive. Participants received praise at the end of the sessions.

Intervention.—During intervention sessions, the electronic control device would record the half-pedaling cycles and activate the favorite stimuli contingent on them (as described above). Other conditions were comparable to those used during baseline.

Results and Discussion

The study lasted about 3.5 months. During the first baseline phase, the participants had mean frequencies of 192 and 327 half-pedaling cycles and zero or one interval with indices of happiness per session (see Figs. 1 and 2). The first intervention phase led to mean frequencies of 248 and 514 half-pedaling cycles and three and two intervals with indices of happiness per

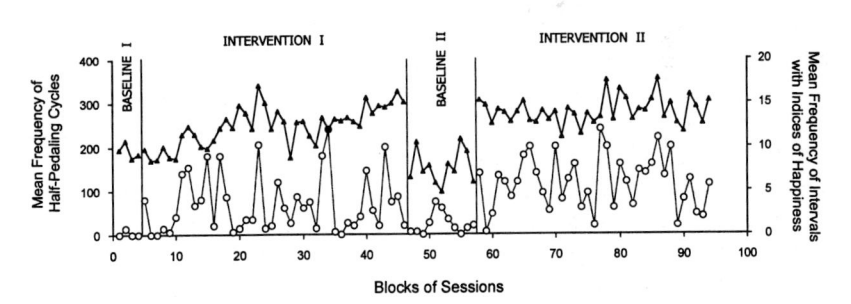

Fig. 1. Emma's data. Data points represent mean frequencies of half-pedaling cycles (▲) and intervals with indices of happiness (○) over blocks of three sessions. Blocks of two sessions may occur only at the end of a baseline or intervention phase.

session. The second baseline and intervention phases were similar to the previous (corresponding) ones for both participants. The Kolmogorov-Smirnov test (Siegel & Castellan, 1988) showed that the increases in pedaling during

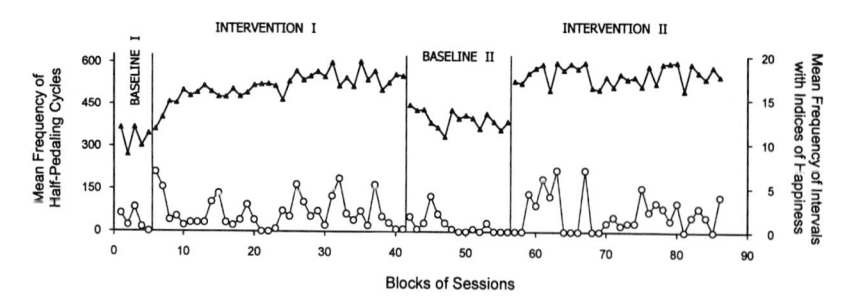

FIG. 2. Lori's data plotted as those in Fig. 1

the intervention phases were significant ($p < .05$) for both participants. The increases in intervals with indices of happiness were significant only for Emma.

These data indicate that the availability of favorite stimuli had a positive impact on the participants' motor performance, thus supporting previous findings (Lancioni, *et al.*, 2003). No checks were conducted about possible benefits of the increased motor performance (also in view of the relatively short duration of the study). One may hypothesize, however, that increasing motor output could eventually be beneficial for general physical conditions such as blood circulation and muscle strength (Linderman & Stewart, 1999). The fact that the increases in indices of happiness were statistically significant only for one of the participants may indicate that (a) only modest mood changes occurred for the second participant or (b) meaningful changes occurred also for this participant but were not displayed among the basic range of behaviors observed. In the latter case, one should take new initiatives to improve the assessment, e.g., using electrophysiological measures (Ritz, Alatupa, Thoens, & Dahme, 2002).

In view of these findings and the previous ones, the combination of simple exercise tools and automatically delivered stimulation appears to be highly suitable in terms of practicality (staff's time requirement) and effects. The three immediate questions that one may put forward for further investigation are whether (a) the effects of the stimulation are due to its occurrence *per se* or to its contingency value, i.e., to its specific connection with the participant's pedaling, (b) rules can be found to identify the participants who are more likely to benefit from this type of intervention program, and (c) new types of measures can be successfully adopted to improve the assessment of indices of happiness.

REFERENCES

CAOUETTE, M., & REID, G. (1991) Influence of auditory stimulation on the physical work output of adults who are severely retarded. *Education and Training in Mental Retardation*, 26, 43-52.

Center, J., Beange, H., & McElduff, A. (1998) People with mental retardation have an increased prevalence of osteoporosis: a population study. *American Journal on Mental Retardation*, 103, 19-28.

Crawford, M. R., & Schuster, J. W. (1993) Using microswitches to teach toy use. *Journal of Developmental and Physical Disabilities*, 5, 349-368.

Green, C. W., & Reid, D. H. (1996) Defining, validating, and increasing indices of happiness among people with profound multiple disabilities. *Journal of Applied Behavior Analysis*, 29, 67-78.

Lancioni, G. E., Gigante, A., O'Reilly, M. F., Oliva, D., & Montironi, L. (2000) Indoor travel and simple tasks as physical exercise for people with profound multiple disabilities. *Perceptual and Motor Skills*, 91, 211-216.

Lancioni, G. E., Singh, N. N., O'Reilly, M. F., Oliva, D., Campodonico, F., & Groeneweg, J. (2003) Assessing the effects of automatically delivered stimulation on the use of simple exercise tools with students with multiple disabilities. *Research in Developmental Disabilities*, 24, 475-483.

Linderman, T. M., & Stewart, K. B. (1999) Sensory integrative-based occupational therapy and functional outcomes in young children with pervasive developmental disorders: a single-subject study. *American Journal of Occupational Therapy*, 53, 207-213.

Richards, S. B., Taylor, R. L., Ramasamy, R., & Richards, R. Y. (1999) *Single subject research: applications in educational and clinical settings*. London: Wadsworth.

Ritz, T., Alatupa, S., Thoens, M., & Dahme, B. (2002) Effects of affective picture viewing and imagery on respiratory resistance in nonasthmatic individuals. *Psychophysiology*, 39, 86-94.

Siegel, S., & Castellan, N. J. (1988) *Nonparametric statistics*. (2nd ed.) New York: McGraw-Hill.

Sparrow, S. S., Balla, D. A., & Cicchetti, D. V. (1984) *Vineland Adaptive Behavior Scales*. Circle Pines, MN: American Guidance Services.

Wagemans, A. M., Fiolet, J. F., van der Linden, E. S., & Menheere, P. P. (1998) Osteoporosis and intellectual disability: is there any relation? *Journal of Intellectual Disability Research*, 42, 370-374.

Accepted April 23, 2004.

VELOCITY OF A TENNIS SERVE AND MEASUREMENT OF ISOKINETIC MUSCULAR PERFORMANCE: BRIEF REVIEW AND COMMENT[1]

T. S. ELLENBECKER AND E. P. ROETERT

Physiotherapy Associates, Scottsdale Sports Clinic
USA Tennis High Performance, Key Biscayne, Florida

Summary.—Isokinetic strength testing provides objective and reliable muscular performance data on elite tennis players; however, such data are not highly correlated with performance on a multiple-joint kinetic chain activity such as the tennis serve. In this brief review, an overview of the muscular performance characteristics generated through isokinetic testing for elite tennis players is presented. Application of population specific isokinetic strength profiles in specific populations for rehabilitation and performance enhancement is recommended.

Developing an isokinetic profile of tennis players' strength can be extremely useful not only in the enhancement of performance but also in the prevention and rehabilitation of injury. Clearly both upper and lower body strength are important characteristics of a tennis athlete who is successful and injury free. In a recent article, Pugh, *et al.* (13) have outlined an excellent case for both upper and lower body strength. In addition to the findings presented there, we point out some practical implications and areas for potential investigation.

Ellenbecker and Roetert (8) measured knee-extension flexion strength in elite junior tennis players and found the legs had equal strength. The critical role leg strength plays in tennis serve has recently been reported (4), noting that players using more than 14° knee flexion during the service motion had significantly lower elbow and shoulder torques with similar serve velocities. Therefore, leg strength appears to be important for tennis players, as it helps provide high velocities in the strokes (particularly the serve) with a relatively small loading profile in the shoulder and elbow (3, 4).

Kibler (11) stressed that physical preparation must encompass all sections of the body in the kinetic chain. The forces produced from the ground up through the lower body, have to be transferred effectively and efficiently to the upper body. Ellenbecker and Roetert (9) stated that muscular activity not only stabilizes the trunk but also links upper and lower extremity segments. Proper trunk strength (flexion, extension, and rotation) is therefore imperative for producing successful tennis strokes (14) in addition to upper

---

[1]Address enquiries to T. S. Ellenbecker, Physiotherapy Associates, Scottsdale Sports Clinic, 90th Street, Suite 100, Scottsdale, AZ 85258 & USA Tennis High Performance, 7310 Crandon Blvd., Key Biscayne, FL 33149.

and lower body strength. Roetert, et al. (14) tested elite junior tennis players ages 14–17 years for whom greater abdominal strength than trunk extension strength was noted, the exact opposite of trunk flexion and extension strength relationships reported for the normal population (15). Adaptations in muscular strength such as greater abdominal strength may lead to muscular imbalances between pairings of agonist and antagonist muscles, with testing of isokinetic muscular performance being a primary method used to assess dynamic muscle strength.

Any torque greater than 50 Nm in the upper extremity was significant in loading that area of the body (2), so the upper limb and shoulder are subject to high loads particularly during the serve (4). These movements, if repeated may times, may have the potential to cause an overuse injury. Study of the internal and external rotators of the glenohumeral joint (1, 5, 6, 7, 9, 10) indicate that, despite increases in accurate first serve velocity after six weeks of concentric internal and external rotation strength training (7, 12), no significant correlation was found between internal rotation muscular strength and serve velocity. Significantly greater internal rotation strength for the dominant arm has been consistently documented for elite players but no significant difference between extremities in glenohumeral external rotation (1, 5, 6, 7, 9, 10).

The multijoint kinetic chain inherent in the tennis serve requires optimal strength, timing, and coordination of many segments of the human body. Further research developing both isokinetic and biomechanical profiles of normal characteristics in elite players should provide additional evidence for clinicians and scientists who treat and try to prevent injuries as well as enhance performance of tennis players.

REFERENCES

1. CHANDLER, T. J., KIBLER, W. B., STRACENER, E. C., ZIEGLER, A. K., & PACE, B. (1992) Shoulder strength, power and endurance in college tennis players. *American Journal of Sports Medicine*, 20, 455-458.
2. DILLMAN, C. J., SCHULTHEIS, J. M., HINTERMEISTER, R. A., & HAWKINS, R. J. (1995) What do we know about body mechanics involved in tennis skills? In H. Krahl, H. Pieper, B. Kibler, & P. Renstrom (Eds.), *Tennis: sports medicine and science*. Auglage: Society for Tennis Medicine and Science. Pp. 6-11.
3. ELIOTT, B. (2003) Technique effects on upper limb loading in the tennis serve. *Journal of Science and Medicine in Sport*, 6, 76-87.
4. ELIOTT, B., MESTER, J., KLEINODER, H., & YUE, Z. (2003) Loading and stroke production. In B. Eliot, M. Reid, & M. Crespo (Eds.), *Biomechanics of advanced tennis*. Washington, DC: International Tennis Federation. Pp. 93-107.
5. ELLENBECKER, T. S. (1991) A total arm strength isokinetic profile of highly skilled tennis players. *Isokinetics and Exercise Science*, 1, 9-21.
6. ELLENBECKER, T. S. (1992) Shoulder internal and external rotation strength and range of motion in highly skilled junior tennis players. *Isokinetics and Exercise Science*, 2, 1-8.
7. ELLENBECKER, T. S., DAVIES, G. J., & ROWINSKI, M. (1988) Concentric vs. eccentric isokinetic strengthening of the rotator cuff: objective data vs. functional test. *American Journal of Sports Medicine*, 16, 64-69.

8. ELLENBECKER, T. S., & ROETERT, E. P. (1995) Concentric isokinetic quadriceps and hamstring strength in elite junior tennis players. *Isokinetics and Exercise Science*, 5, 3-6.
9. ELLENBECKER, T. S., & ROETERT, E. P. (2000) Isokinetic testing and training in tennis. In L. Brown (Ed.), *Isokinetics in human performance*. Champaign, IL: Human Kinetics. Pp. 358-377.
10. ELLENBECKER, T. S., & ROETERT, E. P. (2003) Age specific isokinetic glenohumeral internal and external rotation strength in elite junior tennis players. *Journal of Science and Medicine in Sports*, 6, 63-70.
11. KIBLER, W. B. (1995) Biomechanical analysis of the shoulder during tennis activities. *Clinics in Sports Medicine*, 14, 79-85.
12. MONT, M. A., COHEN, D. B., CAMPBELL, K. R., GRAVARE, K., & MATHUR, S. K. (1992) Isokinetic concentric versus eccentric training of the shoulder rotators with functional evaluation of performance enhancement in elite tennis players. *American Journal of Sports Medicine*, 22, 513-517.
13. PUGH, S. F., KOVALESKI, J. E., HEITMAN, R. J., & GILLEY, W. F. (2003) Upper and lower body strength in relation to ball speed during a serve by male collegiate tennis players. *Perceptual and Motor Skills*, 97, 867-872.
14. ROETERT, E. P., MCCORMICK, T. J., BROWN, S. W., & ELLENBECKER, T. S.(1996) Relationship between isokinetic and functional trunk strength in elite junior tennis players. *Isokinetics and Exercise Science*, 6, 15-20.
15. TIMM, K. E. (1995) Clinical applications of a normative database for the Cybex TEF and Torso spinal isokinetic dynamometers. *Isokinetics and Exercise Science*, 5, 43-49.

Accepted April 30, 2004.

THE STROOP STRATEGY TEST: INVESTIGATION OF A COMPUTERISED VERSION OF THE STROOP TEST FOR CLASSIFYING SWEDISH MILITARY SERVICEMEN [1]

ROLF FEDERMANN, MARTIN BÄCKSTRÖM, AND ROBERT W. GOLDSMITH

University of Lund, Sweden

Summary.—A computerised test termed the Stroop Strategy Test, utilising the Stroop effect, is described. To assess the test's usefulness and discriminant power, it was given to three military groups adjudged on the basis of interview and a test of intelligence to differ in their qualifications (61 men of Level 1, 41 of Level 2, and 17 of Level 3, in descending order) and a group of 16 men imprisoned or put in detention school for violent behaviour. In a discriminant analysis in which the eight measures the test provided were included and the four groups were compared yielded a discriminant power of 52.6% for the group as a whole, highest (56%) for the military Level 1 group. The potential usefulness of the test is discussed.

The present study deals with a preliminary version of a computerised test the first author has developed, termed the Stroop Strategy Test, and the question of how useful the test could be for selection and placement purposes when used in connection with other assessment tests, in a military context in particular. The test aims at comparing individual differences in speed and patterns of coping with what Stroop (1935) referred to as the "interference effect", later called the "Stroop effect". This effect occurs when a longer time is required for naming the colour in which each of a series of words is printed if the words represent colour names and if each word is printed in a colour different from the colour the word designates, for example, the word "red" printed in green. Thus, there is a conflict between the more accustomed task of reading the words and the task given of naming the colour of each word. The discrepancy or incongruence between the actual and the more expected task, leading to the interference effect, affects individuals differently in the time required for the task. Stroop (1935) reported that the interference effect was negatively related to the forming of associations and to flexible adaptation to new situations. The effect has been examined extensively in both cognitive and personality psychology, relationships between individuals' susceptibility to the effect and a wide variety of behavioral correlates having been shown.

The Stroop Strategy Test employs two series of words designating colours, the words being shown one at a time on a computer screen. The tasks in the first series are easy to perform, the colour in which a word appears

---

[1]Address enquiries to R. Federmann, Murarevägen, ·3a, 22 730 Lund, Sweden.

and the colour it denotes being the same (congruent series). The tasks in the second series are much more difficult, given the incongruence between the colour a word designates and the colour in which it appears (incongruent series). In both series, the subject is to react as quickly as possible when the word is shown on the computer screen, using a computer mouse to mark a neutrally coloured square containing the colour name corresponding to the colour in which the word is printed (and in the first series corresponding as well to the meaning of the word).

The practical background to developing the Stroop Strategy Test was to fulfill a need felt in the Swedish armed forces for a test that could complement in a useful way other sources of information utilised in the placement of recruits. Ever since 1969, an intelligence test and an interview by a psychologist had been used for placement purposes (see Lothigius, 1995, for a historical review). Such problems as fatalities caused by mistakes by boat commanders and the failure of many elite soldiers to qualify after being accepted led to the desire for a test which would specify presence or absence of certain characteristics that elite soldiers were expected to possess, a test that could nevertheless be completed quickly. A computerised test based on the Stroop effect was considered a possibility.

In most investigations of the Stroop effect the subject is provided a sheet of paper on which the words in question are printed, the subject giving answers aloud. The test administrator records as accurately as possible any errors the subject makes and the time required for completing the task. In one approach to testing described below, the times needed for completing successive task segments are also recorded.

The Stroop Paradigm

Interference comes about due to response competition between parallel processes, those of reading and of naming, each of which tends to give rise to a response (cf. Morton & Chambers, 1973). Posner and Snyder (1975) noted that word reading is faster than colour naming and that printed words tend to facilitate vocal output, a phenomenon they referred to as the relative speed of processing hypothesis. MacLeod (1991) and MacLeod and Dunbar (1988) indicated that word reading and colour naming differ in terms of automaticity, word reading being more automatic and therefore more difficult to control, so that it interferes with colour naming, a point borne out by MacLeod's finding (1991) that people who are bilingual show greater interference when using their dominant language. More elaborate models based on parallelism and automaticity (e.g., McClelland, 1979; Logan, 1980) have been developed as well.

Two of the many tests that have been used to measure the Stroop effect are Thurstone's test (1944) and the Serial Colour Word Test developed by

Smith, Nyman, and Kragh in the 1950s (see Smith, Nyman, & Hentschel, 1986). On both tests, the subject responds vocally. Thurstone's test contains one incongruent and two congruent series. In the incongruent series, the colour names blue, red, green, and yellow are placed randomly on the test sheet in 10 rows of 10 words each, each word printed in a colour differing from the colour of the word it designates. The other two tasks, both of them congruent, involve naming colours shown in the form of coloured spots and reading names of colours printed in black. The differences between the time required for the first task and for each of the latter two tasks are regarded as measures of the ability to deal with the incongruence inherent in the first task and the problems of interference produced. The ability to deal with interference is assumed to be greater when these differences are small. In using this method to study U.S. Naval officers, Thurstone (1944) found a high correlation between good performance on the test (smaller time differences) and positive reports by superior officers regarding the ability of the men involved to perform their duties.

Development of the Serial Colour Word Test (S-CWT) by Smith, Nyman, and Kragh was based on percept-genetic theory as formulated in psychological terms by Kragh and Smith (1970) and in psychiatric terms by Nyman (see Smith, et al., 1986). They were also influenced both by Thurstone's work and by certain perceptual experiments conducted by Jaensch in 1929 and by Cattell in 1886 concerning time differences between reading words designating colours and naming the colours in which the words were printed.

In taking the S-CWT, participants name the colour in which each of 100 colour words is printed, a procedure repeated five times. For each of the five trials, the reading time for each successive set of 20 words is measured. This provides five measures for each 100-word task. These are used to assess what are termed "primary strategies," the term "strategies" being used to designate approaches people take, regardless of whether these are consciously selected or unconsciously adhered to. In addition, the total times for the separate administrations of the test are used to measure overall performance, involving what are called "secondary strategies." Speed as such is not considered important, but the variation in times is, both within each 100-words trial and among the five trials.

Four primary adaptation strategies are distinguished, defined in terms of the subject's typical performance during the test. The key factors involved are the variance and the regression of the times required, as defined in strict statistical terms, the latter also being denoted in literature on the S-CWT as slope. The different strategies, as presented briefly below, are defined as representing specific combinations of these factors:

1. A stabilised strategy, in which both the variance and regression are

low. This implies the subject's not being appreciably disturbed by the incongruent stimuli. It is considered the most adaptive and flexible strategy of all (Nyman & Smith, 1959; Smith, et al., 1986).

2. A cumulative strategy, in which there is low variance and steep regression. This is a strategy in which the subject appears to find the task increasingly difficult over time. Scores have been related to obsessional-compulsive disorders in clinical groups (Nyman & Smith, 1959; Smith, et al., 1986).

3. A dissociative strategy, in which variations in performance are large but regression is low. In clinical groups this strategy has been associated with difficulties in adapting to new situations and also with the hysteroid personality type (Nyman & Smith, 1959; Smith, et al., 1986).

4. A cumulative-dissociative strategy, which represents a combination of the two styles just mentioned, involving both high regression and variance. This strategy has been associated with serious personality disorders, such as psychoses of different types, and to be infrequent in the normal population (Nyman & Smith, 1959; Smith, et al., 1986). Showing this strategy or Strategies 2 or 3 has also been associated with state anxiety and with trait anxiety (Smith, et al., 1986).

Whereas Thurstone's test involves basically a straightforward use of the Stroop effect, the Serial Colour Word Test is concerned with changes over time in how effectively interference is dealt with. The Stroop Strategy Test with which the present study is concerned involves elements of both.

Correlates of the Stroop Effect

In personality research concerning the Stroop effect, attention has been directed in part at clinical groups, various behavioral patterns and such states as anxiety, depression, and phobia being of concern (e.g., MacLeod, 1991) and in part at reactions to stress (e.g., MacLeod, 1991; Carlsson, Amnèr, & Smith, 1996; Fauvel, Bernard, Laville, Daoud, Pozet, & Zech, 1996; Renaud & Blondin, 1997; André-Petersson, Hagberg, Hedblad, Janzon, & Steen, 1999).

No clear sex differences appear in Stroop interference (MacLeod, 1991; Daniel, Pelotte, & Lewis, 2000). Regarding age effects, MacLeod (1991) found that interference begins in the early school years and rises to its peak about Grade 2 or 3, declining thereafter, but begins to rise again at about the age of 60, whereas in a metastudy Verhaeghen and De Meersman (1998) found no significant age differences in interference in adults.

Regarding personality characteristics related to various S-CWT strategies, in clinical groups a stabilised strategy points to the individual's being more flexible and functioning better, results at the opposite extreme being correlated with mental disturbances (see Smith, et al., 1986). Carlsson, et al.

(1996) have argued, however, that such apparently suboptimal performance on the test is not necessarily negative in all contexts, appearing in some cases to be reflective of a creative or emotional way of dealing with the task at hand.

Williams, Watts, MacLeod, and Mathews (1988, 1997; see Eysenck, 1992, 1997) applied the Stroop-type paradigm to words associated either with anxiety or with negative feelings in general, extending the paradigm's area of application. In line with this, Masia, McNeil, Cohn, and Hope (1999) reported that words other than colour names can acquire emotion-eliciting functions, people who suffered from social phobia reacting with anxiety when confronted with such words as "speech" or "conversation." Barker and Robertson (1997), in using a computerised Stroop test, found that people afraid of spiders were significantly slower in naming the colours in which sets of words representing the physical attributes of spiders were printed, interference being associated only with words concerning spiders and not with other words. Mathews and Sebastian (1993) found a similar relationship between fear of snakes and interference connected with words associated with snakes, and the same for spiders and words associated with them. At the same time, they showed that, if the threatening object was present but was under control (having a snake or a spider visible in a glass cage in the same room as the participant), the fear-provoking words no longer affected reaction times. The experience of fear thus appeared to be related to certain expectations or ideas of lacking control, which disappeared when the threat became visible but was held under control.

Hartston and Swerdlow (1999) stated that people who suffered from obsessive-compulsive disorders showed greater interference in the Stroop task than controls. Similarly, McNeil, Tucker, Miranda, Lewin, and Nordgren (1999) found that the interference connected with colour words and with words related to people was greater in people suffering from obsessive-compulsive disorder, posttraumatic stress disorder, or major depressive disorder, who also showed slower responses both to stimuli representing general anxiety or depression and to incongruent colour words as compared with their reactions to neutral stimuli.

Relations to various physiological states and to medical problems have also been reported. André-Petersson, *et al.* (1999), using S-CWT to investigate hypertensive men born in 1914 who had been examined medically in 1982-1983, found in a follow-up study that men showing primarily a Cumulative-Dissociative strategy had a three-fold greater risk of cardiac difficulties. Fauvel, *et al.* (1996), employing a computerised Stroop test as a source of stress in examining biological and cardiovascular adaptation to mental stress in normotensive and in hypertensive persons, found both groups showed a significant increase in blood pressure, heart rate, and various other biological parameters while taking the test. Renaud and Blondin (1997) likewise found the use of a computerised version of the Stroop test was an effective laboratory stressor, showing that during the test session both heart rate and self-reported anxiety increased.

To explain cognitively a wide variety of relationships reported in the literature between the Stroop effect and other behavioral characteristics, Goldsmith (1968) employed the terms "long" and "short sampling" adapted from Broadbent (1958). Long samplers, defined as those people showing a marked Stroop effect, were assumed generally to "process information from a wide area as regards content, space and time span" (p. 135), whereas short samplers (people showing a weak Stroop effect) did the opposite. He emphasised certain advantages to each of these tendencies. Many practical military tasks, one can note, require a particular focus on certain important information, perhaps especially in the case of commanders and other people who bear considerable responsibility or are given highly demanding tasks. At the same time, measures of change or stability in performance over time, such as are obtained on the Stroop Strategy Test or on the Serial Colour Word Test on which it is partly based, may provide considerable information of relevance to practical performance both in military and in other contexts.

Aim of the Study

The specific aim of the present study was to investigate the extent to which the Stroop Strategy Test could correctly classify four groups of men. Three of the groups consisted of men belonging to the Swedish armed forces. The fourth group consisted of men convicted of one or more serious crimes. The deeper aim was to assess the usefulness of the test, conceived for use in conjunction with other suitable instruments, for selection and placement purposes generally. In addition, insight into those aspects of the test of particular importance in differentiating between the groups that were tested was sought.

Method

The Stroop Strategy Test

The Stroop Strategy Test can be described as follows. The test utilises Stroop tasks in two series of 185 colour words each, the tasks in the first series being congruent and those in the second series incongruent. The specific results for both series were of interest and also were compared with each other. The test is fully computerised, including each of the individual tasks and the instructions specific to it (see Fig. 1), together with the initial instructions for each of the two series. The subject uses the computer mouse to indicate his answer in solving each of the tasks and is completely free to use the leading hand here, left or right. The position on the screen of the response boxes designating the four colours remains the same throughout. Each series begins with several practice tasks that the subject must successfully complete before beginning the test. The procedure differs, therefore, from the original Stroop test, Thurstone's version, and the S-CWT, in each of which the participant reads colour words or names colours that appear on a printed sheet. In the Stroop Strategy Test, four measures are obtained in each series: mean time, variance, regression, and number of errors, giving eight measures (4 × 2) altogether. This differs from the S-CWT, which makes use of only variance and regression, and Thurstone's version of the Stroop test, which makes use of only total time. The greater difficulty of performing in the second series could be expected to affect all four measures. Although the Stroop Strategy Test and S-CWT provide information about changes in performance over time, the Stroop Strategy Test is far more exact and allows small and momentary fluctuations in speed of performance to be recorded.

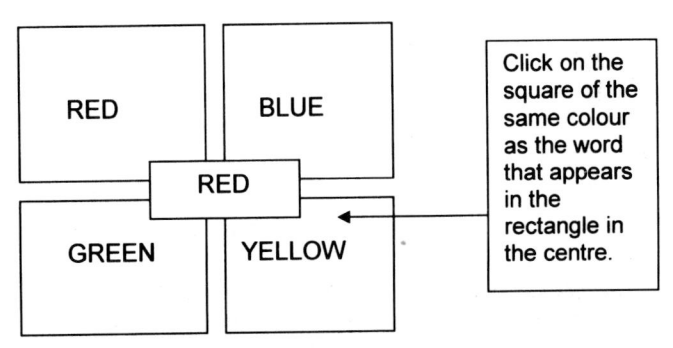

FIG. 1. Example of what appears on the screen in the Stroop Strategy Test

Participants

The four groups of men who were tested were chosen with the idea of their differing ability to act quickly and effectively in the performance of demanding tasks of a military character, tasks involving strong cognitive demands, clear elements of stress and strong elements of conflict, and the need of remaining emotionally stable under pressure. The three military groups, defined in terms of the types of military service to which the different subgroups of which they were composed were assigned, are designated as the Level-1, Level-2, and Level-3 groups. Level 1 was conceived on *a priori* grounds as being highest and Level 3 as being lowest in terms of the men possessing the characteristics just referred to. With the exception of one of the subgroups, a group of military pilots, assigned to their job by a special selection service within the Swedish Air Force, assignment of the men to the military service categories to which they belonged was based on their qualifications as adjudged by military authorities on the basis of results of an intelligence test and an interview by a psychologist. The intelligence test was a computerised test of general intelligence specially developed for the Swedish armed forces and taking about an hour to complete. The interview concerned social skills, emotional stability, success in school and at work, free-time activities, and many other matters. Because of the need of safeguarding the validity of both the test and the interview for continued military selection purposes, more exact details about them are not presented here.

No testing or interviews of members of the group convicted of crimes of violence (termed here the Prisoners group) were carried out prior to the investigation. Although members of that group appeared far from homogeneous, the group was assumed to be inferior in terms of the qualifications referred to above. One can also note that, although Sweden has compulsory military service (with civilian alternatives for conscientious objectors to military service), belonging to the armed forces is closed for men who have committed serious crimes.

The following is a summary of how the various groups, comprising 135 persons altogether, were constituted and of the numbers of persons in each:

1. Level-1 group: 61 men, 20 paratroopers and 20 marines, all age 19 years, and 21 military pilots ages 22–35. The paratroopers and marines, who can be seen as belonging to the most select category at the age levels and within the service subcategories involved, had a group average of about Stanine 8 on their intelligence scores, with a range of 7–9, and were at a level of 7 or above on a 9-level scale in their rating on the interview. The pilots, assigned on *a priori* grounds to Level 1, had selected the airforce as a profession. The paratroopers and marines were doing compulsory military duty.

2. Level-2 group: 41 men, consisting of 20 officer trainees 20 years of age preparing to become professional officers, and 21 combat boat commanders 19 years of age doing compulsory military duty. These men were above average both on the intelligence test (group average of about Stanine 6 with a range of 5–7) and on results of the interview.

3. Level-3 group: 17 men, all age 19 years, doing compulsory military duty as tank gunners. These were ordinary soldiers with approximately average scores on both the intelligence test (group average of about Stanine 5 with a range of 4–6) and the interview.

4. Prisoners: 16 men, 16 to 40 years of age, imprisoned or put in detention school for violent behavior. They had been convicted of manslaughter, assault and battery, and other crimes of violence against persons, and had been given sentences of between several years and life. Many of them had also been described as being emotionally unstable.

Taking the Stroop Strategy Test would obviously be inappropriate for persons with certain degrees and types of colour blindness. None of the participants or potential participants were, in fact, colour blind.

Procedure

Participation of all the subjects was voluntary. Those in the military groups appeared to experience the testing situation as a positive break in their ordinary duties and those in the Prisoners group to experience it as a welcome change in what they were doing. All subjects were tested individually. Initial instructions were oral, and further instructions were presented on the computer screen.

Statistical Analysis

Statistical analysis of the results included initial descriptive measures of means of the eight test variables and of their intercorrelations, and use of multiple discriminant analysis, followed by classification of the subjects into the four groups on the basis of the discriminant functions obtained. This enabled the classification to be compared with actual group membership.

Although practical use of the test could involve obtaining Stroop-effect scores, i.e., the difference between the conflict and nonconflict conditions in the mean-time measures, such scores are not included in the multiple discriminant analysis, since they would add nothing to the results obtained there using simply the eight test variables.

The aim in combining, as was done here, groups representing different categories of military service, to form larger groups (or levels) expected to differ from one another and from the Prisoners group in terms of their Stroop Strategy Test scores, was to investigate as adequately as possible the ability of the test to distinguish accurately between differing groups in this context, which could not be investigated as adequately with use of a large number of considerably smaller groups. Finding the statistical approach described to show a clear differentiation among these levels, as well as between these and the Prisoners group, would provide support for the combinations formed being reasonable ones in terms of the characteristics assumed to be typical for the men involved. It would also provide support for the correctness of the assumptions made regarding what the test measures, as well as for the potential usefulness of the test in a military context.

Results

The means for the separate groups on the eight different test measures are presented in Table 1. As can be seen, the scores of the Prisoners group on the mean, variance, and regression variables were higher on the average than those of the other three groups under both the conflict and the non-

TABLE 1
DESCRIPTIVE STATISTICS FOR FOUR GROUPS AND TOTAL GROUP

Group	Conflict				Nonconflict			
	Errors	M	σ^2	Regression	Errors	M	σ^2	Regression
Prisoners	3.00	1.49	.33	.00053	.00	1.29	.180	.00048
Level 3	4.47	1.25	.18	.00027	.00	1.05	.070	.00023
Level 2	3.20	1.24	.18	.00034	.85	1.05	.063	.00016
Level 1	2.72	1.21	.18	.00013	.44	1.02	.065	.00014
Total	3.12	1.26	.20	.00026	.46	1.06	.079	.00020

conflict conditions, whereas the average error rate appeared to be about the same for the Prisoners group as for the other three groups under the conflict conditions but was lower than that of all the other groups except the Tank Gunners under the nonconflict conditions. These results are purely descriptive but can contribute to an interpretation of certain of the multiple discriminant analysis results to be presented. The making of errors should probably not be considered as representing error proneness in any general sense, since it can be the result of simply attempting to carry out a task as quickly as possible.

Examining the correlations between the eight variables as shown in Table 2 indicates that in the nonconflict series there was a high correlation between mean time and variance (.76) and between variance and regression (.73), as well as a moderately high correlation between mean time and regression (.57), and that in the conflict series there was a high correlation between mean time and variance (.80). There was also a high between-series correlation of the respective mean time measures (.73). The correlations between many of the variables, on the other hand, were rather low.

TABLE 2
PEARSON CORRELATION MATRIX FOR EIGHT VARIABLES CONTAINED IN TWO SERIES

	Nonconflict				Conflict			
	1	2	3	4	1	2	3	4
Nonconflict								
1. Errors		−.02	.02	−.04	.26†	.05	.19*	−.16
2. Mean	−.02		.76†	.57†	−.04	.73†	.42†	.20*
3. Variance	.02	.76†		.73†	−.03	.41†	.22†	.17*
4. Regression	−.04	.57†	.73†		−.08	.20*	−.01	.14
Conflict								
1. Errors	.26†	−.04	−.03	−.08		.19*	.38†	−.04
2. Mean	.05	.73†	.41†	.20*	.19*		.80†	.12
3. Variance	.19*	.42†	.22†	−.01	.38†	.80†		.10
4. Regression	−.16	.20*	.17*	.14	−.04	.12	.10	

*p = .05 (2-tailed). †p = .01 (2-tailed).

Table 3 presents the univariate F ratio for each of the eight variables. The largest F value (18.34) was found for the mean times in the nonconflict series, the same measure in the conflict series having the next-largest F value (10.42). All the differences except for errors under the conflict conditions were statistically significant. One can note that the level of discrimination obtained is somewhat higher under the nonconflict than under the conflict conditions for all the variables except the regression variable, a somewhat unexpected result.

TABLE 3
UNIVARIATE STATISTICS FOR FACTORS INCLUDED IN DISCRIMINANT ANALYSIS

	Wilks λ	F	df_1	df_2	p
Conflict					
Errors	.95	2.23	3	131	ns
Mean	.81	10.42	3	131	<.001
Variance	.87	6.30	3	131	<.001
Regression	.87	6.80	3	131	<.001
Nonconflict					
Errors	.94	2.97	3	131	.03
Mean	.70	18.34	3	131	.001
Variance	.82	9.45	3	131	.001
Regression	.91	4.12	3	131	.008

To assess these differences further, multiple discriminant analysis was done to obtain a set of discriminant functions based on the four groups (see Table 4). Three independent discriminant functions could be extracted. These separated the groups in three different ways.

TABLE 4
STRUCTURE MATRIX OF DISCRIMINANT FUNCTIONS BASED ON ALL FOUR GROUPS

Index	Function 1	Function 2	Function 3
Mean: Nonconflict	.839*	−.022	.094
Mean: Conflict	.633*	−.015	.006
Variance: Nonconflict	.594*	−.209	−.012
Variance: Conflict	.483*	−.172	.081
Regression: Nonconflict	.393*	−.025	−.146
Regression: Conflict	.426	.543*	.173
Errors: Nonconflict	−.175	.255	.593*
Errors: Conflict	.022	.395	−.489*

*Largest absolute correlation for each variable with any of the discriminant functions.

For the first function, the clearly dominant one (Wilks Lambda = 0.489 [for the first through third function]; $\chi^2_{24} = 91.53$, $p < .001$; see Table 5), a clear positive relationship to all the Stroop Strategy Test variables except the wrong-response variables was found (see Table 4). The Prisoners group had the highest mean values on that function (2.039) and differed on it markedly from all of the other groups (see Table 6), the Level-1 group being the one most distant from the Prisoners group in terms of it with a value of −.412.

TABLE 5
WILKS LAMBDA FOR THREE FUNCTIONS OBTAINED IN DISCRIMINANT ANALYSIS

Test of Function(s)	Wilks λ	χ^2	df	p
1 through 3	.489	91.53	24	.001
2 through 3	.780	31.76	14	.004
3	.898	13.82	6	.03

The second discriminant function was also significant (Wilks Lambda = 0.780 [for the second and third functions together]; $\chi^2_{14} = 31.76$, $p < .004$; see Table 5). This function had a moderately high positive correlation with regression in the conflict series (.543) and correlated to a certain extent with wrong responses in both series (.395 and .255 for the nonconflict and conflict series, respectively; see Table 4). It separated the Level-2 and Level-3 groups from the Level-1 group and to a lesser extent from the Prisoners group (see Table 6).

TABLE 6
UNSTANDARDIZED CANONICAL DISCRIMINANT FUNCTIONS EVALUATED AS GROUP MEANS

Group Variable	Function 1	2	3
Prisoners	2.039	.179	.045
Level 3	−.058	.377	−.812
Level 2	−.159	.458	.300
Level 1	−.412	−.366	.013

The third discriminant function was significant as well (Wilks Lambda = .898; $\chi^2_6 = 13.82$, $p < .03$; see Table 5). It separated subjects with a large number of wrong responses in the nonconflict series and a small number of wrong responses in the conflict series from those with the opposite pattern (see Table 4). In terms of the groupings here, the function separated the Level-3 from the Level-2 group (see Table 6), the Level-3 group members having a larger number of wrong responses in the conflict series but a smaller number in the nonconflict series than Level-2 group members (see Tables 1 and 6).

The subjects were also classified into groups on the basis of the three discriminant functions as a whole (see Table 7). When the probability of inclusion in these new groups was set to being equal for all of the original four groups (25% probability for each), 52.6% of the subjects were classified in accord with their prior group membership.

The correct-classification rate can be seen as reasonably good for each of the groups, despite the Level-2 group having a correct-classification rate of somewhat less than 50%, since on the basis of chance one would expect a correct-classification rate of only 25%. Computing group classification on the basis of the actual size of each group resulted in a slightly higher correct-classification rate (55.6%).

TABLE 7
CLASSIFICATION FOR FOUR GROUPS BASED ON DISCRIMINANT ANALYSIS

Group Variable	Predicted Group Membership					Second-best Function
	Prisoners	Level 3	Level 2	Level 1	Total	
Prisoners	8	2	4	2	16	6
Level 3	1	9	2	5	17	4
Level 2	1	8	20	12	41	15
Level 1	2	13	12	34	61	16

In discriminating between more than two groups on the basis of the discriminant functions just referred to, one can rank order each subject over the various groups in terms of probability of membership. Note that six of the eight misclassified Prisoners group members were classified as having that group as their second most probable membership group (see the right-hand column in Table 7). For the Level-3 group, in turn, 4 of the 8 misclassified subjects were classified as having their own group as their second most probable membership group, the comparable figures for the Level-2 and Level-1 groups, respectively, being 15 out of the 21 and 16 out of 27. In addition, of the 119 subjects who were military personnel, only four were classified as the Prisoners group's being the one they most likely belonged to and only seven as its being their second most probable membership group.

DISCUSSION

In this study of a computerised test involving the Stroop effect, the test measures employed were those of variance and regression, as used in the S-CWT as well as of mean response times and wrong responses. All four measures were obtained both for the conflict and the nonconflict series, providing a total of eight different measures. Although discriminating between the three military groups was of primary interest, the Prisoners group was also included to facilitate a better understanding of the test. The general expectation was that the four groups would differ on their Stroop Strategy Test measures.

The significant discriminant functions were used to discriminate among groups. Three such functions were obtained. The first was related most strongly to mean response times in both series, and was related strongly as well to variance and regression measures in both series. The second function loaded highest on regression in the conflict series alone. The third function was related in particular to the extent to which the number of wrong responses was small in the nonconflict series and large in the conflict series.

The test discriminated among the four groups rather well in view of the slightly over 50% correct classification rate obtained being considerably higher than the roughly 25% to be expected by chance. These results also provide empirical support for the assumption that the combinations of military groups decided upon in forming Levels 1, 2, and 3 were reasonable ones in terms of reflecting appreciable differences in the Stroop Strategy Test measures. One should not ignore the possibility that there may have been major personality differences other than those assessed by the Stroop Strategy Test between the different military groups, such as between the professional soldiers (or the pilots) and the short-term recruits, and that certain age differences were found as well (the pilots being oldest).

Discrimination was best between the Prisoners group and the three military groups. The Prisoners group had the highest mean value on the first discriminant function, presumably reflecting their higher mean times, greater increase in response times (positive regression), and greater variance (variation in response times) in both the conflict and nonconflict series. These results point in the same direction as earlier S-CWT studies (S-CWT manual; Smith, *et al.*, 1986), provided one assumes that the behaviour of the Prisoners group approximates that of various of the clinical groups studied earlier.

According to findings of the military enrollment office, tank-gunners (Group 3) tend to resemble the normal population rather closely. The results for the first discriminant function indicated that this group was located between the Level-1 group and the Prisoners group. The Level-2 group, in turn, was located on this first discriminant function between the Level-1 and the Level-3 groups, the Level-1 group having the lowest value on it. This is in line with the expectations of emotional stability and stress tolerance placed upon this most select group.

The second discriminant function, likewise distinguishing between the three military groups, involved in part regression in the conflict series and wrong responses. The results suggest that, despite the rather modest differences between these groups found in terms of mean time and variance (as reflected by the group means on the first function), the conflict series tended to result in greater difficulties for the lower-level groups, in terms both of errors and of decrease in performance over time.

Results for the third discriminant function suggest that wrong responses can be useful in making fine distinctions between, above all, the Level-2 and

Level-3 groups. The three discriminant functions together presented a rather complex pattern of group differences. In examining these differences, one can note that each of the four measures the Stroop Strategy Test provides—mean, variance, regression, and error rate—contributed to an appreciable extent to distinguishing between the groups. This can be seen as a clear advantage as compared to the S-CWT, which only makes use of variance and regression, and both the conventional Stroop test and Thurstone's verison of it, which only make use of total time.

The results as a whole suggest that the Stroop Strategy Test has certain promise for selection and placement purposes for use in conjunction with other instruments of an appropriate type. The results in rank ordering each subject's classifications in accordance with the discriminant functions obtained illustrate how the discriminant power of the test in a classification context can be increased substantially if the second-best classifications are likewise taken into account. In developing the test it might be fruitful to add a third series, one more difficult to perform, with the idea of increasing the test's discriminative power. The somewhat better discrimination obtained for three of the four basic variables under the nonconflict than under the conflict conditions is a matter to investigate further. It is important in addition to study systematically what personality and behavioral traits are related to the variables the test provides and to different patterns of these variables or functions that are based on them and what relations there are between the test results and general intelligence. The applicability of the test in a clinical context could be explored as well, particularly in view of earlier findings there.

REFERENCES

ANDRÉ-PETERSSON, L., HAGBERG, B., HEDBLAD, B., JANZON, L., & STEEN, G. (1999) Incidence of cardiac events in hypertensive men related to adaptive behaviour in stressful encounters. *International Journal of Behavioural Medicine*, 6, 331-355.

BARKER, K., & ROBERTSON, N. (1997) Selective processing and fear of spiders: use of the Stroop task to assess interference for spider-related, movement, and disgust information. *Cognition and Emotion*, 11, 331-336.

BROADBENT, D. E. (1958) *Perception and communication*. London: Pergamon.

CARLSSON, I., AMNÈR, G., & SMITH, G. J. W. (1996) *Creativity and working environment on a Swedish airforce base*. Lund, Sweden: Department of Psychology, Univer. of Lund.

DANIEL, B., PELOTTE, M., & LEWIS, J. (2000) Lack of sex differences on the Stroop Color-Word Test across three age groups. *Perceptual and Motor Skills*, 90, 483-484.

EYSENCK, M. W. (1992) *Anxiety: the cognitive perspective*. London: Erlbaum.

EYSENCK, M. W. (1997) *Anxiety and cognition: a unified theory*. Hove, UK: Psychology Press.

FAUVEL, J. P., BERNARD, N., LAVILLE, M., DAOUD, S., POZET, N., & ZECH, P. (1996) Reproducibility of the cardiovascular reactivity to a computerised version of the Stroop stress test in normotensive and hypertensive subjects. *Clinical Autonomic Research*, 6(Suppl. 4), 219-224.

GOLDSMITH, R. W. (1968) Persönlichkeitsspezifische Komponenten des Entscheidungsverhaltens: I. Beziehungen zwischen der Interferenzneigung und dem Entscheidungsverhalten. *Psychologische Forschung*, 32, 135-168.

HARTSTON, H. J., & SWERDLOW, N. R. (1999) Visuospatial priming and Stroop performance in patients with obsessive compulsive disorder. *Neuropsychology*, 13, 447-457.
KRAGH, U., & SMITH, G. J. W. (1970) *Perceptgenetic analysis*. Lund: Berlingska Boktryckeriet.
LOGAN, G. D. (1980) Attention and automaticity in Stroop and priming tasks: theory and data. *Cognitive Psychology*, 12, 523-553.
LOTHIGIUS, J. (1995) *VIP manual*. Karlstad, Sweden: National Service Administration (Pliktverket).
MACLEOD, C. M. (1991) Half a century of research on the Stroop effect: an integrative review. *Psychological Bulletin*, 109, 163-203.
MACLEOD, C. M., & DUNBAR, K. (1988) Training and Stroop-like interference: evidence for a continuum of automaticity. *Journal of Experimental Psychology: Learning, Memory, and Cognition*, 14, 126-135.
MASIA, C. L., MCNEIL, D. W., COHN, L. G., & HOPE, D. A. (1999) Exposure to social anxiety words: treatment for social phobia based on the Stroop paradigm. *Association for Advancement of Behaviour Therapy*, 6, 248-257.
MATHEWS, A., & SEBASTIAN, S. (1993) Suppression of emotion Stroop effects by fear-arousal. *Cognition and Emotion*, 7, 517-524.
MCCLELLAND, J. L. (1979) On the time relations of mental processes: an examination of systems of processes in cascade. *Psychological Review*, 86, 287-330.
MCNEIL, D. W., TUCKER, P., MIRANDA, R., LEWIN, M. R., & NORDGREN, J. C. (1999) Response to depression and anxiety Stroop stimuli in posttraumatic stress disorder, obsessive-compulsive disorder, and major depressive disorder. *Journal of Nervous and Mental Disease*, 187, 512-515.
MORTON, J., & CHAMBERS, S. M. (1973) Selective attention to words and colours. *Quarterly Journal of Experimental Psychology*, 25, 387-397.
NYMAN, G. E., & SMITH, G. J. W. (1959) A contribution to the definition of psychopathic personality: clinical variants and serial test behaviour in a sample of young female delinquents. *Lunds Universitets årsskrift*, 55(Whole No. 10).
POSNER, M. I., & SNYDER, C. R. R. (1975) Attention and cognitive control. In R. L. Solso (Ed.), *Information processing and cognition: the Loyola symposium*. Hillsdale, NJ: Erlbaum. Pp. 55-85.
RENAUD, P., & BLONDIN, J. P. (1997) The stress of Stroop performance: physiological and emotional responses to color-word interference, task pacing, and pacing speed. *International Journal of Psychophysiology*, 27, 87-98.
SMITH, G. J. W., NYMAN, G. E., & HENTSCHEL, U. (1986) *CWT manual*. Stockholm: Psykologiförlaget.
STROOP, J. R. (1935) Studies of interference in serial verbal reactions. *Journal of Experimental Psychology*, 18, 643-661.
THURSTONE, L. L. (1944) *A factorial study of perception*. Chicago, IL: Univer. of Chicago Press.
VERHAEGHEN, P., & DE MEERSMAN, L. (1998) Aging and the Stroop effect: a meta-analysis. *Psychology and Aging*, 13, 120-126.
WILLIAMS, J. M. G., WATTS, F. N., MACLEOD, C., & MATHEWS, A. (1988) *Cognitive psychology and emotional disorders*. Chichester, UK: Wiley.
WILLIAMS, J. M. G., WATTS, F. N., MACLEOD, C., & MATHEWS, A. (1997) *Cognitive psychology and emotional disorders*. (2nd ed.) Chichester, UK: Wiley.

Accepted April 26, 2004.

FALSE RECOGNITION WITH THE DEESE-ROEDIGER-McDERMOTT-REID-SOLSO PROCEDURE: A QUANTITATIVE SUMMARY[1]

STUART J. McKELVIE

Bishop's University

Summary.—In the Deese-Roediger-McDermott-Read-Solso (DRMRS) procedure, participants study lists of words associated with central concepts (critical themes) that are not on the lists, then their memory is tested. Based on 224 estimates, the rate of False Recognition of the nonstudied critical themes was .59 (95% confidence interval of .56 to .61), which is smaller than the Hit rate of .75 for correct recognition of studied items (95% confidence interval of .73 to .77) but greater than various rates of False Alarms for other nonstudied items (ranging from .13 to .19). Ratings of subjective confidence were similar on Hits and on False Recognitions but higher than on False Alarms, confirming that false recognition was more like correct recognition than like other errors. The results from judgments of feeling of remembering or knowing, from the effects of intervening activities (particularly recall) between study and test, and from the effects of age suggest that False Recognition occurs because the critical theme is activated along with studied items during list presentation and perhaps also during recall. Invoking fuzzy trace theory, it is argued Hits are based on verbatim traces whereas False Recognition is based on gist traces and a failure of source memory. Proposals are made for research.

Beginning in the mid-1990s, many studies investigated memory performance using the Deese-Roediger-McDermott-Read-Solso procedure (DRMRS or "Drummers"; McKelvie, 2001) in which participants study lists of words associated with central concepts that do not themselves appear. For example, *bed, rest, awake, dream,* and *snooze* could be words on the list associated with *sleep.* Extending the original work of Deese (1959), who tested recall of such lists, Roediger and McDermott (1995) examined both recall and recognition, with particular attention to false memory for the nonstudied central concepts (often referred to as "critical themes").

Bruce and Winograd (1998) stated that this procedure became popular because it was linked to the controversial topic of false versus recovered memory of sexual abuse, and Roediger and McDermott (1995) themselves open their paper by wondering whether certain therapeutic practices might lead to false memories being reported. Although remembering words in the laboratory does not share obvious features with remembering trauma in real

---

[1]This article was supported in part by a grant from the Bishop's University Publications Committee. Send correspondence to Stuart J. McKelvie, Department of Psychology, Bishop's University, Lennoxville, Quebec J1M 1Z7, Canada or e-mail (smckelvi@ubishops.ca).

life (Freyd & Gleaves, 1996), the results may be interesting in their own right as phenomena of memory. Furthermore, as Mook (1983) pointed out, specific laboratory findings may not generalize, but experiments can reveal principles that are externally valid. In this case, the *mechanism* that generates false memory in the laboratory may also operate in real life.

Following a recent quantitative summary and review of the results with recall (McKelvie, 2003), the present report provides a quantitative summary of the results with recognition, which Roediger and McDermott (1995) also investigated in their seminal research. The first question here is whether the amount of incorrect recognition of the nonstudied critical themes (False Recognition) would be more like correct recognition of studied items (Hits) or more like incorrect recognition of other nonstudied items (False Alarms). Following Thapar and McDermott (2001), the second question is whether the effects of independent variables on False Recognition would be similar to their effects on Hits. From the answers to these questions, it was hoped to clarify the mechanism that underlies False Recognition.

Theoretical Considerations and Predictions

Roediger and McDermott (1995) speculated that False Recognition might occur because the nonstudied critical theme becomes familiar through spreading of activation in the associative network of memory. That is, because the central concept was related to all the items on a list, its memory strength might be increased, and participants would falsely recognize it as having been studied. The notion of spreading activation is similar to fuzzy trace theory, which a number of authors have invoked to explain false memory. According to this theory (Brainerd & Reyna, 1998), information in memory is stored in terms of surface characteristics (a verbatim trace) and semantic characteristics (a gist trace). When applied to the DRMRS procedure, it is assumed that studied items are differentiated from each other on the basis of verbatim traces. However, because each of them is related to the central concept, it is activated as a gist trace. Spreading activation and fuzzy trace theory predict that False Recognition would be higher than False Alarms and perhaps almost as high as Hits.

Judgments of remembering and of knowing.—Roediger and McDermott (1995) also argued that, when a studied item was presented on the recognition-memory test and recognized as familiar, it would most likely be accompanied by a vivid experience of explicitly "remembering" that it had been encountered before. Using Brainerd and Reyna's terminology (1998), this would occur on the basis of the verbatim trace. In contrast, Roediger and McDermott suggested that, when a critical theme was presented on the recognition test and recognized as familiar, it might be accompanied only by a feeling of "knowing" that it had been encountered before. Using Brainerd and Reyna's terminology (1998), this would occur on the basis of the gist trace. In fact, Roediger and McDermott pointed out that previous work on recognition memory had shown that correct recognitions were accompanied more often by judgments of remembering than of knowing, whereas False Alarms were more often accompanied by judgments of knowing than of remembering. Because False Recognitions are errors, they might also be accompanied more often by judgments of knowing than of remembering.

On the other hand, Roediger and McDermott observed that the critical theme might occur to participants while they were initially studying the related items. That is, the gist trace might be activated so strongly that the person consciously thought of the critical theme. Subsequently, when the theme is presented on a recognition test, they might remember that they experienced it but falsely recognize the item as having been on the list. This would be a failure of source memory—the person remembered the item but misattributed its source to the external list rather than to their internal experience. In this case, False Recognition might be accompanied more often by judgments of remembering than by judgments of knowing, just like memory for studied items (Hits). Indeed, experiencing the critical theme might even result in a partially-verbatim trace. This matter was investigated by examining the frequency of judgments of remembering or of knowing for each kind of response.

Judgments of confidence.—Another kind of subjective experience that accompanies memory is confidence. Roediger and McDermott (1995) stated that remember judgments do not simply reflect higher confidence than know judgments because the two kinds of judgments are affected by different variables. The relationship between confidence and accuracy has been a controversial question in recognition-memory research, particularly with eyewitnessing because people have sometimes been extremely confident in their decision that an item had been presented when it had not (Deffenbacher, 1980). Therefore, a practical question here is whether confidence would follow the pattern of Hits, False Recognitions, and False Alarms. If so, it might provide a guide to a person's accuracy. In particular, if confidence on False Recognitions is lower than confidence on Hits, it might be possible to establish a level of confidence that would indicate that their response was a false memory.

Effect of prior recall.—In Roediger and McDermott's experiments (1995), some participants recalled the list items before taking the recognition test, and others engaged in an arithmetic filler task. This provides an opportunity to examine whether the independent variable of prior recall had the same effect on Hits and on False Recognitions. If it did, this would suggest that the False Recognitions were based on a similar mechanism to Hits. In particular, if prior recall increased both Hits and False Recognitions, this might mean that the nonstudied critical theme was generated during recall along with the studied items (Roediger & McDermott, 1995). This could occur because the gist trace for the critical theme had been activated during initial list presentation. However, it is also possible that the gist trace was only activated during recall.

Because a number of studies followed Roediger and McDermott's procedure with prior recall and arithmetic conditions, this matter was investigated here. However, many studies included a control condition without arithmetic between list presentation and recognition test. Because the delay was usually filled with test instructions and did not provide an opportunity for recall or rehearsal, it was predicted that, if prior recall enhanced Hits and False Recognition compared to that of the arithmetic condition, it would also do so compared to this no activity condition.

It was argued above that Hits would be accompanied more often by judgments of remembering than of knowing, and that False Recognitions might be accompanied more often by judgments of knowing *or* of remembering. However, recall might enhance the feeling of remembering on the recognition test. This would mean that the difference between judgments of remembering and of knowing on Hits would be greater following recall than following arithmetic or no activity. This would also apply to False Recognitions if remembering was more frequent than knowing after arithmetic or no activity. However, if remembering was less frequent than knowing in these conditions, the increase in remembering judgments following recall might bring them up to the same level as judgments of knowing.

Age and recognition.—Age of participants has been included in a number of studies of false memory. If the strength of studied items in memory (verbatim trace) is weaker for older people than for younger people, old and new items would be more similar in memory strength for older people, leading them to have fewer Hits and more False Alarms. The prediction for False Recognitions depends on whether spreading activation differs in the two groups. If it is less for older people, they would have weaker gist traces, and fewer False Recognitions than younger people. If it is similar, the two groups would have a similar number of False Recognitions; however, if spreading activation was greater for older people, they would have stronger gist traces and more False Recognitions than younger people. It is also possible that older people have poorer source memory than younger people (LaVoie & Mulstrom, 1998). If False Recognition is based on a failure of source memory, False Recognition would again be higher for older people.

METHOD

For details of how the studies were located, see McKelvie (2003). Briefly, the PsycLIT data base, Current Contents (Social and Behavioral Sciences), and the reference sections of retrieved papers were searched from 1994 to 1999. For recognition memory, 27 papers were found. In some cases, authors were contacted for details of their results.

In the recognition tests, participants were presented with items from the lists (studied items), the nonstudied central concept for each list (critical theme), and other new items that had not been presented (other nonstudied items). These other nonstudied items were usually of two kinds: (a) unrelated to items on the studied lists but selected from different lists that had been constructed around other central concepts so items were related to each other and (b) the other central concepts. In some studies, the other nonstudied items were unrelated to items on any list and were the only distractors presented.

Participants judged whether each item was "old" (had been on a list) or "new" (had not been on a list). They may also have given a rating to indicate how confident they were in this response or asked for a judgment about remembering or knowing, where "remembering" means that they felt that the original experience was reinstated (like episodic memory) and "knowing" means that they felt only generally familiar with the item (like semantic memory) (Roediger & McDermott, 1995; Anastasi, Rhodes, & Burns, 2000).

The experiments contained a number of independent variables, but the only two that occurred sufficiently often to be included in the present analyses were prior activity in which recognition was preceded by a recall test, by an arithmetic filler task, or by no test at all, and age where participants were younger adults (usually university students) or older adults.

As in the quantitative analysis of false recall (McKelvie, 2003), two sets of descriptive statistics were calculated for both the general recognition-memory data and for data that separated the remember or know judgments. In the Complete Set, results from all experiments were included. These data were used for the major analyses and to examine the effects of prior activity and of age. In the Standard Set, only results from the most popular combination of conditions were retained: young participants (usually university students), blocked presentation of word lists, at least four lists, at least 10 list items, at least a 1-sec. exposure time per item, no special encoding or forewarning instructions, test reasonably soon after all lists (usually the time taken to give instructions), and no special test instructions. These data were not analyzed in detail, but are provided for archival purposes (see also Westerberg & Marsolek, 2003). Here, they constitute a data base that can serve as norms for researchers who use this procedure. It represents the basic conditions in Roediger and McDermott's seminal work (1995).

Positive ("old") responses were either correct (hits) or incorrect (false positives), but the latter were coded into four categories yielding five categories of response corresponding to the five kinds of item described above:

Hits (correctly judging studied items as old), False Recognitions (incorrectly judging the nonstudied critical themes as old), Hit False Alarms (incorrectly judging nonstudied items as old but these items were selected from the different lists constructed around other central concepts), False Recognition False Alarms (incorrectly judging the other central concepts as old), and General False Alarms (incorrectly judging nonstudied items as old but these items were the only distractors). Hit False Alarms were compared to Hits, and False Recognition False Alarms were compared to False Recognitions.

Data for all five responses are reported. However, to remove the effect of a possible positive response bias towards classifying any item as "old," which would artificially inflate the number of old responses to studied items, hits on a recognition-memory test are often corrected, for example, by subtracting false alarms (e.g., McKelvie, 1990). This adjustment, which is known as the two-high-threshold measure of sensitivity, assumes that the positive responses to new items are guesses, and that a similar number of the positive responses to old items are also guesses (Snodgrass & Corwin, 1988). Therefore, to obtain a true measure of sensitivity, the hits are corrected by subtracting the false alarms. Here, Hits and False Recognitions were each corrected by subtracting their corresponding false alarms. This means that False Recognitions were treated as a kind of "hit." If the only distractors were new items that were not paired with studied items or with critical lures, both Hits and False Recognitions were corrected by subtracting the General False Alarms. Although the strategy of taking false alarm rates into account when evaluating hit rates is routinely followed in signal-detection experiments and in recognition-memory experiments, it is less frequent in studies of false recognition. However, it has been demonstrated that the two-high-threshold measure is particularly sensitive to changes in discriminative capacity (Snodgrass & Corwin, 1988; Seamon, Luo, Kopecky, Price, Rothschild, Fung, & Schwartz, 2002) and has consequently been chosen as the best method to correct Hits and False Recognitions (Seamon, Goodkind, Dumey, Dick, Aufseeser, Strickland, Woulfin, & Fung, 2003).

Confidence data were sparse, but were examined. However, many studies included judgments about remembering or knowing, giving a good basis for quantitative analysis.

Results

Alpha was set at .05 for all standard inferential statistics. Analyses were conducted with SPSS Version 7.5.

General Recognition Memory

Original Responses

Comparison of Hits, False Recognitions, and False Alarms.—Table 1 shows the mean proportions for the five kinds of response for the Standard

Set and for the Complete Set of data. In both cases, all means were significantly greater than zero, as evident in single-sample t tests (not reported). However, Hits were highest (.78, .75, respectively), followed by False Recognitions (.70, .59). The other three false alarm rates were lowest (between .11 and .19).

TABLE 1
General Recognition Memory: Original Responses

	Hits	Hit False Alarms	General False Alarms	False Recognition False Alarms	False Recognitions
Standard Set					
n	57	31	14	29	58
M	.78	.14	.11	.19	.70
SD	.08	.07	.07	.09	.13
Complete Set					
n	227	128	38	126	224
M	.75	.15	.13	.19	.59
SD	.13	.01	.01	.12	.22
95% Confidence Intervals for Hits and False Recognitions					
	.73 to .77				.56 to .61
Prior Activity					
Recall					
n	34	9	12	9	35
M	.81	.18	.01	.23	.69
SD	.01	.01	.01	.10	.14
Arithmetic					
n	14	4		4	14
M	.67	.12		.19	.74
SD	.11	.00		.08	.01
No Activity					
n	171	107	26	107	167
M	.74	.16	.16	.19	.54
SD	.14	.01	.01	.12	.22
Age					
Younger					
n	151	84	30	82	151
M	.74	.16	.13	.21	.57
SD	.13	.01	.01	.12	.22
Older					
n	64	33	8	33	61
M	.78	.01	.13	.12	.60
SD	.14	.01	.01	.10	.22
Studies With Both Younger People and Older People					
Younger					
n	50	22		22	47
M	.80	.08		.11	.42
SD	.09	.06		.09	.25
Older					
n	50	22		22	47
M	.75	.12		.16	.56
SD	.13	.07		.09	.23

For the Complete Set, the Hit False Alarms and General False Alarms (.15, .13) were not significantly different, but both were lower than False Recognition False Alarms (.59; $t_{350} = 2.99$, $p < .01$; $t_{164} = 2.70$, $p < .01$, respectively). Omitting General False Alarms, for which the sample size was much smaller than for the other four responses, a one-way within-groups analysis of variance on Hits, Hit False Alarms, False Recognition False Alarms, and False Recognitions was significant ($F_{2,229} = 515.58$, $p < .001$). *Post hoc* Neuman-Keuls tests showed that the means were ordered as follows: Hits > False Recognitions > False Recognition False Alarms > Hit False Alarms (.75, .59, .19, .15).

Effect of prior activity.—For the Complete Set, the effects of prior activity were examined with between-groups one-way analyses of variance. The effect was significant for Hits ($F_{2,216} = 6.91$, $p < .005$), for General False Alarms ($F_{1,35} = 5.20$, $p < .02$), and for False Recognitions ($F_{2,213} = 12.22$, $p < .001$). Hits (.81) were significantly higher after recall than after no activity (.74) or after arithmetic (.67), but the latter two did not differ from each other. General False Alarms were lower after no activity than after recall (.01, .16). Given insufficient numbers, there was no arithmetic condition here. False Recognitions did not differ significantly between arithmetic and recall (.74, .69), but both were significantly higher than after no activity (.54).

Effect of age.—The effect of age was significant for Hit False Alarms ($t_{115} = 3.73$, $p < .001$), and for False Recognition False Alarms ($t_{113} = 3.59$, $p < .001$). In both cases, False Alarms were higher for younger adults than for older adults. Hits tended to be higher for older than for younger participants, but the trend was not significant at the .05 level ($t_{213} = 1.80$, ns).

However, one problem with this analysis is that some of the studies with only younger participants had difficult encoding conditions, such as short exposure times. A second analysis was conducted on the studies of both younger and older participants, which ensured that they were both exposed to comparable conditions. Here, Hits were lower for older than for younger participants ($t_{98} = 2.39$, $p < .02$), and False Recognitions were higher for older than for younger participants ($t_{92} = 2.85$, $p < .01$). There were also trends towards more Hit False Alarms and more False Recognition False Alarms for older than for younger participants, but they were not significant at the .05 level ($t_{42} = 1.74$, 1.86, ns, respectively). Mean scores are shown in Table 1 above.

The tendency for older people to have slightly more hits (first analysis) and more false positives on the three kinds of new item than younger people might mean that the older people were generally more biased towards saying "old." To examine this possibility, older and younger participants were compared on the two-high-threshold measure of response bias towards saying old (Snodgrass & Corwin, 1988). The formula is $B_r = FA/[1 - (H - FA)]$, where B_r = response bias, FA = false alarm rate, and H = hit rate. If the percentage correct on Hits and False Alarms is equal, there is no bias, giving a value of .5. For example, if Hits were .80 and False Alarms were .20, B_r = .20/[1 – (.80 – .20)] = .50. Values above .50 indicate a liberal bias towards "old", and values below .50 indicate a conservative bias away from "old."

A 2 × 2 (Age of Participant × Response) mixed model analysis of variance showed that there were significant main effects for age of participant ($F_{1,86}$ = 8.52, $p < .01$) and of response ($F_{1,86}$ = 22.50, $p < .001$). Bias was higher for older people than for younger people and was also higher on Hits than on False Recognitions. Means and standard deviations in the four conditions were .27 (.16) for Hits by younger people, .35 (.18) for Hits by older people, .17 (.16) for False Recognitions by younger people, and .29 (.20) for False Recognitions by older people. Given this age difference in bias, it is particularly important to examine the effect of age on recognition accuracy on the corrected response measure (see below).

Confidence judgments.—Participants were not usually asked to rate how confident they were in their responses but, using the complete data, there were eight estimates for confidence with Hits, with General False Alarms, and with False Recognitions. Because the number of points on the rating scale varied across studies, the data were transformed to proportions of the maximum rating. For example, if the mean rating for correct responses was 4.2 on a 5-point scale, the mean became .84 (McKelvie, 2003). A one-way within-groups analysis of variance showed that there was a significant effect of response ($F_{2,14}$ = 22.89, $p < .001$). The mean confidence for the three responses were .80 (SD = .01) for Hits, .49 (SD = .13) for General False Alarms, and .73 (SD = .01) for False Recognitions. *Post hoc* Newman-Keuls comparisons showed that the confidence did not differ significantly between Hits and False Recognitions, but it was higher for both of them than for General False Alarms.

Corrected Responses

Comparison of Hits and False Recognitions.—Table 2 shows the mean proportions for Hits and for False Recognitions. For the Standard Set, Hits were significantly higher than False Recognitions (.65, .55; t_{55} = 5.29, $p < .001$). The same result occurred for the Complete Set (.61, .42; t_{219} = 12.46, $p < .001$).

Effect of prior activity.—For the Complete Set, a 3 × 2 (Prior Activity × Response) mixed model analysis of variance showed significant effects of prior activity ($F_{2,209}$ = 8.72, $p < .001$), response ($F_{1,209}$ = 23.49, $p < .001$), and their interaction ($F_{2,209}$ = 8.96, $p < .001$). Hits were generally higher than False Recognitions, but this difference was only significant after recall (.69, .54; t_{32} = 5.78, $p < .01$) and after no activity (.60, .38; t_{164} = 16.59, $p < .01$), but not after arithmetic (.51, .53). Hits were also higher after recall than after arith-

TABLE 2
General Recognition Memory: Corrected Responses
(Two-high-threshold Measure of Sensitivity)

Measure	Hits n	M	SD	False Recognitions n	M	SD
Standard Set	56	.65	.11	56	.53	.16
Complete Set	220	.61	.19	220	.42	.21
95% Confidence Intervals		.59 to .64			.39 to .45	
Prior Activity						
Recall	33	.69	.14	33	.54	.18
Arithmetic	14	.51	.16	14	.53	.13
No Activity	165	.60	.20	165	.38	.21
Age of Participant						
Younger	147	.60	.19	147	.40	.21
Older	61	.67	.17	61	.47	.21
Studies With Both Younger People and Older People						
Age of Participant						
Younger	44	.72	.12	44	.34	.23
Older	44	.63	.15	44	.41	.20

metic (.69, .51; $t_{209}=3.02$, $p<.01$) and higher after recall than after no activity (.69, .60; $t_{209}=2.58$, $p<.01$), but they did not differ significantly between arithmetic and no activity (.51, .60). In contrast, False Recognitions were higher after recall and arithmetic than after no activity (.54, .53, .38; $t_{209}=4.33, 2.85$, $ps<.01$) but did not differ significantly between recall and arithmetic.

Effect of age.—For the Complete Set that included studies with younger *or* older participants, conditions were not equivalent, but the analysis is reported for completeness. A 2 × 2 (Age of Participant × Response) mixed-model analysis of variance showed a significant main effect of age of participant ($F_{1,206}=8.69$, $p<.001$) and of response ($F_{1,206}=127.40$, $p<.001$), but the interaction was not significant. Older people had more Hits and more False Recognitions than younger people, and Hits were higher than False Recognitions for both groups.

However, for studies that had *both* younger *and* older participants, there were significant effects of response ($F_{1,86}=162.49$, $p<.001$) and of the interaction between age of participant and response ($F_{1,86}=13.06$, $p<.002$). Hits were more frequent than False Recognitions for both groups, but Hits were lower for older people than for younger people (.63, .72; $t_{86}=2.78$, $p<.01$), and False Recognitions were higher for older people than for younger people (.41, .34; $t_{86}=2.02$, $p<.05$).

Judgements of Remembering or Knowing

Original Responses

Comparison of Hits, False Recognitions, and False Alarms.—Table 3 shows the mean proportions for the five kinds of response with the standard and complete sets of data. For the Complete Set, paired-sample t tests showed that remember judgments were significantly higher than know judgments for Hits (.51, .21; $t_{67}=11.50$, $p<.001$) and for False Recognitions (.40, .26; $t_{67}=5.50$, $p<.001$) but significantly lower for False Recognition False Alarms (.08, .12; $t_{39}=3.60$, $p<.002$) and for Hit False Alarms (.06, .10; $t_{40}=3.81$, $p<.001$). Remember and know judgments also showed this trend for General False Alarms, but the difference was not significant at the .05 level ($t_{10}=2.00$, ns).

TABLE 3
JUDGMENTS OF REMEMBERING (R) OR KNOWING (K): ORIGINAL RESPONSES

	Hits R	Hits K	Hit False Alarms R	Hit False Alarms K	General False Alarms R	General False Alarms K	False Recognition False Alarms R	False Recognition False Alarms K	False Recognition R	False Recognition K
Standard Set										
n	25	25	14	14	5	5	13	13	25	25
M	.51	.24	.07	.11	.04	.10	.07	.13	.41	.30
SD	.11	.08	.05	.04	.03	.03	.05	.04	.10	.11
Complete Set										
n	68	68	41	41	11	11	40	40	68	68
M	.51	.21	.06	.10	.07	.13	.08	.12	.40	.26
SD	.15	.09	.05	.06	.05	.07	.06	.08	.15	.12
Complete Set: Without General False Alarms, Within Subjects										
n	40	40	40	40			40	40	40	40
M	.54	.21	.06	.09			.08	.12	.39	.24
SD	.15	.08	.04	.06			.06	.08	.16	.10
Prior Activity										
Recall										
n	12	12	12	12			12	12	12	12
M	.53	.21	.05	.09			.08	.12	.53	.25
SD	.10	.04	.04	.04			.07	.06	.09	.06
Arithmetic										
n	12	12	12	12			12	12	12	12
M	.42	.23	.05	.09			.08	.12	.45	.29
SD	.12	.06	.04	.04			.07	.06	.15	.10
No Activity										
n	39	39	39	39			39	39	39	39
M	.53	.21	.07	.11			.08	.12	.33	.24
SD	.16	.11	.05	.07			.06	.08	.15	.14

Because there were not many studies with General False Alarms, a 4 × 2 (Response × Judgment) within-groups analysis of variance was conducted on the other four responses in the Complete Set ($n=40$, see Table 3). All three effects were significant: response ($F_{3,117}=212.02$, $p<.001$), judgment ($F_{1,39}=39.50$, $p<.001$), and their interaction ($F_{3,117}=84.663$, $p<.001$). Using

Newman-Keuls tests for remember judgments, Hits were higher than False Recognitions (.54, .39), and False Recognitions were higher than the two False Alarm responses (.39, .06, .08). For know judgments, none of the comparisons was significant. Again, remember judgments were more frequent than know judgments for Hits and for False Recognitions, whereas remember judgments were less frequent than know judgments for Hit False Alarms and for False Recognition False Alarms.

Effects of age and of prior activity.—Unfortunately, there were insufficient cases to examine the effect of age with judgments of remembering and of knowing.

However, for prior activity, a 3 × 4 × 2 (Prior Activity × Response × Judgment) mixed-model analysis of variance was conducted. The main effects of response ($F_{3,180} = 370.24$, $p < .001$) and of judgment ($F_{1,60} = 28.10$, $p < .001$) were significant. There were also some significant interactions, the most important of which was the interaction among all three factors ($F_{6,180} = 4.54$, $p < .001$). Remember judgments were generally higher than know judgments, but this occurred only for Hits (recall $t_{11} = 6.46$, $p < .01$; arithmetic $t_{11} = 3.80$, $p < .01$; no activity $t_{38} = 11.87$, $p < .01$), and for False Recognitions (recall $t_{11} = 5.77$, $p < .01$, arithmetic $t_{11} = 3.09$, $p < .01$, no activity $t_{38} = 3.48$, $p < .01$). None of the comparisons for Hit False Alarms or for False Recognition False Alarms was significant. Hits were also generally higher than False Recognitions, but this was only significant in one condition: for remember judgments after no activity ($t_{38} = 15.98$, $p < .01$). However, in two other conditions, Hits were lower than False Recognitions ($t_{11} = 2.88$, $p < .05$), for know judgments after arithmetic ($t_{38} = 2.79$, $p < .01$) and for know judgments after no activity. The results for Newman-Keuls tests for remember and for know judgments are reported above.

Of most interest here, *post hoc* tests were also conducted on the effect of prior activity for each score with remember and with know judgments. With remember judgments, Hits were higher after recall than after arithmetic (.53, .42; $t_{180} = 3.78$, $p < .01$) and after no activity than after arithmetic (.53, .42; $t_{180} = 5.96$, $p < .01$), but there were no significant differences for know judgments. For Hit False Alarms and for General False Alarms, prior activity had no effects with remember or with know judgments. With remember judgments, False Recognitions were higher after recall than after arithmetic (.53, .45; $t_{180} = 3.79$, $p < .01$), and after arithmetic than after no activity (.45, .33; $t_{180} = 5.98$, $p < .01$). One comparison was significant with know judgments: False Recognitions were higher after arithmetic than after no activity (.29, .24; $t_{180} = 2.91$, $p < .01$).

Corrected Responses

Comparison of Hits and False Recognitions.—In a 2 × 2 (Response ×

Judgment) within-groups analysis of variance on the Standard Set of data, there were significant effects of response ($F_{1,24} = 6.23$, $p < .03$), of judgment ($F_{1,24} = 54.48$, $p < .001$), and of their interaction ($F_{1,24} = 28.29$, $p < .001$). A similar pattern occurred for the Complete Set, with significant effects of response ($F_{1,67} = 18.88$, $p < .001$), judgment ($F_{1,67} = 182.24$, $p < .001$), and their interaction ($F_{1,67} = 36.35$, $p < .001$). First, Table 4 shows that remember judgments were higher than know judgments for both Hits (.45, .11; $t_{67} = 7.62$, $p < .01$) and for False Recognitions (.32, .13; $t_{67} = 4.19$, $p < .01$), but the difference was greater for Hits (.34, .19). Second, hits were more frequent than False Recognitions for remember judgments (.45, .32; $t_{67} = 10.4$, $p < .01$) but not for know judgments (.11, .13) for which the difference was not significant.

TABLE 4
JUDGMENTS OF REMEMBERING OR KNOWING: CORRECTED RESPONSES
(TWO-HIGH-THRESHOLD MEASURE OF SENSITIVITY)

| | Hits |||||| | False Recognitions ||||||
| | Remembering ||| Knowing ||| Remembering ||| Knowing |||
	n	M	SD	n	M	SD	n	M	SD	n	M	SD
Standard Set	25	.46	.10	25	.14	.09	25	.35	.11	25	.18	.12
Complete Set	68	.45	.16	68	.11	.01	68	.32	.14	68	.13	.11
Prior Activity												
Recall	12	.48	.12	12	.12	.06	12	.45	.10	12	.13	.10
Arithmetic	12	.37	.13	12	.14	.08	12	.37	.14	12	.17	.13
No Activity	39	.46	.18	39	.10	.09	39	.25	.12	39	.12	.11

Effect of prior activity.—A 3 × 2 × 2 (Prior Activity × Response × Judgment) mixed-model analysis of variance was also conducted on the Complete Set. There were significant main effects of prior activity ($F_{1,60} = 4.89$, $p < .02$) and of judgment ($F_{1,60} = 130.23$, $p < .001$), and they were accompanied by a number of significant interactions, the most important of which was the three-way interaction ($F_{2,60} = 7.56$, $p < .005$). First, remember judgments were significantly higher than know judgments for both Hits and False Recognitions in all three conditions (all *post hoc t*s, $p < .01$). However, the differences for Hits and for False Recognitions were similar after recall (.36, .33) and after arithmetic (.23, .20), but greater for Hits than for False Recognitions after no activity (.35, .14). Second, for remember judgments, Table 4 shows that Hits were significantly higher than False Recognitions after no activity (.46, .25; $t_{38} = 7.30$, $p < .01$) but were very similar to False Recognitions after recall (.48, .45) and after arithmetic (.37, .37). However, for know judgments, Hits were somewhat fewer than False Recognitions in all three prior activity conditions, although none of the three comparisons was statistically significant.

Finally, a comparison of performance among the three prior activity conditions showed the following results for *remember* judgments: Hits were not significantly different between recall and no activity, but both were higher than after arithmetic (recall $t_{180}=2.24$, $p<.05$; no activity $t_{180}=2.31$, $p<.05$); False Recognitions were not significantly different between recall and arithmetic, but both were higher than after no activity (recall $t_{180}=3.00$, $p<.01$; arithmetic $t_{180}=2.84$, $p<.01$). None of the comparisons for know judgments was significant. This means that the higher number of False Recognitions for know judgments after arithmetic than after no activity with original responses did not appear when the False Recognitions were corrected by False Recognition False Alarms.

Discussion

This discussion considers the two major questions of whether False Recognitions would more closely resemble Hits or False Alarms and whether False Recognitions and Hits would be affected in a similar way by independent variables (judgments of remembering or knowing, prior activity, age of participants). Using these results, theoretical accounts of the false recognition effect were examined.

General Comparisons

Accuracy.—Considering all five categories of response, Hits were more frequent than the four kinds of error (Hit False Alarms, General False Alarms, False Recognition False Alarms, and False Recognitions). However, False Recognitions (.59) were clearly higher than the three false alarms (.15, .13, .19) and were almost as high as Hits (.75). Thus, although the critical themes were not studied, they were often mistaken for items that were studied. In this sense, they were more like Hits than like False Alarms. The 95% confidence intervals were .73 to .77 for Hits and .56 to .61 for False Recognitions. For False Recognitions, the standardized effect size d (Cohen, 1977) was 2.70, which far exceeds Cohen's guideline of 0.80 for a large effect.

An unexpected result was that False Recognition False Alarms were higher than both Hit False Alarms and General False Alarms, which did not differ from each other. Because the items for Hit False Alarms were drawn from nonstudied lists that were formulated around central concepts, they shared some semantic relationships, but this did not increase the likelihood that they would be incorrectly identified as old when compared with items completely unrelated to each other. However, participants were more likely to identify mistakenly central concepts *that were not associated with any studied items*. Perhaps these central concepts were generally more familiar than the other nonstudied items that were chosen to be on the lists. Unfortunately, this creates a problem for the estimate of False Recognitions. The fact that False Recognition False Alarms were higher than both the Hit False

Alarms and General False Alarms implies that Hits and False Recognitions are not strictly comparable because participants may be more biased towards saying "old" in the second case.

To allow for this, the Hits and False Recognitions were each corrected by subtracting their respective False Alarms (the two-high-threshold measure). Hits remained higher than False Recognitions, the corrected estimates being .61 and .42, respectively, rather than .75 and .59. Nevertheless, a false recognition rate of .42 is not far below the hit rate of .61 and demonstrates the strength of the false recognition effect. The corrected 95% confidence intervals were .59 to .64 for Hits and .39 to .45 for False Recognitions. The standardized effect size for False Recognitions was $d=2.0$, which is again extremely large according to Cohen's 0.80 guideline.

Notably, in the recent quantitative review of false *recall*, the corresponding mean rates were .37 for recall of critical themes, .57 for recall of studied items, and .08 for other recall errors (McKelvie, 2003). Therefore, both False Recognition and false recall were considerably higher than other errors. In addition, although the value of .37 for false recall of critical themes is just below the present False Recognition confidence interval, the standardized effect size for false recall was $d=2.3$, which is just above the value of 2.0 for corrected False Recognition. Clearly, both kinds of error are extremely large.

Confidence.—Some investigators have examined the phenomenological experience of their participants in memory studies, particularly whether a person's confidence reflects their accuracy. In the present studies, confidence data were not collected very often, but the analysis showed that subjective confidence was rated higher for Hits and for False Recognitions than for General False Alarms. This demonstrates that the experience of participants on False Recognitions was more like their experience on Hits than on General False Alarms and is consistent with the fact the rate for False Recognition rate was closer to the rate for Hits than to the rates for other False Alarms.

These confidence results show how strongly people believed in their false recognition responses, but they do not support the suggestion that confidence ratings might be helpful for discriminating Hits from False Recognitions. Hits themselves were significantly higher than False Recognitions, but this was not reflected in the confidence judgments. This supports previous evidence that confidence and accuracy are not strongly related (Deffenbacher, 1980), but it is inconsistent with the results from recall studies (McKelvie, 2003), where confidence ratings followed objective responses precisely: correct recall was higher than false recall of critical themes, and both were higher than false recall of unrelated items. Confidence ratings might be helpful for identifying false recall, but they do not seem to be useful for identifying false recognition.

Together, the results on accuracy and confidence demonstrate that False Recognitions were more similar to Hits than to other False Alarms. This is consistent with the theory of spreading activation, according to which the critical theme is activated from memory during list presentation (Roediger & McDermott, 1995). Because False Recognitions are not identical to Hits, they are also consistent with fuzzy trace theory according to which studied items are represented as verbatim traces and critical themes are represented as gist traces.

Judgments of Remembering or Knowing and the Effect of Prior Activity

Judgments of remembering or knowing.—Many investigators of false recognition have examined the phenomenological experiences of remembering and knowing. In both cases, participants are confident that they recognize an item, but remembering means a mental reliving of the original experience whereas knowing does not (Roediger & McDermott, 1995; Anastasi, *et al.*, 2000). We would expect that accurate responses would be associated with remembering rather than knowing and that inaccurate responses would be associated with knowing rather than remembering (Anastasi, *et al.*, 2000). In fact, Roediger and McDermott (1995) stated that judgments of remembering are more frequent than judgments of knowing for Hits whereas judgments of knowing are more frequent than judgments of remembering for False Alarms. The interesting question here was how judgments of remembering and of knowing would differ for False Recognitions.

Considering all five categories of response, the present analysis replicates previous findings (Roediger & McDermott, 1995) that judgments of remembering were more frequent than judgments of knowing for Hits whereas judgments of knowing were more frequent than judgments of remembering for False Alarms. This occurred for both Hit False Alarms and for False Recognition False Alarms, and there was a similar trend for General False Alarms that was not statistically significant. In contrast, the phenomenological experience on False Recognitions was similar to that on Hits, not to that on False Alarms: when participants falsely recognized critical themes, judgments of remembering were more frequent than judgments of knowing. This confirms that False Recognitions are not the same as other kinds of recognition-memory error. The pattern of judgments for remembering or knowing was more like Hits than False Alarms.

In addition, judgments of remembering were also more frequent than judgments of knowing for corrected Hits and for corrected False Recognitions, which is consistent with Roediger and McDermott's suggestion (1995) that the critical theme was consciously experienced along with the studied items during list preparation. This implies that False Recognition is an error of source memory: participants mistakenly attribute their memory for their internal experience of the critical theme to its appearance on the list. At the same time, the difference between the judgments of remembering and judgments of knowing was greater on Hits (.45 − .11 = .34) than on False Recognitions (.32 − .13 = .19). Perhaps this is due to the fact that Hits are based on verbatim traces whereas False Recognitions are based on gist traces, which are not so likely to generate a vivid experience.

Effect of prior activity.—Considering all five categories of response, both Hits and False Recognitions were higher after recall than after no activity. This is not due to a tendency to simply respond "old" more often after recall because there was no significant effect of prior activity on Hit False Alarms or on False Recognition False Alarms, and General False Alarms were actually *lower* after no activity than after recall. It is not clear why prior activity would affect only General False Alarms, but they reinforce the interpretation that the results with Hits and False Recognitions are not due to response bias. Indeed, with corrected scores, both Hits and False Recognitions were higher after recall than after no activity. These results support Roediger and McDermott's suggestion (1995) that the critical theme might be generated along with studied items during recall.

In addition, the results show again that an independent variable affects Hits and False Recognitions in a manner that is similar but different from the effect on False Alarms.

What about the intervening activity of arithmetic, which Roediger and McDermott (1995) compared to recall? As predicted, Hits were higher after recall than after no activity or arithmetic, and performance did not differ significantly between the latter two. However, both uncorrected and corrected Hits were absolutely *lower* after arithmetic than after no activity (corrected values of .51 and .60, respectively). Indeed, the difference between Hits in these two conditions (.09) was the same as the difference between recall and no activity (.69 − .60 = .09). One reason that the first difference is not significant is that the number of cases with arithmetic was only 14, whereas it was 33 with recall and 165 with no activity.

In contrast, False Recognitions were higher for both recall and arithmetic than for no activity (corrected scores of .54, .53, .38, respectively), and False Recognitions were just as high as Hits after arithmetic (.53, .54, respectively). Therefore, the intervening activity of arithmetic had a different effect on Hits and on False Recognitions: it tended to decrease Hits, and it increased False Recognitions. A possible explanation is arithmetic may not only have prevented rehearsal of studied items, it might also have *interfered* with their *verbatim* traces. Arithmetic may also have prevented rehearsal of critical themes but *without* interfering with their *gist* traces. If arithmetic had interfered with gist traces, False Recognitions should have shown the same downward trend as Hits. The increase in False Recognitions following arithmetic compared to no activity may have occurred because it *interfered* with *source memory* for the critical theme. This matter should be investigated by including all three prior activity conditions in the same experiment.

Judgments of remembering or knowing and effects of prior activity.—It was speculated that the intervening task of recall might not only enhance both Hits and False Recognitions but might also increase the feeling of remembering more than the feeling of knowing. Thus, if judgments of remembering were already more frequent than judgments of knowing after arithmetic and after no activity, this difference might be exaggerated after recall.

This is essentially what happened with False Recognition. Judgments of remembering were higher than judgments of knowing after no activity (.25, .12, giving a difference of .13), but the difference was greater after recall (.45, .13, difference = .32). Notably, and in line with the general effect of recall in False Recognitions reported above, judgments of remembering were higher after arithmetic than after no activity (.37, .25), yielding a difference between judgments of remembering and of knowing after arithmetic of .20 (.37 − .17). However, the difference after recall (.32) was greater still.

The effect of intervening activity on judgments of remembering had a somewhat different effect in Hits than on False Recognitions. As with False Recognitions, judgments of remembering were higher than judgments of knowing after no activity (.46, .10, giving a difference of .36). However, unlike False Recognitions, they were very similar to this after recall (.48, .12, giving a difference of .36). In particular, judgments of remembering on Hits did *not* increase after recall compared to no activity (.48, .46). This stands in contrast to the *general* effect of recall on Hits. As noted above, Hits increased from .60 with no activity to .69 with recall. Because this result is based on all studies, some of which did not obtain judgments of remembering and of knowing, it is possible that the effect of recall on recognition is not the same when these judgments are given and when they are not. This should be experimentally investigated by comparing the effects of prior activity on Hits and on False Alarms with and without the request to provide judgments of remembering and knowing.

There was another difference between the results on Hits with all studies, and with those on judgments of remembering. In the first case, it was also observed that Hits were somewhat but not significantly lower after arithmetic than after no activity (.51, .60). However, with judgments of remembering, this difference was significant (.37, .46), so that Hits were significantly lower after arithmetic than after recall *and* after no activity. Because it is assumed that judgments of remembering reflect a conscious experience of the studied item during initial list presentation, this result supports the suggestion that arithmetic interferes with verbatim traces of studied items.

In the general analysis of Hits and False Recognitions discussed above,

Hits were higher. This also occurred with judgments of remembering after no activity. However, with judgments of knowing in all intervening activity conditions, Hits and False Recognitions did not differ significantly. Similarly, with judgments of remembering after recall, Hits and False Recognitions were not significantly different (.48, .45) because Hits did not change and False Recognitions rose compared to no activity. Furthermore, for judgments of remembering after arithmetic, Hits and False Recognitions were identical because Hits fell and False Recognitions rose compared to no activity. The loss of the advantage of Hits over False Recognitions for judgments of remembering after arithmetic and after recall provides further evidence that recognition responses are affected by the task of judging feelings of remembering and of knowing.

Effect of Age

The discussion is confined to the results from studies in which the conditions were comparable. Hits were significantly lower for older people than for younger people, and there was a trend towards more Hit False Alarms and False Recognition False Alarms for older people than for younger people. This is generally consistent with the possibility that verbatim traces would be weaker for older people than for younger people, leading older people to confuse studied and nonstudied items more than younger people.

However, uncorrected and corrected False Recognitions were significantly higher for older people than for younger people. This is consistent with the idea that spreading activation is greater for older people, leading them to have stronger gist traces than younger people. However, it is also consistent with the idea that older people have poorer source memory. It is also possible that older people have stronger gist traces and poorer source memory than younger people. Unfortunately, it is not possible to discriminate among these ideas from the present results, but research should be designed to do so.

There was a trend towards more "old" responses by older than by younger people on all three kinds of nonstudied items (those paired with Hits, those paired with False Recognitions, and the critical themes). This suggests that older people may have had a more lenient response bias towards saying "old" than younger people. This was examined by calculating the two-high-threshold measure of response bias, where a value of .50 means neutral bias, and values greater than .50 and less than .50 mean a liberal and a conservative bias, respectively (Snodgrass & Corwin, 1988). The values for both younger and older people on Hits and on False Recognitions were all less than .50, indicating a generally conservative bias. However, for both Hits and for False Recognitions, values were higher for older than for younger people, indicating that older people were *less conservative* (had a lower criterion for saying "old") than younger people. A similar trend has been observed in research on eyewitnessing (Wells & Olson, 2003).

CONCLUSION

This quantitative summary has demonstrated that False Recognition, like false recall (McKelvie, 2003), is a robust phenomenon. In particular, the False Recognition in terms of performance and of subjective confidence was more similar to correct recognition (Hits) than to other incorrect recognition (False Alarms). Indeed, under some conditions (with know judgments, and after arithmetic or after recall with remember judgments), False Recognitions were not significantly different from Hits. Similarly, when performance on remember and know judgments was compared, False Recognitions often showed the same pattern as Hits. In addition, when the effects of prior activity are considered, the False Recognitions were more similar to Hits than to False Alarms. In fact, of 15 comparisons among False Recognitions, Hits, and False Alarms, False Recognitions were closer to Hits than to False Alarms in four cases and showed similar results as Hits in 11 cases.

It was also observed that False Recognition False Alarms were consistently higher than Hit False Alarms. That is, nonstudied central concepts were more likely to be thought of as familiar than general nonstudied list items. This implies that the original False Recognition rate might be an overestimate and that studies of False Recognition should routinely include both kinds of nonstudied item so that the False Recognition and Hits rates can be corrected to render them comparable. The two-high-threshold measure is recommended for this purpose. It is sensitive to changes in discrimination capacity and is simple to calculate. Many studies have included corresponding nonstudied items for studied items and for critical themes, but some have only included a single set of nonstudied items. In the present study, positive responses to these were General False Alarms.

While False Recognitions were more similar to Hits than to other False Alarms, it is argued here that Hits are based on verbatim traces and that False Recognitions are based on gist traces formed via spreading activation during list presentation and a failure of source memory. It is suggested that the role of verbatim and gist traces be examined further by experimentally comparing the effects of recall, arithmetic, and no activity on Hits and on False Recognitions.

REFERENCES

ANASTASI, J. S., RHODES, M. G., & BURNS, M. C. (2000) Distinguishing between memory illusions and actual memories using phenomenological measurements and explicity warnings. *American Journal of Psychology*, 113, 1-26.

ARNDT, J., & HIRSHMAN, E. (1998) True and false recognition in MINERVA2: explanations from a global matching perspective. *Journal of Memory and Language*, 39, 371-379.*

---

*References marked with an asterisk indicate studies included in the quantitative summary. Not all may have been cited in the text.

BRAINERD, C. J., & REYNA, V. F. (1998) When things that were never experienced are easier to "remember" than things that were. *Psychological Science*, 9, 484-489.*
BRUCE, D., & WINOGRAD, E. (1998) Remembering Deese's 1959 articles: the Zeitgeist, the sociology of science, and false memories. *Psychonomic Bulletin & Review*, 5, 615-624.
COHEN, J. (1977) *Statistical power analysis for the behavioral sciences*. (Rev. ed.) New York: Academic Press.
DEESE, J. (1959) On the prediction of occurrence of particular verbal intrusions in immediate recall. *Journal of Experimental Psychology*, 58, 17-22.
DEFFENBACHER, K. A. (1980) Eyewitness accuracy and confidence: can we infer anything about the relationship? *Law and Human Behavior*, 4, 243-260.
FREYD, J. J., & GLEAVES, D. H. (1996) "Remembering" words not presented in lists: relevance to the current recovered/false memory controversy. *Journal of Experimental Psychology: Learning, Memory, and Cognition*, 22, 811-813.
GALLO, D. A., ROBERTS, M. J., & SEAMON, J. G. (1997) Remembering words not presented on lists: can we avoid creating false memories? *Psychonomic Bulletin & Review*, 4, 271-276.*
INTONS-PETERSON, M. J., ROCCHI, P., WEST, T., MCLELLAN, K., & HACKNEY, A. (1999) Age, testing at preferred or nonpreferred times (testing optimality), and false memory. *Journal of Experimental Psychology: Learning, Memory, and Cognition*, 25, 23-40.*
ISRAEL, L., & SCHACHTER, D. L. (1997) Pictorial encoding reduces false recognition of semantic associates. *Psychonomic Bulletin & Review*, 4, 577-581.*
KENSINGER, E. A., & SCHACHTER, D. L. (1999) When true memories suppress false memories: effects of aging. *Cognitive Neuropsychology*, 16, 399-415.*
KOUTSAAL, W., & SCHACHTER, D. L. (1997) Gist-based recognition of pictures in older and younger adults. *Journal of Memory and Language*, 37, 555-583.*
KOUTSAAL, W., SCHACHTER, D. L., GALLUCCIO, L., & STOFER, K. A. (1999) Reducing gist-based false memories in older adults: encoding and retrieval manipulations. *Psychology and Aging*, 14, 220-237.*
LAMPINEN, J. M., NEUSCHATZ, J. S., & PAYNE, D. G. (1999) Source attributions and false memories: a test of the demand characteristics account. *Psychonomic Bulletin & Review*, 6, 130-135.*
LAVOIE, D. J., & MULSTROM, T. (1998) False recognition effects in young and older adults' memory for text passages. *Journal of Gerontology*, 53B, P255-P262.
MATHER, M., HENKEL, L. A., & JOHNSON, M. K. (1997) Evaluating characteristics of false memories: remember/know judgments and memory characteristics questionnaire compared. *Memory & Cognition*, 25, 826-837.*
MCDERMOTT, K. B., & ROEDIGER, H. L. III. (1998) Attempting to avoid illusory memories: robust false recognition of associates persists under conditions of explicit warning and immediate testing. *Journal of Memory and Language*, 39, 508-520.*
MCKELVIE, S. J. (1990) Effects of exposure time and inversion on the confidence-accuracy relationship in facial memory: a test of the optimality hypothesis. *Perceptual and Motor Skills*, 71, 32-34.
MCKELVIE, S. J. (2001) Effect of free and forced retrieval instructions on false recall and recognition. *The Journal of General Psychology*, 128, 261-278.*
MCKELVIE, S. J. (2003) False recall with the DRMRS ("Drummers") procedure: a quantitative summary and review. *Perceptual and Motor Skills*, 97, 1011-1030.
MILLER, M. B., & WOLFORD, G. L. (1999) Theoretical commentary: the role of criterion shift in false memory. *Psychological Review*, 106, 398-405.*
MOOK, D. G. (1983) In defense of external invalidity. *American Psychologist*, 38, 379-387.
NORMAN, K. A., & SCHACHTER, D. L. (1997) False recognition in younger and older adults: exploring the characteristics of illusory memories. *Memory & Cognition*, 25, 838-848.*
PAYNE, D. G., ELIE, C. J., BLACKWELL, J. M., & NEUSCHATZ, J. S. (1996) Memory illusions: recalling, recognizing, and recollecting events that never occurred. *Journal of Memory and Language*, 35, 261-285.*
PLATT, R. D., LACEY, S. C., IOBST, A. D., & FINKELMAN, D. (1998) Absorption, dissociation, and fantasy-proneness as predictors of memory distortion in autobiographical and laboratory-generated memories. *Applied Cognitive Psychology*, 12, S77-S89.*

ROBINSON, K. J., & ROEDIGER, H. L. III. (1997) Associative processes in false recall and false recognition. *Psychological Science*, 8, 231-237.*

ROEDIGER, H. L. III, & McDERMOTT, K. B. (1995) Creating false memories: remembering words not presented on lists. *Journal of Experimental Psychology: Learning, Memory, and Cognition*, 21, 803-814.*

SCHACHTER, D. L., ISRAEL, L., & RACINE, C. (1999) Suppressing false recognition in younger and older adults: the distinctiveness heuristic. *Journal of Memory and Language*, 40, 1-24.*

SCHACHTER, D. L., VERFAELLIE, M., AMES, M. D., & RACINE, C. (1998) When true recognition suppresses false recognition: evidence from amnesic patients. *Journal of Cognitive Neuroscience*, 10, 668-679.*

SCHACHTER, D. L., VERFAELLIE, M., & PRADRE, D. (1996) The neuropsychology of memory illusions: false recall and recognition in amnesic patients. *Journal of Memory and Language*, 35, 319-334.*

SEAMON, J. G., GOODKIND, M. S., DUMEY, A. D., DICK, E., AUFSEESER, M. S., STRICKLAND, S. E., WOULFIN, J. R., & FUNG, N. S. (2003) "If I didn't write it, why would I remember it?" Effects of encoding, attention, and practice on accurate and false memory. *Memory & Cognition*, 31, 455-457.*

SEAMON, J. G., LUO, C. R., & GALLO, D. A. (1998) Creating false memories of words with or without recognition of list items: evidence for nonconscious processes. *Psychological Science*, 9, 20-26.*

SEAMON, J. G., LUO, C. R., KOPECKY, J. J., PRICE, C. A., ROTHSCHILD, L., FUNG, N. S., & SCHWARTZ, M. A. (2002) Are false memories more difficult to forget than accurate memories? The effect of retention interval on recall and recognition. *Memory & Cognition*, 30, 1054-1064.

SNODGRASS, J. G., & CORWIN, J. (1988) Pragmatics of measuring recognition memory: applications to dementia and amnesia. *Journal of Experimental Psychology: General*, 117, 34-50.

STADLER, M. A., ROEDIGER, H. L. III, & McDERMOTT, K. B. (1999) Norms for word lists that create false memories. *Memory & Cognition*, 27, 494-500.*

THAPAR, A., & McDERMOTT, K. B. (2001) False recall and false recognition induced by presentation of associated words: effects of retention interval and level of processing. *Memory & Cognition*, 29, 424-432.

TUN, P. A., WINGFIELD, A., ROSEN, M. J., & BLANCHARD, L. (1998) Response latencies for false memories: gist-based processes in normal aging. *Psychology and Aging*, 13, 230-241.*

TUSSING, A. A., & GREENE, R. L. (1997) False recognition of associates: how robust is the effect? *Psychonomic Bulletin & Review*, 4, 572-576.*

WELLS, G. L., & OLSON, E. A. (2003) Eyewitness testimony. *Annual Review of Psychology*, 54, 277-295.

WESTERBERG, C. E., & MARSOLEK, C. J. (2003) Sensitivity reductions in false recognition: a measure of false memories with stronger theoretical implications. *Journal of Experimental Psychology: Learning, Memory, and Cognition*, 29, 747-759.

WINOGRAD, E., PELUSO, J. P., & GLOVER, T. A. (1998) Individual differences in susceptibility to memory illusions. *Applied Cognitive Psychology*, 12, S5-S27.*

Accepted April 28, 2004.

SAILING EXPERIENCE AND SEX AS CORRELATES OF SPATIAL ABILITY[1]

ANN SLOAN DEVLIN

Connecticut College

Summary.—The relationship between sailing experience and men's and women's spatial ability was examined by assessing the sailing history and Mental Rotations Test scores of 230 participants. The 102 men and 128 women came from three groups: college sailors ($n=65$), members of the general student body ($n=110$), and college crew team members ($n=55$). Participants completed the Vandenberg and Kuse Mental Rotations Test and Lawton's Way-finding Strategy Scale and Spatial Anxiety Scale. Demographic variables and sailing experience were also assessed. Men scored significantly higher on the Mental Rotations Test than did women, and sailing team members scored significantly higher on that test than did student body members and crew team members. Results are discussed in terms of current explanations for sex differences in spatial ability.

Although men are consistently reported to have higher scores on tests of spatial ability, particularly mental rotation (e.g., Harris, 1978, 1981; Hyde, 1981, 1990; Halpern, 1986; Masters & Sanders, 1993; Collins & Kimura, 1997; Dabbs, Chang, Strong, & Milun, 1998; Nordvik & Amponsah, 1998; Voyer, Nolan, & Voyer, 2000; Malinowski, 2001), the contribution to these scores of participation in activities with a spatial component, such as sailing, remains unclear. Explanations for this sex difference in spatial ability have been offered from neurological, hormonal, and sociocultural perspectives, among others (McGee, 1979, 1982; Geschwind & Galaburda, 1985, 1987; Halpern, 1986; Thomas & Kail, 1991; Galea & Kimura, 1993; Hassler, 1993; Richardson, 1994; Buss, 1995; Neisser, Boodoo, Bouchard, Boykin, Brody, Ceci, Halpern, Loehlin, Perloff, Sternberg, & Urbina, 1996; James & Kimura, 1997; McBurney, Gaulin, Devineni, & Adams, 1997; Masters, 1998). A meta-analysis by Linn and Petersen (1985) indicated that the effect size for mental rotation was the largest of the spatial ability factors, and that the Vandenberg and Kuse Mental Rotations Test (1978) produced the largest effect size (weighted estimate was $d=.94$). The efficiency, speed, and caution with which the stimuli are processed may all contribute to the documented sex differences (Linn & Petersen, 1985). A more recent meta-analysis on sex differences in spatial abilities (Voyer, Voyer, & Bryden, 1995) also showed

---

[1]Thanks to Jeff Bresnahan, Eva Kovach, Zack Leonard, and Ric Ricci for making practice time available for this study. Please address correspondence to Ann Sloan Devlin, Ph.D., Department of Psychology, Box 5448, Connecticut College, 270 Mohegan Avenue, New London, CT 06320.

that the largest effect size continued to be for mental rotation, mean weighted $d = .56$, and these differences were not significantly smaller in more recent studies, indicating that the gap between the sexes on this particular measure of spatial ability has not narrowed.

While genetic, neurological, and hormonal influences are difficult to assess and offer few opportunities for intervention, the sociocultural domain offers fruitful ground for study. The focus of these studies on spatial ability in the sociocultural domain has been the role of differential experience, primarily the role of toy play, activities such as sports, and, more recently, computer use. A number of studies have looked at the role of activities vis-à-vis spatial ability (Lunneborg, 1982; Newcombe, Bandura, & Taylor, 1983; Lunneborg & Lunneborg, 1984; Olson, Eliot, & Hardy, 1988; Nordvik & Amponsah, 1998; Voyer, et al., 2000). In general these studies suggest that there is some relationship between time spent in spatial activities and spatial ability scores, although the relationship is not always clear-cut.

Following research by Nash (1975) indicating a relationship of sex-role attitudes to spatial competence, Newcombe, et al. (1983) developed a spatial activity questionnaire, in which 81 activities were judged as requiring spatial ability or not and as traditionally male or female. More skills that involved spatial components were considered more masculine, and more men than women participated in such activities. In a second study, men were significantly more likely to have participated in the spatial activities judged to be masculine, e.g., building model planes; ice hockey, whereas women were significantly more likely to have participated in the spatial activities judged to be feminine, e.g., pottery; figure skating. Although the sociocultural explanation of sex differences in spatial ability has support, it should also be noted that there is also evidence for the role that hormones play (e.g., Reinisch, 1981; Berenbaum & Hines, 1992; Kimura & Hampson, 1993; Hausmann, Slabbekoorn, Van Goozen, Cohen-Kettenis, & Gunturkun, 2000; McCormick & Teillon, 2001). Although not all research is supportive (e.g., Gordon & Lee, 1993; Rosenberg & Park, 2002), there is some evidence that spatial performance in women, at least on three-dimensional items, may be related to hormonal fluctuations in the menstrual cycle (e.g., Phillips & Silverman, 1997). Women's performance on the Vandenberg and Kuse test was significantly higher during the menstrual period phase, a time when estrogen levels, compared to other phases of the cycle, are at their lowest (Silverman & Phillips, 1993).

Thus, with multiple explanations for the sex difference in spatial ability, the role of experience is unclear, and its effect is important to assess and understand. Professions such as architecture stress visuospatial abilities (Peterson & Lansky, 1983), and women are significantly underrepresented in this profession for a variety of reasons (Ahrentzen & Groat, 1992), one of which may relate to spatial ability. A better understanding of the role of experience in spatial ability may lead to approaches to enhance spatial competence.

One finding from Voyer, et al. (2000) relevant to the current study is that the Mental Rotations Test may be susceptible to environmental influences, as indicated by the fact that people who preferred spatial toys as children had higher scores. Arguably, boys and girls are exposed to different kinds of social pressures, and toy availability and selection are but two examples of the difference (Unger & Crawford, 1992). Research indicates that differential exposure to toys and activities with a spatial emphasis is related to spatial ability. Girls and boys who engage in climbing, block building, and vehicle play score higher on a spatial ability test than those who select more feminine-typed objects such as dolls and housekeeping items (Serbin & Connor, 1979). When young children (3½ to 4 years of age) are exposed to training on toys described as boys' (blocks, tinker toys), their spatial ability scores may be higher (Sprafkin, Serbin, Denier, & Connor cited in Unger & Crawford, 1992).

Taken together, the research on retrospective accounts of toy play and spatial activities suggests that experience is related to mental rotation, although few studies have linked mental rotation performance to real-world tasks. In one study that made this connection, mental rotation ability was related to performance on an orienteering way-finding task in a group of military students (Malinowski, 2001). Using a 6-km orienteering course, a significant relationship between mental rotation scores on the Vandenberg and Kuse test and orienteering performance in terms of total points and time to complete the course was observed.

The current study is an attempt to understand better how experience relates to spatial ability by including sailing experience, a real-world activity that arguably places a considerable emphasis on mental rotation. Sailors, particularly those who race, are constantly recalibrating the distance and direction vectors required to reach a particular buoy to be rounded ("make the mark" or "hit the lay line"). They also must consider (imagine) what the shape of the sail will be on the next tack or the position of the spinnaker pole, much like aspects of the rotation involved in the Vandenberg and Kuse task. In the context of giving directions, Ward, Newcombe, and Overton (1986) suggested that some of the sex differences they observed, e.g., greater use of cardinality and mileage estimates by men than women, may be tied to the higher involvement of men than women in sailing, using a compass, or other activities such as orienteering.

Beyond the assessment of sailing history and completion of the Vandenberg and Kuse Mental Rotations Test, a number of other measures were included in this study. These included Lawton's Spatial Anxiety Questionnaire

(1994) and her Way-finding Strategy Scale (1994). These tests were included to better understand the relationship between a spatial activity like sailing and other way-finding preferences and perceptions. Sex differences in spatial behavior with implications for real-world activities include the kind of strategies people use to orient in the world and the anxiety they may feel about way-finding activities. Lawton's Spatial Anxiety Scale measures how uncomfortable people feel in situations presumed to require spatial skills. The Way-finding Strategy Scale differentiates between an emphasis on routes to navigate or a use of what she calls an orientation strategy, in which the individual monitors self "relative to points of reference in the environment" (p. 769). In her research, she reported that women have higher scores on spatial anxiety and more typically report use of a route strategy. Men, on the other hand, reported more use of the orientation strategy. Lawton also reported that spatial anxiety was negatively correlated with the orientation strategy.

To summarize, there is a decided advantage for men over women on the Vandenberg and Kuse Mental Rotations Test. The relationship between participation in spatial activities and performance on the Mental Rotations Test is evident but weak, and training on spatial tasks can improve performance by both women and men (McClurg & Chaille, 1987; DeLisi & Cammarano, 1996). Most of the research examining the relationship between mental rotation performance and spatial activities has used retrospective assessments.

The current study extends the literature by comparing college students who are members of college sailing teams to those who come from the student body at large. In addition, a third group, members of men's and women's crew teams, was added because it provides a comparison in terms of sports team membership, on the one hand, but without the emphasis on spatial orientation that sailing requires. It thus permits a comparison of the spatial nature of the sport while controlling for issues of competitiveness and expectancies of success (Voyer, *et al.*, 2000).

Based on the literature, the following hypotheses were formulated: (1) Men would score higher on the Mental Rotations Test than would women. (2) Sailing team members would score higher on the Mental Rotations Test than would nonsailing team students, both students at large and crew team members. (3) There would be an interaction between sailing team membership and sex, in that the difference between sailing and nonsailing participants would be greater for women than for men. (4) Sailing team members would score lower on spatial anxiety than nonsailing team students. (5) Sailing team members would report significantly greater use of orientation strategies than would nonsailing team students.

Method

Participants

There were 230 college participants in the study, 65 members of college sailing teams (48 from one institution and an additional 17 recruited from another school to obtain a larger sample), and 165 other students who came from the initial institution. Of these 165, 99 were from the general student body, 11 were a class of chemistry students who were asked to participate and returned all questionnaires, and 55 were members of the men's and women's crew teams. There were 102 men (33 of whom were sailors) and 128 women (32 of whom were sailors). The mean age for men was 19.8 yr. ($SD=1.3$, $n=102$), and the mean age for women was 19.7 yr. ($SD=2.1$, $n=128$). Of the 220 who indicated their class year, almost 90% of the students came from the freshman, sophomore, and junior classes. Of the 220 who reported their race, 92.3% were Euro-American.

Tests

The study included the Mental Rotations Test (Vandenberg & Kuse, 1978), a 20-item measure of mental rotation frequently used in literature. The test is given in two timed sections of 3 min. each (10 items per section). The test was scored following the recommendations of Vandenberg and Kuse (1978), which build in a correction for guessing; the maximum score is 40 points.

Lawton's Spatial Anxiety Scale (1994) and Way-finding Strategy Scale (1994) were both given. The Spatial Anxiety Scale consists of eight items that may cause anxiety, e.g., "Trying a new route that you think will be a shortcut without the benefit of a map." Participants respond to a scale where the intensity of anxiety is rated on anchors of 1 = not at all and 5 = very much (scores range from 8–40). Lawton (1994) reported a Cronbach alpha of .80 for this scale. The Way-finding Strategy Scale is a 14-item measure divided into nine questions involving Orientation strategies (scores range from 9–45) and five questions involving Route strategies (scores range from 5–25). Participants respond on a scale to anchors of 1 = not at all typical of me and 5 = extremely typical of me, and scores range from 9–45 for the Orientation strategy scale and 5–25 for the Route strategy scale. Cronbach alpha for the Orientation scale was .73, and for the Route scale .65 (Lawton, 1994). For the Route strategy questions, the emphasis seems to be on landmarks and turns, whereas the Orientation strategy questions place more emphasis on mileage indicators, cardinal directions, and perception of self in relationship to the larger environment.

A survey also asked participants a variety of questions related to their sailing experience, e.g., age they started sailing.

Procedure

Participants were recruited from the Psychology Department's Participant Pool at one school and from students in a chemistry class at that school who were asked to participate. Further, the sailing team members at this and another school were asked to participate at afternoon practice. To gather more data from sailors, the sailing team at the initial school was approached in two different seasons (two years apart) to complete the survey questions. Only those students who had not participated in earlier data collection were then added to the sample. Further, to strengthen the study, another athletic team from the school that was the primary source of participants was added for comparison in a sport with less emphasis on spatial skills. Members of the men's and women's crew teams at that school were asked to participate prior to an afternoon practice. For all participants except the chemistry students, the researcher administered the survey at one session, with the timed Mental Rotations Test administered first, followed by the remainder of the survey completed at the students' own pace. The time of day (afternoon) at which the scales were administered to the sailing and crew teams was dictated by availability within their training schedule. Further, the Mental Rotations Test was always administered first because it is a timed test that requires everyone start together and capitalized on subjects' attention at the beginning of the research session. For the chemistry students, the timed Mental Rotations Test was administered by the researcher at the beginning of class, and then students were asked to return the remaining portion of their surveys through campus mail, as sufficient class time could not be set aside for this purpose.

Analyses

Hypotheses 1, 2, and 3, that men would have higher Mental Rotation scores than would women (H_1), that sailing team members would have higher Mental Rotation scores than would students in other categories (general student body, crew team) (H_2), and that there would be an interaction between sex and sailing team membership (H_3), were evaluated in one analysis of variance. Hypotheses 4 and 5, that sailing team members would report lower Anxiety than the other two student groups (H_4), and more use of way-finding strategies that incorporated Orientation as opposed to Route emphases than the other two student groups (H_5), were evaluated using a multivariate analysis of variance. Anxiety, Orientation strategy, and Route strategy were the dependent variables. Finally, Spearman correlations were done separately for the sailing team, members of the general student body, and members of the crew team to examine the relationship between age at which people began sailing and scores on the Mental Rotations Test.

RESULTS

Results indicated full or partial support for four of the hypotheses. Results supported both Hypothesis 1, that men would have higher Mental Rotations Test scores than would women, and Hypothesis 2, that sailing team members would have higher Mental Rotations Test scores than would students in the other categories. Analyses of variance indicated a significant main effect for sex, with men having significantly higher Mental Rotations Test scores than women ($F_{1,224} = 28.06$, $p < .01$; $\eta^2 = .11$) and a significant main effect for students' category (sailing team, crew team, and general student body; $F_{2,224} = 3.20$, $p < .05$; $\eta^2 = .03$). Tukey *post hoc* tests indicated that sailing team members had significantly higher Mental Rotations Test scores than either students at large ($p < .05$) or crew team members ($p < .05$). The Mental Rotations Test scores of crew team members and student body members did not differ significantly ($p > .05$). There was no interaction ($F_{2,224} = 0.19$, $p > .05$), thereby giving no support to Hypothesis 3, which postulated that the difference between sailing team and nonsailing team participants would be greater for women than for men (see Table 1 for means and standard deviations).

TABLE 1
MEANS AND STANDARD DEVIATIONS OF MENTAL ROTATIONS TEST SCORES BY SEX AND STUDENTS' CATEGORY

Students' Category	Men M	SD	n	Women M	SD	n	Category Total M	SD	n
Total Sample	21.7	9.6	102	15.7	6.8	128	18.3	8.7	230
Sailing Team	24.2	8.4	33	17.4	7.3	32	20.9	8.5	65
Student Body	20.5	10.7	46	15.2	6.7	64	17.4	8.9	110
Crew Team	20.6	8.3	23	14.8	6.4	32	17.2	7.7	55

It was also hypothesized that sailing team members would report lower Anxiety than the other two student groups (Hypothesis 4) and more use of way-finding strategies that incorporated Orientation as opposed to Route emphases than the other two student groups (Hypothesis 5). To investigate these hypotheses, a multivariate analysis of variance was conducted with Anxiety, Orientation strategy, and Route strategy as the dependent variables. The analysis indicated a significant multivariate effect for students' category (Wilks lambda = .87; $F_{6,436} = 5.36$, $p < .01$; $\eta^2 = .07$) and a significant multivariate effect for sex (Wilks lambda = .88; $F_{3,218} = 9.67$, $p < .01$; $\eta^2 = .12$). The interaction was not significant ($p > .05$).

For students' category, univariate tests indicated significant differences for Anxiety ($F_{2,220} = 6.26$, $p < .01$; $\eta^2 = .05$) and for Orientation strategy ($F_{2,220} = 8.52$, $p < .01$; $\eta^2 = .07$). There was no significant difference for the Route strategy ($p<.05$). On the Anxiety scale, Tukey *post hoc* tests indicated a significant difference between sailing team members and the members of the general student body ($p<.01$). For Orientation strategy, Tukey *post hoc* tests also indicated a significant difference between members of the sailing team and the general student body ($p<.01$) and between crew team members and members of the general student body ($p<.05$). Sailing team members reported significantly lower Anxiety and greater use of Orientation strategy for way-finding than did members of the general student body. There were no group differences for the Route Strategy scores (see Table 2 for means and standard deviations). Crew team members also reported significantly greater use of Orientation strategy than did members of the general student body. There was thus partial support for Hypothesis 4 in that sailing team members reported less Anxiety than members of the general student body, but their scores were not significantly lower than those of crew team members. Similarly, there was partial support for Hypothesis 5 in that sailing team members reported significantly greater use of Orientation strategy for way-finding than did members of the general student body but not significantly more than crew team members.

TABLE 2
Means and Standard Deviations of Spatial Anxiety Scale and Way-finding Strategy Subscales (Orientation, Route) by Sex and Students' Category

Subscale	Men ($n=101$) M	SD	Women ($n=125$) M	SD	Sailing Team ($n=63$) M	SD	Student Body ($n=108$) M	SD	Crew Team ($n=55$) M	SD
Anxiety	18.2	5.0	20.2	5.8	17.6	5.2	20.5	5.5	18.9	5.5
Orientation	25.6	5.7	24.3	6.5	27.0	6.2	23.2	5.5	25.7	6.6
Route	17.2	3.6	19.1	3.0	17.5	3.3	18.7	3.4	18.5	3.6

For sex, univariate tests indicated significant effects for Anxiety ($F_{1,220}=9.18$, $p<.01$; $\eta^2=.04$) and for Route ($F_{1,220}=17.00$, $p<.01$; $\eta^2=.07$). The difference for use of Orientation strategy was not significant ($p>.05$). Women reported more Anxiety and greater use of Route strategy for way-finding than did men (see Table 2 for means and standard deviations).

Using Mental Rotations Test scores and a question regarding that age at which the individual began sailing, Spearman correlations were separately done for the sailing team, members of the general student body, and members of the crew team. There were no significant relationships between age when sailing started and Mental Rotation scores for sailing team members ($r_{15}=-.09$), crew team members ($r_{17}=-.22$), or students at large ($r_{64}=-.11$). To explore associations between sex and sailing experience, an analysis was conducted to compare whether men and women on the sailing team differed in their sailing roles. A chi-squared analysis indicated that men were significantly more likely to be skippers (81.8%) than crews (18.2%), whereas women were more likely to be crews (74.2%) than skippers [25.8%; χ_1^2 ($N = 64$) = 20.24, $p < .01$]; one participant did not indicate her role. This analysis showed that there were only eight women skippers and six men who served as crews. The small sample argued against further analyses.

DISCUSSION

The results of this study show that college sailors performed better on a test of spatial ability, the Vandenberg and Kuse Mental Rotations Test (1978), than members of the general student body or crew team members. As a group, sailors also reported lower spatial anxiety and more reliance on an orientation strategy when navigating than did members of the general student body but not significantly so than did crew team members. The findings here also reinforce the often-reported result that men score better on the Vandenberg and Kuse Mental Rotations Test than do women.

The fact that there was no interaction between sailing team membership and sex on the Mental Rotations Test scores is reminiscent of earlier findings. As in the cases of Nordvik and Amponsah (1998) and Quaiser-Pohl and Lehmann (2002), an educational track or practice (in this case, sailing) may be related to the performance of participants (technology students in the case of Nordvik and Amponsah, or computational visualistics students in the case of Quaiser-Pohl and Lehmann), but men's scores on the Mental Rotations Test are higher than women's scores nevertheless.

Also worthy of comment is the fact that the correlation between the age at which sailing began and Mental Rotations Test scores was not significant. It is possible that beyond a certain number of years of sailing experience, Mental Rotations Test scores do not increase incrementally, leading to this nonsignificant relationship. Another explanation is self-selection; that is, individuals who may excel at mental rotation tasks may be drawn to the sport. Also, most students who sail started around the age of eight, leading to a restriction of range of scores.

Beyond the spatial ability findings, this study shows that there is a relationship between participating on a sailing team and way-finding correlates. As a group, sailing team members reported less spatial anxiety and were more likely to adopt an orientation strategy in way-finding than were members of the general student body. This outcome is consistent with the notion that sailing emphasizes what the orientation strategy measures—"monitoring position of self relative to points of reference in the environment" (Lawton, 1994, p. 769). In this instance, the driving involves a boat, not an automobile, but the findings suggest that the fundamental principle is the same. The similarity seems especially clear when you consider some of the items on the orientation dimension such as "I kept track of the relationship between where I was and the next place where I had to change direction" or "I kept track of the direction (north, south, east, or west) in which I was going." These are activities that are essential to sailing.

The fact that the spatial anxiety of sailing team members was not significantly different from those of crew team members may be related to a number of factors such as the expectation of success (Voyer, *et al.*, 2000) among athletes and the reticence to acknowledge anxiety. These expectations of success may contribute to lower spatial anxiety. The reported use of the orientation strategy by sailing team members was also not significantly greater than it was for crew team members. Crew team members also reported greater use of this strategy than did members of the general student body. One possible reason for the lack of significant difference between sailors and crew team members on this variable is the fact that crew team members practice either in the very early morning (before classes) or late in the day and may be aware of the angle of the sun in the sky; they may also be aware of the direction they are heading on the river. A number of questions on the Orientation Strategy Scale involve this kind of awareness.

In interpreting these results, it should be noted that even the largest estimates of the magnitude of the effects were small. The largest estimates were for sex differences on the Mental Rotations Test scores and the multivariate effect dealing with sex differences on the Anxiety, Orientation strategy, and Route strategy scores. The fact that the largest differences involved sex is consistent with the literature on sex differences in spatial ability, particularly differences involving mental rotation; however, the meaningfulness of these differences should be interpreted with some caution.

In this study, the sailing roles of men and women on the college sailing team differed significantly, with relatively few women skippering and relatively few men crewing. College skippers "drive" the boat and make tactical and strategic decisions. College sailing typically involves championship events for single-handed boats in the fall (separately for men and women) and for double-handed boats in the spring (for co-ed and women's teams, separately). Thus, there is a need for women skippers for the women's events (single- and double-handed). Yet there were only eight women's skippers across the sailing teams of two colleges with nationally ranked sailing teams.

One explanation for the significantly larger percentage of male skippers is that sailing may be a male sex-typed activity; another explanation is that the emphasis on spatial components in sailing (an explanation which the higher Mental Rotations Test scores by sailing team members than nonsailing team members reinforces) is better suited to men. Men are more likely to have better mental rotation ability and this, according to the bent twig theory (Sherman, 1978), makes it more likely that they will continue in the sport and excel as their experience reinforces this ability. This explanation is consistent with the work of Newcombe and Dubas (1992). In their longitudinal study of adolescent females, spatial ability at Age 11 predicted spatial activity at Age 16, suggesting a kind of self-selection. Also, Halpern and Wright (1996) have looked at sex differences from the standpoint of information-processing patterns. They argue that men are better at tasks emphasizing the use of information in working memory, whereas women will do better at tasks requiring access to stored information, such as those involving verbal fluency. Sailboat racing is an activity wherein being able to respond to rapidly changing conditions, such as wind shifts, gives a competitor a distinct advantage. Using the Halpern and Wright model, men might succeed because of their superiority at tasks involving the manipulation of information in working memory.

However, the gender schema argument, making becoming a skipper by women more difficult because it is a cross-sex-typed activity (e.g., Cecil, Paul, & Olines, 1973; Glick, Zion, & Nelson, 1988; Devlin, 1997), deserves careful consideration. At the most competitive levels, sailing is a sex-typed masculine activity, and girls have few role models in this regard. Almost all head coaches of competitive college sailing teams are men, as are the vast majority of coaches at the youth championship events. As an example, at the 2002 Youth Championships in San Diego, 11 of the 13 official coaches were men. Further, of the 113 skippers at this event, 20 (17.7%) were girls, actually an overestimate because 10 of those 20 sailed one class of boat, the Europe Dinghy, sailed only by women at this regatta.

Researchers might expand the sample of women who are skippers and men who are crews to examine potential differences in their sailing histories that may be related to spatial ability. Research could also include a retrospective assessment of spatial toy play (e.g., Voyer, et al., 2000), an assessment of spatial activity (Newcombe, et al., 1983), and personality measures related to masculinity and femininity and sex-typed interests (Newcombe & Dubas, 1992). These steps would provide a more wide-ranging and complex assessment of experiential factors that may be related to spatial ability.

REFERENCES

Ahrentzen, S., & Groat, L. N. (1992) Rethinking architectural education: patriarchal conventions and alternative visions from the perspectives of women faculty. *Journal of Architectural and Planning Research*, 9, 95-111.

Berenbaum, S. A., & Hines, M. (1992) Early androgens are related to childhood sex-typed toy preferences. *Psychological Science*, 3, 203-206.

Buss, D. M. (1995) Psychological sex differences: origins through sexual selection. *American Psychologist*, 50, 164-168.

Cecil, E. A., Paul, R. J., & Olines, R. A. (1973) Perceived importance of selected variables used to evaluate male and female job applicants. *Personnel Psychology*, 26, 397-404.

Collins, D. W., & Kimura, D. (1997) A large sex difference on a two-dimensional mental rotation task. *Behavioral Neuroscience*, 111, 845-849.

Dabbs, J. M., Chang, E-L., Strong, R. A., & Milun, R. (1998) Spatial ability, navigation strat-

egy, and geographic knowledge among men and women. *Evolution and Human Behavior*, 19, 89-98.
DeLisi, R., & Cammarano, D. M. (1996) Computer experience and gender differences in undergraduate mental rotation performance. *Computers in Human Behavior*, 12, 351-361.
Devlin, A. S. (1997) Architects: gender-role and hiring decisions. *Psychological Reports*, 81, 667-676.
Galea, L. A., & Kimura, D. (1993) Sex differences in route-learning. *Personality and Individual Differences*, 14, 53-65.
Geschwind, N., & Galaburda, A. M. (1985) Cerebral lateralization: biological mechanisms, associations, and pathology: I. A hypothesis and a program for research. *Archives of Neurology*, 42, 428-459.
Geschwind, N., & Galaburda, A. M. (1987) *Cerebral lateralization.* Cambridge, MA: MIT Press.
Glick, P., Zion, C., & Nelson, C. (1988) What mediates sex discrimination in hiring decisions? *Journal of Personality and Social Psychology*, 55, 178-186.
Gordon, H. W., & Lee, P. L. (1993) No differences in cognitive performance between phases of the menstrual cycle. *Psychoneuroendocrinology*, 18, 521-531.
Halpern, D. F. (1986) *Sex differences in cognitive abilities.* Hillsdale, NJ: Erlbaum.
Halpern, D. F., & Wright, T. M. (1996) A process oriented model of cognitive sex differences. *Learning and Individual Differences*, 8, 3-24.
Harris, L. J. (1978) Sex differences in spatial ability: possible environmental, genetic, and neurological factors. In M. Kinsbourne (Ed.), *Asymmetrical functions of the brain.* Cambridge, UK: Cambridge Univer. Press. Pp. 405-522.
Harris, L. J. (1981) Sex-related variations in spatial skill. In L. S. Liben, A. H. Patterson, & N. Newcombe (Eds.), *Spatial representation and behavior across the life span.* New York: Academic Press. Pp. 83-125.
Hassler, M. (1993) Anomalous dominance, immune parameters, and spatial ability. *International Journal of Neuroscience*, 68, 145-156.
Hausmann, M., Slabbekoorn, D., Van Goozen, S. H. M., Cohen-Kettenis, P. T., & Gunturkun, O. (2000) Sex hormones affect spatial abilities during the menstrual cycle. *Behavioral Neuroscience*, 114, 1245-1250.
Hyde, J. S. (1981) How large are cognitive gender differences? *American Psychologist*, 36, 892-901.
Hyde, J. S. (1990) Meta-analysis and the psychology of gender differences. *Signs*, 16, 55-73.
James, T. W., & Kimura, D. (1997) Sex differences in remembering the locations of objects in an array: location-shifts versus location exchanges. *Evolution and Human Behavior*, 18, 155-163.
Kimura, D., & Hampson, E. (1993) Neural and hormonal mechanisms mediating sex differences in cognition. In P. A. Vernon (Ed.), *Biological approaches to the study of human intelligence.* Norwood, NJ: Ablex. Pp. 375-397.
Lawton, C. A. (1994) Gender differences in way-finding strategies: relationship to spatial ability and spatial anxiety. *Sex Roles*, 20, 765-779.
Linn, M. C., & Petersen, A. C. (1985) Emergence and characterization of sex differences in spatial ability: a meta-analysis. *Child Development*, 56, 1479-1498.
Lunneborg, C. E., & Lunneborg, P. W. (1984) Contribution of sex-differentiated experience to spatial and mechanical reasoning abilities. *Perceptual and Motor Skills*, 59, 107-113.
Lunneborg, P. W. (1982) Sex differences in self-assessed everyday spatial abilities. *Perceptual and Motor Skills*, 55, 200-202.
Malinowski, J. C. (2001) Mental rotation and real-world wayfinding. *Perceptual and Motor Skills*, 92, 19-30.
Masters, M. S. (1998) The gender difference on the Mental Rotations Test is not due to performance factors. *Memory & Cognition*, 26, 444-448.
Masters, M. S., & Sanders, B. (1993) Is the gender difference in mental rotation disappearing? *Behavior Genetics*, 23, 337-341.
McBurney, D. H., Gaulin, S. J. C., Devineni, T., & Adams, C. (1997) Superior spatial memory of women: stronger evidence for the gathering hypothesis. *Evolution and Human Behavior*, 18, 165-174.

McClurg, P. A., & Chaille, C. (1987) Computer games: environments for developing spatial cognition. *Journal of Educational Computing Research*, 3, 95-111.

McCormick, C. M., & Teillon, S. M. (2001) Menstrual cycle variation in spatial ability: relation to salivary cortisol levels. *Hormones and Behavior*, 39, 29-38.

McGee, M. G. (1979) *Human spatial abilities: sources of sex differences.* New York: Praeger.

McGee, M. G. (1982) Spatial abilities: the influence of genetic factors. In M. Potegal (Ed.), *Spatial abilities: development and physiological foundations.* New York: Academic Press. Pp. 199-222.

Nash, S. C. (1975) The relationship among sex-role stereotyping, sex-role preference, and the sex difference in spatial visualization. *Sex Roles*, 1, 15-32.

Neisser, U., Boodoo, G., Bouchard, T. J., Jr., Boykin, A. W., Brody, N., Ceci, S. J., Halpern, D. F., Loehlin, J. C., Perloff, R., Sternberg, R., & Urbina, S. (1996) Intelligence: knowns and unknowns. *American Psychologist*, 51, 77-101.

Newcombe, N., Bandura, M. M., & Taylor, D. G. (1983) Sex differences in spatial ability and spatial activities. *Sex Roles*, 9, 377-386.

Newcombe, N., & Dubas, J. S. (1992) A longitudinal study of predictors of spatial ability in adolescent females. *Child Development*, 63, 37-46.

Nordvik, H., & Amponsah, B. (1998) Gender differences in spatial abilities and spatial activity among university students in an egalitarian educational system. *Sex Roles*, 38, 1009-1023.

Olson, D. M., Eliot, J., & Hardy, R. C. (1988) Relationships between activities and sex-related differences in performance on spatial tests. *Perceptual and Motor Skills*, 67, 223-232.

Peterson, J. M., & Lansky, L. M. (1983) Success in architecture: a research note. *Perceptual and Motor Skills*, 57, 222.

Phillips, K., & Silverman, I. (1997) Differences in the relationship of menstrual cycle phase to spatial performance on two- and three-dimensional tasks. *Hormones and Behavior*, 32, 167-175.

Quaiser-Pohl, C., & Lehmann, W. (2002) Girls' spatial abilities: charting the contributions of experiences and attitudes in different academic groups. *British Journal of Educational Psychology*, 72, 245-260.

Reinisch, J. (1981) Prenatal exposure to synthetic progestins increases potential for aggression in humans. *Science*, 211, 1171-1173.

Richardson, J. T. E. (1994) Gender differences in mental rotation. *Perceptual and Motor Skills*, 78, 435-448.

Rosenberg, L., & Park, S. (2002) Verbal and spatial functions across the menstrual cycle in healthy young women. *Psychoneuroendocrinology*, 27, 835-841.

Serbin, L. A., & Connor, J. M. (1979) Sex-typing of children's play preferences and patterns of cognitive performance. *Journal of Genetic Psychology*, 134, 315-316.

Sherman, J. A. (1978) *Sex-related cognitive differences: an essay on theory and evidence.* Springfield, IL: Thomas.

Silverman, I., & Phillips, K. (1993) Effects of estrogen changes during the menstrual cycle on spatial performance. *Ethology & Sociobiology*, 14, 257-270.

Thomas, H., & Kail, R. (1991) Sex differences in speed of mental rotation and the X-linked genetic hypothesis. *Intelligence*, 15, 17-32.

Unger, R., & Crawford, M. (1992) *Women and gender: a feminist psychology.* New York: McGraw-Hill.

Vandenberg, S., & Kuse, A. (1978) Mental rotation: a group test of three-dimensional spatial visualization. *Perceptual and Motor Skills*, 47, 599-604.

Voyer, D., Nolan, C., & Voyer, S. (2000) The relation between experience and spatial performance in men and women. *Sex Roles*, 43, 891-915.

Voyer, D., Voyer, S., & Bryden, M. P. (1995) Magnitude of sex differences in spatial abilities: a meta-analysis and consideration of critical variables. *Psychological Bulletin*, 117, 250-270.

Ward, S. L., Newcombe, N., & Overton, W. F. (1986) Turn left at the church, or three miles north: a study of direction giving and sex differences. *Environment and Behavior*, 18, 192-213.

Accepted April 28, 2004.

RELIABILITY AND STABILITY OF A DREAM RECALL FREQUENCY SCALE[1]

MICHAEL SCHREDL

Central Institute of Mental Health, Mannheim

Summary.—Dream recall frequency varies widely between people as well as within individuals. To explore the relationship between dream recall frequency and trait variables such as personality dimensions, a measure of stable interindividual differences is necessary. In the present study ($N = 198$ patients with sleep disorders; 115 women, 83 men; M age $= 45.8 \pm 15.3$ yr.) a high retest reliability of the 7-point Dream Recall Frequency scale developed by Schredl in 2002a was found. If the participants' focus was not directed explicitly towards dream recall when the scale was presented within a general sleep questionnaire, the hitherto-reported increase of dream recall due to measuring dream recall frequency did not occur. In conclusion, the present scale is well suited for measuring interindividual differences in dream recall frequency reliably.

Dream recall frequency varies widely between people as well as within individuals (cf. Schredl, 1999). To relate dream recall frequency to trait variables such as personality dimensions, a measure of stable interindividual differences is necessary. Measures should possess high reliability indices, especially high retest reliability. For measuring dream recall frequency in a home setting, two methods are commonly applied, questionnaires and dream diaries. Scores for these two methods are very often highly correlated ($r = .56$, $p < .0001$, $N = 285$; Schredl, 2002b). The retest reliability (over intervals ranging from 2 to 3 months) of a 4-point frequency scale with anchors of often, on occasion, rarely, never was .59 ($N = 106$; Bernstein & Belicki, 1995–96). In a pilot study ($N = 39$), a markedly higher coefficient of .83 was obtained for a 7-point rating scale (Schredl, 2002a) including absolute categories, e.g., about once a month (see Appendix, p. 1426) compared to the above-mentioned scale with relative categories. This seems plausible since the meaning of "on occasion", for example, may vary among subjects as well as between two measurements.

For dream diaries, it is possible to compute the internal consistency (one morning with or without dream recall as a dichotomous item) serving as a reliability coefficient. A 14-day diary yielded a value of .74 ($N = 444$; Schredl, Wittmann, Ciric, & Götz, 2003). Extending the measurement period to 4 wk., the internal consistency increased to .90 (Schredl & Fulda, in press), indicating that measurement intervals of two to four weeks are suffi-

---

[1]Send correspondence to M. Schredl, Ph.D., Sleep Laboratory, Central Institute of Mental Health, P.O. Box 12 21 20, 68072 Mannheim, Germany or e-mail (Schredl@zi-mannheim.de).

cient to equalize day-to-day fluctuations in dream recall. The retest study of Bernstein and Belicki (1995–96) yielded a correlation of .67 ($N = 106$) for a dream diary which has been applied twice two or three months apart. Since in classical test theory the critical value of .80 is considered as sufficient and acceptable reliability (Groth-Marnat, 1990), the initial results of the pilot study by Schredl (2002a) are promising, and the present study investigated the retest reliability of the 7-point dream recall frequency scale with a larger sample to extend the findings.

In addition to the issue of stable interindividual differences in dream recall frequency (high retest reliability), it is of equal interest to investigate whether frequency varies with time. Within this context, the findings regarding the effect of participating in a dream study should be taken into consideration. Several studies (Redfering & Keller, 1974; Halliday, 1992; Schredl, Brenner, & Faul, 2002) have indicated a marked increase in dream recall frequency during the study period if dream recall frequency was measured by a single item or question at the beginning of the study, indicating that measuring dream recall frequency influences the variable under consideration. On the other hand, the frequency decreases over time if dream content was additionally elicited (Belicki & Bernstein, 1995–96; Schredl, Funkhouser, Cornu, Hirsbrunner, & Bahro, 2001), although retest reliability was high in these studies. Since there was no decrease in a study applying sleep and dream diaries without eliciting dream reports over longer time periods (over 100 days) (Schredl & Fulda, in press), it seems likely that the decrease is attributable to motivational factors. In the present study, the dream recall frequency scale was presented within a general sleep questionnaire, i.e., the focus of the participants was not drawn towards dreams. It was hypothesized that dream recall frequency is not affected and, thus, means do not differ between the two measurements.

Method

Measure

The Dream Recall Frequency scale (Schredl, 2002a) a 7-point rating scale (anchors of 0 = never, 1 = less than once a month, 2 = about once a month, 3 = twice or three times a month, 4 = about once a week, 5 = several times a week, and 6 = almost every morning), measuring dream recall frequency of the previous months, was presented within the LISST sleep questionnaire (Weeß, Schürmann, & Steinberg, 1997). This sleep questionnaire has 75 items measuring sleep quality, daytime sleepiness, occurrence of 'restless legs' symptoms, etc. The Dream Recall Frequency scale was presented as Item 51. A translation of the German scale can be found in the Appendix (p. 1426). To obtain units of mornings per week, scores were converted using averaged values for each category (see Appendix, p. 1426).

Participants and Procedure

The participants were patients with sleep disorders who were referred by their physicians to the sleep laboratory of the Central Institute of Mental Health, Mannheim, Germany. Routinely, the LISST questionnaire was sent out to patients who were asked to complete the questionnaire shortly prior to the first contact in the outpatient department of the sleep laboratory. Within this first contact, which includes a thoroughly carried out anamnesis, or diagnostic interview about current sleep problems, sleep history, medication, concomitant disorders, of about one hour duration, it was decided whether a polysomnographic recording over two nights was necessary for final diagnosis. Within this procedure, the LISST questionnaire was presented a second time prior to the first laboratory night. Based on the anamnestic and polysomnographic data, a diagnosis according to the ICD–10 [Deutsches Institut für Medizinische Dokumentation und Information (DIMDI), 1994] was made.

Of 214 patients who completed the LISST questionnaire at both times, only 198 (111 women, 83 men) could be included in the analysis given missing values at t_1 or t_2. The mean age was 45.8 yr. ($SD = 15.3$). The largest diagnostic groups were: primary insomnia ($n = 71$), restless legs syndrome ($n = 42$), depression/dysthymia ($n = 25$), primary hypersomnia ($n = 11$), parasomnias ($n = 10$), narcolepsy ($n = 9$), and sleep-related breathing disorders ($n = 6$). The remaining patients were those with anxiety disorder, drug abuse, posttraumatic stress disorder, personality disorder, compulsive disorder, phase-delayed sleep pattern, schizophrenia, and attention deficit disorder. The mean retest interval was 54.8 days ($SD = 44.8$).

Results and Discussion

The Pearson correlation of the scores on the Dream Recall Frequency scale measured at t_1 and t_2 was .85 ($p < .0001$, $N = 198$). The absolute value of the difference between dream recall frequency measured at both times did not substantially correlate with the duration of the retest interval ($r = -.05$, ns). Similarly, no difference in mean values at t_1 and t_2 emerged (t_1: $M = 1.67$, $SD = 2.09$; t_2: $M = 1.62$, $SD = 2.05$; $t = -0.7$, ns). The patients recalled dreams on average of one to two mornings per week.

These results were consistent with the findings of the pilot study (Schredl, 2002a) regarding the high retest reliability of the 7-point Dream Recall Frequency scale. This rating scale, which includes absolute answer categories and refers to a time interval of several months, should be given preference over the 4-point scale of Bernstein and Belicki (1995–96) with its lower retest reliability of .59. The nonsignificant correlation between retest interval and the change in dream recall frequency further indicates that dream recall frequency is very stable over time; otherwise longer retest intervals would be associated with larger differences. In conclusion, the present scale investigated is well suited for measuring interindividual differences in Dream Recall Frequency reliably.

As expected no mean differences between dream recall frequency between t_1 and t_2 were found. If the participants' focus was not directed explicitly toward dream recall, the hitherto reported increase in dream recall frequency when being measured did not occur. This is congruent with the finding of Schredl and Fulda (in press) whose subjects kept sleep/dream diaries consisting mostly of questions about sleep and daytime activities.

Within this context, the following finding is interesting. Mean dream recall frequency was slightly but significantly higher if the present scale was given within a dream questionnaire than within a general sleep questionnaire (retest interval of two days on maximum; Schredl, *et al.*, 2003). These results indicate that repeated measurements of dream recall frequency are valid only if the scale is part of a more general questionnaire, e.g., about sleep, so participants' focus is not directed towards dreams. Otherwise, participating in a dream study or motivational factors, e.g., when dream reports are elicited, affect dream recall frequency markedly. It will be desirable to extend studies of reliability to all methods of measuring dream recall, e.g., recall rates obtained by awakenings in the sleep laboratory.

REFERENCES

BERNSTEIN, D. M., & BELICKI, K. (1995–96) On the psychometric properties of retrospective dream content questionnaires. *Imagination, Cognition and Personality*, 15, 351-364.

DEUTSCHES INSTITUT FÜR MEDIZINISCHE DOKUMENTATION UND INFORMATION (DIMDI). (1994) *Internationale statistische Klassifikation der Krankheiten und verwandter Gesundheitsprobleme (ICD–10)*. Bern: Hans Huber.

GROTH-MARNAT, G. (1990) *Handbook of psychological assessment*. New York: Wiley.

HALLIDAY, G. (1992) Effect of encouragement on dream recall. *Dreaming*, 2, 39-44.

REDFERING, D. L., & KELLER, J. N. (1974) Influence of differential instruction on the frequency of dream recall. *Journal of Clinical Psychology*, 30, 268-271.

SCHREDL, M. (1999) Dream recall: research, clinical implications and future directions. *Sleep and Hypnosis*, 1, 72-81, A2-A4.

SCHREDL, M. (2002a) Messung der Traumerinnerung: siebenstufige Skala und Daten gesunder Personen. *Somnologie*, 6, 34-38.

SCHREDL, M. (2002b) Questionnaires and diaries as research instruments in dream research: methodological issues. *Dreaming*, 12, 17-26.

SCHREDL, M., BRENNER, C., & FAUL, C. (2002) Positive attitude towards dreams: reliability and stability of a ten-item scale. *North American Journal of Psychology*, 4, 343-346.

SCHREDL, M., & FULDA, S. (in press) Reliability and stability of dream recall frequency. *Dreaming*.

SCHREDL, M., FUNKHOUSER, A. T., CORNU, C. M., HIRSBRUNNER, H-P., & BAHRO, M. (2001) Reliability in dream research: a methodological note. *Consciousness and Cognition*, 10, 496-502.

SCHREDL, M., WITTMANN, L., CIRIC, P., & GÖTZ, S. (2003) Factors of home dream recall: a structural equation model. *Journal of Sleep Research*, 12, 133-141.

WEESS, H. G., SCHÜRMANN, T., & STEINBERG, R. (1997) *Landecker Inventar zur Erfassung von Schlafstörungen*. Klingenmünster: Unveröffentlicher Fragebogen des Schlafmedizinischen Zentrums.

Accepted April 26, 2004.

APPENDIX

Seven-point Rating Scale Measuring Dream Recall Frequency

How often have you recalled your dreams recently (in the past several months)?	Original Scores	Recoded Scores
almost every morning	6	6.50
several times a week	5	3.50
about once a week	4	1.00
two or three times a month	3	0.63
about once a month	2	0.25
less than once a month	1	0.13
never	0	0.00

REPORT ORDER AND IDENTIFICATION OF MULTIDIMENSIONAL STIMULI: A STUDY OF EVENT-RELATED BRAIN POTENTIALS [1]

KONG-KING SHIEH AND I-HSUAN SHEN

Department of Industrial Management
National Taiwan University of Science and Technology

Summary.—An experiment was conducted to investigate the effect of order of report on multidimensional stimulus identification. Subjects were required to identify each two-dimensional symbol by pushing corresponding buttons on the keypad on which there were two columns representing the two dimensions. Order of report was manipulated for the dimension represented by the left or right column. Both behavioral data and event-related potentials were recorded from 14 college students. Behavioral data analysis showed that order of report had a significant effect on response times. Such results were consistent with those of previous studies. Analysis of event-related brain potentials showed significant differences in peak amplitude and mean amplitude at time windows of 120–250 msec. at Fz, F3, and F4 and of 350–750 msec. at Fz, F3, F4, Cz, and Pz. Data provided neurophysiological evidence that reporting dimensional values according to natural language habits was appropriate and less cognitively demanding.

The problems in designing displays have been among the most important topics in human factors engineering. Compacting information into a single multidimensional stimulus can be an effective way of utilizing limited display space and reducing clutter (Tsang & Bates, 1990). It may also facilitate integration of information (Wickens & Andre, 1990; Wickens & Carswell, 1995) and reduce mental workload (Duncan, 1984; Carswell & Wickens, 1996). If operators search the dimensions in a particular order in a multidimensional stimulus identification task, it implies that search performance is determined by the specific order in which dimensions are examined (Fisher & Tanner, 1992). To develop an optimal symbol set, the designer must take into account the order of the search through the dimensions.

In a multidimensional display, the order of reporting dimensional values may play an important role in the accuracy and speed of identifying targets. Allport (1971), Egeth and Pachella (1969), Lappin (1967), and Lawrence and LaBerge (1956) also found that the order of report had a significant effect on accuracy. In the study of Harris and Haber (1963), it has been shown that the attribute encoded first was shown to have a higher accuracy rate. However, if subjects reported the stimulus attributes in ways that con-

---

[1]Address requests for reprints to K-K. Shieh, Department of Industrial Management, National Taiwan University of Science and Technology, 43, Sec 4, Keelung Road, Taipei 106, Taiwan, R.O.C. or e-mail (kks@im.ntust.edu.tw).

flicted with long-standing habits based on standard English word order, the accuracy dropped sharply. Recently, Shieh and his colleagues (Shieh, Lai, & Ellingstad, 1996; Shieh & Chen, 2002) investigated the effects of order of report on the speed and accuracy of identifying multidimensional stimuli. They found that the order of report affected the speed and accuracy of identification. Subjects responded faster and more accurately if there was a natural language-appropriate order of reporting the dimensional attributes. Their interpretation was based on the assumption that people tend to report stimulus attributes in ways consistent with their long-standing language habits.

However, all reaction time investigations must make inferences about the processes between stimulus and response by looking at the final product of the response. To augment this mental chronometry, the event-related brain potential (ERP) has been used to provide a direct estimate of the timing of processes up to the intermediate stage of stimulus categorization (Donchin, 1981; Gratton, Coles, Sirevaag, Eriksen, & Donchin, 1988). The ERP is a series of voltage oscillations or components that are recorded from the scalp to indicate the brain's electrical response to discrete stimulus events. The "report-order effect" has been repeatedly demonstrated in behavioral studies, but event-related brain potentials effects related to this effect have not been reported. Kutas and Hillyard (1980) reported that semantically inappropriate words, for example, 'He spread the warm bread with socks', elicited a large-amplitude negative ERP component with peak latency of 400 msec. (N400 component), relative to the ERPs elicited by semantically appropriate words, e.g., 'It was his first day at work'. Similarly, several studies have shown N400-like effects to pairs of related and unrelated pictures (Barrett & Rugg, 1990; Holcomb & McPherson, 1994). The present study investigates the relationships between reaction times and ERP components for various report orders. The aim is to support the observed effects of report order with ERP evidence. It is hypothesized that subjects reporting dimensional values not according to natural language habits would elicit a larger N400.

Method

Subjects

Fourteen male college students between 20 and 26 years old ($M = 20.1$ yr., $SD = 4.6$) were tested. All had 18/20 corrected visual acuity or better and normal color vision. The subjects were paid for their participation.

Stimuli

A subset of the Naval Tactical Display System (NTDS) symbols was used as the stimulus set (see Fig. 1). This representative sample of basic symbols and modifiers has been described in detail by Osga (1982) and presented in Shieh, et al.'s study (1996). Each of the nine symbols used in this study was encoded with two basic dimensions. The first dimension, "shape," was circular, square, or angular. The second dimension, "part," was upper half, full, or lower half. Nine stimuli were used and those nine symbols were white. The background against which a shape was presented was black. The height and width of the stimuli were 1 cm by 1 cm for full shapes and 0.5 cm by 1 cm for the half shapes. The luminance of display symbols was about 35 cd/m^2 on a black background.

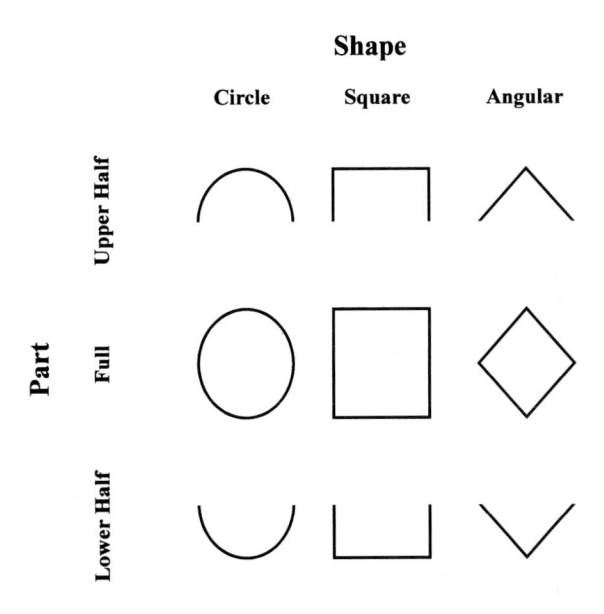

FIG. 1. Nine symbols defined by shape and part dimensions. Each dimension had three values.

Design

The study evaluated one independent variable, order of report, with two levels. In Order Part/Shape, subjects were instructed to report the "part" dimension first and the "shape" dimension second. In Order Shape/Part, the order of report was reversed. Shieh, et al. (1996) found that subjects responded faster and more accurately to Order Part/Shape. For example, reporting a whole circular shape as "full circular" was more natural than reporting it as "circular full." Such results were consistent with the findings of Harris and Haber (1963) that the performance based on "adjective then noun" order is better than that based on the reverse order. A between-subject design was conducted with 14 male subjects randomly assigned to the two order conditions. There were seven subjects in each treatment group. A block consisted of five random presentations of the nine symbols. Subjects completed four blocks of 45 trials in the experiment. There was a 2-min. break between blocks. The first blocks were used as a training period, and Blocks 2–4 served as the data set for analysis.

Procedure

The symbols were presented one per trial at the center of the display during the identification task. Viewing distance between the subject and display was approximately 60 cm. The symbols were presented till the subject completed the response. Before each trial, subjects were asked to fixate their vision on a small cross on the middle of the screen. A warning tone sounded 1.5 sec. just before each stimulus presentation to direct the subject's attention to the display. Each symbol could be identified on two dimensions according to the instructed order of report for the particular experimental conditions. The subjects were instructed to identify the symbol presented during each trial by pressing the buttons that defined the symbols. Two columns on the keyboard, three buttons in each column, were labeled with the descriptive names. The two columns represented the two stimulus dimensions, and the three buttons in each column represented the three values of that dimension. The order of report was manipulated by the dimension the left or right column represented.

Electrophysiological Methods

The electroencephalogram was recorded with Ag/AgCl electrodes monopolarly from three midline positions (Fz, Cz, Pz) and one pair of lateral electrodes (F3 and F4) according to the International 10–20 System. The right mastoid served as reference. Bipolar electrooculogram (EOG) was recorded between electrodes situated at the outer right canthus and below the right eye. The use of EOG recording was to remove the eye-movement artifacts in the data analysis. Electroencephalograms (EEGs) were recorded with a bandpass of 0.25–70 Hz and digitized at 1000 Hz. A notch filter was used to remove 60-Hz interference. Interelectrode impedances were below 10 Kohm.

Data Analysis

Behavioral and ERP data were averaged separately for each order of report condition. Four behavioral measures were collected. Response time for the first stimulus dimension (RT_1) was the time between the presentation of a symbol and the subject's correct response to the first dimension. Response time for the second stimulus dimension (RT_2) was the time between the subject's identification of the first dimension and the correct response to the second dimension. Response time total (RT_T) was the sum of RT_1 and RT_2. Total percentage correct was 100 times the number of symbols correctly identified divided by the number of symbols presented under each experimental treatment. The mean response times and percentage correct were collected in Blocks 2 to 4 for each subject. An analysis of variance was conducted for the four dependent measures.

ERP data on all trials were scanned offline for artifact contamination (eye blinks or movements, uncorrected responses, electrode drift, and excessive muscular activity). After artifact rejection, EEG epochs of 900 msec. length were averaged using stimulus onset as trigger for each report order. The prestimulus epoch (baseline) was 100 msec. long, the poststimulus epoch 800 msec. P120–250 was defined as a major positive wave that occurred between 120–250 msec. following the stimulus onset. N2 was the major negative deflection between 250–350 msec. N400 was the major negative deflection between 350–750 msec. after stimulus onset. Peak latency, peak amplitude, and mean amplitude were measured in the three time windows.

Results

Behavioral Data

Table 1 shows mean response times for the first and second dimensions, total response time, and total percentage correct for each order of report. The overall mean of response time for the first dimension was 880 msec. Analysis of variance showed that order of report had significant effect on response time for the first dimension (RT_1). Response time for the first dimension for Order Part/Shape (783 msec.) was significantly shorter ($F_{1,12} = 7.39$, $p < .05$) than Order Shape/Part (978 msec.). The overall mean of response time for the second dimension (RT_2) was 337 msec., much shorter than for the first dimension. Response times for the second dimension were 309 msec. and 365 msec. for Order Part/Shape and Order Shape/Part. However, these differences were not significant. The overall mean total response time (RT_T) was 1218 msec.

TABLE 1
Means and Standard Deviations (msec.) For Four Behavior Measures For Each Report Order

Experimental Condition	n	RT_1 M	SD	RT_2 M	SD	RT_T M	SD	% Correct M	SD
Order Part/Shape	7	783	133	309	93	1092	207	95.9	1.6
Order Shape/Part	7	978	135	365	117	1343	197	94.1	2.6
Grand Mean	14	880	164	337	105	1218	233	94.9	2.3

Analysis of variance showed that order of report had significant effect on total response time. Total response time for Order Part/Shape (1092 msec.) was significantly shorter ($F_{1,12} = 5.37$, $p < .05$) than Order Shape/Part

(1342 msec.). Apparently, response time for the first dimension was the more important component for total response time than response time for the second dimension. The overall percentage correct was 94.9, 95.8% for Order Part/Shape and 94.1% for Order Shape/Part. Analysis of variance performed on the percentage correct showed no significant effect.

Electrophysiological (ERP) Data

Fig. 2 shows the grand average of ERPs for correct response trials, for Order Part/Shape and Shape/Part at Fz, F3, F4, Cz, and Pz. The plots showed ERPs for Order Part/Shape and Order Shape/Part were different. ERPs of Order Shape/Part were more positive-going than those of Order Part/Shape in the time-window of 120–250 msec. following the onset of the

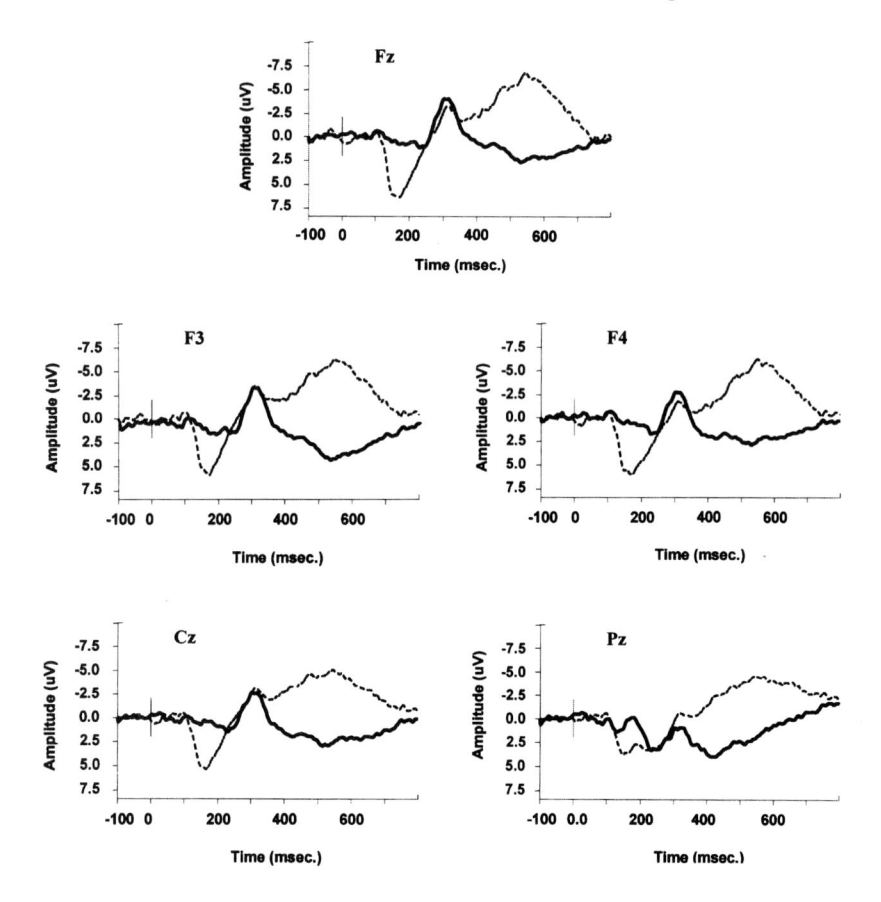

FIG. 2. Event-related potential waveform recorded in the experimental condition (———: Part/Shape Order; – – –: Shape/Part Order) at Fz, F3, F4, Cz, and Pz electrode sites. Vertical dotted lines indicate symbol presentation.

stimulus. In the time-window of 250–350 msec., ERPs showed a similar waveform for both report orders. Further, ERPs of Order Shape/Part were negative-going and Order Part/Shape were positive-going in the time-window of 350–750 msec. following the onset of stimulus. For each ERP component, a separate analysis of variance was computed for peak latency, peak amplitude, and mean amplitude.

Peak Latency

Peak latency (msec.) at each electrode site for P125–250, N2, and N400 components for each report order are shown in Table 2. Analysis of variance indicated in the P120–250 components no significant effects of order of report and none in the N2 component or the N400 component.

TABLE 2
Peak Latency (msec.) at Each Electrode Site For P125–250, N2, and N400 Components For Each Report Order

Component	Fz	F3	F4	Cz	Pz
P125–250					
Order Part/Shape	208	204	212	201	210
Order Shape/Part	172	174	200	175	196
N2					
Order Part/Shape	305	361	304	301	302
Order Shape/Part	316	321	321	314	325
N400					
Order Part/Shape	498	527	498	469	460
Order Shape/Part	549	550	572	588	602

Peak Amplitude

Peak amplitude (μV) at each electrode site for P125–250, N2, and N400 components for each report order are shown in Table 3. An analysis of variance indicated for P120–250 components, peak amplitude for Order

TABLE 3
Peak Amplitude (μV) at Each Electrode Site For P125–250, N2, and N400 Components For Each Report Order

Component	Fz	F3	F4	Cz	Pz
P125–250					
Order Part/Shape	2.80	2.79	3.05	3.59	4.43
Order Shape/Part	8.15	6.20	6.47	7.15	7.07
N2					
Order Part/Shape	−4.67	−4.48	−3.61	−3.43	−0.03
Order Shape/Part	−4.52	−4.64	−3.08	−4.11	−1.42
N400					
Order Part/Shape	5.13	5.75	5.53	5.66	6.24
Order Shape/Part	−10.22	−9.89	−9.18	−7.57	−6.69

Shape/Part (8.15 µV, 6.20 µV, and 6.47 µV) was significantly larger than for Order Part/Shape at Fz ($F_{1,14}=9.10$, $p<.05$), F3 ($F_{1,14}=9.25$, $p<.05$), and F4 ($F_{1,14}=9.69$, $p<.01$). Peak amplitude for Order Shape/Part was larger than for Order Part/Shape at Cz and Pz. But the differences were not statistically significant. For the N2 component, peak amplitude at each electrode site showed no significant effect of order of report. For the N400 component, peak amplitudes for Order Shape/Part were negative compared with those of Order Part/Shape at Fz, F3, F4, Cz, and Pz. Analysis of variance at each electrode site showed that there were significant main effects of report order at Fz ($F_{1,14}=20.46$, $p<.001$), F3 ($F_{1,14}=22.74$, $p<.001$), F4 ($F_{1,14}=23.69$, $p<.001$), Cz ($F_{1,14}=27.05$, $p<.001$), and Pz ($F_{1,14}=47.89$, $p<.001$).

Mean Amplitude

Mean Amplitudes (µV) at each electrode site of the P120–250, N2, and N400 of ERPs under report order were shown in Table 4. Analysis of variance yielded for the P120–250 component, mean amplitudes for Order Shape/Part larger than for Order Part/Shape at Fz, F3, and F4. Analysis of variance showed significant main effects of report order at Fz ($F_{1,14}=10.83$, $p<.01$), F3 ($F_{1,14}=7.42$, $p<.05$), and F4 ($F_{1,14}=10.71$, $p<.01$). The differences at other sites were not statistically significant. For the N2 component, the mean amplitude at each electrode site gave no significant effect of order of report. For the N400 component, mean amplitudes for Order Shape/Part were negative compared with those of Order Part/Shape at Fz, F3, F4, Cz, and Pz. An analysis of variance showed significant main effects of report order at Fz ($F_{1,14}=6.38$, $p<.05$), F3 ($F_{1,14}=7.62$, $p<.05$), F4 ($F_{1,14}=6.96$, $p<.05$), Cz ($F_{1,14}=7.84$, $p<.05$), and Pz ($F_{1,14}=10.96$, $p<.01$).

TABLE 4
MEAN AMPLITUDE (µV) AT EACH ELECTRODE SITE OF THE 120–250, 251–350, AND 351–750 MSEC. LATENCY REGIONS OF EVENT-RELATED POTENTIALS EVOKED BY DIFFERENT REPORT ORDER

Latency Region	Fz	F3	F4	Cz	Pz
120–250					
Order Part/Shape	0.62	0.58	0.82	0.76	1.35
Order Shape/Part	4.05	3.50	4.19	3.19	3.06
251–350					
Order Part/Shape	−2.41	−2.30	−1.32	−1.42	1.80
Order Shape/Part	−1.77	−2.06	−0.47	−1.87	0.81
351–750					
Order Part/Shape	1.36	1.93	1.82	1.82	1.51
Order Shape/Part	−3.70	−3.59	−3.20	−3.24	−3.13

DISCUSSION

This study was designed to examine the physiological evidence of the effect of order of report on multidimensional stimulus identification. Shieh, *et al.* (1996) suggested that subjects responded faster and more accurately if the order of reporting stimulus dimension was naturally language-appropriate. The behavioral data showed that response time for the first stimulus dimension (RT_1) and response time total (RT_T) for Order Part/Shape were significantly shorter than Order Shape/Part. These results support findings by Shieh, *et al.* (1996) and Shieh and Lai (1996, 1997) that the response times for the first dimension were smaller if subjects reported the part dimension first and the shape dimension second than if they reported dimensions in the opposite order. They suggested that the former order of report fit the Chinese "adjective then noun" grammar.

Stimulus features as well as the attentional demands posed by a visual discrimination task may affect the amplitude, voltage topography across the scalp, and latency of ERP components (Hillyard, Mangun, Woldorff, & Luck, 1995). Traditionally, the ERP waveform has been conveniently divided into exogenous (stimulus characteristic) and endogenous (cognitive and decision making) components. The three components P120–250, N2, and N400 have been associated with endogenous parameters (Kenemans, Kok, & Smulders, 1993; Coles & Rugg, 1995; Smid, Jakob, & Heinze, 1999). P120–250 concerns a slow endogenous positive shift, which may be called frontal selection positivity in other studies (Kenemans, *et al.*, 1993; Smid, *et al.*, 1999). The frontal selection positivity is thought to be related to prefrontal or subcortical selective processing (Aine & Harter, 1986). In the studies of Smid, *et al.* (1999) and Kenemans, Smulders, and Kok (1995), the frontal selection positivity reflects a mechanism associated with a selection-for-action on the actual trial behavior. The ERP data in this study indicated the P120–250 component had significantly higher peak amplitude for Order Shape/Part than Order Part/Shape at Fz, F3, and F4. The mean amplitudes showed significant differences between Order Part/Shape and Order Shape/Part at Fz, F3, and F4 and a difference at Cz and Pz which fell just short of significance. It seems that subjects processed more effortfully during the selection for dimensions in Order Shape/Part than in Order Part/Shape.

There were no peak latency, peak amplitude, and mean amplitude differences of N2 component in each electrode site for the two report orders. Ritter, Simson, and Vaughan (1983) proposed that the N2 reflects the process of stimulus classification, while Näätänen (1992), O'Donnell, Swearer, Smith, Hokama, and McCarley (1997), Potts, Liotti, Tucker, and Posner (1996), and Ritter, Simson, Vaughan, and Friedman (1979) identified N2 as being a signature of target detection. The N2 amplitude in this study showed no significant effect of order of report. It might reflect there were no differences in detection for report orders.

The N400 component was the major negative deflection between 350–750 msec. after stimulus onset. Kutas and Hillyard (1980) speculated that the N400 might be an "electrophysiological" sign of the "reprocessing" of semantically anomalous information. Van Petten and Kutus (1987) suggested that highly activated words elicit a small N400, while less-activated words elicit a larger N400. The results of their study gave a larger N400 to contextually inappropriate targets than to contextually appropriate targets, suggesting that the contextually appropriate meanings of the words were selectively activated in memory. In this study, the mean N400 amplitudes at Fz, F3, F4, Cz, and Pz all showed significant effects of report order. Order Part/Shape is a natural language order in Chinese. Reporting a whole circular shape by "full circular" was more natural than reporting it by "circular full." Hence, Order Part/Shape elicited a smaller N400 compared with Order Shape/Part.

This research is an early electrophysiological study examining the effect of order of report on multidimensional stimulus identification. These results suggest that the neural activities under Order Shape/Part and Order Part/Shape are different, and it seems plausible that subjects put more effort into selection and showed more related semantic activation in Order Shape/Part than in Order Part/Shape. Both behavioral and physiological data showed that it is more appropriate and less demanding if people report stimulus attributes in ways consistent with their long-standing language habits.

REFERENCES

AINE, C. J., & HARTER, M. R. (1986) Visual event-related potentials to colored patterns and color names: attention to features and dimensions. *Electroencephalography and Clinical Neurophysiology*, 54, 228-245.

ALLPORT, D. A. (1971) Parallel encoding within and between elementary stimulus dimensions. *Perception & Psychophysics*, 10, 104-108.

BARRETT, S. E., & RUGG, M. D. (1990) Event-related potentials and the semantic matching of pictures. *Brain and Cognition*, 14, 201-212.

CARSWELL, C. M., & WICKENS, C. D. (1996) Mixing and matching lower-level codes for object displays: evidence for two sources of proximity compatibility. *Human Factors*, 38, 1-23.

COLES, M. G. H., & RUGG, M. D. (1995) Event-related brain potentials: an introduction. In M. D. Rugg & M. G. H. Coles (Eds.), *Electrophysiology of mind: event-related brain potential and cognition*. New York: Oxford Univer. Press. Pp. 1-26.

DONCHIN, E. (1981) Surprise! . . . surprise! *Psychophysiology*, 18, 493-513.

DUNCAN, J. (1984) Selective attention and the organization of visual information. *Journal of Experimental Psychology: General*, 118, 13-42.

EGETH, H. E., & PACHELLA, R. (1969) Multidimensional stimulus identification. *Perception & Psychophysics*, 5, 341-346.

FISHER, D. L., & TANNER, N. S. (1992) Optimal symbol set selection: a semiautomated procedure. *Human Factors*, 34, 79-95.

GRATTON, G., COLES, M. G. H., SIREVAAG, E., ERIKSEN, C. W., & DONCHIN, E. (1988) Pre- and post-stimulus activation of response channels: a psychophysiological analysis. *Journal of Experimental Psychology: Human Perception and Performance*, 14, 331-344.

HARRIS, C. S., & HABER, R. N. (1963) Selective attention and coding in visual perception. *Journal of Experimental Psychology*, 65, 328-333.

HILLYARD, S. A., MANGUN, G. R., WOLDORFF, M. G., & LUCK, S. J. (1995) Neural systemsec. mediating selective attention. In M. S. Gazzaniga (Ed.), *The cognitive neurosciences*. Cambridge, MA: MIT Press. Pp. 665-681.

HOLCOMB, P. J., & MCPHERSON, W. B. (1994) Event-related brain potentials reflect semantic priming in an object decision task. *Brain and Cognition*, 24, 259-276.

Kenemans, J. L., Kok, A., & Smulders, F. T. Y. (1993) Event-related potentials to conjunctions of spatial frequency and orientation as a function of stimulus parameters and response requirements. *Electroencephalography and Clinical Neurophysiology*, 88, 51-63.

Kenemans, J. L., Smulders, F. T. Y., & Kok, A. (1995) Selective procession of two-dimensional visual stimuli in young and old subjects: an electrophysiological analysis. *Psychophysiology*, 32, 108-120.

Kutas, M., & Hillyard, S. A. (1980) Reading senseless sentences: brain potentials reflect semantic incongruity. *Science*, 207, 203-205.

Lappin, J. S. (1967) Attention in the identification of stimulus in complex visual displays. *Journal of Experimental Psychology*, 75, 321-328.

Lawrence, D. H., & LaBerge, D. L. (1956) Relationship between recognition accuracy and order of reporting stimulus dimensions. *Journal of Experimental Psychology*, 51, 12-18.

Näätänen, R. (1992) *Attention and brain function*. Hillsdale, NJ: Erlbaum.

O'Donnell, B. F., Swearer, J. M., Smith, L. T., Hokama, H., & McCarley, R. W. (1997) A topographic study of ERP elicited by visual feature discrimination. *Brain Topography*, 10, 133-143.

Osga, G. (1982) *An evaluation of identification performance for Raster Scan generated NTDS symbology*. (Final Report) San Diego, CA: Naval Ocean System Center.

Potts, G. F., Liotti, M., Tucker, D. M., & Posner, M. I. (1996) Frontal and inferior temporal cortical activity in visual target detection: evidence from high spatially sampled event-related potential. *Brain Topography*, 9, 3-14.

Ritter, W., Simson, R., & Vaughan, H. G. (1983) Event-related potential correlated of two stages of information processing in physical and semantic discrimination tasks. *Psychophysiology*, 20, 168-179.

Ritter, W., Simson, R., Vaughan, H. G., & Friedman, D. (1979) A brain event related to the making of a sensory discrimination. *Science*, 203, 1358-1361.

Shieh, K-K., & Chen, F. F. (2002) Effects of report order and stimulus type on multidimensional stimulus identification. *Perceptual and Motor Skills*, 95, 783-794.

Shieh, K-K., & Lai, C. J. (1996) Effects of practice on the identification of multidimensional stimulus. *Perceptual and Motor Skills*, 83, 435-448.

Shieh, K-K., & Lai, C. J. (1997) Multidimensional stimulus identification: instructing subjects in the order of reporting stimulus dimension. *Perceptual and Motor Skills*, 84, 995-1008.

Shieh, K-K., Lai, C. J., & Ellingstad, V. S. (1996) Effects of report order, identification method, and stimulus characteristics on multidimensional stimulus identification. *Perceptual and Motor Skills*, 82, 99-111.

Smid, H. G. O. M., Jakob, A., & Heinze, H-J. (1999) An event-related brain potential study of visual selective attention to conjunctions of color and shape. *Psychophysiology*, 36, 264-279.

Tsang, P. S., & Bates, W. E. (1990) Resource of allocation and object displays. In *Proceedings of the Human Factors Society 34th Annual Meeting*. Santa Monica, CA: Human Factors Society. Pp. 1484-1488.

van Petten, C., & Kutas, M. (1987) Ambiguous words in context: an event-related potential analysis of the time course of meaning activation. *Journal of Memory and Language*, 26, 188-208.

Wickens, C. D., & Andre, A. D. (1990) Proximity compatibility and information display: effects of color, space, and objectness on information integration. *Human Factors*, 32, 61-77.

Wickens, C. D., & Carswell, C. M. (1995) The proximity compatibility principle: its psychological foundation and relevance to display design. *Human Factors*, 37, 473-494.

Accepted April 23, 2004.

SEASONS IN DREAMS [1]

MICHAEL SCHREDL

Central Institute of Mental Health, Mannheim, Germany

Summary.—Based on the continuity hypothesis of dreaming, whether season-related themes are more often found in five dreams collected over a 2-wk. period in particular seasons was examined for 376 women and 68 men. Whereas for winter-related themes the continuity hypothesis was supported, the percentage of summer-related themes did not differ between dream samples collected in the winter or summer months, respectively. Researchers should include the amount of time spent with season-related activities, conversations, and films to test whether in dreams the relation is direct between waking life and dreaming about seasons.

The continuity hypothesis of dreaming which states that waking-life experiences are reflected in dreams is widely accepted in dream research (cf. Schredl, 2003). The hypothesis in its general form, however, is vague. It seems fruitful to take a closer look at the exact relationship between waking and dreaming and to identify factors which might affect this relationship. Hartmann (2000) and Schredl and Hofmann (2003), for example, found that focused cognitive activities such as reading, writing, and calculating are incorporated into dreams less often than other activities like talking with friends, walking outdoors, and sexuality, indicating that the type of the waking-life experience mediated the likelihood of incorporation into subsequent dreams. Another example is the research on the effect of trauma on dreams; an emotionally intense experience can exhibit a strong effect on a person's dreams (cf. Barrett, 1996).

In the present study, the hypothesis was tested that season-related dream contents are more often found in dreams that were dreamt, recalled and reported in the corresponding season. This characteristic was chosen to complement previous research focused on more central themes in dreams (cf. Schredl, 2003).

METHOD

The participants kept a standardized dream diary over a 2-wk. period. If able to recall at least one dream, they were asked to record their dreams(s) as completely as possible (on a maximum of five mornings per person). The dream reports were typed, randomized, and scored along scales measuring the occurrence of summer themes (hot weather, swimming, etc.) and winter themes (snow, skiing, Christmas, etc.).

---

[1]Send correspondence to M. Schredl, Dr. phil., Schlaflabor, Zentralinstitut für Seelische Gesundheit, Postfach 12 21 20, 68072 Mannheim, Germany.

Overall, 444 persons (376 women, 68 men) participated. Their mean age was 23.5 yr. ±5.7. Participants were students at the universities of Mannheim, Heidelberg, and Landau. For a detailed description of the study's design, see Schredl, Wittmann, Ciric, and Götz (2003). During the months May, June, and July 814 dreams were reported, whereas 796 dreams were elicited in November and December. Mean length was 155 ± 130 words (range: 5 to 1320 words). The "winter" dreams were on the average slightly longer than the "summer" dreams (163 ± 147 words vs 148 ± 111 words; $t =$ 2.4, $p = .02$). Dreams (50 dreams with season-related themes and 50 dreams without season-related themes) were coded by a second judge to assess interrater agreement.

Results and Discussion

Summer-related themes were coded in 110 dreams, winter-related themes in 54 dream reports (including 8 dreams with summer and winter themes coded). A statistical test showed that summer themes were coded significantly more often than winter themes ($\chi^2 = 5.6$, $p = .02$). The exact agreement for the summer scale and the winter scale were 88% and 94%, respectively. Controlling the comparison for dream length by computing logistic regressions with the independent variables of season (winter vs summer) and word count, the summer themes did not differ between the dreams of the two recording periods [5.5% (summer) vs 8.2% (winter); season: $\chi^2 = 2.7$, ns; dream length: $\chi^2 = 27.5$, $p < .0001$]. But for winter themes, the expected result was obtained [2.0% (summer) vs 3.8% (winter); season: $d = 0.11$ (effect size), $\chi^2 = 7.5$, $p = .003$; dream length: $\chi^2 = 14.3$, $p = .0002$].

Overall, season-related themes were present in 9.7% of the dream reports indicating that this theme is not uncommon in dreams. The higher percentage of summer themes and related activities might be explained by a corresponding higher priority in waking-life, a testable hypothesis. Another option would be to collect dreams from regions with longer winter periods (snow, cold weather) than Germany to test whether these dream samples incorporate more winter themes.

Although the effect is small, winter-related themes were found in dreams reported in the winter more often than in dreams reported in the summer. This finding, thus, supports the continuity hypothesis. The nonsignificant finding (assuming a small effect size, the power of this statistical test was 0.98) regarding summer-related themes raises the question whether actual experience during the day is the only factor influencing subsequent incorporation into dreams. Strauch and Meier (1996), for example, emphasized the importance of including also thoughts about waking-life experiences as a factor to affect dream content. The hypothesis whether the higher occurrence of summer-related themes in the winter months might be explained by higher occurrence of summer themes in thoughts, conversations, or even media presentations should be investigated.

REFERENCES

BARRETT, D. (Ed.) (1996) *Trauma and dreams*. Cambridge, MA: Harvard Univer. Press.

HARTMANN, E. A. (2000) We do not dream of the 3 R's: implications for the nature of dream mentation. *Dreaming*, 10, 103-110.

SCHREDL, M. (2003) Continuity between waking and dreaming: a proposal for a mathematical model. *Sleep and Hypnosis*, 5, 38-52.

SCHREDL, M., & HOFMANN, F. (2003) Continuity between waking activities and dream activities. *Consciousness and Cognition*, 12, 298-308.

SCHREDL, M., WITTMANN, L., CIRIC, P., & GÖTZ, S. (2003) Factors of home dream recall: a structural equation model. *Journal of Sleep Research*, 12, 133-141.

STRAUCH, I., & MEIER, B. (1996) *In search of dreams: results of experimental dream research*. Albany, NY: State Univer. of New York Press.

Accepted April 24, 2004.

AUDITORY EVENT-RELATED POTENTIALS IN PARKINSON'S DISEASE IN RELATION TO COGNITIVE ABILITY [1]

Z. KATSAROU, S. BOSTANTJOPOULOU,
V. KIMISKIDIS, E. ROSSOPOULOS, AND A. KAZIS

*3rd Department of Neurology
University of Thessaloniki, Thessaloniki*

Summary.—Auditory event-related potentials were evaluated in 45 nondemented patients with mild to moderate Parkinson's disease and 40 matched normal controls. All patients were neuropsychologically assessed by means of the Raven Colored Progressive Matrices, four subtests of the Wechsler Memory Scale (Digit Span Forward, Logical Memory, Visual Memory, Associate Learning), and the Wisconsin Card-sorting Test. The P300 component of the auditory event-related potentials was significantly prolonged in the patients with Parkinson's disease. Correlations between P300 latency and neuropsychological measures showed significant associations with lower performance on the Raven Colored Progressive Matrices and the Wisconsin Card-sorting Test. Our results indicate that for patients with mild to moderate Parkinson's disease subtle changes in cognitive abilities may be reflected as P300 prolongation.

Parkinson's disease is a predominantly motor disorder characterized also by cognitive impairment ranging from mild specific cognitive deficits to overt dementia. Patients with Parkinson's disease even in early stages may have visuospatial impairment, memory deficits, and disturbance of attentional control and executive functions (Levin & Katzen, 1995; Mohr, Mendis, & Grimes, 1995; Hammond-Tooke & Pollock, 1999). Motor impairment may interfere with neuropsychological testing; therefore, reliable motor-free methods of cognitive function evaluation are more suitable for these patients.

Event-related potentials, particularly the P300 component, provide a means of measuring cognitive processing that is independent of motor speed and disability. Although various studies have shown that P300 latency is negatively correlated with mental function in normal and demented subjects (Oken, 1990; Kutas & Dale, 1997), there is still controversy about the actual psychological meaning of P300 parameters, their exact significance, prognostic value, and relation to specific cognitive deficits (Goodin & Aminoff, 1987; Kuegler, Taghavy, & Platt, 1993; Knight & Scabini, 1998). The physiological aspects of P300 in relation to its site of generation and neurotransmitter systems involved are also under investigation (Kuegler, *et al.*, 1993).

---

[1]Address correspondence to Zoe Katsarou, M.D., 3 Ipsilantou st, Gr 55337 Thessaloniki, Greece or e-mail (zoekatmd@otenet.gr) or (bostkamb@spark.net.gr).

The putative involvement of cholinergic and dopaminergic neural networks in the generation of P300 make the study of P300 in patients with Parkinson's disease more relevant (Stanzione, Fattaposta, Giunti, D'Alesio, Tagliati, Afficiano, & Amabile, 1991; Kuegler, et al., 1993). Auditory P300 has been reported to be abnormal in demented patients with Parkinson's disease (Oken, 1990). Nevertheless, the main focus of interest is nondemented patients. P300 abnormalities have been reported even for patients with mild Parkinson's disease and subtle cognitive deficits in some studies (Goodin & Aminoff, 1987; Elwan, Baradah, Madkour, Elwan, Hassan, Elwan, Mahfouz, Ali, & Fahmy, 1996; Green, Woodard, Sirockman, Zakers, Maier, Green, & Watts, 1996; Stanzione, Semprini, Pierantozzi, Santilli, Fadda, Traversa, Peppe, & Bernardi, 1998), while others reported normal findings (Pirtosek, Jahanshahi, Barrett, & Lees, 2001).

The purpose of our study was to investigate whether nondemented patients with Parkinson's disease showed any P300 abnormalities compared to normal matched controls. We hypothesized that a possible P300 abnormality could be related to impairment in cognitive domains known to be influenced by the disease process.

Method

Subjects

Forty-five Greek patients diagnosed with Parkinson's disease (31 men, 14 women) were studied. They had a mean Mini-Mental State Examination (MMSE) score greater than 25, and they were not demented according to the DSM–IV criteria for dementia. Their mean age was 59.3 yr. ($SD = 6.7$), and the mean duration of their disease was 6.1 yr. ($SD = 3.7$). They were in Stage II or III of the disease according to the modified Hoehn and Yahr classification scale (Fahn, Elton, Members of the UPDRS Development Committee, 1987). The three cardinal symptoms of the disease, tremor, rigidity, and bradykinesia were rated using anchors of $0 =$ normal and $4 =$ maximal severity as suggested by the Unified Parkinson's Disease Rating Scale (Fahn, et al., 1987). Mean scores were for tremor 1.2 ($SD = 0.6$); bradykinesia 1.7 ($SD = 0.6$); rigidity 1.6 ($SD = 0.6$). All patients were under treatment with L-dopa and dopaminergic agonists. None were taking anticholinergics or amantadine. They were examined in the morning 1 hr. after taking their first dose of medication.

Forty normal subjects (29 men, 11 women) matched for age and education served as controls for the electrophysiological assessment. All participants gave informed consent for testing.

Electrophysiological Assessment

Auditory event-related potentials were elicited using a standard two-tone discrimination or "oddball" paradigm. Briefly, patients were presented a series of binaural tones at 70-dB sound pressure level (SPL), with a 10-msec. rise/fall and a 100-msec. plateau time. The auditory stimuli were presented in a random sequence with target tones of 2000 Hz occurring 20% of the time and standard tones of 1000 Hz occurring 80% of the time at a rate of 0.5 Hz. Patients were instructed to count the target tones silently and report the total number at the end of the series. Electroencephalographic activity was recorded (filter bandpass: 0.1–50 Hz, analysis time: 1 sec.) from scalp AgCl electrodes at Cz and Pz sites according to the International 10/20 system, referred to linked earlobe electrodes, with a forehead ground. Electrooculography (EOG) was recorded between the outer canthus and the lower eyelid of the right eye. Trials in which the EEG or EOG exceeded ±50 µV were automatically rejected. The electrical activity was digitized (12 bit) at 250 Hz from 0.1 sec. before to 0.9 sec. after stimulus onset. Responses to target and standard tones were averaged separately. Stimuli were presented until 30 artifact-free trials were recorded. Each patient was tested twice to ensure that waveform components were reproducible. Latency and peak-to-peak amplitude of components N1, P2, N2, and P3 were measured in the averaged responses to the target tones. The peak of the components was measured as follows: if the waveform was smooth, the point of maximal amplitude was taken as a peak. Alternatively, the leading and trailing slopes of the waveform were extended, and the intersection point determined. The component N1 was defined as the maximum negativity occurring between 80 and 160 msec. poststimulus, while P2 was the maximum positivity between 150 and 250 msec. The wave N2 was defined as the maximum negativity between 175 and 250 msec. that immediately preceded the P3 wave, and the latter was defined as the maximum positivity between 250 and 600 msec. In subjects with distinct P3a and P3b waves, P3 measures were taken from P3b (Kazis, Kimiskidis, Georgiadis, & Kapinas, 1996).

Neuropsychological Assessment

Patients were neuropsychologically assessed on the following tests: Raven Colored Progressive Matrices (Raven, 1962); four subtests of the Wechsler Memory Scale: Digit Span Forward, Logical Memory, Visual Memory, and Associate Learning (Wechsler, 1945); the Wisconsin Card-sorting Test (Heaton, Chelune, Talley, Kay, & Curtiss, 1993).

Statistical Analysis

Comparisons of auditory event-related potential parameters between patients and controls were performed by means of the Student t test. Relationship between P300 latency and duration of the disease, cardinal symptoms as well as neuropsychological test scores were evaluated using the Pearson correlation coefficient after a logarithmic base 10 transformation of data to reduce skewness. All reported p values are two-tailed.

Results and Discussion

In all subjects, the auditory event-related potentials were recorded successfully. P300 latency was significantly prolonged in patients with Parkinson's disease ($p < .001$), while no other values were affected (cf. Table 1). Neuropsychological assessment scores are presented in Table 2. When patients' scores were compared with standard data from matched normal subjects, their performance was inferior on Logical Memory and three measures of the Wisconsin Card-sorting Test.

TABLE 1
Auditory Event-related Potentials: Parameters in Patients and Controls (ns = 45)

Parameter	Patients M	Patients SD	Controls M	Controls SD	t
Amplitude, µV					
N1	9.1	3.5	8.2	3.6	1.16
P2	11.4	5.0	13.0	4.7	−1.52
N2	7.7	4.3	8.4	5.7	−0.58
P300	12.8	6.9	13.7	6.2	−0.63
Latency, µsec.					
N1	101.9	10.7	96.4	17.3	1.74
P2	175.6	14.2	70.2	11.1	1.99
N2	241.4	25.3	37.7	15.2	0.83
P300	388.5	37.4	355.1	35.1	4.24

*$p < .001$.

Correlation between P300 latency and neuropsychological findings showed a significant association between scores on Raven Colored Progressive Matrices ($r = -.35$, $p < .02$) and the following measures of the Wisconsin Card-sorting Test: total number of errors, percentage of errors, perseverative responses and errors, percent perseverative responses and errors as well as number of categories completed. Correlation for all other test scores were not significant (Table 3). Correlations between P300 latency and disease parameters such as duration, stage, and motor symptoms were not significant.

The P300 component of the auditory event-related potentials is a long latency waveform considered to reflect high cognitive processing (Polich, 1998). P300 is characterized by its amplitude and latency; however, the interpretation of the functional meaning of P300 is not an easy task. Various psychophysiological theories have been proposed to explain the relationship between P300 parameter changes and cognitive function (Kuegler, et al., 1993; Kutas & Dale, 1997; Knight & Scabini, 1998; Polich, 1998).

According to theorists, P300 amplitude probably reflects the processing

TABLE 2
Neuropsychological Assessment of Patients With
Parkinson's Disease and Controls ($ns = 45$)

Test	Patients M	Patients SD	Controls M	Controls SD	t
Raven Colored Progressive Matrices	24.5	5.4	26.5	6.0	1.60
Weschler Memory Scale					
Digit Span	5.5	0.8	5.9	0.7	−1.20
Logical Memory	6.5	2.7	9.3	3.1	−4.10†
Visual Memory	8.6	3.5	9.8	3.0	−1.70
Associate Learning	14.0	3.8	15.3	3.4	−1.70
Wisconsin Card Sorting Test					
Number of trials administered	95.6	18.8	86.2	14.2	2.60*
Total number correct	73.5	9.8	69.8	7.9	1.92
Total number of errors	20.6	11.9	16.4	9.2	1.83
Percent errors	20.6	7.9	18.3	4.2	1.65
Perseverative responses	20.0	14.8	13.6	6.1	2.70*
Percent perseverative responses	19.7	10.6	15.0	5.7	2.60*
Perseverative errors	12.7	9.8	9.3	5.1	1.95
Percent perseverative errors	12.6	7.1	10.3	4.2	1.84
Number of categories completed	5.8	0.4	5.9	0.1	−1.70

Note.—Significance has been calculated by comparisons between patients' scores and data from a sample of normal matched population. *$p < .02$. †$p < .001$.

of incoming information when it is incorporated into memory representations of the stimulus and the context in which the stimulus occurs (Knight & Scabini, 1998; Polich, 1998). The P300 latency is particularly sensitive to stimulus evaluation relative to response selection and execution processes. Therefore, it has been considered as the upper limit of the time required to reach the perceptual decision that an informative event has occurred (Kutas & Dale, 1997; Polich, 1998). P300 latency is negatively correlated with mental function in normal individuals; shorter latencies are associated with superior cognitive performance. Accordingly, demented patients have significant prolongation of P300 latency corresponding to the severity of their dementia (Polich, 1998).

In general, although P300 amplitude and latency may be linked behaviorally to a range of cognitive processes, it is still controversial whether their changes can accurately represent discrete cognitive functions or whether they should be viewed as an indirect index of global cognitive capacity (Goodin & Aminoff, 1987; Knight & Scabini, 1998). Furthermore, in the interpretation of P300, physiological data should be taken into consideration. Various neural generators of P300 have been proposed, with the hippocampal and inferior parietal sites being the most important (Green, et al., 1996). However, there is also a significant contribution from other brain areas, such as the frontal lobe, basal ganglia, and the thalamus that cannot be ignored (Velasco, Velasco, Velasco, Almanza, & Olvera, 1986; Tachibana, Aragane, Kawabata, & Sugita, 1997). These findings argue in favor of an extended neural network involvement in P300 generation and are in line with the assumption that P300 is much more sensitive to general cognitive impairment than specific neuropsychological deficits (Kuegler, et al., 1993).

TABLE 3
CORRELATIONS BETWEEN P300 LATENCY AND NEUROPSYCHOLOGICAL TEST PERFORMANCE FOR PATIENTS WITH PARKINSON'S DISEASE

Test	Pearson r	p
Raven Colored Progressive Matrices	−.35	.019*
Weschler Memory Scale		
Digit Span	−.03	ns
Logical Memory	.26	ns
Visual Memory	−.30	ns
Associate Learning	−.13	ns
Wisconsin Card Sorting Test		
Total number correct	.12	ns
Total number of errors	.44	.002†
Percent errors	.45	.003†
Perseverative responses	.49	.001‡
Percent perseverative responses	.49	.001‡
Perseverative errors	.38	.008†
Percent perseverative errors	.33	.03*
Number of categories completed	−.37	.01*

*$p<.05$. †$p<.01$. ‡$p<.001$.

In various studies involving nondemented patients with Parkinson's disease, P300 latency was either normal (Green, et al., 1996; Raudino, Gadavaglia, Beretta, & Pellegrini, 1997; Pirtosek, et al., 2001) or prolonged (Goodin & Aminoff, 1987; Hayashi, Hanyk, Shindo, Tamaru, & Yanagisawa, 1993; Elwan, et al., 1996; Sohn, Kim, Huh, & Kim, 1998). Amplitude was normal (Pirtosek, et al., 2001), decreased (Raudino, et al., 1997), or elevated (Green, et al., 1996). Controversy appears also in studies exploring the relationship of P300 latency and neuropsychological test scores for nondemented patients with Parkinson's disease. Pang, Borod, Hernandez, Bodis-Wollner, Raskin, Mylin, Coscia, and Yahr (1990) found that P300 latency correlated negatively with scores on Logical Memory and Visual Perception but not with general cognitive ability. A relationship between P300 prolongation and inferior performance on the modified Wisconsin Card-sorting Test was postulated by Iizima, Osawa, Iwata, Miyazaki, and Tei (2000). Other studies have not yielded a correlation between P300 latency and achievement on tests of general cognitive ability (Rumbach, Tranchant, Viel, & Warter, 1993; Elwan, et al., 1996; Hayashi, Hanyk, Kurashima, Tokutake, & Yanagisawa, 1996; Stanzione, et al., 1998).

Our results showed that nondemented patients with Parkinson's disease had a significantly prolonged P300 latency compared to normal matched controls. In our patients, a prolongation of P300 latency was related to decreased performance on the Raven Colored Progressive Matrices, a test indicative of general cognitive ability. It is noteworthy that, although our patients were not demented, they had subtle deficits in the domains of memory and executive functions. Correlation between P300 latency and memory tests did not show an association. However, most measures of the Wisconsin Card-sorting Test correlated with P300 prolongation. Although correlations among scores on multiple neuropsychological tests increase the probability of Type I error, most correlations concerning the measures of the Wisconsin Card-sorting Test yielded strong correlation coefficients of comparatively satisfactory significance.

In Parkinson's disease, cognitive impairment sometimes leading to dementia in the advanced stages of the disease is a well-established clinical finding (Hammond-Tooke & Pollock, 1999; Starkstein & Merello, 2002). One can hypothesize that in early stages of Parkinson's disease, subtle changes in cognitive abilities may be reflected in P300 prolongation. However, further longitudinal studies are required to assess the clinical utility of P300 in cognitive function evaluation of patients with Parkinson's disease as well as its prognostic value in early detection of patients at risk for developing dementia.

REFERENCES

Elwan, O. H., Baradah, O. H., Madkour, O., Elwan, H., Hassan, A. A. H., Elwan, H., Mahfouz, M., Ali, A., & Fahmy, M. (1996) Parkinson's disease cognition and aging: clinical, neuropsychological, electrophysiological and cranial computerized tomographic assessment. *Journal of Neurological Sciences*, 143, 64-71.

Fahn, S., Elton, R. L., & Members of UPDRS Development Committee. (1987) Unified Parkinson's Disease Rating Scale. In S. Fahn, C. D. Marsden, D. Calne, & M. Goldstein (Eds.), *Recent developments in Parkinson's disease*. Florham Park, NJ: Macmillan Healthcare Information. Pp. 153-163.

Goodin, D. S., & Aminoff, M. J. (1987) Electrophysiological differences between demented and nondemented patients with Parkinson's disease. *Annals of Neurology*, 21, 90-94.

Green, J., Woodard, J. L., Sirockman, B. S., Zakers, G. O., Maier, C. L., Green, R. C., & Watts, R. L. (1996) Event-related potential P3 change in mild Parkinson's disease. *Movement Disorders*, 11, 32-42.

Hammond-Tooke, G. D., & Pollock, M. (1999) Depression, dementia and Parkinson's disease. In A. B. Joseph & R. R. Young (Eds.), *Movement disorders in neurology and neuropsychiatry*. Malden, MA: Blackwell Science. Pp. 195-204.

Hayashi, R., Hanyk, N., Kurashima, T., Tokutake, T., & Yanagisawa, N. (1996) Relationship between cognitive impairments, event-related potentials and motor disability scores in patients with Parkinson's disease: 2-yr. follow-up study. *Journal of Neurological Sciences*, 141, 45-48.

Hayashi, R., Hanyk, N., Shindo, M., Tamaru, F., & Yanagisawa, N. (1993) Event-related potentials, reaction time and cognitive state in patients with Parkinson's disease. *Advances in Neurology*, 60, 429-433.

Heaton, R. K., Chelune, G. J., Talley, J. L., Kay, G., & Curtiss, G. (1993) *Wisconsin Card-sorting Test manual: revised and expanded*. Odessa, FL: Psychological Assessment Resources.

Iizima, M., Osawa, M., Iwata, M., Miyazaki, A., & Tei, H. (2000) Topographic mapping of P300 and frontal cognitive function in Parkinson's disease. *Behavioural Neurology*, 12, 143-148.

Kazis, A., Kimiskidis, V., Georgiadis, G., & Kapinas, K. (1996) Cognitive event-related potentials and magnetic resonance imaging in myotonic dystrophy. *Neurophysiologie Clinique*, 26, 75-78.

Knight, R. T., & Scabini, D. (1998) Anatomic bases of event-related potentials and their relationship to novelty detection in humans. *Journal of Clinical Neurophysiology*, 15, 3-13.

Kugler, C., F. A., Taghavy, A., & Platt, D. (1993) The event-related P300 potential analysis of cognitive human brain aging: a review. *Gerontology*, 39, 283-303.

Kutas, M., & Dale, A. (1997) Electrical and magnetic readings of mental functions. In M. D. Rugg (Ed.), *Cognitive neuroscience*. Hove East Sussex, UK: Psychology Press. Pp. 197-242.

Levin, B. E., & Katzen, H. L. (1995) Early cognitive changes and nondementing behavioral abnormalities in Parkinson's disease. *Advances in Neurology*, 65, 85-95.

Mohr, E., Mendis, T., & Grimes, J. D. (1995) Late cognitive changes in Parkinson's disease with an emphasis in dementia. *Advances in Neurology*, 65, 97-113.

Oken, B. S. (1990) Endogenous event-related potentials. In K. Chiappa (Ed.), *Evoked potentials in clinical medicine*. (2nd ed.) New York: Raven. Pp. 563-592.

Pang, S., Borod, J. C., Hernandez, A., Bodis-Wollner, I., Raskin, S., Mylin, L., Coscia, L., & Yahr, M. D. (1990) The auditory P300 correlates with specific cognitive deficits in Parkinson's disease. *Journal of Neural Transmission (P-D Section)*, 2, 249-264.

Pirtosek, Z., Jahanshahi, M., Barrett, G., & Lees, A. (2001) Attention and cognition in bradykinetic-rigid syndromes: an event-related potential study. *Annals of Neurology*, 50, 567-573.

Polich, J. (1998) P300 clinical utility and control of variability. *Journal of Clinical Neurophysiology*, 15, 14-33.

Raudino, F., Gadavaglia, P., Beretta, S., & Pellegrini, G. (1997) Auditory event-related potentials in Parkinson's disease. *Electromyography and Clinical Neurophysiology*, 37, 409-413.

Raven, J. C. (1962) *Coloured Progressive Matrices*. London: H. K. Lewis.

Rumbach, L., Tranchant, C., Viel, J. F., & Warter, J. M. (1993) Event-related potentials in Parkinson's disease. *Journal of Neurological Sciences*, 116, 148-151.

Sohn, Y. K., Kim, G. W., Huh, K., & Kim, J. S. (1998) Dopaminergic influences on the P300 abnormality in Parkinson's disease. *Journal of Neurological Sciences*, 158, 83-87.

Stanzione, P., Fattaposta, F., Giunti, P., D'Alesio, C., Tagliati, M., Afficiano, C., & Amabile, G. (1991) P300 variations in parkinsonian patients before and during dopaminergic monotherapy: a suggested dopamine component in P300. *Electroencephalography and Clinical Neurophysiology*, 80, 446-453.

Stanzione, P., Semprini, R., Pierantozzi, M., Santilli, A. M., Fadda, L., Traversa, R., Peppe, A., & Bernardi, G. (1998) Age and stage dependency of P300 latency alterations in nondemented Parkinson's disease patients without therapy. *Electroencephalography and Clinical Neurophysiology*, 108, 80-91.

Starkstein, S. E., & Merello, M. (2002) *Psychiatric and cognitive disorders in Parkinson's disease*. Cambridge, UK: Cambridge Univer. Press. Pp. 55-87.

Tachibana, H., Aragane, K., Kawabata, K., & Sugita, M. (1997) P3 latency change in aging and Parkinson's disease. *Archives of Neurology*, 54, 296-302.

Velasco, M., Velasco, F., Velasco, A. L., Almanza, X., & Olvera, A. (1986) Subcortical correlates of the P300 potential complex in man to auditory stimuli. *Electroencephalography and Clinical Neurophysiology*, 64, 199-210.

Wechsler, D. (1945) A standardized memory scale for clinical use. *Journal of Psychology*, 19, 87-95.

Accepted April 27, 2004.

THROWING ACCURACY DURING PRISM ADAPTATION: MALE ADVANTAGE FOR THROWING ACCURACY IS INDEPENDENT OF PRISM ADAPTATION RATE[1]

LAURIE SYKES TOTTENHAM AND DEBORAH M. SAUCIER

Department of Psychology
University of Saskatchewan

Summary.—Previous studies have found that men are more accurate at throwing an object at a target than are women, independent of experience. However, these studies' results are based on average scores from multiple trials. As such, it is unknown whether the male advantage results from superior throwing accuracy or from a superior ability to calibrate subsequent throws. This study examined whether men can calibrate repeated throws more quickly and accurately than women. 25 men and 30 women were required to throw velcro-covered balls at a carpet-covered target, both with and without 10-diopter prism lenses. Participants had multiple trials in both conditions. Analyses examined whether there was a sex difference in the rate of adaptation to the prism lenses (as indicated by calibration of subsequent throws), instead of simply averaging all throwing accuracy scores and looking for an overall sex difference. Men threw the balls significantly more accurately than women, both with and without the prism lenses. However, there was no significant sex difference found on the rate of prism adaptation, as measured by improvement across the trials, i.e., calibration. Although men were more accurate at throwing balls overall, there was no sex difference in calibration of subsequent throws in adapting to the prism lenses, therefore indicating that the male advantage in throwing accuracy does not result from superior ability to calibrate subsequent throws but rather from superior throwing accuracy overall.

Men are typically more accurate at throwing an object at a target than are women, independent of sports history (Watson & Kimura, 1991; Hall & Kimura, 1995) or style of throwing, i.e., overhand or underhand throwing of balls, or throwing of darts (Jardine & Martin, 1983; Watson & Kimura, 1989, 1991; Hall & Kimura, 1995). However, the reason for this advantage is unknown.

Most studies examining throwing accuracy use the distance between the position where a thrown object hit and the location of the target as the score. However, these studies usually average multiple throws (e.g., Jardine & Martin, 1983; Watson & Kimura, 1989, 1991; Hall & Kimura, 1995). Throwing is a skill that yields feedback, as the participants can see how far the thrown object was from the target as well as the direction in which they erred. As such, participants can correct or calibrate subsequent throws, perhaps affecting overall accuracy. Studies that examine sex differences by using average scores do not document whether the sex difference is due to

---

[1]Address correspondence to Deborah Saucier, Ph.D., Department of Psychology, University of Saskatchewan, 9 Campus Drive, Saskatoon, SK S7N 5A5 Canada

overall throwing accuracy or differences in calibration of subsequent throws. Thus it is possible that the typical male advantage for throwing accuracy results from men being superior in calibrating subsequent throws more accurately rather than a superior ability to hit individual targets.

Prism lenses create a situation in which the visual scene is displaced from the actual position of the objects. When neurologically normal participants wear prism lenses while performing a throwing task, their initial throwing accuracy is displaced—although they can rapidly compensate for this (Gauthier, Hofferer, Hoyt, & Stark, 1979; Weiner, Hallett, & Funkenstein, 1983; Thach, Goodkin, & Keating, 1991). Presumably correcting for the visual deviation is reliant on cerebellar function, as patients with cerebellar lesions do not adapt to the prism lenses and do not calibrate subsequent throws, despite equivalent initial accuracy without the prism lenses. Thus, the purpose of the present study was to examine whether the sex differences seen in throwing accuracy result from differences between the sexes in calibration or in throwing accuracy.

In the present study participants performed a throwing task while wearing lenses that had either plain lenses or prism lenses (10-diopter), thereby allowing us to observe the process of calibration. When wearing the prism lenses, participants' throwing accuracy is initially displaced and then gradually corrected. Fernandez-Ruiz and Diaz (1999) found that calibration is not instantaneous, rather it required a mean of six throws to return to a prior accuracy. Throwing accuracy in the present study was measured as the distance between where the ball hit and where the target actually was for each trial. As such, a lower score indicated greater accuracy. In accordance with previous findings (e.g., Jardine & Martin, 1983; Watson & Kimura, 1989, 1991; Hall & Kimura, 1995), it was predicted that men would outperform women on the throwing task when it was done without the prism lenses. No predictions were made regarding sex differences in throwing balls at a target while wearing prism lenses, and no predictions were made regarding sex differences in the rate of adaptation to the prism lenses, reflected by calibration and consequent improved accuracy over a number of trials.

Additionally, the present study required participants to complete a Mental Rotations task (Vandenberg & Kuse, 1978). This was done to test the sample for the expected male advantage that is typically seen on this task (e.g., Linn & Petersen, 1985), thereby confirming that the sample was representative of the population. As well, correlational analysis was done to check whether participants' mental rotation performance was related to their throwing accuracy, as both are spatial skills typically demonstrating a male advantage. However, as neither Saucier and Kimura (1998) nor Watson and Kimura (1991) observed a significant relationship among similar tasks, no significant correlation was predicted.

Method

Participants

Twenty-five men and 30 women were recruited from a university participant pool for psychology classes. All participants were between the ages of 18 and 26 years (age: men, $M = 20.4$ yr., $SD = 2.2$; women, $M = 21.1$ yr., $SD = 2.9$). Participants were awarded credit toward their grade in introductory psychology. All participants were right-handed based on a questionnaire (Kimura, 1973) that required participants to mime eight unimanual tasks. Participants were classified as right-handed if they performed at least seven of the tasks with the right hand, with the stipulation that writing had to be one of the seven tasks performed with the right hand. Initial recruitment of participants excluded participants with extensive sports experience, including either recreational or competitive participation in sports that involved extensive throwing skill, e.g., darts, or sports that involve underhand throws, e.g., softball. No participants indicated that they participated in sports more than once per month.

Tasks and Procedure

All participants were individually tested by the same researcher. The testing sessions began with the participants providing informed consent, followed by the completion of a questionnaire containing questions regarding demographic information, handedness, and sports history. However, as noted above, participants were prescreened and excluded for sports history. Following completion of the questionnaire participants performed the throwing task with one hand. Then participants performed four distractor tasks and the Mental Rotations Test (Vandenberg & Kuse, 1978), which took approximately 15 minutes. The testing sessions ended with the participants performing the throwing task with the hand that had not yet been used; thus participants performed the throwing task with both the right and left hands. Order of the tasks and the hand used first in the throwing task were counterbalanced among the participants.

The throwing task was the same as that reported by Saucier and Kimura (1998). Participants threw a velcro-covered ball at a carpet-covered target that was 285 cm from where they stood. The target was a 6.5-cm × 6.5-cm square placed in the middle of a 145-cm × 145-cm carpet backdrop. The target was elevated 150 cm above the floor.

Participants performed an underhanded throw at the target both with and without binocular prism lenses (10-diopter lenses). Participants performed five trials without the prism lenses, 10 trials with the prism lenses, and then an additional five trials without the prism lenses. This sequence was performed with both the left and right hands.

RESULTS

Repeated-measures analyses of variance were performed on the participants' throwing accuracy, with separate analyses for the first five trials (without lenses), the next 10 trials (with prism lenses), and the last five trials (without lenses). For each analysis, the within-subjects measures were trial number and hand used to throw, and the between-subjects measure was sex. The dependent measure was the deviation (cm) between the 'hit' point and the closest edge of the target for each trial. A one-way analysis of variance was performed on participants' Mental Rotations Test scores, with sex as the between-subjects measure and number correct as the dependent measure. A Pearson correlation was performed on the throwing accuracy scores and Mental Rotations scores.

Throwing

First five trials (trials prior to wearing prism lenses).—An analysis of variance indicated that, as predicted, men ($M = 12.8$, $SD = 4.3$) outperformed women [$M = 15.5$, $SD = 5.6$; $F_{1,53} = 3.75$ (Pillai's Trace), $p = .06$, $\eta^2 = .07$]. Further, performance with the right hand ($M = 12.7$, $SD = 5.9$) was significantly more accurate than performance with the left hand [$M = 15.9$, $SD = 7.1$; $F_{1,53} = 8.89$ (Pillai's Trace), $p = .004$, $\eta^2 = .15$]. However, it is the interaction of trial by sex which is of particular interest here, as it indicates whether there was a sex difference in the rate of change over the trials. The interaction of trial by sex did not reach significance [$F_{4,50} = 2.06$ (Pillai's Trace), $p = .10$, $\eta^2 = .14$]; see Fig. 1. All participants significantly improved over the course of the five trials [$F_{4,50} = 6.86$ (Pillai's Trace), $p < .001$, $\eta^2 = .35$].

Middle 10 trials (trials while wearing prism lenses).—An analysis of variance indicated that, as predicted, men ($M = 12.2$, $SD = 4.4$) outperformed women [$M = 15.9$, $SD = 4.9$; $F_{1,53} = 8.88$ (Pillai's Trace), $p = .004$, $\eta^2 = .14$]. Further, performance with the right hand ($M = 13.1$, $SD = 6.3$) was significantly more accurate than performance with the left hand [$M = 15.3$, $SD = 6.2$; $F_{1,53} = 4.42$ (Pillai's Trace), $p = .04$, $\eta^2 = .08$]. However, as above, the interaction of trial by sex did not reach significance [$F_{9,45} = 0.46$ (Pillai's Trace), ns, $\eta^2 = .09$]; see Fig. 1. All participants significantly improved over the course of the 10 trials [$F_{9,45} = 4.57$ (Pillai's Trace), $p = .001$, $\eta^2 = .48$].

Final five trials (trials following the wearing of prism lenses).—An analysis of variance indicated that, as predicted, men ($M = 11.7$, $SD = 5.0$) outperformed women [$M = 14.9$, $SD = 4.7$; $F_{1,53} = 5.91$ (Pillai's Trace), $p = .02$, $\eta^2 = .10$]. Further, performance with the right hand ($M = 11.5$, $SD = 5.9$) was significantly more accurate than performance with the left hand [$M = 15.3$, $SD = 6.8$; $F_{1,53} = 13.03$ (Pillai's Trace), $p = .001$, $\eta^2 = .20$]. However, as above, the interaction of trial by sex was not significant [$F_{4,50} = 0.48$ (Pillai's Trace), ns, $\eta^2 = .04$]; see Fig. 1. All participants significantly improved over the course of the five trials [$F_{4,50} = 2.58$ (Pillai's Trace), $p = .05$, $\eta^2 = .17$].

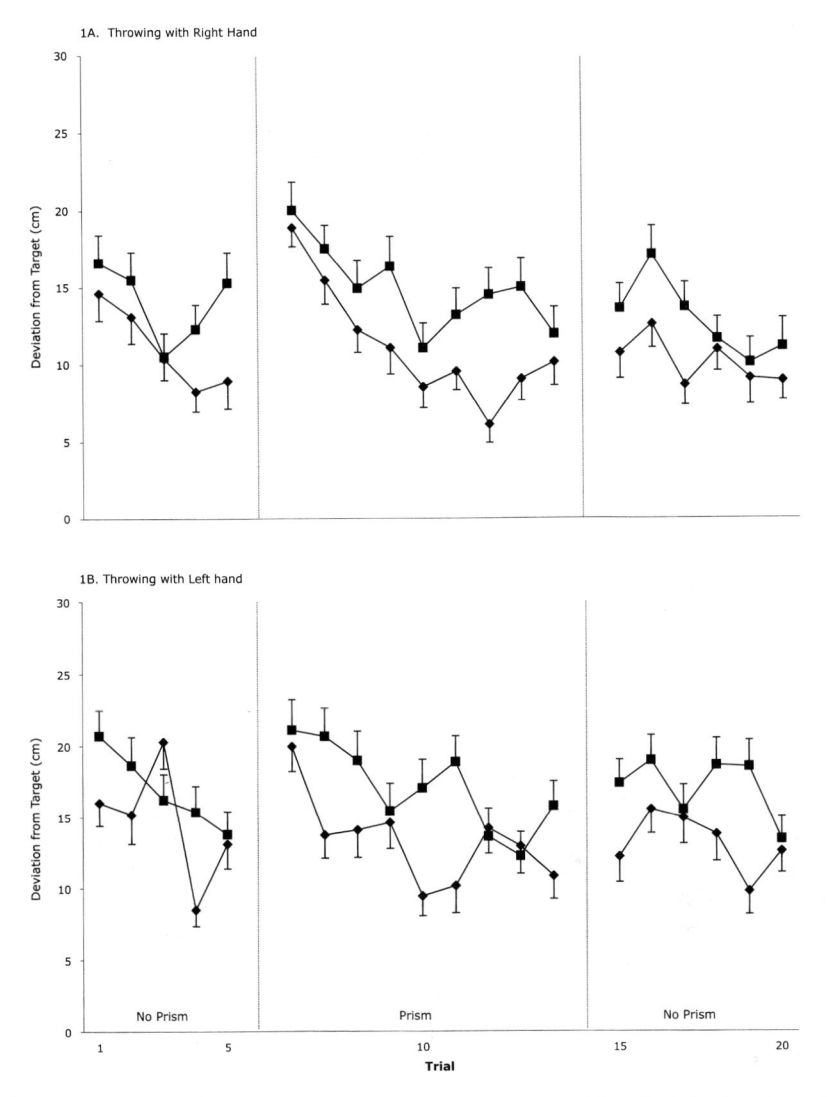

FIG. 1. The distance between the target and hit point for each trial of the throwing tasks for men (♦ $n=25$) and women (■ $n=30$), both with and without the prism lenses

Mental Rotations Test

As predicted, analysis of variance indicated that men ($M=10.8$, $SD=5.1$) outperformed women [$M=6.8$, $SD=3.6$; $F_{1,53}=11.46$ (Pillai's Trace), $p=.001$, $\eta^2=.18$]. Consistent with previous research (e.g., Watson & Kimura, 1991; Saucier & Kimura, 1998), there were no significant correlations found between the spatial abilities; in this study, throwing accuracy (for either the right or left hand) and performance of mental rotations were not significantly correlated (all correlations were less than .19).

Discussion

In all instances, men were significantly more accurate at hitting the target than women, both with and without the prism lenses. This confirms and extends previous findings indicating a male advantage for throwing accuracy (Jardine & Martin, 1983; Watson & Kimura, 1989, 1991; Hall & Kimura, 1995). However, we did not find that men were able to adapt to the prism lenses and thus to calibrate subsequent throws any faster or more accurately than women. Further, as participants had to re-adjust to visual feedback after wearing the prism lenses (final five trials), we confirmed the participants' ability to calibrate their throws twice. Neither time was there significant interaction for trial by sex.

This suggests that the sex difference in throwing accuracy is not based on differences in calibration of motor movements. As adaptation to prism lenses is hypothesized to be related to cerebellar mechanisms (Thach, Goodkin, & Keating, 1992), it is not likely that sex differences in cerebellar control of motor movement required for calibration of throwing can account for this sex difference in throwing accuracy. However, as we did not directly measure cerebellar function, we cannot preclude a role for other aspects of cerebellar control implicated in sex differences that could influence throwing accuracy.

As there was no interaction of sex by trial, either with or without the prism lenses present, our results are consistent with the position that men and women are equally proficient at calibrating their visual gaze and that men are more skilled at throwing accurately. Our data suggest that, although women can adapt to the prismatic visual distortion as quickly and accurately as men, they did not throw as accurately. This implies that there is another factor in throwing accuracy which underlies the observed sex difference.

REFERENCES

Fernandez-Ruiz, J., & Diaz, R. (1999) Prism adaptation and aftereffect: specifying the properties of a procedural memory system. *Learning and Memory*, 6, 47-53.

Gauthier, G. M., Hofferer, J. M., Hoyt, W. F., & Stark, L. (1979) Visual-motor adaptation: quantitative demonstration in patients with posterior fossa involvement. *Archives of Neurology*, 36, 155-160.

Hall, J., & Kimura, D. (1995) Sexual orientation and performance on sexually dimorphic motor tasks. *Archives of Sexual Behavior*, 24, 395-407.

Jardine, R., & Martin, N. G. (1983) Spatial ability and throwing accuracy. *Behavior Genetics*, 13, 331-340.

Kimura, D. (1973) Manual activity during speaking: left handers. *Neuropsychologia*, 11, 51-55.

Linn, M. C., & Petersen, A. C. (1985) Emergence and characterization of sex differences in spatial ability: a meta-analysis. *Child Development*, 56, 1479-1498.

SAUCIER, D. M., & KIMURA, D. (1998) Intrapersonal motor but not extrapersonal targeting skill is enhanced during the midluteal phase of the menstrual cycle. *Developmental Neuropsychology*, 14, 385-398.

THACH, W. T., GOODKIN, H. P., & KEATING, J. G. (1991) Inferior olive disease in man prevents learning of novel eye-hand synergies. *Society for Neuroscience Abstracts*, 17, 1380.

THACH, W. T., GOODKIN, H. P., & KEATING, J. G. (1992) The cerebellum and the adaptive coordination of movement. *Annual Reviews of Neuroscience*, 15, 403-442.

VANDENBERG, S. G., & KUSE, A. R. (1978) Mental rotations, a group test of three-dimensional spatial representation. *Perceptual and Motor Skills*, 47, 599-604.

WATSON, N. V., & KIMURA, D. (1989) Right-hand superiority for throwing but not for intercepting. *Neuropsychologia*, 27, 1399-1414.

WATSON, N. V., & KIMURA, D. (1991) Nontrivial sex differences in throwing and intercepting: relation to psychometrically-defined spatial functions. *Personality and Individual Differences*, 12(5), 375-385.

WEINER, M. J., HALLETT, M., & FUNKENSTEIN, H. (1983) Adaptation to lateral displacement of vision in patients with lesions of the central nervous system. *Neurology*, 54, 231-244.

Accepted April 29, 2004.

CHECKLIST FOR ORDERING RECENT MATERIALS IN PSYCHOLOGY

ADLER, J. R. (Ed.) *Forensic psychology: concepts, debates and practice.* Portland, OR: Willan, 2004. Pp. xviii + 333. $65.00.

ALLOTT, R. *The great mosaic eye: language and evolution.* Sussex, UK: The Book Guild Ltd., 2001. Pp. xiv + 228. £30.00.

ALLOTT, R. *The natural origin of language: the structural inter-relation of language, visual perception and action.* Herts., UK: Able Publ., 2001. Pp. iv + 267.

AZIMA, F. J. C., & GRIZENKO, N. (Eds.) *Immigrant and refugee children and their families: clinical, research, and training issues.* Madison, CT: International Universities Press, 2002. Pp. xvii + 238. $24.95.

BARAB, S. A., KLING, R., & GRAY, J. H. (Eds.), *Designing for virtual communities in the service of learning.* New York: Cambridge Univer. Press, 2004. Pp. xxv + 451. $75.00 hdc; 28.00 pbk.

BLASS, T. *The man who shocked the world: the life and legacy of Stanley Milgram.* New York: Basic Books, 2004. Pp. xxiv + 360. $26.00.

BOGDASHINA, O. *Sensory perceptual issues in autism and Asperger Syndrome: different sensory experiences different perceptual worlds.* New York: Jessica Kingsley/Taylor & Francis, 2003. Pp. 217. $23.95.

CATTANACH, A. *Introduction to play therapy.* New York: Taylor & Francis/Routledge, 2003. Pp. 200. $23.95.

CORNOLDI, C., & VECCHI, T. *Visuo-spatial working memory and individual differences.* New York: Psychology Press, 2003. Pp. vii + 169. $47.95.

DAVIDSON, J. E., & STERNBERG, R. J. (Eds.) *The psychology of problem solving.* New York: Cambridge Univer. Press, 2003. Pp. xi + 394. $75.00 hdc; 27.00 pbk.

DAVIDSON, R. J., SCHERER, K. R., & GOLDSMITH, H. H. (Eds.) *Handbook of affective sciences.* New York: Oxford Univer. Press, 2003. Pp. xvii + 1199. $165.00.

DIXON, T. *From passions to emotions: the creation of a secular psychological category.* New York: Cambridge Univer. Press, 2003. Pp. x + 287. $60.00.

DOMHOFF, G. W. *The scientific study of dreams: neural networks, cognitive development, and content analysis.* Washington, DC: American Psychological Assn, 2003. Pp. ix + 209. $39.95.

DONOGHUE, D. *Speaking of beauty.* New Haven, CT: Yale Univer. Press, 2003. Pp. xi + 209. $24.95.

DOOLEY, D., & PRAUSE, J. *The social costs of underemployment: inadequate employment as disguised unemployment.* New York: Cambridge Univer. Press, 2004. Pp. ix + 274. $65.00.

DUANMU, S. *The phonology of standard Chinese.* New York: Oxford Univer. Press, 2000. Pp. xv + 308. $74.00.

DUNLAP, J. C., LOROS, J. J., & DECOURSEY, P. J. (Eds.) *Chronobiology: biological timekeeping.* Sunderland, MA: Sinauer, 2004. Pp. xix + 406. $74.95.

EDINGER, E. F. (Transc. & Ed. J. D. Blackmer) *The sacred psyche: a psychological approach to the Psalms.* Toronto, ON: Inner City Books, 2004. Pp. 158. $18.00.

ELISON, J., & MCGONIGLE, C. *Liberating losses: when death brings relief.* Cambridge, MA: Perseus, 2003. Pp. xxiv + 214. $16.95.

FELDMAN, R. M., & STALL, S. *The dignity of resistance: women residents' activism in Chicago public housing.* New York: Cambridge Univer. Press, 2004. Pp. xx + 388. $75.00.

FLASHER, L. V., & FOGLE, P. T. *Counseling skills for speech-language pathologists and audiologists.* Clifton Park, NY: Thomson/Delmar Learning, 2004. Pp. xviii + 326.

FORGAS, J. P., WILLIAMS, K. D., & VON HIPPEL, W. (Eds.) *Social judgments: implicit and explicit processes.* New York: Cambridge Univer. Press, 2003. Pp. xxi + 417. $80.00.

GEE, J. P. *What video games have to teach us about learning and literacy.* New York: St. Martin's Press/Palgrave Macmillan, 2003. Pp. 225. $26.95.

GREENWOOD, J. D. *The disappearance of the social in American social psychology.* New York: Cambridge Univer. Press, 2004. Pp. xii + 315. $65.00.

HAYWARD, C. (Ed.) *Gender differences at puberty.* New York: Cambridge Univer. Press, 2003. Pp. xix + 337. $75.00 hdc; 27.00 pbk.

HUETTEL, S. A., SONG, A. W., & MCCARTHY, G. *Functional magnetic resonance imaging.* Sunderland, MA: Sinauer, 2004. Pp. xviii + 492. $79.95.

KING, R. A., NEUBAUER, P. B., ABRAMS, S., & DOWLING, A. S. (Eds.) *The psychoanalytic study of the child.* Vol. 58. New Haven, CT: Yale Univer. Press, 2003. Pp. vii + 311. $65.00.

LANG, F. R., & FINGERMAN, K. L. (Eds.) *Growing together: personal relationships across the lifespan.* New York: Cambridge Univer. Press, 2004. Pp. xv + 414. $75.00.

LEIGHTON, J. P., & STERNBERG, R. J. (Eds.) *The nature of reasoning.* New York: Cambridge Univer. Press, 2004. Pp. x + 470.

LUTHAR, S. S. (Ed.) *Resilience and vulnerability: adaptation in the context of childhood adversities.* New York: Cambridge Univer. Press, 2003. Pp. xxxi + 574. $90.00 hdc; 32.00 pbk.

MARCUS, G. *The birth of the mind: how a tiny number of genes creates the complexities of human thought.* New York: Basic Books, 2004. Pp. ix + 278. $26.00.

MARKOVÁ, I. *Dialogicality and social representations: the dynamics of mind.* New York: Cambridge Univer. Press, 2003. Pp. xviii + 224. $70.00.

MASATAKA, N. *The onset of language.* New York: Cambridge Univer. Press, 2003. Pp. xi + 281. $70.00.

MATTHEWS, G., DREARY, I. J., & WHITEMAN, M. C. *Personality traits.* (2nd ed.) New York: Cambridge Univer. Press, 2003. Pp. xxiv + 493. $85.00 hdc; 30.00 pbk.

MCDANIELS, T., & SMALL, M. J. (Eds.) *Risk analysis and society.* New York: Cambridge Univer. Press, 2004. Pp. ix + 468. $85.00 hdc; 30.00 pbk.

NASTASI, B. K., MOORE, R. B., & VARJAS, K. M. *School-based mental health services: creating comprehensive and culturally specific programs.* Washington, DC: American Psychological Assn, 2004. Pp. xv + 232. $49.95.

NODDINGS, N. *Happiness and education.* New York: Cambridge Univer. Press, 2003. Pp. vii + 308. $30.00.

NORMAN, D. A. *Emotional design: why we love (or hate) everyday things.* New York: Basic Books, 2004. Pp. x + 257. $26.00.

OLSON, D. R. *Psychological theory and educational reform: how school remakes mind and society.* New York: Cambridge Univer. Press, 2003. Pp. xiv + 343. $70.00 hdc; 24.00 pbk.

PERERA, S. B. *The Irish bull god: image of multiform and integral masculinity.* Toronto, ON: Inner City Books, 2004. Pp. 155. $18.00.

PERRET-CLERMONT, A-N., PONTECORVO, C., RESNICK, L. B., ZITTOUN, T., & BURGE, B. (Eds.) *Joining society: social interaction and learning in adolescence and youth.* New York: Cambridge Univer. Press, 2004. Pp. xvii + 342. $75.00 hdc; 25.00 pbk.

PHELPS, R. P. *Kill the messenger: the war on standardized testing.* New Brunswick, NJ: Transaction, 2003. Pp. xix + 331. $34.95.

PLAKE, B. S., IMPARA, J. C., & SPIES, R. A. (Eds.) *The fifteenth mental measurements yearbook.* Lincoln, NE: Buros Institute, 2003. Pp. xvii + 1143.

PLANTE, T. G. (Ed.) *Sin against the innocents: sexual abuse by priests and the role of the Catholic church.* Westport, CT: Praeger, 2004. Pp. xxvii + 226. $39.95.

RADOCY, R. E., & BOYLE, J. D. *Psychological foundations of musical behavior.* (4th ed.) Springfield, IL: Thomas, 2003. Pp. xiv + 449. $75.95 hdc; 55.95 pbk.

RESNIK, S. (R. Alcorn, Transl.) *The delusional person: bodily feelings in psychosis.* New York: H. Karnac (Books), 2001. Pp. xii + 250. $29.95.

RITCHEY, D. *The H.I.S.S. of the A.S.P.: understanding the anomalously sensitive person.* Terra Alta, WV: Headline Books, Inc., 2003. Pp. xviii + 390.

ROAZEN, P. *Cultural foundations of political psychology.* New Brunswick, NJ: Transaction, 2003. Pp. xv + 295. $49.95.

SALTER, A. C. *Predators: pedophiles, rapists, & other sex offenders.* Cambridge, MA: Perseus/Basic Books, 2003. Pp. xvi + 272. $14.95.

SAWCHUK, P. H. *Adult learning and technology in working-class life.* New York: Cambridge Univer. Press, 2003. Pp. xviii + 252. $55.00.

SCHEPARD, A. I. *Children, courts, and custody: interdisciplinary models for divorcing families.* New York: Cambridge Univer. Press, 2004. Pp. xvi + 224. $70.00 hdc; 25.00 pbk.

SCHNEIDER, S. L., & SHANTEAU, J. (Eds.) *Emerging perspectives on judgment and decision research.* New York: Cambridge Univer. Press, 2003. Pp. xxii + 713. $95.00 hdc; 35.00 pbk.

SCHORE, A. N. *Affect dysregulation and disorders of the self.* New York: Norton, 2003. Pp. xvii + 403. $45.00.

SCHORE, A. N. *Affect regulation and the repair of the self.* New York: Norton, 2003. Pp. 363. $45.00.

SCHWARTZ, M. S., & ANDRASIK, F. (Eds.) *Biofeedback: a practitioner's guide.* (3rd ed.) New York: Guilford, 2003. Pp. xiv + 930. $75.00.

SHERMER, M. *In Darwin's shadow: the life and science of Alfred Russel Wallace.* New York: Oxford Univer. Press, 2002. Pp. xx + 422. $35.00.

SOLES, D. *The essentials of academic writing.* Boston/New York: Houghton Mifflin, 2005. Pp. xix + 347.

SQUIRE, L. R., & SCHACTER, D. L. (Eds.) *Neuropsychology of memory.* (3rd ed.) New York: Guilford, 2002. Pp. xviii + 519. $75.00 hdc; 42.00 pbk.

STAUB, E. *The psychology of good and evil.* New York: Cambridge Univer. Press, 2003. Pp. xvi + 592. $80.00 hdc; 27.00 pbk.

STERNBERG, R. J. (Ed.) *The anatomy of impact: what makes the great works of psychology great.* Washington, DC: American Psychological Assn, 2003. Pp. x + 241. $29.95.

STERNBERG, R. J. (Ed.) *International handbook of intelligence.* New York: Cambridge Univer. Press, 2004. Pp. xi + 496. $95.00 hdc; 35.00 pbk.

STERNBERG, R. J. *Wisdom, intelligence, and creativity synthesized.* New York: Cambridge Univer. Press, 2003. Pp. xviii + 227. $35.00.

STROUS, M. *Racial sensitivity and multicultural training.* Westport, CT: Praeger, 2003. Pp. xii + 161. $64.95.

TOMASELLO, M. *Constructing a language: a usage-based theory of language acquisition.* Cambridge, MA: Harvard Univer. Press, 2003. Pp. viii + 388. $45.00.

UMBERSON, D. *Death of a parent: transition to a new identity.* New York: Cambridge Univer. Press, 2003. Pp. viii + 255. $28.00.

URSANO, R. J., FULLERTON, C. S., & NORWOOD, A. E. (Eds.) *Terrorism and disaster: individual and community mental health interventions.* New York: Cambridge Univer. Press, 2003. Pp. xii + 349. $150.00 hdc; 55.00 pbk.

VAN DEN BERG, H., WETHERELL, M., & HOUTKOOP-STEENSTRA, H. (Eds.) *Analyzing race talk: multidisciplinary approaches to the interview.* New York: Cambridge Univer. Press, 2003. Pp. xv + 317. $75.00 hdc; 27.00 pbk.

WADE, N. J. *Destined for distinguished oblivion: the scientific vision of William Charles Wells (1757-1817).* New York: Kluwer Academic/Plenum, 2003. Pp. xi + 310. $95.00.

WALLACE, P. *The internet in the workplace: how new technology is transforming work.* New York: Cambridge Univer. Press, 2004. Pp. xiii + 301. $28.00.

WAXMAN, H. C., THARP, R. G., & HILBERG, R. S. (Eds.) *Observational research in U.S. classrooms: new approaches for understanding cultural and linguistic diversity.* New York: Cambridge Univer. Press, 2004. Pp. xii + 284. $65.00 hdc; 25.00 pbk.

PERCEPTUAL AND MOTOR SKILLS
ISSN 0031-5125

CONTENTS OF VOLUME 98, FEBRUARY–JUNE 2004

SENIOR EDITORS   R. B. Ammons and C. H. Ammons   *Ammons Scientific, Ltd.*

EDITORS   Bruce Ammons, Douglas Ammons, S. A. Isbell

ASSOCIATE EDITORS

Marian Annett
University of Leicester

Clark D. Ashworth
NE Washington Family Counseling

Richard W. Bohannon
University of Connecticut

Willard L. Brigner
Appalachian State University

Josef Brožek
St. Paul, MN

Peter Brugger
University Hospital Zurich

Ross H. Day
La Trobe University, Bundoora

Robert Didden
Katholieke Universiteit Nijmegen

G. William Domhoff
University of California, Santa Cruz

Christopher C. Dunbar
Brooklyn College of CUNY

John Eliot
University of Maryland, College Park

H. J. Eysenck
University of London

Ann M. Filinger
Hagerstown, MD

Bernard Fine
Weston, MA

Robert Fudin
Long Island University

David M. Furst
San Jose State University

Richard Gajdosik
The University of Montana

K. O. Götz
Kunstakademie Düsseldorf

E. Rae Harcum
The College of William & Mary

Julian Hochberg
Columbia University

Alan S. Kaufman
Yale University School of Medicine

Johannes Kingma
University Hospital Groningen

Marcel Kinsbourne
Boston University

Muriel Lezak
Oregon Health Sciences University

Paul Naitoh
San Diego, California

Kent B. Pandolf
U.S. Army Research Institute

J. Timothy Petersik
Ripon College

Paul Roodin
SUNY College at Oswego

Leon E. Smith
St. Thomas University, Miami

Arthur E. Stamps III
Institute of Environmental Quality

D. L. Streiner
Baycrest Center for Geriatric Care

Stephan Swinnen
Katholieke Universiteit Leuven

Üner Tan
Karadeniz Technical University

James M. Vanderplas
Washington University

Min Q. Wang
University of Maryland

Paul R. Yarnold
Northwestern Univer. Medical School

Published bimonthly by Perceptual and Motor Skills, Box 9229, Missoula, Montana; printed by Ammons Scientific, Ltd., 1911-17 South Higgins Avenue, Missoula, Montana 59801-1911. Please address correspondence and changes of address to Box 9229, Missoula, Montana 59807-9229. POSTMASTER: Send address changes to *Perceptual and Motor Skills*, P.O. Box 9229, Missoula, Montana 59807-9229.

Copyright 2004   Perceptual and Motor Skills

CONSULTING READERS FOR 2004

During the past several months of 2004, some papers seemed to call for additional review by persons highly competent in specific areas. The Editors and Associate Editors wish to acknowledge valuable assistance by the following consulting readers:

A. M. Abdel-Khalek
Liza Abraham-Murali
Valery V. Abramov
John P. Aggleton
David P. Agle
Benigno E. Aguirre
Lewis R. Aiken, Jr.
Varol Akman
Mark S. Aldenderfer
Gary Lynn Allen
Karen M. Allen
Susan L. Andersen
Craig A. Anderson
Luigi Anolli
Mark H. Anshel
William Anthony
Alessandro Antonietti
Theodore A. Avtgis
Brooke Ayars
Michelle A. Bachus
Bruno Baldaro
John D. Ball
Bruce Barber
John E. Barbuto, Jr.
William R. Barfield
John Andrew Bargh
Julie H. Barlow
Anne M. C. Barnfield
Thorsten Barnhofer
William B. Barr
Paul T. Barrett
Suzanne B. Bausch
Annett L. Beautrais
Gilbert Becker
Elisardo Becoña
John R. Beech
Russell W. Belk
Aaron Belkin
Matthias Berger
Ennis A. Berker

Kenneth J. Berry
John B. Best
Carl O. Bickel
Erin D. Bigler
Ian M. Bisset
Shelia Black
John N. I. Bohannon III
Richard W. Bohannon
Frank G. Bolton, Jr.
Boni B. Boswell
Aaron R. Boyson
Sharon Bradley-Johnson
Frank Brady
Gérard Brand
James Robert Brašić
William G. Braud
Jack W. Brehm
David A. Brodie
Charles I. Brooks
Alfred L. Brophy
Michael B. Brown
Lowell L. Brubaker
Stephen Bruehl
Janet Buckworth
Susan Bullard
Kevin L. Burke
Christopher D. B. Burt
Darrell L. Butler
Stephen A. Butterfield
William S. Cain
Wayne J. Camara
Paul Cameron
Alfredo Campos
Chris Cantor
Maurizio Cardaci
Bradley J. Cardinal
Kevin Casebolt
James H. Cauraugh
Tony Cellucci
Timmen L. Cermak

Zack Z. Cernovsky
Catherine A. Chambliss
Edward C. Chang
Paul H. Chappell
Richard A. Charter
Jean-Charles Chebat
Denise Chen
Peter Y. Chen
Weiyun Chen
William L. Chovan
John W. Chow
Usha Chowdhary
Larry B. Christensen
Russell D. Clark III
Theodore Coladarci
Amy Elizabeth Colbert
Andrew M. Colman
Jorge Conesa
Jeffrey M. Conte
John R. M. Copeland
Germaine Cornélissen
Judith E. Courtney
Gloria Cowan
William F. Cox, Jr.
Ashley R. Craig
Robert James Craig
Canice Crerand
Patricia M. Crittenden
Salvatore Cullari
Brechtje J. Daams
H. A. M. Daanen
Jess Dancer
Henry Davis IV
Mark H. Davis
Greg E. Dear
Carolyn H. Declerck
Jerry L. Deffenbacher
Charmaine DeFrancesco
J. Scott Delaney
Paul Delfabbro

(continued on next page)

CONSULTING READERS FOR 2004

Regan DelPrione
Patricia R. DeLucia
William N. Dember
John Jesse DeMello
Craig Demmer
Martin Dempster
Valerian John Derlega
Stephen I. Deutsch
Dale DeVoe
David M. Diamond
Edward Diener
Don A. Dillman
Kathleen M. Dillon
Sherry Dingman
Richard A. Dodder
Stephen J. Dollinger
Joseph W. Donnelly
Richard L. Doty
Jerrold L. Downey
John Duckitt
Ron P. Dumont
Robert M. Duncan
Randall B. Dunham
Shimon Edelman
Phil Edwards
Howard Eichenbaum
Martin E. Eigenberger
Nancy Eisenberg
Hillary Anger Elfenbein
Gary D. Ellis
David G. Elmes
Veikko Eloranta
Iris Engelhard
George M. Engelhardt
Ruth C. Engs
Carol J. Erdwins
David M. Erlanger
Ann Erling
Bryan Lee Euler
Frank E. Eyetsemitan
Bruno Facon
Frank H. Farley
Richard F. Farmer
Diane Fassel
John F. Feldhusen
David M. Fergusson
Pere-Joan Ferrando Piera
F. Figura
Joan E. Finegan

Gerhard H. Fischer
Robert J. Fletcher
Douglas H. Flint
Kory Floyd
Robert L. Folmer
James J. Forest
Carol Ann Fowler
Richard J. Fox
Leslie J. Francis
B. Don Franks
Karin S. Frey
Matthew J. Friedman
James R. Friedrich
William Norman Friedrich
Donald J. Fucci
Katsuo Fujiwara
Kazuhiko Fukuda
Adrian Furnham
Bernadette M. Gadzella
Gary C. Galbraith
David L. Gallahue
Ge Gao
James C. Garbutt
Rick M. Gardner
Stephen M. Gavazzi
William F. Gayton
Randall F. Gearhart, Jr.
Michael E. Geisser
Hans-Georg Geissler
Betholyn F. Gentry
Claire Gérard
Roseann Giarrusso
Karel Gijsbers
Diane L. Gill
Kathleen Martin Ginis
Arthur P. Ginsburg
Amedeo Giorgi
Michel Girodo
Carol L. Gohm
Scott B. Going
John F. Golding
Marion Golenia
Paula Goolkasian
Judith D. Goss
William Drew Gouvier
Steve Graham
Philippe Grandjean
Abraham P. Greeff
J. Matt Green

Marsha L. Green
James N. Gribble
Michael Grunebaum
Nicolas Guéguen
Eleanora Gullone
Gary W. Guyot
Ilse Hakvoort
Donald M. Hall
Judith A. Hall
Kellie Green Hall
Gordon Halliday
Hallgeir Halvari
Donald D. Hammill
W. Rodney Hammond
Peter A. Hancock
David W. Harder
Clive G. Harper
Christian L. Hart
Wolfgang Hartje
James E. Hartley
Anita H. Hartmann
John H. Harvey
Robin L. Harwood
Peter Hassmén
Takeshi Hatta
Mitsuo Hayashi
Ryoichi Hayashi
Keikichi Hayashibe
Leslie Alec Hayduk
Harlene Hayne
Ronald D. Hays
Kathleen M. Haywood
Tim B. Heaton
Michelle (Mikki) Rae Hebl
W. Harvey Hegarty
Lora K. Heisler
Ronald I. Herning
Bradley R. Hertel
Robert A. Hicks
Clara E. Hill
Marc Hillbrand
Terence M. Hines
Mikio Hirano
Michael A. Hitt
Albert F. Hodapp
Paul R. Hoffman
Geert Hofstede
John D. Hogan
Robert T. Hogan

(continued on next page)

CONSULTING READERS FOR 2004

Robert L. P. J. Hogenraad
Mohammadreza Hojat
John L. Holland
Cooper B. Holmes
Diane M. Horm-Wingerd
Thelma S. Horn
Yoko Hoshi
James Houran
J. Daniel House
John M. Houston
Johannes E. Hovens
Aimee Howley
Shulan Hsieh
Kenneth Hugdahl
Leon A. Hyer
Ronald J. Iannotti
Yuichi Iizuka
Kazunari Ikeda
Mitsuo Ikeda
Larry D. Isaacs
Seppo E. Iso-Ahola
Allen E. Ivey
Sumiko Iwao
Edgar L. Jackson
Piotr Jaśkowski
Leonard A. Jason
Gerald J. Jerome
H. Durell Johnson
Stephen E. Johnson
Brick Johnstone
Anupama Joshi
Charles E. Joubert
Toivo Jürimäe
Boris Kabanoff
Inga Kadish
Mirja Kalliopuska
Michael A. Kamins
Randy W. Kamphaus
Kázmér Karádi
Costas I. Karageorghis
Ragnheidur Karlsdottir
Tatsuya Kasai
Howard Kassinove
Zoe Katsarou
James C. Kaufman
Göran Kecklund
Patricia C. Keith-Spiegel
Michael Kellmann
James P. Kelly

Sandra Kelly
David A. Kenny
Brett Kessler
Sara B. Kiesler
William D. Scott Killgore
Angus D. Kindley
Bruce M. King
Cheryl A. King
E. Kioumourtzoglou
Bruce D. Kirkcaldy
Martha Kirkpatrick
Stuart T. Klapp
Eric Klinger
Tracy A. Knight
Duane V. Knudson
Mladen Koljatic
Małgorzata Kossowska
Vikki Krane
David R. Krathwohl
Leonard Kravitz
Stanley Krippner
Daryl G. Kroner
Arie W. Kruglanski
Klaus D. Kubinger
V. K. Kumar
Ute Kunzmann
Susan M. Labott
Reinhold G. Laessle
Kristen M. Lagally
Matt A. Lambon Ralph
Giulio E. Lancioni
Ronald S. Landis
Andrew M. Lane
Rael T. Lange
Rense Lange
Robert E. Larzelere
Don Latham
Adrienne Y. Lee
Antoon A. Leenaars
Paul R. Lees-Haley
Paul M. Lehrer
Robert Lemieux
Richard M. Lerner
Henry R. Lesieur
David Lester
Peter M. Lewinsohn
Ronald Ley
Filip Lievens
Per Lindqvist

William R. Lindsay
Mary M. Livingston
Gerald M. Long
Robert Loo
Thomas R. Lord
Geoff Lowe
Christopher M. Lowery
Richard Lynn
David P. Mackinnon
Richard A. Magill
Noreen E. Mahon
Joseph L. Mahoney
J. John Mann
Jacobus G. Maree
Kevin Marjoribanks
William T. Markham
David Markland
Elizabeth W. Markson
Herbert W. Marsh
Maryanne Martin
David R. Matsumoto
J. Douglas Maxwell
Richard E. Mayer
Rebecca J. McCauley
Teresa McCormack
Penny McCullagh
Mark G. McGee
Conor McGuckin
John W. McHoskey
Elspeth McKay
Wilbert J. McKeachie
Stuart J. McKelvie
Terry McMorris
Douglas M. McNair
John R. McNamara
Harry J. Meeuwsen
Christian A. Meissner
Beverley K. Mendelson
Mario F. Mendez
Harald Merckelbach
Peter F. Merenda
M. Vicenta Mestre
John Peter Meyer
Paul W. Mielke, Jr.
Jeffrey A. Miles
Jeremy N. V. Miles
Craig S. Miller
Lisa F. Miller
Scott Richard Millis

(continued on next page)

Alma Mintu-Wimsatt
John Mirowsky
Philip H. Mirvis
Mitsumasa Miyashita
Andile Mji
F. Gerard Moeller
Robert L. Montgomery
James P. Morgan, Jr.
Michael J. Morgan
Alain Morin
Craig S. Morrison
Gabriel Moser
Naoyasu Motomura
Robert R. Mowrer
Ronald L. Moy
Peter E. Mudrack
Robert L. Muelleman
Brian Mullen
Mark B. Muraven
Bennet B. Murdock, Jr.
Luigi Murri
Keiko Nakano
Gosaku Naruse
Jack L. Nasar
Jan Naughton
Janet Davis Neal
Herbert L. Needleman
Andrew B. Newberg
Aaron J. Newman
Robert G. Newman
Audrey Newton
Maria Newton
Karen A. Nolan
Hilmar Nordvik
Adrian C. North
Vincent Nougier
Stephen Nowicki, Jr.
Paul D. Nussbaum
Michael S. Nystul
Shinga Oda
Mark Onslow
Arturo Orsini
Patricia A. Oswald
Paul E. Panek
Charlambos Papaxanthis
David Pargman
Andrew C. Parrott
Jérôme Patron
Gordon L. Paul

Thomas Pechmann
Darhl M. Pedersen
Guido Peeters
Robert J. Pellegrini
Larry H. Percy
Lawrence C. Perlmuter
Michael A. Persinger
Herbert L. Petri
Linda Petrosino
Vicky Phares
Colin Phillips
Chris Piotrowski
Zvezdan Pirtosek
Kenneth H. Pitetti
Thomas G. Plante
Richard D. Platt
Robert Plutchik
John Polich
Anne-Marie Polimeni
Ovide F. Pomerleau
Joseph G. Ponterotto
Jeffrey A. Potteiger
Hillel Pratt
Felicia Pratto
John Predebon
Fred H. Previc
Ian R. Price
Robert F. Priest
James O. Prochaska
Thomas J. Pujol
Frank W. Putnam
Stanley J. Rachman
Fred M. Rafilson
David W. Rainey
Lynda B. Ransdell
Sarah Ransdell
Taina Rantanen
Shulamit Raviv
John R. Reddon
T. Gilmour Reeve
Marianne Regard
Gregory Reid
Michael Reiß
Ralph M. Reitan
Robert E. Reys
John T. E. Richardson
Dennis R. Ridley
L. Douglas Ried
Shirley Rietdyk

Arthur J. Riopelle
Gary E. Roberts
Jonathan E. Roberts
Maxwell J. Roberts
Robert E. Roberts
Robert J. Robertson
James D. Roff
Peter A. Rogerson
Stephen P. R. Rose
Elliott D. Ross
Miriam Rothman
James G. Rotton
Bruce J. Rounsaville
David C. Rubin
I. Alex Rubino
Ellen Bouchard Ryan
Joseph F. Rychlak
David A. Sabatino
Susan J. Sachsenmaier
Paul R. Sackett
Seyed-Hossein Salimi
R. K. Salokangas
William A. Sands
Darcy A. Santor
Gary L. Sapp
Eleni Sarlani
Klaus-Steffen Saternus
Muriel D. Saunders
Russell Schachar
Charles E. Schaefer
K. Warner Schaie
Wilmar B. Schaufeli
Margaret Schenkman
Thomas R. Schill
Klaus Schneewind
Marlene Schommer-Aikins
David J. Schretlen
Petra B. Schuler
Shalom Hillel Schwartz
Ralf Schwarzer
Karl Schweizer
Anthony Scioli
R. Michael Scott
H. A. M. Seelen
David R. Segal
Ola A. Selnes
Thomas J. Sheeran
Roy J. Shephard
Roberta B. Shepherd

(continued on next page)

Claudine Sherrill
Mark E. Shevlin
Naoki Shibahara
Eva Hanski Shinar
Kenneth I. Shulman
David M. Siegel
Michael Siegrist
Steven B. Silvern
John R. Sirard
Emmanouil K. Skordilis
Gary S. Skrinar
Elissa L. Slanger
Andrew P. Smith
Jonathan C. Smith
Ronald E. Smith
Michael Sol
Eric R. Spangenberg
Chris Spatz
Norman E. Spear
Janet T. Spence
David Spiegel
Brian H. Spitzberg
Otfried Spreen
Susan Sprich
Steven Stack
Robert E. Stadulis
Kenneth M. Steele
Robert A. Steer
Jürgen M. Steinacker
Dawn E. Stephens
Michael J. Stevens
Paul Stevens
Heather A. Stewart
Michael J. Stewart
Eugene F. Stone-Romero
Andrew Stuart
Alice F. Stulmacher
Masatomo Suetsugi
Michael W. Suleiman
Heikki Summala
Jerry J. Sweet
Toshiaki Tachibana
Hideoki Tada
Kazuo Takai
Jasmine Tata
Douglas N. Taylor
Janet L. Taylor
John G. Taylor
Richard Glenn Tedeschi
Ali İzzet Tekcan
Hasan Gürkar Tekman

Shirley Telles
Gershon Tenenbaum
Elisabeth M. TenVergert
Michael A. Thalbourne
Stephen G. Tibbetts
Marika Tiggemann
Joaquín Tomás-Sábado
Phillip D. Tomporowski
Terence J. G. Tracey
John W. Trinkaus
A. Stewart Truswell
Warren W. Tryon
Haralambos Tsorbatzoudis
Reuven Tsur
Fernando Tusell
Takeshi Ueda
James S. Uleman
Rolf Ulrich
Carlo Umiltá
Paul M. Valliant
Henry VandeWalle
Yves Vanlandewijck
Jacques H. A. van Rossum
T. van Strien
Katalin Varga
Ruut Veenhoven
Paul Verhaeghen
Madhubalan Viswanathan
Vish C. Viswesvaran
Filippos M. Vlachos
Brent Alan Vogt
Martin Voracek
Daniel Voyer
Jiří Wackermann
Thomas A. Wadden
Edwin E. Wagner
Michael B. Walker
Stephen A. Wallace
Daniel L. Wann
Catherine L. Ward
Joel S. Warm
Rebecca M. Warner
Margo C. Watt
Charles N. Weaver
Michael A. Webster
Daniel M. Wegner
Naomi Weintraub
Cynthia M. Whissell
Frank W. Wicker
David Wilkinson
Geoffrey C. Williams

J. Mark G. Williams
John G. Williams
Kenneth C. Williams
Anne E. Wilson
Y. K. Wing
Piotr Winkielman
Roselle L. Wissler
Karsten Witt
Leo Wolmer
Edward F. Wright
Craig A. Wrisberg
J. Michael Wyss
Toshiyuki Yamashita
Elleen M. Yancey
Bijou Yang
Wei-Jun Jean Yeung
Michael J. Zajano
Carlos P. Zalaquett
Lucia Zanuttini
Christine Zaza
Li-fang Zhang
Betty Zimmerberg
Vasiliki Zisi
Machiel J. Zwarts

CONTENTS OF VOLUME 98, FEBRUARY–JUNE 2004

ABEL, E. L., AND KRUGER, M. L. Relation of handedness with season of birth of professional baseball players revisited 44
ADAMS, R. D. See LEE, H.
ÅKERSTEDT, T. See LANDSTRÖM, U.
ALBERS, C. See DICERBO, K. E.
ALKHATEEB, H. M. Spatial visualization of undergraduate education majors classified by thinking styles 865
AMBROSI-RANDIĆ, N., AND TOKUDA, K. Perceptions of body image among Japanese and Croatian children of preschool age 473
ANDO, S., KIDA, N., AND ODA, S. Retention of practice effects on simple reaction time for peripheral and central visual fields 897
ANDREWS, M. W. See BRANNON, E. M.
ANNESI, J. J., WESTCOTT, W. W., AND GANN, S. Preliminary evaluation of a 10-wk. resistance and cardiovascular exercise protocol on physiological and psychological measures for a sample of older women 163
ANTONINI PHILIPPE, R., SEILER, R., AND MENGISEN, W. Relationships of coping styles with type of sport 479
ANTONIOU, P. See BEBETSOS, E.
ARENDASY, M., AND SOMMER, M. Measuring perceptual speed in complex everyday situations 615
ARNAS, Y. A., SIĞIRTMAÇ, A. D., AND GÜL, E. D. A study of 60- to 89-mo.-old children's skill at writing numerals 656
ARNAU, J., AND BONO, R. Evaluating effects in short time series: alternative models of analysis 419
BÄCKSTRÖM, M. See FEDERMANN, R.
BALLON, F. See PAPAIOANNOU, A.
BALSAMO, M. See SAGGINO, A.
BARTOW, R. E., JR. See MCBRIDE, S. A.
BARUCH, C., PANISSAL-VIEU, N., AND DRAKE, C. Preferred perceptual tempo for sound sequences: comparison of adults, children, and infants 325
BATAVIA, M. See GIANUTSOS, J. G.
BEBETSOS, E., ANTONIOU, P., KOULI, O., AND TRIKAS, G. Knowledge and information in prediction of intention to play badminton 1210
BERRY, K. J. See JOHNSTON, J. E.
BERRY, K. J., JOHNSTON, J. E., AND MIELKE, P. W., JR. Exact goodness-of-fit tests for unordered equiprobable categories 909
BIGAND, E. See TILLMANN, B.
BJÖRKQVIST, K. See VARHAMA, L. M.
BLANCHARD, J. See DICERBO, K. E.
BÖHM, J. See STRENGE, H.
BONO, R. See ARNAU, J.
BONOTI, F. See VLACHOS, F.
BORNHOLT, L. J. See BRAKE, N. A.
BOSTANTJOPOULOU, S. See KATSAROU, Z.
BRADLEY, M. T., AND STOICA, G. Diagnosing estimate distortion to significance testing in literature on detection of deception 827
BRAKE, N. A., AND BORNHOLT, L. J. Personal and social bases of children's self-concepts about physical movement 711
BRAND, G., MILLOT, J-L., JACQUOT, L., THOMAS, S., AND WETZEL, S. Left:right differences in psychophysical and electrodermal measures of olfactory thresholds and their relation to electrodermal indices of hemispheric asymmetries 759
BRANNON, E. M., ANDREWS, M. W., AND ROSENBLUM, L. A. Effectiveness of video of conspecifics as a reward for socially housed bonnet macaques (*Macaca radiata*) 849
BRIDGES, F. S., AND KUNSELMAN, J. C. Gun availability and use of guns for suicide, homicide, and murder in Canada 594
BRIDGES, F. S., AND PEARSON, L. C. Use of the same and a longer time series to replicate David Lester's study of suicide and birth rates in Canada 1090
BROCHARD, R. See DUFOUR, A.

BROUSARD, K. T. See BURDA, A. N.
BROXON-HUTCHERSON, A. See SCHULER, P. B.
BRUGGER, P. See PROIOS, H.
BURDA, A. N., HAGEMAN, C. F., BROUSARD, K. T., AND MILLER, A. L. Dementia and identification of words and sentences produced by native and nonnative English speakers 1359
BYSTRÖM, M. See LANDSTRÖM, U.
CAMERON, E. M., AND FERRARO, F. R. Body satisfaction in college women after brief exposure to magazine images 1093
CAMPBELL, J. L., GADZICHOWSKI, K. M., AND PASNAK, R. Mastery of number conservation by a man with severe cognitive disabilities 1283
CAMPODONICO, F. See LANCIONI, G. E.
CAN, Ş. See DANE, Ş.
CAPILOUTO, G. J., MCCLENAGHAN, B., WILLIAMS, H. G., DICKERSON, J., AND HUSSEY, J. R. Performance of able-bodied subjects on a text-typing task using a head-operated device and expanded membrane cursor keys 147
CASEBOLT, K., AND RIZZO, T. L. Concurrent evidence of physical educators' attitude toward teaching individuals with disabilities 366
CELSE, C. See OLIVIER, G.
CEPICKA, L. Stepnicka's modification of the Brace Test: an investigation of dimensionality 171
CERBONE, M. R. See SAGGINO, A.
CHAN, A. H. S. See YU, R-F.
CHASSE, J-L. See ROYET, J-P.
CHENG, T-S., AND LEE, T-H. Human pulling strengths in different conditions of exertion 542
CHERNEY, I. D., AND NEFF, N. L. Role of strategies and prior exposure in mental rotation 1269
CHIERCHIE, S. See LANCIONI, G. E.
CHUNG, P-K. See LEUNG, R. W.
CLARK, R. D. III. On the independence of golf scores for professional golfers 675
CLOUGH, P. J. See CRUST, L.
CLOUTIER, G. See FAIGENBAUM, A. D.
COBB, Y. See SHAUNESSY, E.
COHEN, J. M. See GIANUTSOS, J. G.
COKER, C. A. Bilateral symmetry in coincident timing: a preliminary investigation 359
COLLET, C. See GUILLOT, A.
CONTI, M. A. See CONTI, R. P.
CONTI, R. P., AND CONTI, M. A. Mock jurors' perceptions of facial hair on criminal offenders 1356
CORBALLIS, M. C. See GUTNIK, B. J.
COSTIGAN, E. M. See LAGALLY, K. M.
CRAFT, B. B. See SZALDA-PETREE, A. D.
CRESSWELL, S., AND HODGE, K. Coping skills: role of trait sport confidence and trait anxiety 433
CREWS, D. J., LOCHBAUM, M. R., AND LANDERS, D. M. Aerobic physical activity effects on psychological well-being in low-income Hispanic children 319
CREWS, T. R. See GREEN, J. M.
CRIBBIE, R. A. See SANTARCANGELO, M.
CRUST, L. Carry-over effects of music in an isometric muscular endurance task 985
CRUST, L., CLOUGH, P. J., AND ROBERTSON, C. Influence of music and distraction on visual search performance of participants with high and low affect intensity 888
DANE, Ş. Review of some sex-related effects of forced unilateral nostril breathing on the autonomic nervous system 736
DANE, Ş., CAN, S., GÜRSOY, R., AND EZİRMİK, N. Sport injuries: relations to sex, sport, injured body region 519
DANE, Ş., ERSÖZ, M., GÜMÜŞTEKIN, K., POLAT, P., AND DAŞTAN, A. Handedness differences in widths of right and left craniofacial regions in healthy young adults 1261
DASÍ, C. See RUIZ, J. C.
DAŞTAN, A. See DANE, Ş.
DAVLIN, C. D. Dynamic balance in high level athletes 1171
DEDITIUS-ISLAND, H. K. See SZALDA-PETREE, A. D.
DEMIRHAN, G. See KOCA, C.
DEMURA, S. See IKEMOTO, Y.
DEMURA, S. See NAGASAWA, Y.

DEMURA, S. See NODA, M.
DESPRÉS, O. See DUFOUR, A.
DEVLIN, A. S. Sailing experience and sex as correlates of spatial ability 1409
DHALIWAL, H. S. See TORIOLA, A. L.
DICERBO, K. E., OLIVER, J., ALBERS, C., AND BLANCHARD, J. Effects of reducing attentional demands on performance of reading comprehension tests by third graders 561
DICKERSON, J. See CAPILOUTO, G. J.
DITTMAR, A. See GUILLOT, A.
DOTY, R. L. See WUDARSKI, T. J.
DRAKE, C. See BARUCH, C.
DUFOUR, A., BROCHARD, R., DESPRÉS, O., SCHEIBER, C., AND ROBERT, C. Perceptual encoding of fingerspelled and printed alphabet by deaf signers: an fMRI study 971
DUGAS, J. P. See HAMPSON, D. B.
DUPONT, M. J., MCKAY, B. E., PARKER, G., AND PERSINGER, M. A. Geophysical variables and behavior: XCIX. Reductions in numbers of neurons within the parasolitary nucleus in rats exposed perinatally to a magnetic pattern designed to imitate geomagnetic continuous pulsations: implications for Sudden Infant Death 958
DURAND, M. See HAUW, D.
EDWARDS, S. D. See PILLAY, A. L.
EHNINGER, G. See NAUMANN, R.
EID, J. See PALLESEN, S.
EINSLE, F. See NAUMANN, R.
EISELE, P. Judgment and decision-making: experts' and novices' evaluation of chess positions 237
ELLENBECKER, T. S., AND ROETERT, E. P. Velocity of a tennis serve and measurement of isokinetic muscular performance: brief review and comment 1368
ERSÖZ, M. See DANE, Ş.
EZİRMİK, N. See DANE, Ş.
FAIGENBAUM, A. D., MILLIKEN, L. A., CLOUTIER, G., AND WESTCOTT, W. L. Perceived exertion during resistance exercise by children 627
FAURE, S. See OLIVIER, G.
FEDERMANN, R., BÄCKSTRÖM, M., AND GOLDSMITH, R. W. The Stroop Strategy Test: investigation of a computerised version of the Stroop test for classifying Swedish military servicemen 1371
FERRARO, F. R. See CAMERON, E. M.
FÉRY, Y-A. See GOLOMER, E.
FINLEY, P. S., AND HALSEY, J. J. Determinants of PGA tour success: an examination of relationships among performance, scoring, and earnings 1100
FITZPATRICK, R. E., AND PERSINGER, M. A. Weekly treatments with a burst-firing magnetic field alters behavior in the elevated plus maze after two sessions 983
FOLEY, A. J., MICHALUK, L. M., AND THOMAS, D. G. Pace alteration and estimation of time intervals 291
FORNS, M. See PEREDA, N.
FOURNIER, N. M., AND PERSINGER, M. A. Geophysical variables and behavior: C. Increased geomagnetic activity on days of commercial air crashes attributed to computer or pilot error but not mechanical failure 1219
FRAWLEY, W. See GREENE, E.
FUDIN, R., AND LEMBESSIS, E. The Mozart effect: questions about the seminal findings of Rauscher, Shaw, and colleagues 389
GADZICHOWSKI, K. M. See CAMPBELL, J. L.
GALIC, M. A. Elevated nociceptive thresholds in rats with multifocal brain damage induced with single subcutaneous injections of lithium and pilocarpine 825
GALIC, M. A., AND PERSINGER, M. A. Geomagnetic activity during the previous day is correlated with increased consumption of sucrose during subsequent days: is increased geomagnetic activity aversive? 1126
GANN, S. See ANNESI, J. J.
GIANUTSOS, J. G., COHEN, J. M., AND BATAVIA, M. Test-retest reliability in performance of persons with hemiparesis tracking by means of compatibly displayed myoelectric feedback derived from upper limb muscles 19
GIOTAKOS, O. Handedness and hobby preference 869
GOLDBERG, E. See GOLDFARB, R.
GOLDFARB, R., AND GOLDBERG, E. Communicative responsibility and semantic task in the language of adults with dementia 1177

GOLDSMITH, R. W. See FEDERMANN, R.
GOLOMER, E., KELLER, J., FÉRY, Y-A., AND TESTA, M. Unipodal performance and leg muscle mass in jumping skills among ballet dancers 415
GÓMEZ-BENITO, J. See TOMÁS-SÁBADO, J.
GREEN, J. M., CREWS, T. R., PRITCHETT, R. C., MATHFIELD, C., AND HALL, L. Heart rate and ratings of perceived exertion during treadmill and elliptical exercise training 340
GREENE, E., AND FRAWLEY, W. Modeling judgments of linear extent 1049
GRIECO, A. See SAGGINO, A.
GRIMSHAW, P. See MARQUES-BRUNA, P.
GROENEWEG, J. See LANCIONI, G. E.
GROUIOS, G. Motoric dominance and sporting excellence: training versus heredity 53
GUIDO, G., AND PROVENZANO, M. R. Abstractness and emotionality values for 398 English words 1265
GUILLOT, A., AND COLLET, C. Field dependence–independence in complex motor skills 575
GUILLOT, A., COLLET, C., MOLINARO, C., AND DITTMAR, A. Expertise and peripheral autonomic activity during the preparation phase in shooting events 371
GÜL, E. D. See ARNAS, Y. A.
GÜMÜŞTEKIN, K. See DANE, Ş.
GÜRSOY, R. See DANE, Ş.
GUTNIK, B. J., CORBALLIS, M. C., AND NICHOLSON, J. Lateralized regular spatial patterns in oscillating drawing arm movements of right-handed young women 249
HAGEMAN, C. F. See BURDA, A. N.
HALL, L. See GREEN, J. M.
HALSEY, J. J. See FINLEY, P. S.
HAMPSON, D. B., ST CLAIR GIBSON, A., LAMBERT, M. I., DUGAS, J. P., LAMBERT, E. V., AND NOAKES, T. D. Deception and perceived exertion during high-intensity running bouts 1027
HANSEN, A. See PALLESEN, S.
HATAYAMA, M. See HATAYAMA, T.
HATAYAMA, T., HATAYAMA, M., AND KIKUCHI, N. A mobile device for measuring sensorimotor timing in synchronized tapping 1327
HAUW, D., AND DURAND, M. Elite athletes' differentiated action in trampolining: a qualitative and situated analysis of different levels of performance using retrospective interviews 1139
HIRAI, T. See NARUSE, K.
HIROKAWA, K., YAGI, A., AND MIYATA, Y. Comparison of blinking behavior during listening to and speaking in Japanese and English 463
HOAG, J. See SCHMELKIN, L. P.
HODGE, K. See CRESSWELL, S.
HOLT, D. T. See LAUDENSLAGER, M. S.
HUBBARD, A. S. E. See SANTARCANGELO, M.
HUGDAHL, K. See PALLESEN, S.
HUNTER, G. R. See MCLAFFERTY, C. L., JR.
HUSSEY, J. R. See CAPILOUTO, G. J.
ICHIKAWA, N., AND OHIRA, H. Eyeblink activity as an index of cognitive processing: temporal distribution of eyeblinks as an indicator of expectancy in semantic priming 131
IGBOKWE, N. U. See TORIOLA, A. L.
IKEMOTO, Y., AND DEMURA, S., AND YAMAJI, S. Relations between the inflection point on the force-time curve and force-time parameters during static explosive grip 507
IMANAKA, K. See YAMAUCHI, K.
INOMATA, K. See WAKAYAMA, H.
IRWIN, J. D. Prevalence of university students' sufficient physical activity: a systematic review 927
ISOSAARI, R. M. See SCHULER, P. B.
JACOBSON, J. M., NIELSEN, N. P., MINTHON, L., WARKENTIN, S., AND WIIG, E. H. Multiple rapid automatic naming measures of cognition: normal performance and effects of aging 739
JACQUOT, L. See BRAND, G.
JAEGER, T., AND LANG, J. Contrast influences perceived duration of brief time intervals 682
JANSEN, S. See KALB, R.
JANßEN, J. P. Evaluation of empirical methods and methodological foundations of human left-landedness 487
JEFFRIES, K. J. See LIU, Y-C.
JOHNSEN, B. H. See PALLESEN, S.

CONTENTS OF VOLUME 98, FEBRUARY–JUNE 2004

JOHNSON, R. F. See MCBRIDE, S. A.
JOHNSTON, J. E. See BERRY, K. J.
JOHNSTON, J. E., BERRY, K. J., AND MIELKE, P. W., JR. A measure of effect size for experimental designs with heterogeneous variances ... 3
JORASCHKY, P. See NAUMANN, R.
KAIS, K., AND RAUDSEPP, L. Cognitive and somatic anxiety and self-confidence in athletic performance of beach volleyball ... 439
KALB, R., JANSEN, S., REULBACH, U., AND KALB, S. Sex differences in simple reaction tasks ... 793
KALB, S. See KALB, R.
KARNES, F. A. See SHAUNESSY, E.
KASHIWAGI, T. See MASUMOTO, K.
KATSAROU, Z., BOSTANTJOPOULOU, S., KIMISKIDIS, V., ROSSOPOULOS, E., AND KAZIS, A. Auditory event-related potentials in Parkinson's disease in relation to cognitive ability ... 1441
KAUFMAN, A. M. See SCHMELKIN, L. P.
KAZIS, A. See KATSAROU, Z.
KEATING, T. M., KENDLER, B. S., AND MERRIMAN, W. Evaluation of a possible proximity effect of Aspartame and Vitamin C on muscular strength ... 100
KEENER, J. See MILLSLAGLE, D.
KELLER, J. See GOLOMER, E.
KENDLER, B. S. See KEATING, T. M.
KHURSHID, A. See PILOTTI, M.
KIDA, N. See ANDO, S.
KIKUCHI, N. See HATAYAMA, T.
KIMATA, H. Differential effects of laughter on allergen-specific immunoglobulin and neurotrophin levels in tears ... 901
KIMISKIDIS, V. See KATSAROU, Z.
KITABAYASHI, T. See NAGASAWA, Y.
KITABAYASHI, T. See NODA, M.
KOCA, C., AND DEMIRHAN, G. An examination of high school students' attitudes toward physical education with regard to sex and sport participation ... 754
KOENIG, O. See ROYET, J-P.
KÖLLNER, V. See NAUMANN, R.
KONDRICHIN, S. V. See LESTER, D.
KOULI, O. See BEBETSOS, E.
KRUGER, M. L. See ABEL, E. L.
KUDADJIE-GYAMFI, E. Effects of random outcomes on choice behavior ... 1296
KUGLER, J. See NAUMANN, R.
KUNSELMAN, J. C. See BRIDGES, F. S.
KUNTO, S. See THOMPSON, G. L.
KVÅLSETH, T. O. On a general class of chi-squared goodness-of-fit statistics ... 967
LABIALE, G. See OLIVIER, G.
LAGALLY, K. M., AND COSTIGAN, E. M. Anchoring procedures in reliability of ratings of perceived exertion during resistance exercise ... 1285
LAMBERT, E. V. See HAMPSON, D. B.
LAMBERT, M. I. See HAMPSON, D. B.
LANCIONI, G. E., SINGH, N. N., O'REILLY, M. F., CAMPODONICO, F., OLIVA, D., AND GROENEWEG, J. Effects of automatically delivered stimulation on persons with multiple disabilities during their use of a stationary bicycle ... 1363
LANCIONI, G. E., SINGH, N. N., O'REILLY, M. F., AND OLIVA, D. A microswitch program including words and choice opportunities for students with multiple disabilities ... 214
LANCIONI, G. E., SINGH, N. N., O'REILLY, M. F., OLIVA, D., MONTIRONI, G., AND CHIERCHIE, S. Assessing a new response-microswitch combination with a boy with minimal motor behavior ... 459
LANDERS, D. M. See CREWS, D. J.
LANDSTRÖM, U., ÅKERSTEDT, T., BYSTRÖM, M., NORDSTRÖM, B., AND WIBOM, R. Effect on truck drivers' alertness of a 30-min. exposure to bright light: a field study ... 770
LANG, J. See JAEGER, T.
LAUDENSLAGER, M. S., HOLT, D. T., AND LOFGREN, S. T. Understanding Air Force members' intentions to participate in pro-environmental behaviors: an application of the theory of planned behavior ... 1162

LEE, H., NICHOLSON, L. L., AND ADAMS, R. D. Sensitivity to differences in the extent of neck-retraction and -rotation movements made with and without vision 1081
LEE, I H. See LIU, Y.-C.
LEE, L-C. See LIU, Y.-C.
LEE, T-H. See CHENG, T-S.
LEGRAND, S. See VENEZIANO, C.
LEHTO, J. E. A test for children's goal-directed behavior: a pilot study 223
LEMBESSIS, E. See FUDIN, R.
LESTER, D. The fragmented self 1326
LESTER, D., AND KONDRICHIN, S. V. Finno-Ugrians, blood types, and suicide: comment on Voracek, Fisher, and Marusic 814
LEUNG, M-L. See LEUNG, R. W.
LEUNG, R. W., LEUNG, M-L., AND CHUNG, P-K. Validity and reliability of a Cantonese-translated Rating of Perceived Exertion scale among Hong Kong adults 725
LIEBLING, D. E. See SCHMELKIN, L. P.
LIN, F-T. Optimal handle angle of the fencing foil for improved performance 920
LIN, K-C. See LIU, Y.-C.
LIU, Y.-C., YANG, Y. K., LIN, K-C., LEE, I H., JEFFRIES, K. J, AND LEE, L-C. Eye-hand preference in schizophrenia: sex differences and significance for hand function 1225
LOCHBAUM, M. R. See CREWS, D. J.
LOFGREN, S. T. See LAUDENSLAGER, M. S.
LOHMAN, P. Comparison of two training methods to enhance awareness of the oral cavity 525
LORANT, J. See REYNES, E.
MARINO, F. E. See PATERSON, S.
MARMORATO, M. S. See ORSINI, A.
MARQUES-BRUNA, P., AND GRIMSHAW, P. Reliability of gait parameters in children under two years of age 123
MARTIN, L. M. See SZALDA-PETREE, A. D.
MASUMOTO, K., TAKAI, T., TSUNETO, S., AND KASHIWAGI, T. Influence of motoric encoding on forgetting function of memory for action sentences in patients with Alzheimer's disease 299
MATHFIELD, C. See GREEN, J. M.
MATI-ZISSI, H. See ZAFIROPOULOU, M.
MAYER, J. M. See UDERMANN, B. E.
MCBRIDE, S. A., JOHNSON, R. F., MERULLO, D. J., AND BARTOW, R. E., JR. Effects of the periodic administration of odor or vibration on a 3-hr. vigilance task 307
MCCLENAGHAN, B. See CAPILOUTO, G. J.
MCHALE, M. A. See WOLACH, A. H.
MCKAY, B. E. See DUPONT, M. J.
MCKELVIE, S. J. False recognition with the Deese-Roediger-McDermott-Reid-Solso procedure: a quantitative summary 1387
MCLAFFERTY, C. L., JR., WETZSTEIN, C. J., AND HUNTER, G. R. Resistance training is associated with improved mood in healthy older adults 947
MENGISEN, W. See ANTONINI PHILIPPE, R.
MERRIMAN, W. See KEATING, T. M.
MERULLO, D. J. See MCBRIDE, S. A.
MICHALUK, L. M. See FOLEY, A. J.
MIELKE, P. W., JR. See BERRY, K. J.
MIELKE, P. W., JR. See JOHNSTON, J. E.
MILLER, A. L. See BURDA, A. N.
MILLIKEN, L. A. See FAIGENBAUM, A. D.
MILLOT, J-L. See BRAND, G.
MILLSLAGLE, D., RUBBELKE, S., MULLIN, T., KEENER, J., AND SWETKOVICH, R. Effects of foot-pedal positions by inexperienced cyclists at the highest aerobic level 1074
MINTHON, L. See JACOBSON, J. M.
MIYATA, Y. See HIROKAWA, K.
MOLINARO, C. See GUILLOT, A.
MONTIRONI, G. See LANCIONI, G. E.
MULLIN, T. See MILLSLAGLE, D.

CONTENTS OF VOLUME 98, FEBRUARY–JUNE 2004

Murai, G. See Wakayama, H.
Murray, N. P. See Tennant, L. K.
Murray, S. R. See Udermann, B. E.
Nagasawa, Y., Demura, S., and Kitabayashi, T. Concurrent validity of tests to measure the coordinated exertion of force by computerized target pursuit 551
Nakayama, M. See Yamauchi, M.
Naruse, K., Sakuma, H., and Hirai, T. Effect of slow movement execution on cognitive function 35
Naumann, R., Köllner, V., Einsle, F., Schneider, E., Ehninger, G., Joraschky, P., and Kugler, J. Pain perception in patients undergoing bone marrow puncture—a pilot study 116
Neff, N. L. See Cherney, I. D.
Nicholson, J. See Gutnik, B. J.
Nicholson, L. L. See Lee, H.
Nielsen, N. P. See Jacobson, J. M.
Nishizawa, S. See Yamauchi, M.
Nittono, H. See Wada, K.
Noakes, T. D. See Hampson, D. B.
Noda, M., Demura, S., Yamaji, S., and Kitabayashi, T. Influence of alcohol intake on the parameters evaluating the body center of foot pressure in a static upright posture 873
Nordström, B. See Landström, U.
Oda, S. See Ando, S.
Ohira, H. See Ichikawa, N.
Ohira, H. See Takagi, S.
Ohira, H. Social support and salivary secretory Immunoglobulin A response in women to stress of making a public speech 1241
Oliva, D. See Lancioni, G. E.
Oliver, J. See DiCerbo, K. E.
Olivier, G., Velay, J. L., Labiale, G., Celse, C., and Faure, S. Mental rotation and simulation of a reaching and grasping manual movement 1107
Olsen, T. See Pallesen, S.
O'Reilly, M. F. See Lancioni, G. E.
Orsini, A., Simonetta, S., and Marmorato, M. S. Corsi's block-tapping test: some characteristics of the spatial path which influence memory 382
Pallesen, S., Johnsen, B. H., Hansen, A., Eid, J., Thayer, J. F., Olsen, T., and Hugdahl, K. Sleep deprivation and hemispheric asymmetry for facial recognition reaction time and accuracy 1305
Panissal-Vieu, N. See Baruch, C.
Papaioannou, A., Ballon, F., Theodorakis, Y., and Vanden Auweele, Y. Combined effect of goal setting and self-talk in performance of a soccer-shooting task 89
Parker, G. See Dupont, M. J.
Pasnak, R. See Campbell, J. L.
Paterson, S., and Marino, F. E. Effect of deception of distance on prolonged cycling performance 1017
Paugam-Moisy, H. See Royet, J-P.
Pearson, L. C. See Bridges, F. S.
Pereda, N., and Forns, M. Psychometric properties of the Spanish version of the Self-perception Profile for Children 685
Persinger, M. A. See Dupont, M. J.
Persinger, M. A. See Fitzpatrick, R. E.
Persinger, M. A. See Fournier, N. M.
Persinger, M. A. See Galic, M. A.
Persinger, M. A. Students' perceptions of dangerousness to public safety of paraphrases from the Koran, New Testament, Book of Mormon, Tibetan Book of the Dead, and Egyptian Book of the Dead presented as patients' beliefs 1345
Persinger, M. A. Weak-to-moderate correlations between global geomagnetic activity and reports of diminished pleasantness: a nonspecific source for multiple behavioral correlates? 78
Pfeffer, K., and Wilson, B. Children's perceptions of dangerous substances 700
Philipp, S. F. See Schuler, P. B.
Philipp, S. F., and Schuler, P. B. Differences in African-American and Euro-American athletes' perceptions of treatment by coaches 1333
Pillay, A. L., and Edwards, S. D. Interrater reliability in professional psychology student selection ... 86

PILOTTI, M., AND KHURSHID, A. Semantic satiation effect in young and older adults ... 999
POLAT, P. See DANE, Ş.
PREDEBON, J. Influence of the Poggendorff illusion on manual pointing ... 47
PRITCHETT, R. C. See GREEN, J. M.
PROIOS, H., AND BRUGGER, P. Influence of color on number perseveration in a serial addition task ... 944
PROVENZANO, M. R. See GUIDO, G.
PUZENAT, D. See ROYET, J-P.
RAUDSEPP, L. See KAIS, K.
RAVIELE, N. N. See SAGGINO, A.
REDSTONE, P. See WEST, J. F.
REULBACH, U. See KALB, R.
REYNES, E., AND LORANT, J. Competitive martial arts and aggressiveness: a 2-yr. longitudinal study among young boys ... 103
RICHARDS, L. See VENEZIANO, C.
RIZZO, T. L. See CASEBOLT, K.
ROBERT, C. See DUFOUR, A.
ROBERTSON, C. See CRUST, L.
ROBINSON, D. See SCHULER, P. B.
RODWAY, P. Stimulus array onset as a preparatory signal in attentional selection ... 599
ROETERT, E. P. See ELLENBECKER, T. S.
ROSENBLUM, L. A. See BRANNON, E. M.
ROSSOPOULOS, E. See KATSAROU, Z.
ROYET, J-P., KOENIG, O., PAUGAM-MOISY, H., PUZENAT, D., AND CHASSE, J-L. Levels-of-processing effects on a task of olfactory naming ... 197
RUBBELKE, S. See MILLSLAGLE, D.
RUIZ, J. C., SOLER, M. J., AND DASÍ, C. Study time effects in recognition memory ... 638
RYAN, S. See SCHULER, P. B.
SAGENDORF, K. See UDERMANN, B. E.
SAGGINO, A., BALSAMO, M., GRIECO, A., CERBONE, M. R., AND RAVIELE, N. N. Corsi's block-tapping task: standardization and location in factor space with the WAIS–R for two normal samples of older adults ... 840
SAKUMA, H. See NARUSE, K.
SAKURAGI, T. Association of culture with shyness among Japanese and American university students ... 803
SANTARCANGELO, M., CRIBBIE, R. A., AND HUBBARD, A. S. E. Improving accuracy of veracity judgment through cue training ... 1039
SAUCIER, D. M. See SYKES TOTTENHAM, L.
SCHEIBER, C. See DUFOUR, A.
SCHMELKIN, L. P., HOAG, J., LIEBLING, D. E., AND KAUFMAN, A. M. Effects of expectations about evaluation and peer recommendations on students' ratings ... 643
SCHNEIDER, E. See NAUMANN, R.
SCHREDL, M. Reliability and stability of a Dream Recall Frequency scale ... 1422
SCHREDL, M. Seasons in dreams ... 1438
SCHULER, P. B. See PHILIPP, S. F.
SCHULER, P. B., BROXON-HUTCHERSON, A., PHILIPP, S. F., RYAN, S., ISOSAARI, R. M., AND ROBINSON, D. Body-shape perceptions in older adults and motivations for exercise ... 1251
SEILER, R. See ANTONINI PHILIPPE, R.
SHAUNESSY, E., KARNES, F. A., AND COBB, Y. Assessing potentially gifted students from lower socioeconomic status with nonverbal measures of intelligence ... 1129
SHEN, I-H. See SHIEH, K-K.
SHIEH, K-K., AND SHEN, I-H. Report order and identification of multidimensional stimuli: a study of event-related brain potentials ... 1427
SIĞIRTMAÇ, A. D. See ARNAS, Y. A.
SIMONETTA, S. See ORSINI, A.
SINGH, N. N. See LANCIONI, G. E.
SOHMIYA, S. Explanation for neon color effect of chromatic configurations on the basis of perceptual ambiguity in form and color ... 272
SOLER, M. J. See RUIZ, J. C.
SOMMER, M. See ARENDASY, M.

CONTENTS OF VOLUME 98, FEBRUARY–JUNE 2004

STAMPS, A. See ZACHARIAS, J.
STANKARD, W. Test of an alternative explanation for effects of arousal gradient on cognitive performance 992
ST CLAIR GIBSON, A. See HAMPSON, D. B.
STOICA, G. See BRADLEY, M. T.
STRENGE, H., AND BÖHM, J. Random number generation in native and foreign languages 1153
SWETKOVICH, R. See MILLSLAGLE, D.
SYKES TOTTENHAM, L., AND SAUCIER, D. M. Throwing accuracy during prism adaptation: male advantage for throwing accuracy is independent of prism adaptation rate 1449
SZALDA-PETREE, A. D., CRAFT, B. B., MARTIN, L. M., AND DEDITIUS-ISLAND, H. K. Self-control in rhesus macaques (*Macaca mulatta*): controlling for differential stimulus exposure 141
TAKAGI, S., AND OHIRA, H. Effects of expression and inhibition of negative emotions on health, mood states, and salivary secretory Immunoglobulin A in Japanese mildly depressed undergraduates 1187
TAKAI, T. See MASUMOTO, K.
TARLEA, A. See WOLACH, A. H.
TENNANT, L. K., MURRAY, N. P., AND TENNANT, L. M. Effects of strategy use on acquisition of a motor task during various stages of learning 1337
TENNANT, L. M. See TENNANT, L. K.
TESTA, M. See GOLOMER, E.
THAYER, J. F. See PALLESEN, S.
THEODORAKIS, Y. See PAPAIOANNOU, A.
THOMAS, D. G. See FOLEY, A. J.
THOMAS, S. See BRAND, G.
THOMPSON, G. L., AND KUNTO, S. From phonemes to meaning: John Steinbeck's work examined 785
TILLMANN, B., AND BIGAND, E. Further investigation of harmonic priming in long contexts using musical timbre as surface marker to control for temporal effects 450
TOKUDA, K. See AMBROSI-RANDIĆ, N.
TOMÁS-SÁBADO, J., AND GÓMEZ-BENITO, J. Death anxiety and death obsession in Spanish students 31
TORIOLA, A. L., TORIOLA, O. M., DHALIWAL, H. S., AND IGBOKWE, N. U. Relationship between physical education students' achievements in a French badminton service test and expert ratings of technique quality 406
TORIOLA, A. L., TORIOLA, O. M., AND IGBOKWE, N. U. Validity of specific motor skills in predicting table-tennis performance in novice players 584
TORIOLA, O. M. See TORIOLA, A. L.
TRIKAS, G. See BEBETSOS, E.
TSUNETO, S. See MASUMOTO, K.
UDERMANN, B. E., MURRAY, S. R., MAYER, J. M., AND SAGENDORF, K. Influence of cup stacking on hand-eye coordination and reaction time of second-grade students 409
VANCE, D. E. Cortical and subcortical dynamics of aging with HIV infection 647
VANDEN AUWEELE, Y. See PAPAIOANNOU, A.
VAN ROSSUM, J. H. A. Perceptions of determining factors in athletic achievement: an addendum to Hyllegard, *et al.* (2003) 81
VARHAMA, L. M., AND BJÖRKQVIST, K. Conflicts, burnout, and bullying in a Finnish and a Polish company: a cross-national comparison 1234
VELAY, J. L. See OLIVIER, G.
VENEZIANO, C., VENEZIANO, L., LEGRAND, S., AND RICHARDS, L. Neuropsychological executive functions of adolescent sex offenders and nonsex offenders 661
VENEZIANO, L. See VENEZIANO, C.
VLACHOS, F., AND BONOTI, F. Handedness and writing performance 815
WADA, K., AND NITTONO, H. Cancel and rethink in the Wason selection task: further evidence for the heuristic–analytic dual process theory 1315
WAKAYAMA, H., WATANABE, E., MURAI, G., AND INOMATA, K. Development of the Sport Achievement Orientation Questionnaire for Japanese athletes by exploratory factor analysis 533
WARKENTIN, S. See JACOBSON, J. M.
WATANABE, E. See WAKAYAMA, H.
WEST, J. F., AND REDSTONE, F. Alignment during feeding and swallowing: does it matter? A review 349
WESTCOTT, W. L. See FAIGENBAUM, A. D.
WESTCOTT, W. W. See ANNESI, J. J.

WETZEL, S. See BRAND, G.
WETZSTEIN, C. J. See MCLAFFERTY, C. L., JR.
WHISSELL, C. "The sound must seem an echo to the sense": Pope's use of sound to convey meaning in his translation of Homer's Iliad ---- 859
WHISSELL, C. Using computer-scored measures of emotion and style to discriminate among disputed and undisputed Pauline and non-Pauline epistles ---- 1117
WIBOM, R. See LANDSTRÖM, U.
WIIG, E. H. See JACOBSON, J. M.
WILLIAMS, H. G. See CAPILOUTO, G. J.
WILSON, B. See PFEFFER, K.
WOLACH, A. H., MCHALE, M. A., AND IARLEA, A. Numerical Stroop effect ---- 67
WUDARSKI, T. J., AND DOTY, R. L. Comparison of detection threshold values determined using glass sniff bottles and plastic squeeze bottles ---- 192
YAGI, A. See HIROKAWA, K.
YAMAJI, S. See IKEMOTO, Y.
YAMAJI, S. See NODA, M.
YAMAUCHI, M., IMANAKA, K., NAKAYAMA, M., AND NISHIZAWA, S. Lateral difference and interhemispheric transfer on arm-positioning movement between right and left handers ---- 1199
YANG, Y. K. See LIU, Y-C.
YU, R-F., AND CHAN, A. H. S. Comparative research on response stereotypes for daily operation tasks of Chinese and American engineering students ---- 179
ZACHARIAS, J., AND STAMPS, A. Perceived building density as a function of layout ---- 777
ZAFIROPOULOU, M., AND MATI-ZISSI, H. A cognitive-behavioral intervention program for students with special reading disabilities ---- 587

Lateral Difference and Interhemispheric Transfer on Arm-positioning Movement Between Right and Left Handers: Masaki Yamauchi, Kuniyasu Imanaka, Masao Nakayama, and Sho Nishizawa 1199

Knowledge and Information in Prediction of Intention to Play Badminton: Evangelos Bebetsos, Panagiotis Antoniou, Olga Kouli, and Georgios Trikas 1210

Geophysical Variables and Behavior: C. Increased Geomagnetic Activity on Days of Commercial Air Crashes Attributed to Computer or Pilot Error But Not Mechanical Failure: N. M. Fournier and M. A. Persinger 1219

Eye-Hand Preference in Schizophrenia: Sex Differences and Significance For Hand Function: Yi-chia Liu, Yen Kuang Yang, Keh-chung Lin, I Hui Lee, Keith J Jeffries, and Li-Ching Lee 1225

Conflicts, Burnout, and Bullying in a Finnish and a Polish Company: a Cross-national Comparison: Lasse M. Varhama and Kaj Björkqvist 1234

Social Support and Salivary Secretory Immunoglobulin A Response in Women to Stress of Making a Public Speech: Hideki Ohira 1241

Body-shape Perceptions in Older Adults and Motivations For Exercise: Petra B. Schuler, Amanda Broxon-Hutcherson, Steven F. Philipp, Stuart Ryan, Robert M. Isosaari, and Destini Robinson 1251

Handedness Differences in Widths of Right and Left Craniofacial Regions in Healthy Young Adults: Şenol Dane, Mustafa Ersöz, Kenan Gümüştekin, Pinar Polat, and Ali Daştan 1261

Abstractness and Emotionality Values For 398 English Words: Gianluigi Guido and Maria Rosaria Provenzano 1265

Role of Strategies and Prior Exposure in Mental Rotation: Isabelle D. Cherney and Nicole L. Neff 1269

Mastery of Number Conservation by a Man With Severe Cognitive Disabilities: Jessica Lynn Campbell, K. Marinka Gadzichowski, and Robert Pasnak 1283

Anchoring Procedures in Reliability of Ratings of Perceived Exertion During Resistance Exercise: Kristen M. Lagally and Elizabeth M. Costigan 1285

Effects of Random Outcomes on Choice Behavior: Elizabeth Kudadjie-Gyamfi 1296

Sleep Deprivation and Hemispheric Asymmetry For Facial Recognition Reaction Time and Accuracy: Ståle Pallesen, Bjørn Helge Johnsen, Anita Hansen, Jarle Eid, Julian F. Thayer, Trond Olsen, and Kenneth Hugdahl 1305

Cancel and Rethink in the Wason Selection Task: Further Evidence For the Heuristic–Analytic Dual Process Theory: Kazushige Wada and Hiroshi Nittono 1315

The Fragmented Self: David Lester 1326

A Mobile Device For Measuring Sensorimotor Timing in Synchronized Tapping: Toshiteru Hatayama, Misako Hatayama, and Naoko Kikuchi 1327

Differences in African-American and Euro-American Athletes' Perceptions of Treatment by Coaches: Steven F. Philipp and Petra B. Schuler 1333

Effects of Strategy Use on Acquisition of a Motor Task During Various Stages of Learning: L. Keith Tennant, Nicholas P. Murray, and Laurie M. Tennant 1337

Students' Perceptions of Dangerousness to Public Safety of Paraphrases From the Koran, New Testament, Book of Mormon, Tibetan Book of the Dead, and Egyptian Book of the Dead Presented as Patients' Beliefs: M. A. Persinger 1345

Mock Jurors' Perceptions of Facial Hair on Criminal Offenders: Richard P. Conti and Melanie A. Conti 1356

Dementia and Identification of Words and Sentences Produced by Native and Nonnative English Speakers: Angela N. Burda, Carlin F. Hageman, Kelly T. Brousard, and Andrea L. Miller 1359

Effects of Automatically Delivered Stimulation on Persons With Multiple Disabilities During Their Use of a Stationary Bicycle: G. E. Lancioni, N. N. Singh, M. F. O'Reilly, F. Campodonico, D. Oliva, and J. Groeneweg 1363

Velocity of a Tennis Serve and Measurement of Isokinetic Muscular Performance: Brief Review and Comment: T. S. Ellenbecker and E. P. Roetert 1368

The Stroop Strategy Test: Investigation of a Computerised Version of the Stroop Test For Classifying Swedish Military Servicemen: Rolf Federmann, Martin Bäckström, and Robert W. Goldsmith 1371

False Recognition With the Deese-Roediger-McDermott-Reid-Solso Procedure: a Quantitative Summary: Stuart J. McKelvie 1387

Sailing Experience and Sex as Correlates of Spatial Ability: Ann Sloan Devlin 1409

Reliability and Stability of a Dream Recall Frequency Scale: Michael Schredl 1422

Report Order and Identification of Multidimensional Stimuli: a Study of Event-related Brain Potentials: Kong-King Shieh and I-Hsuan Shen 1427

Seasons in Dreams: Michael Schredl 1438

Auditory Event-related Potentials in Parkinson's Disease in Relation to Cognitive Ability: Z. Katsarou, S. Bostantjopoulou, V. Kimiskidis, E. Rossopoulos, and A. Kazis 1441

Throwing Accuracy During Prism Adaptation: Male Advantage For Throwing Accuracy is Independent of Prism Adaptation Rate: Laurie Sykes Tottenham and Deborah M. Saucier 1449

NOTICE

June issues of PERCEPTUAL AND MOTOR SKILLS and PSYCHOLOGICAL REPORTS for 2004 are in two parts. The special issue appears as Part 2 for June. Pages are consecutive with those in Part 1 and articles appear in the indexes for the first volumes of 2004.

THE EDITORS